Infectious Diseases: A Case-Based Approach

Infectious Diseases: A Case-Based Approach

Editor: Marcel Soto

AMERICAN
MEDICAL PUBLISHERS
www.americanmedicalpublishers.com

AMERICAN
MEDICAL PUBLISHERS
www.americanmedicalpublishers.com

Cataloging-in-Publication Data

Infectious diseases : a case-based approach / edited by Marcel Soto.
p. cm.
Includes bibliographical references and index.
ISBN 979-8-88740-209-3
1. Infection. 2. Communicable diseases. 3. Infection--Case studies.
4. Communicable diseases--Case studies. I. Soto, Marcel.
RC111 .I543 2023
616.9--dc23

American Medical Publishers,
41 Flatbush Avenue,
1st Floor, New York,
NY 11217, USA

ISBN 979-8-88740-209-3 (Hardback)

Contents

Preface

Infectious diseases are the diseases caused by microorganisms such as bacteria, viruses, fungi, or protozoans. The transmitters of infection can be classified into various categories depending on size, biochemical characteristics, or the way in which they interact with the human host. Some common signs of infectious diseases include fever, fatigue, diarrhea, muscle aches and coughing, but usually depend on the organism causing the infection. The two modes of transmission of infectious diseases are through direct contact and indirect contact. Direct contact such as person-to-person, animal-to-person, and mother-to-unborn child may result in spread of infectious diseases. Consumption of contaminated food and insect bites may also lead to transmission of pathogens. Infectious diseases such as pneumonia, AIDS, and meningitis may prove to be fatal, if left untreated. Infections with human papillomavirus, Helicobacter pylori, and Hepatitis B and C are a few infections associated to an increased risk of cancer. Preventive measures such as washing hands, vaccination, safe sex, and healthy habits can decrease the risk of infection. This book provides comprehensive insights into the field of infectious diseases. Coherent flow of topics, student-friendly language, and extensive use of examples make this book an invaluable source of knowledge. It is a vital tool for all researching or studying these diseases as it gives incredible insights into emerging trends of their management and diagnosis.

This book is the end result of constructive efforts and intensive research done by experts in this field. The aim of this book is to enlighten the readers with recent information in this area of research. The information provided in this profound book would serve as a valuable reference to students and researchers in this field.

At the end, I would like to thank all the authors for devoting their precious time and providing their valuable contribution to this book. I would also like to express my gratitude to my fellow colleagues who encouraged me throughout the process.

Editor

1

Selective Engagement of FcγRIV by a M2e-Specific Single Domain Antibody Construct Protects Against Influenza A Virus Infection

Dorien De Vlieger[1,2,3], Katja Hoffmann[4], Inge Van Molle[5,6], Wim Nerinckx[1,3], Lien Van Hoecke[1,2], Marlies Ballegeer[1,2,3], Sarah Creytens[1,2,3], Han Remaut[5,6], Hartmut Hengel[4], Bert Schepens[1,2] and Xavier Saelens[1,2,3]**

[1] VIB-UGent Center for Medical Biotechnology, VIB, Ghent, Belgium, [2] Department of Biomedical Molecular Biology, Ghent University, Ghent, Belgium, [3] Department of Biochemistry and Microbiology, Ghent University, Ghent, Belgium, [4] Institute of Virology, Medical Center, Faculty of Medicine, University of Freiburg, Freiburg, Germany, [5] Structural Biology Brussels, Vrije Universiteit Brussel, Brussels, Belgium, [6] VIB-VUB Center for Structural Biology, Brussels, Belgium

***Correspondence:**
Bert Schepens
bert.schepens@vib-ugent.be
Xavier Saelens
xavier.saelens@vib-ugent.be

Lower respiratory tract infections, such as infections caused by influenza A viruses, are a constant threat for public health. Antivirals are indispensable to control disease caused by epidemic as well as pandemic influenza A. We developed a novel anti-influenza A virus approach based on an engineered single-domain antibody (VHH) construct that can selectively recruit innate immune cells to the sites of virus replication. This protective construct comprises two VHHs. One VHH binds with nanomolar affinity to the conserved influenza A matrix protein 2 (M2) ectodomain (M2e). Co-crystal structure analysis revealed that the complementarity determining regions 2 and 3 of this VHH embrace M2e. The second selected VHH specifically binds to the mouse Fcγ Receptor IV (FcγRIV) and was genetically fused to the M2e-specific VHH, which resulted in a bi-specific VHH-based construct that could be efficiently expressed in *Pichia pastoris*. In the presence of M2 expressing or influenza A virus-infected target cells, this single domain antibody construct selectively activated the mouse FcγRIV. Moreover, intranasal delivery of this bispecific FcγRIV-engaging VHH construct protected wild type but not $Fc\gamma RIV^{-/-}$ mice against challenge with an H3N2 influenza virus. These results provide proof of concept that VHHs directed against a surface exposed viral antigen can be readily armed with effector functions that trigger protective antiviral activity beyond direct virus neutralization.

Keywords: influenza, matrix protein 2 ectodomain, single domain antibody, Fcγ receptor, effector functions

INTRODUCTION

Influenza A virus infections are a major recurrent cause of seasonal respiratory tract infections. The best way to prevent influenza disease is considered to be vaccination. However due to the accumulation of point mutations in the viral hemagglutinin (HA) and neuraminidase (NA) genes, human influenza vaccines need to be reformulated and administered regularly based on the prediction of the circulating strains (1). The variable effectiveness and the long manufacturing timeline encourage the development of more broadly protective vaccines. Antivirals, such as oseltamivir and baloxavir marboxil, have been licensed for the prophylaxis and treatment of uncomplicated influenza, but the risk of selecting drug resistant viruses limits their widespread use (2, 3).

The 23 amino acid residues long M2 ectodomain (M2e) is highly conserved among the different influenza A virus subtypes and thus represents an attractive target for broadly protective prophylactic vaccine strategies as well as for antibody-based antiviral biologicals [reviewed in Saelens (4)] (4, 5). Various studies using different vaccine formats have demonstrated that M2e-based vaccination can provide broad protection in animal models of influenza A and that this protection is antibody mediated (6–9). Next to vaccines, a therapeutic intervention with an intravenously administered recombinant human IgG1 monoclonal antibody directed against the M2 N-terminus was found to reduce the symptoms in human volunteers that had been infected with an H3N2 virus (10). Furthermore, this phase 2a trial showed that the antibody treatment was associated with a trend toward reduced viral shedding from the nasal mucosa, and no anti-M2e escape mutants could be detected. Finally, intravenous administration of engineered, so called bi-specific T cell engagers that comprise a M2e-specific single chain variable fragment that is linked to a CD3ε-specific single chain variable fragment, could protect mice against an otherwise lethal influenza A virus challenge (11).

Fc gamma receptor (FcγR) interactions are essential for the protective activity of M2e-specific antibodies (12–14). FcγRs are type I membrane proteins that are expressed on different innate immune cells, including macrophages, neutrophils, natural killer cells and dendritic cells (15, 16). In mice, FcγRs are characterized by the presence of an immunoreceptor tyrosine-based activation motif (ITAM) in the cytoplasmic portion of the common γ chain that is associated with the activating FcγRI, FcγRIII and FcγRIV, or by an immunoreceptor tyrosine-based inhibition motif (ITIM) in the cytoplasmic portion of the inhibitory FcγRIIb (17–19). These receptors differ in their affinities for the different IgG isotypes (16, 20). Previously, we have shown that protection by M2e-specific mouse IgG1 requires FcγRIII while IgG2a isotypes can protect by any of the three activating FcγRs (13).

Since the reported discovery of heavy chain-only antibodies in camelids in 1993, recombinant single domain proteins comprising the variable domain of these antibodies (VHHs also known as Nanobodies®) have been used in numerous therapeutic applications (21). In the context of viral infections, various virus-neutralizing VHHs have been described that can interfere with different steps in the viral life cycle (22). Due to their outstanding stability and solubility, as well as their small size (~15 kDa), ease of production and formatting flexibility, they are highly versatile building blocks for the development of new antivirals. Next to a direct antiviral effect, VHHs can also easily be formatted (e.g., by generating Fc fusions) to recruit host effector functions (23). These features, combined with the possibility to deliver therapeutic VHHs into the lung environment, and maintained stability after prolonged storage, make VHH-based anti-influenza biologicals especially attractive for epidemic as well as pandemic preparedness plans (24–27).

In this study we explored a new strategy to engage host cell effector functions to combat influenza A. This strategy is based on a tail-to-head genetic fusion of two VHHs, one that selectively binds to FcγRIV and a second one that is specific for M2e. The resulting bi-specific construct can be efficiently expressed in *Pichia pastoris* cells and protects mice against an otherwise lethal influenza A virus infection by simple intranasal delivery.

MATERIALS AND METHODS

Cell Lines and Culture Conditions

HEK293T cells (a gift from Dr M. Hall, University of Birmingham, Birmingham, UK) and HEK293T cells stably transfected with influenza M2 (28) were cultured in Dulbecco's modified Eagle's medium supplemented with 10% of fetal calf serum, 2 mM of L-glutamine, 0.4 mM of Na-pyruvate, non-essential amino acids, 100 U/ml of penicillin and 10 μM amantadine for the M2 expressing HEK cells. Madin-Darby canine kidney (MDCK) cells were cultured in Dulbecco's modified Eagle's medium supplemented with 10% of fetal calf serum, 2 mM of L-glutamine, non-essential amino acids and 100 U/ml of penicillin. Mf4/4 cells (an immortalized cell line of spleen macrophages derived from C57BL/6 mice) were grown in RPMI 1640 medium, supplemented with 10% of fetal calf serum, 2 mM of L-glutamine, 0.4 mM of Na-pyruvate, non-essential amino acids, 50 mM 2-mercaptoethanol, 25 mM Hepes and 100 U/ml of penicillin (29). Cloning of FcγR-ζ constructs, the generation of FcγR-ζ BW5147 reporter cells and the culture conditions were similar as reported previously (30, 31).

Production of Recombinant Mouse FcγRIV Protein

Recombinant FcγRIV protein was produced by transient transfection of subconfluently grown FreesStyle^{TM}293-F cells (ThermoFisher scientific) with pCAGGs expression vectors encoding the ectodomain of FcγRIV (amino acids 1-201) coupled to a C-terminal 6XHis tag. Recombinant FcγRIV protein was purified from the supernatant 6 days after transfection, using a 1 ml HisTrap HP column (GE Healthcare). Fractions containing FcγRIV protein were pooled and concentrated with a Vivaspin column (5 kDa cutoff, GE Healthcare) and then further purified by gel filtration on a Superdex 75 column. Fractions containing FcγRIV protein were pooled and concentrated. Purity was evaluated by SDS-PAGE followed by Coomassie blue staining.

Isolation of M2e-Binding, VHH-Displaying Phages

A llama was immunized 6 times at weekly intervals subcutaneously with 150 μg M2e-tGCN4 (28) in the presence of Gerbu LQ#3000 adjuvant. Immunizations and handling of the llama were performed according to directive 2010/63/EU of the European parliament for the protection of animals used for scientific purposes and approved by the Ethical Committee for Animal Experiments of the Vrije Universiteit Brussel (permit No. 13-601-1). Five days after the last immunization, blood was collected and lymphocytes were prepared. Total RNA was extracted and used as template for the first strand cDNA synthesis with oligodT primer. The VHH encoding sequences were amplified from the cDNA and cloned into the *Pst*I and *Not*I sites of the phagemid vector pMECS. In this vector, the VHH coding sequence is followed by a linker, an HA- and 6xHis tag (AAAYPYDVPDYGSHHHHHH).

Electro-competent *E.coli* TG1 cells were transformed with the recombinant pMECS vector resulting in a VHH library of about 10^8 independent transformants. A library of VHH-presenting phages was obtained after infection with VCS M13 helper phages. Two different panning strategies were used. In the first strategy, phages were added to 20 μg of immobilized M2e-tGCN4 in panning round 1 and 20 μg of human H3N2 peptide (SLLTEVETPIRNEWGCRCNDSSD) in panning round 2. In the second strategy, phages were first added to 25 × 10^6 HEK293T cells to deplete potential binders to determinants on these cells. The unbound phages were next added to 25 × 10^6 HEK293T cells stably transfected with influenza M2, to enrich for M2-specific phages. To avoid internalization of the target antigen, all steps were performed at 4°C. After washing, retained phages were eluted by pH elution with TEA-solution (14% triethylamine (Sigma) pH 10) for 10 min. A solution of 1 M Tris-HCl pH 8 was used to lower the pH of the eluted phage solution. The enrichment relative to panning on the negative control antigen, was determined by infecting TG1 cells with 10-fold serial dilutions of the phages after which the bacteria were plated on LB agar plates with 100 μg/ml ampicillin and 1% glucose.

Isolation of FcγRIV-Binding, VHH-Displaying Phages

The FcγRIV specific VHHs were isolated form a library that was part of a study described elsewhere by Deschacht et al. (32). In brief, a llama was immunized six times at weekly intervals with 10^8 immature murine bone marrow-derived dendritic cells. A library of VHH-presenting phages was obtained as described above. FcγRIV specific VHHs were enriched after three panning rounds on 20 μg of immobilized FcγRIV protein.

Periplasmic ELISA Screen to Identify M2e- and FcγRIV-Specific VHHs

After panning, individual pMEC colonies were randomly selected for further analysis by ELISA for the presence of M2e- and FcγRIV-specific VHHs in their periplasm. To prepare periplasmic extract, individual colonies were inoculated in 2 ml of terrific broth (TB) medium with 100 μg/ml ampicillin in 24-well deep well plates. After 5 h incubation isopropyl β-D-1-thiogalactopyranoside (IPTG) (1 mM) was added to induce VHH expression. After overnight incubation at 37°C, bacterial cells were pelleted and resuspended in 200 μl TES buffer (0.2 M Tris-HCl pH 8, 0.5 mM EDTA, 0.5 M sucrose) and incubated at 4°C for 30 min. An osmotic shock was induced by adding 300 μl of water. After 1 h incubation at 4°C followed by centrifugation, the periplasmic extract was collected. VHH-containing periplasmic extracts were then tested for binding to either M2e-tGCN4 (28), human H3N2 M2e peptide (SLLTEVETPIRNEWGCRCNDSSD) or recombinant mouse FcγRIV protein. Briefly, wells of microtiter plates were coated overnight with either 100 ng M2e-tGCN4, 100 ng mouse FcγRIV protein, bovine serum albumin (BSA, Sigma-Aldrich) at 4°C or 100 ng human H3N2 M2e peptide at 37°C. The coated plates were blocked with 5% milk powder in phosphate buffered saline (PBS) and 100 μl of the periplasmic extract was added to the wells. Bound VHHs were detected with anti-HA mAb (1/2000, MMS-101P Biolegend) followed by horseradish peroxidase (HRP)-linked anti-mouse IgG (1/2000, NXA931, GE Healthcare). All periplasmic fractions, which resulted in OD_{450} values of the antigen coated wells that were at least two times higher than the OD_{450} values obtained in BSA coated wells, were selected. DNA of the selected colonies was isolated using the QIAprep Spin Miniprep kit (Qiagen) and sequenced using the primer MP057(5′-TTATGCTTCCGGCTCGTATG-3′).

VHH Expression in *Pichia pastoris*

The VHH encoding sequence was amplified by PCR using the following forward and reverse primer (5′-GGC GGG TAT CTC TCG AGA AAA GGC AGG TGC AGC TGC AGG AGT CTG GG-3′) and (5′- CTA ACT AGT CTA GTG ATG GTG ATG GTG GTG GCT GGA GAC GGT GAC CT GG-3′). The PCR fragments were then cloned between the *Xho*I and *Spe*I sites in the pKai61 expression vector [described by Schoonooghe et al. (33)]. In the vector, the VHHs sequences containing a C-terminal 6XHis tag sequence are under control of the methanol inducible AOX1 promotor and in frame with a modified version of the *S. cerevisiae* α-mating factor prepro signal sequence. The vector contains a Zeocine resistance marker for selection in bacteria as well as in yeast cells. The vectors were linearized by *Pme*I and transformed in the *P. pastoris* strain GS115 using the condensed transformation protocol described by Lin-Cereghino et al. (34) After transformation, the yeast cells were plated on YPD plates (1% (w/v) yeast extract, 2% (w/v) peptone, 2% (w/v) dextrose, and 2% (w/v) agar) supplemented with zeocin (100 μg/ml) for selection.

VHH Production and Purification

The transformed *P. pastoris* clones were first analyzed for VHH expression in 2 ml cultures. On day one, 2–5 clones of each construct were inoculated in 2 ml of YPNG medium (2% pepton, 1% Bacto yeast extract, 1.34% YNB, 0.1 M potassium phosphate pH 6, 1% glycerol) with 100 μg/ml Zeocin (Life Technologies) and incubated at 28°C for 24 h. The next day, the cells were pelleted by centrifugation and the medium was replaced by YPNM medium (2% pepton, 1% Bacto yeast extract, 1.34% YNB, 0.1 M potassium phosphate pH 6.0, 1% methanol). Cultures were incubated at 28°C and 50 μl of 50% methanol was added at 16, 24, and 40 h. After 48 h, the supernatant was collected and the presence of soluble VHHs in the supernatant was verified using SDS-PAGE and subsequent Coomassie Blue staining. Production was scaled up (300 ml) for the transformants with the highest levels of VHH in the medium. Growth and methanol induction conditions and harvesting of medium were similar as mentioned above for the 2 ml cultures. The secreted VHHs in the medium were precipitated by ammonium sulfate $(NH_4)_2SO_4$ precipitation (80% saturation) for 4 h at 4°C. The insoluble fraction was pelleted by centrifugation at 20,000 g and resuspended in 10 ml binding buffer (20 mM NaH_2PO_4 pH 7.5, 0.5M NaCl and 20 mM imidazole pH 7.4). The VHHs were purified from the solution using a 1 ml HisTrap HP column (GE Healthcare). Bound VHHs were eluted with a linear imidazole gradient starting from 20 mM and ending at 500 mM imidazole in binding buffer over a total volume of 20 ml. VHH containing fractions were pooled and concentrated with a Vivaspin column (5 kDa cutoff, GE Healthcare) and then further purified by gel filtration (Superdex 75) in PBS buffer. Fractions containing VHH were again pooled and concentrated. Purity was evaluated by SDS-PAGE followed by Coomassie blue staining.

Enzyme-Linked Immunosorbent Assay

Wells of microtiter plates were coated overnight with either 100 ng M2e-tGCN4, 100 ng BM2e-tGCN4, 100 ng M2e peptide or 100 ng mouse FcγRIV protein. The coated plates were blocked with 5% milk powder in phosphate buffered saline (PBS) and dilution series of the VHHs were added to the wells. In the M2e ELISA, bound VHHs were detected with mouse anti-Histidine Tag antibody (MCA1396, Abd Serotec) followed by horseradish peroxidase (HRP)-linked anti-mouse IgG (1/2000, NXA931, GE Healthcare). In the ELISA with coated recombinant FcγRIV protein, binding was detected with a HRP conjugated rabbit anti-camelid VHH antibody (A01861-200, GenScript). After washing 50 μl of TMB substrate (Tetramethylbenzidine, BD OptETA) was added to every well. The reaction was stopped by addition of 50 μl of 1M H_2SO_4, after which the absorbance at 450 nM was measured with an iMark Microplate Absorbance Reader (Bio Rad).

Crystallization of M2e-VHH-23m in Complex With M2e Peptide

For crystallization, the purified M2e-VHH-23m was concentrated to 20 mg/ml. The M2e peptide was added in a 1.2 times excess. Crystallization screens were set up in sitting drop vapor diffusion at 20°C. Crystals grown in the Jenna Classic screen, in 30% ethanol, 10% PEG6000, 100 mM Na acetate were cryoprotected using fluorosilicone and flash frozen in liquid nitrogen. X-ray data were collected at the i03 beamline of the Diamond Light Source synchrotron facility and processed using XDS.[47]

The structure of the M2e-VHH-23m-M2e peptide complex was solved using the structure of another nanobody (PDB code 5HGG) as search model for molecular replacement, using the Phaser program from the CCP4 crystallographic software suite (35, 36). The M2e-VHH-23m model was built automatically using Autobuild from the Phenix crystallographic software suite (37). The initial model was further built manually in Coot and refined using phenix.refine and Refmac (38–40). Data collection parameters, as well as processing and refinement statistics are shown in **Table 1**. The crystal structure has been deposited in the Protein Data Bank (PDB) and is available with accession code 6S0Y.

TABLE 1 | Data collection statistics and refinement parameters.

Data collection	
Synchrotron	Diamond Light Source
Beamline	i03
Wavelength, Å	0.97965
Data processing	
Space group	P 21 21 2
Cell parameters, Å ($\alpha=\beta=\gamma=90°$)	57.47 94.76 53.06
Resolution, Å (outer shell) [c]	53.06–1.80 (1.83–1.80)
Total reflections	35827 (17918)
No. of unique reflections	27557 (1359)
Completeness	99.97 (100)
Multiplicity	13.0 (13.2)
R_{pim}, %	4.4 (66.6)
$CC_{1/2}$, %	99.8 (57.1)
$<I/\sigma(I)>$	11.0 (1.1)
Mosaicity, °	0.063°
Refinement	
Resolution range, Å	47.38–1.81
No. of reflections	25859
Percentage observed	99.96
R_{cryst},[a] %	18.69
R_{free},[b] %	22.53
RMS	
Bonds, Å	0.01
Angles, °	1.66
Ramachandran Plot	
Most favored, %	95.28
Additionally allowed, %	4.72
Disallowed, %	0
PDB code	6S0Y

[a] $R_{cryst} = \Sigma(|F_{obs}|-|F_{calc}|)/\Sigma|F_{obs}|$, F_{obs} and F_{calc} are observed and calculated structure factor amplitudes.
[b] R_{free} as for R_{cryst} using a random subset of the data excluded from the refinement.
[c] Data in brackets are for the highest resolution shell.

Docking

All water molecules, the ligand, and chain B of the nanobody crystal structure were manually deleted from the pdb-text file. The emptied structure was subjected to a local minimization with the GROMOS96 (43B1 parameter set) implementation within Swiss-PdbViewer 4.1.0 (41), and polar hydrogens were added. The peptide-ligand VETPIRNEWG was 3D-drawn with Avogadro 1.2.0 (42) and minimized with the built-in united force field. The AutoDockTools 1.5.6 suite (43) was used for pdbqt-format conversions and grid-box determination. The grid-box size was x = 22, y = 30 and z = 20 centered at x = 1.9, y = 9.7 and z = 8.3. Docking was performed with Smina (44, 45) with exhaustiveness set at 128. Visualization was with PyMOL 2.3.0 (46).

Isothermal Titration Calorimetry

M2e-VHH-23m was dialyzed overnight against PBS buffer and concentrated using Amicon Ultra 3 kDa cut off centrifugal filter devices. The M2e peptide was resuspended in PBS at a stock concentration of 3 mM, and diluted in PBS to 300 μM. Titrations comprised 26 × 1.5 μL injections of peptide (300 μM) into the protein (30 μM), with 90 s intervals. An initial injection of ligand (0.5 μL) was made and discarded during data analysis. The data were fitted to a single binding site model using the Microcal LLC ITC_{200} Origin software provided by the manufacturer.

Ala Scan Mutagenesis

HEK293T cells were transiently transfected with Flag-tagged M2 wild type (WT) and M2e Ala scan mutants. 24 h after infection the cells were detached, washed and blocked. Cells were stained with 20 μg/ml M2e VHH-23m or 20 μg/ml F-VHH-4 and subsequently fixed with 2% paraformaldehyde. After permeabilization (10× permeabilization buffer diluted in double-distilled water; eBioscience), cells were stained with mouse anti-Histidine tag antibody (MCA1396, Abd Serotec) and rabbit anti-Flag tag antibody (F7425, Sigma-Aldrich). Binding of the primary antibodies was revealed with donkey anti-mouse IgG coupled to Alexa Fluor 647 (1/600; Invitrogen) and donkey anti-rabbit IgG coupled to Alexa Fluor 488 (1/600; Invitrogen). The median fluorescence intensity (MFI) of the cells was determined with an LSRII HTS flow cytometer (BD) and was calculated by subtracting the median fluorescence of binding of M2e-VHH-23m or F-VHH-4 to transfected cells from the median fluorescence of untransfected cells bound by M2e-VHH-23m or F-VHH-4.

VHH Binding to Influenza A Virus Infected Cells

HEK293T cells were mock-infected or infected with A/Puerto Rico/8/1934 (H1N1), A/X47 (H3N2), A/Udorn/307/1972 (H3N2) or A/Swine/Ontario (H3N3) at a MOI of 1. Twenty-four hours after infection the cells were detached, washed and blocked. Cells were stained with 20 μg/ml M2e VHH-23m, 20 μg/ml F-VHH-4 or 10 μg/ml MAb148. To determine the affinity of M2e-VHH-23m on infected cells, 1/3 dilution series of M2e-VHH-23m or F-VHH4 were applied to A/Puerto Rico/8/1934 (H1N1) infected cells. Subsequently, the cells were fixed with 2% paraformaldehyde and stained with mouse anti-Histidine Tag antibody (MCA1396, Abd Serotec) and goat anti-A/Puerto Rico/8/1934 serum (Biodefense and Emerging Infections Resources Repository, NIAID, NIH, V314-511-157) followed by anti-mouse IgG Alexa 488 (Invitrogen) and anti-goat IgG Alexa 647 (Invitrogen). The median fluorescence intensity (MFI) was measured on the LSRII-tubes flow cytometer (BD) and was calculated by subtracting the median fluorescence of binding of M2e-VHH-23m or F-VHH-4 to infected cells from the median fluorescence of uninfected cells bound by M2e-VHH-23m or F-VHH-4.

Plaque Reduction Assay

Different amounts of M2e-VHH-23m (2.5 μM, 1.25 μM or 0.625 μM), 0.333 μM MAb37 or sera of mice infected with A/Puerto Rico/8/1934 (H1N1) virus were incubated for 1 h at 4°C with 10–20 plaque forming units/well of A/Udorn/307/1972 (H3N2) or A/Puerto Rico/8/1934 (H1N1) virus. After incubation, the mixture was added to MDCK cells, seeded in a flat bottom 24-well plate. After 1 h, the cells were overlaid with an equal volume of 1.2% Avicel RC-591 (FMC Biopolymer) supplemented with 2 μg/ml of TPCK-treated trypsin (Sigma). Infection was allowed for 2 days at 37°C in 5% CO_2. The overlay was subsequently removed and the cells were fixed with 4% paraformaldehyde. Viral plaques were stained with convalescent mouse anti- A/Puerto Rico/8/34 or A/Udorn/307/72 serum followed by horseradish peroxidase (HRP)-linked anti-mouse IgG (NXA931, GE Healthcare). Finally, after washing, the plaques were visualized with TrueBlue peroxidase substrate (KPL, Gaithersburg).

VHH Binding to FcγRs Expressing Cells

Human Embryonic Kidney (HEK) 293T cells were transiently transfected with full length mouse FcγRI (MG50086-CF), FcγRIIb (MG50030-CY, SinoBiological Inc.), FcγRIII (MG50326, SinoBiological Inc.) or FcγRIV (MG50036-CF, SinoBiological Inc.) expression constructs along with the common γ-chain for the activating FcγRs (MG50935-CF) by polyethylenimine (PEI)-based transfection. A GFP-reporter plasmid was co-transfected. FcγRIV-VHH-7m and M2e-VHH-23m were directly labeled with the Alexa Fluor™ 647 antibody labeling kit (A20186, ThermoFisher scientific). Of the labeled VHHs, 0.2 μM or ¼ serial dilution series of the VHHs starting from 0.2 μM were added to the transfected cells or Mf4/4 cells (29). Fluorescence was measured on an LSRII flow cytometer (BD). The median fluorescence intensity (MFI) was calculated by subtracting the median fluorescence of binding of M2e-VHH-23m or FcγRIV-VHH-7m to transfected cells from the median fluorescence of untransfected cells bound by M2e-VHH-23m orFcγRIV-VHH-7m.

Construction of Bispecific VHHs

To construct FcγRIV VHH-M2e VHH, FcγRIV VHH-F VHH, and FcγRIIIa VHH-M2e VHH bispecific VHHs, we made use of a GoldenBraid-based cloning strategy (47). The coding information of FcγRIV-VHH-7m or FcγRIIIa VHH [C28 sdAb, described by Behar et al. (48)] was amplified with the following forward (5′- GCG ATG CAG GGT CTC ACT TCA AGG CAG GTG CAG CTG CAG GAG TC-3′) and reverse primer (5′ GGC GAT GGT GGG TCT CAC TTC ATG AGG AGA CGG TGA CCT GGG-3′) that add specific overhangs for their identity as N-terminal VHH together with a *Bsa*I and *Sap*I restriction site. The C-terminal VHHs, M2e-VHH-23m and F-VHH-4 were amplified with a forward (5′-GCG CGA TGC AGG GTC TCA CTT CAC AGG TGC AGC TGC AGG AG TC-3′) and reverse primer (5′-GGG CGA TGG TGG GTC TCA CTT CAA GTC TAG TGA TGG TGA TGG TGG TGG CTG GAG ACG GTG ACC TG GG-3′) that add specific overhangs for their identity as C-terminal VHH together with a *Bsa*I and *Sap*I restriction site. The 15 amino acid long $(Gly_4Ser)_3$ linker was generated with the following forward (5′- GCG ATG CAG GGT CTC ACT TCA TCA GGC GGA GGC GGT AGT GGC GGA GGT GGA TCT GGA GGC GGC GGT AGT CA GT-3′) and reverse primer (5′-GGC GAT GGT GGG TCT CAC TTC ACT GAC TAC CGC CGC CTC CAG ATC CAC CTC CGC CAC TAC CGC CTC CGC CTG AT-3′) that also add a specific overhang together with a *Bsa*I and *Sap*I restriction site. The PCR amplified fragments were each assembled in a pUPD2 entry vector by a *Bsa*I restriction and ligation reaction. Once stored in the pUPD2 vector, the different parts were assembled together in the pKai61 expression vector using a T4 DNA ligase and a *Sap*I restriction enzyme which recognizes the *Sap*I restriction site which was introduced after ligation into the pUPD2 vector.

In vitro FcγR Activation Assay

FcγR activation by MAbs 37 and 65 as well as by different M2e-specific nanobodies was determined using an *in vitro* FcγR activation assay (13, 30, 31). Cloning of FcγR-ζ constructs and the generation of FcγR-ζ BW5147 reporter cells were performed as reported previously (30, 31). Activation of stably transduced FcγR-ζ BW5147 reporter cells by immune complexes results in the production of mouse interleukin-2 (mIL-2), which was quantified by ELISA (30, 31).

HEK293T cells that were stably transfected with an M2 expression vector (28) were cultured in the presence of 10 μM amantadine. The cells were seeded 1 day before the co-culture experiment in 96-well flat-bottom plates, pre-coated with fibronectin purified from human plasma (4 μg/ml diluted in PBS). The next day, serial dilutions of the respective MAbs or VHH fusion constructs (concentrations as indicated ranging from 4 to 0.0625 μg/ml) were added to the HEK293T-M2 and incubated for 30 min at 37°C, followed by the addition of 1.5×10^5 FcγR-ζ BW5147 reporter cells in a total volume of 200 μl RPMI1640 medium with 10% fetal calf serum per well. Target cells and reporter cells were incubated overnight at 37°C in a 5% CO_2 atmosphere to allow mIL-2 production. Supernatants were analyzed by an anti-mIL-2 sandwich ELISA as described using the capture MAb JES6-1A12 and the biotinylated detection MAb JES6-5H4 (BD Pharmingen™, Belgium) (30, 31).

For infection with influenza A/Puerto Rico/8/1934 virus, Madin-Darby canine kidney (MDCK) cells were seeded in 96-well flat-bottom plates and infected with influenza PR8 virus (multiplicity of infection [MOI], 5). After 1 h of incubation at 37°C, unbound virus particles were removed by washing, and serial dilutions of the respective MAbs or VHHs (concentrations ranging from 4 to 0.0625 μg/ml) were added and incubated for 30 min at 37°C, followed by the addition of 1.5×10^5 FcγR-ζ BW5147 reporter cells in a total volume of 200 μl RPMI1640 medium with 10% fetal calf serum per well. Target cells and reporter cells were incubated overnight at 37°C in a 5% CO_2 atmosphere to allow mIL-2 production. Supernatants were analyzed by an anti-IL-2 sandwich ELISA as described (30, 31). If not indicated otherwise, experiments were performed in triplicates.

Challenge Experiments in Mice

All experiments were approved by and performed according to the guidelines of the animal ethical committee of Ghent University (Ethical applications EC2017-66 and EC2018-12). Female BALB/c mice and male and female C57BL/6 mice were purchased from Charles River (France) and *FcγRIV*$^{-/-}$ C57BL/6 mice (49) were bred in-house under specified-pathogen-free conditions. Mice were used at age 6–12 weeks and were SPF-housed with food and water *ad libitum*. Mice were anesthetized with isoflurane for treatment and infection. The mice were treated 4 h before and 24 h after influenza A virus challenge by intranasal administration of 50 μg of the bispecific VHHs in a volume of 50 μl PBS. Mice were challenged with 2xLD_{50} of A/X47 (H3N2) influenza virus. Body weight loss was monitored for 14 days. To determine the lung viral titer, complete lungs were harvested on day 6 after infection and homogenized in 1 ml of PBS with a sterile metal bead on the Mixer Mill MM 200 (Retsch). After clearance by centrifugation at 4°C, the lung homogenates were used for virus titration by plaque assay. The plaque assay was performed as described before, plaques were stained using convalescent mouse anti-X47 serum followed by horseradish peroxidase (HRP)-linked anti-mouse IgG (NXA931, GE Healthcare).

Statistical Analysis

Statistical comparison of the differences in body weight loss was analyzed as repeated measurements data using the residual maximum likelihood (REML) as implemented in Genstat v19. Briefly, a linear mixed model (random terms underlined) of the form y = μ + experiment + treatment + time +treatment.time + mouse.time was fitted to the longitudinal data. The term mouse.time represents the residual error term with dependent errors because the repeated measurements are taken in the same individual, causing correlations among observations. Times of measurement were set as equally spaced, and the autoregressive model of order 1 was selected as the best correlation model based on the Aikake Information Coefficient. Significances of treatment effects across time (i.e., treatment.time) and of pairwise differences between treatment effects across time were assessed by an approximate *F*-test, of which the denominator degrees of freedom were calculated using algebraic derivatives as implemented in Genstat v19.

Survival analysis was performed on the right-censored survival data obtained for the five treatment groups. Groups were compared using the nonparametric log-rank test as implemented in Genstat v19. The two independent experiments were set as different groupings for a stratified test.

For the statistical analysis of the differences in lung viral titers a Hierarchical Generalized Linear Mixed Model (HGLMM; fixed model: poisson distribution, log link; random model: gamma distribution, log link) as implemented in Genstat v19 (see ref below), was fitted to the titer data. Treatment, having five levels, was set as fixed term, while replicate was set as random term. T statistics were used to assess the significance of treatment differences compared with the FcγRIV VHH-F VHH set as reference level (on the log-transformed scale). Estimated mean values and standard errors were obtained as predictions from the HGLMM, formed on the original scale of the response variable.

Conservation of the M2 Ectodomain Sequences in Human H3N2 Influenza A Viruses

All complete M2 protein sequences of human H2N2 viruses, human H3N2 viruses and human H1N1 influenza A viruses circulating between 1933 and 2008 were extracted from the Influenza Research Database (http://www.fludb.org/) on 3th May 2019.

RESULTS

Isolation of M2e-Specific VHHs

To generate M2e-specific VHHs a llama was immunized repeatedly with M2e-tGCN4 protein, a soluble recombinant immunogen that mimics the natural tetrameric M2e conformation, that was previously shown to induce protective M2e-specific IgG antibodies in mice (28, 50). Five days after the last immunization, peripheral blood lymphocytes were isolated from the llama and an immune VHH phagemid library of about 10^8 clones was generated. M2e-specific VHHs were enriched from this library by sequential panning on immobilized M2e-tGCN4 (round 1) and M2e peptide (SLLTEVETPIRNEWGCRCNDSSD, corresponding to M2e of human H3N2 viruses) (round 2). As a second strategy, M2e-specific VHHs were enriched by panning on HEK293T cells that stably express M2. Individual phagemid clones enriched after both panning strategies were randomly selected and tested for binding to M2e-tGCN4 and M2e peptide in ELISA. Sequence analysis of the VHH encoding clones which tested positive for binding to either M2e-tGCN4 or M2e peptide revealed a low sequence diversity. Two clones (M2e-VHH-23m and M2e-VHH-66m) isolated with the first, and one clone (M2e-VHH-10m) isolated with the second panning strategy, were selected for further characterization. These VHHs had a cysteine residue at position 50 in the CDR2 and position 100b in the CDR3 (Kabat numbering), allowing the formation of an additional stabilizing disulfide bound, and were devoid of N-glycosylation sequons (**Figure 1A**) (51). The M2e-specific VHHs and an irrelevant control F-VHH-4 directed against the F protein of human respiratory syncytial virus, were subsequently expressed in *Pichia pastoris* in a secreted format (52). After purification from the yeast medium, the epitope specificity was assessed by ELISA. M2e-VHH-23m and M2e-VHH-66m bound to M2e-tGCN4 with a relatively high affinity, whereas M2e-VHH-10m displayed weaker binding (**Figure 1B**). None of the VHHs bound to purified recombinant influenza B M2 ectodomain fused to tGCN4, suggesting that the VHHs bind to M2e. The three selected VHHs bound to immobilized M2e-peptide in ELISA. Amino-acid residues 10 to 23 of M2(e) display some sequence diversity (50). We therefore tested binding of the VHHs to peptide variants that correspond to M2e from A/Brevig Mission/1918 (H1N1), A/Hong Kong/485/1997 (H5N1) and A/swine/Belgium/1/1998 (H1N1) (**Figure 1B**). None of the purified VHHs bound to these M2e peptides, whereas a control mouse monoclonal antibody (MAb148) that is specific for the extremely conserved amino-terminus of M2 (SLLTEVET) did bind (**Figure 1B**). This indicates that the isolated VHHs can bind to M2 expressed by human H2N2, the majority of human H3N2 strains and the majority of human H1N1 viruses circulating between 1933 and 2008 but are unlikely to recognize M2 of currently circulating human H1N1 viruses or most avian and swine influenza viruses. Remarkably, the isolated VHHs also failed to bind the H1N1 A/Brevig Mission/1/1918 M2e, which suggests that Ile11 in M2e contributes substantially to binding. We selected M2e-VHH-23m to target M2e in the subsequent experiments.

M2e-Specific VHH Clamps M2e Peptide Between Its CDR2 and CDR3

We performed isothermal titration calorimetry (ITC) experiments to determine the binding affinity of M2e-VHH-23m to the human H3N2 M2e peptide. The data revealed a 1:1 biomolecular association between the VHH and the M2e peptide with a K_d value of 730 nM (**Figure 2**). The affinity of the single domain M2e-VHH-23m is thus over a 1,000-fold lower than the previously reported affinities for the M2e-specific mouse monoclonal antibodies MAb65 and MAb37 (13).

To precisely resolve the epitope of M2e-VHH-23m, we determined the crystal structure of this VHH in complex with human H3N2 M2e peptide to 1.81 Å resolution (**Table 1**, PDB code 6S0Y). M2e-VHH-23m binds the M2e N-terminus as a linear epitope (**Figure 3A**, left panel). In the crystal structure, one M2e peptide interacts with three adjacent M2e-VHH-23m molecules at three respective interfaces (**Figure S1**). M2e residues E6 to N13 bind in a shallow groove formed by CDR3, CDR2 and the main body of the VHH formed by β-strands C, C', C", and F (Interface 1; **Figure 3A**). As expected, based on the VHH sequence data, a stabilizing disulfide bridge is observed between the CDR3 and CDR2 (**Figure 3A**). Interface 1 includes hydrogen bonds between the M2e-VHH-23m residues Arg45-Gln46-Gly47 and M2e residues Glu8 and Thr9, M2e-VHH-23m residue Cys100b and M2e residue Ile11, and M2e-VHH-23m residue Glu100 and M2e residues Arg12 and Asn13. In addition, three hydrophobic contacts are formed: (1) M2e residue Val7 binds a shallow pocket lined by residue Phe37, Val100f and Trp103, (2) Pro10 stacks against Tyr100d, and (3) the side chain of M2e residue Ile11 is inserted in a pocket formed by the side chain of Ile58 of the VHH CDR2, and the backbones of Tyr59 (CDR2), Gly47, Val48 and Ser49 (CDR3). De bottom of the latter pocket is formed by the stabilizing disulfide bridge between Cys50 in CDR2 and Cys100b in CDR3 (**Figure 3A**). In interface 2, M2e residues 14 to 19 lie on a surface formed by CDR2 and CDR3. The highly conserved M2e Trp15 side chain is inserted in a deep pocket formed by residues from the 3 CDRs: the side chains of Ile58 and Tyr97, and backbones of Ile51, Gly56, Thr57, Asn98, Val99, and Gly100a. In addition, the imidazole NH of Trp15 is hydrogen bonded to the backbone of Asn98 (Interface 2, **Figure 3B**).

In the crystals, the M2e peptide contacts three adjacent molecules in an interaction reminiscent of domain swapping (53). Closer inspection indeed suggests that ligand swapping occurs between the M2e peptides bound to symmetry related molecules in the crystal (**Figure S2**). Docking experiments using the VETPIRNEWG M2e peptide show that the Interface 1 and 2 regions of the M2e peptide (residues 6–12 and 14–19, respectively) can bind a single M2e-VHH-23m molecule (**Figure 3C**). This is also supported by ITC experiments indicating that in solution M2e-VHH-23m and M2e interact in a 1:1 stoichiometry (**Figure 2**). To validate the relative importance of the two binding interfaces in this interaction, we additionally tested the binding of M2e-VHH-23m to HEK293T cells expressing M2 protein or M2e Ala-mutants by flow cytometry (**Figure 3D**). M2e-VHH-23m did not bind to cell that were transfected with an M2Ile11Ala or M2Trp15Ala expression construct, confirming the involvement of interface 1 and 2 in the interaction with M2e. These findings are also in line with the observation that M2e-VHH-23m fails to bind the H1N1 A/Brevig Mission/1/1918 M2e peptide, which carries a serine instead of an isoleucine residue at position 11 (**Figure 1B**). Reduced binding to cells expressing M2Val7Ala also concurs

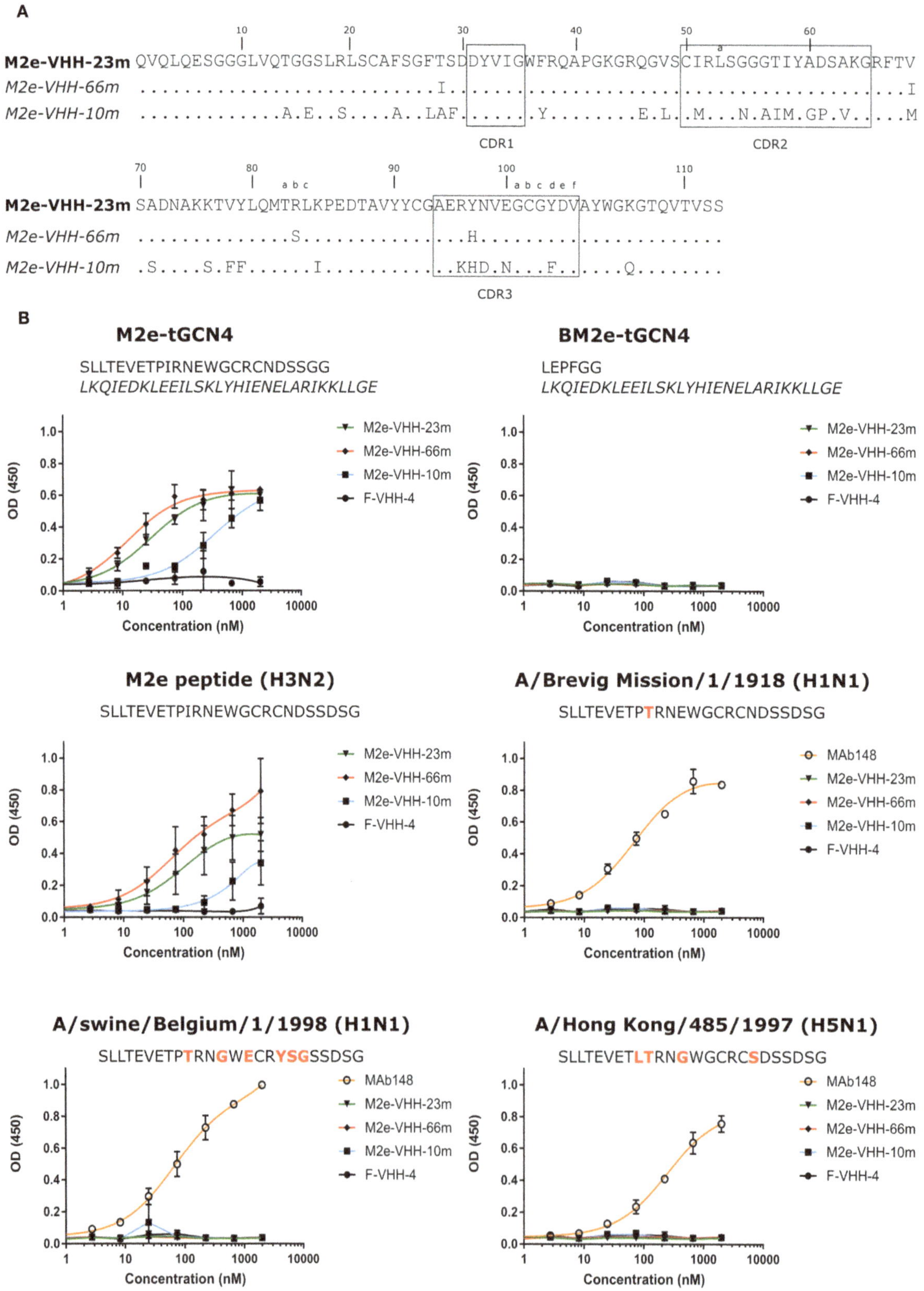

FIGURE 1 | M2e-specific VHHs and their binding specificities. **(A)** Predicted amino acid residue sequences of M2e-VHH-23m and M2e-VHH-66m (isolated after panning on M2e-tGCN4 and human H3N2 M2e peptide) and M2e-VHH-10m (isolated after panning on HEK cells stably expressing M2). Above the sequences the

(Continued)

FIGURE 1 | Kabat numbering is indicated. The complementarity determining regions (CDR) are boxed. **(B)** M2e peptide ELISAs. Wells of microtiter plates were coated with 100 ng M2e-tGCN4, BM2e-tGCN4, or high-performance liquid chromatography (HPLC)-purified M2e peptide. The amino acid residue sequences of the coated proteins or peptides are depicted above the graphs. Amino acid residues that deviate from the consensus human H3N2 M2e sequence are highlighted in red. Dilution series of the indicated VHHs and MAb148 (a mouse monoclonal IgG1 that recognizes the M2e N-terminus) were added to the coated plates. Binding was detected with a mouse anti-His tag MAb, followed by a secondary sheep anti-mouse IgG Ab conjugated to horseradish peroxidase (HRP). Data points represent averages of triplicates and error bars represent standard deviations.

with the co-crystal structure data which show an interaction of M2eVal7 with a shallow hydrophobic pocket on the surface of M1e- VHH-23m (**Figure 3A**).

M2e-VHH-23m Binds to Infected Cells and Does Not Neutralize Influenza A Virus

Next we used flow cytometry to determine if M2e-VHH-m23 could bind to M2e in its natural context, on the surface of influenza A virus infected cells. HEK293T cells were infected with A/Puerto Rico/8/1934 (H1N1) (M2e: SLLTEVETPIRNEWGCRCNGSSD), A/X47 (H3N2) (M2e: SLLTEVETPIRNEWGCRCNDSSD) or A/Udorn/307/1972 (H3N2) (M2e: SLLTEVETPIRNEWGCRCNDSSD) and were subsequently immuno-stained with MAb148, M2e-VHH-23m or F-VHH-4. M2e-VHH-23m could bind to the surface of cells infected with either of the three viruses with a K_d of 13.63 nM for influenza A/Puerto Rico/8/1934 (H1N1) infected cells (**Figure 4A**). In contrast, and as expected, M2e-VHH-23m failed to bind to cells infected with A/Swine/Ontario/42729A/2001 (H3N3) (M2e: SLLTEVETPTRNGWECRCSDSSD) virus. These data confirm that M2e-VHH-23m can bind to M2e sequences that are similar to the H3N2 M2e consensus sequence, recognizes the central part of such M2e sequences and that at least the aspartic acid to glycine substitution at position 21 in A/Puerto Rico/8/1934 M2 is not essential for binding.

It is known that some anti-M2e antibodies can restrict the *in vitro* replication of certain influenza A virus strains such as A/Udorn/307/1972 and A/Hong Kong/8/1968 but not other viruses such as A/Puerto Rico/8/1934 and A/WSN/1933 *in vitro* (54, 55). To address this issue, M2e-VHH-23m or MAb37, a M2e-specific IgG1 antibody with *in vitro* neutralizing activity against A/Udorn/307/1972, were mixed with 10–20 plaque forming units (pfu) of A/Puerto Rico/8/1934 or A/Udorn/307/1972 before infection of MDCK cells (56). As expected, both the plaque size and number of A/Udorn/307/1972, but not of A/Puerto Rico/8/1934 were reduced in the presence of MAb37 (**Figure 4B**). However, unlike MAb37, and even at a concentration of 2.5 μM (30 μg/ml), M2e-VHH-23m did not affect the number and size of A/Udorn/307/1972 plaques (**Figure 4B**).

Isolation of FcγRIV-Specific VHHs

Our next aim was to arm M2e-VHH-23m with a second VHH that targets one of the activating FcγRs such as FcγRIV. We focused on this activating FcγR because of its restricted expression on macrophages, monocytes, neutrophils and dendritic cells but no other myeloid cell population, and because of its very high affinity for IgG2a monoclonal antibodies, which contribute the most protection by non-neutralizing influenza antibodies in the mouse model (13, 20).

To isolate FcγRIV-specific VHHs a phage library obtained from a llama that had been immunized with immature mouse dendritic cells (described by Deschacht *et al.*) was enriched for candidate FcγRIV-specific phagemid clones by three panning rounds using immobilized recombinant mouse FcγRIV extracellular domain protein produced in HEK293T cells (32). Of these candidates, FcγRIV-VHH-7m was selected after a subsequent ELISA screen using the FcγRIV antigen (**Figure 5A**). The binding specificity of purified FcγRIV-VHH-7m was analyzed by flow cytometry using HEK-293 cells that were transiently transfected with GFP and expression vectors coding for mouse FcγRI, FcγRIII or FcγRIV together with a plasmid coding for the common γ-chain, or with an expression vector coding for the inhibitory FcγRIIb. Concentration-dependent binding to cells transfected with the mouse FcγRIV plus the common γ chain was clearly detected (**Figure 5B**). Only at the highest concentration tested, FcγRIV-VHH-7m weakly bound to HEK293T cells that expressed mouse FcγRI, FcγRIIb or FcγRIII (**Figure 5B**). Expression of the FcγRs on the surface of the HEK293T cells was verified by staining with an antibody directed against the tag attached to the FcγRs (**Figure S4**). Clear expression of the mouse FcγRI, FcγRIII and FcγRIV was detected. Expression of the mouse FcγRIIb was less evident, therefore no firm conclusions about the binding of FcγRIV-VHH-7m to the mouse FcγRIIb could be deduced. To evaluate that FcγRIV-VHH-7m was able to bind to cells that express endogenous levels of the mouse FcγRIV, we tested its binding to Mf4/4 cells, a mouse macrophage like cell line (29). Unlike M2e-VHH-M2e, FcγRIV-VHH-7m bound Mf4/4 cells with a deduced K_d value comparable to the K_d value for binding to FcγRIV transfected cells (**Figure 5B**).

Tail-to-Head Fused FcγRIV- and M2e-Specific VHHs Selectively and M2-Dependently Activate FcγRIV

To evaluate the possibility to arm the M2e-specifc VHH with FcγRIV-dependent effector functions, we genetically fused M2e-VHH-23m carboxy-terminal of FcγRIV-VHH-7m by means of a flexible 15 amino acid long $(Gly_4Ser)_3$ linker. As controls M2e-VHH-23m was also fused to a VHH directed against human FcγRIIIa [described by Behar et al. (48)] and FcγRIV-VHH-7m was linked to F-VHH4. The resulting constructs were named FcγRIV VHH-M2e VHH, FcγRIIIa VHH-M2e VHH, and FcγRIV VHH-F VHH, respectively, and were produced in transformed *Pichia pastoris* shake flask cultures (**Figure 6A**). FcγRIV VHH-M2e VHH could bind to M2e peptide and coated soluble FcγRIV protein in ELISA (**Figure 6A**). Next, we evaluated the potency of the bispecific constructs to activate individual

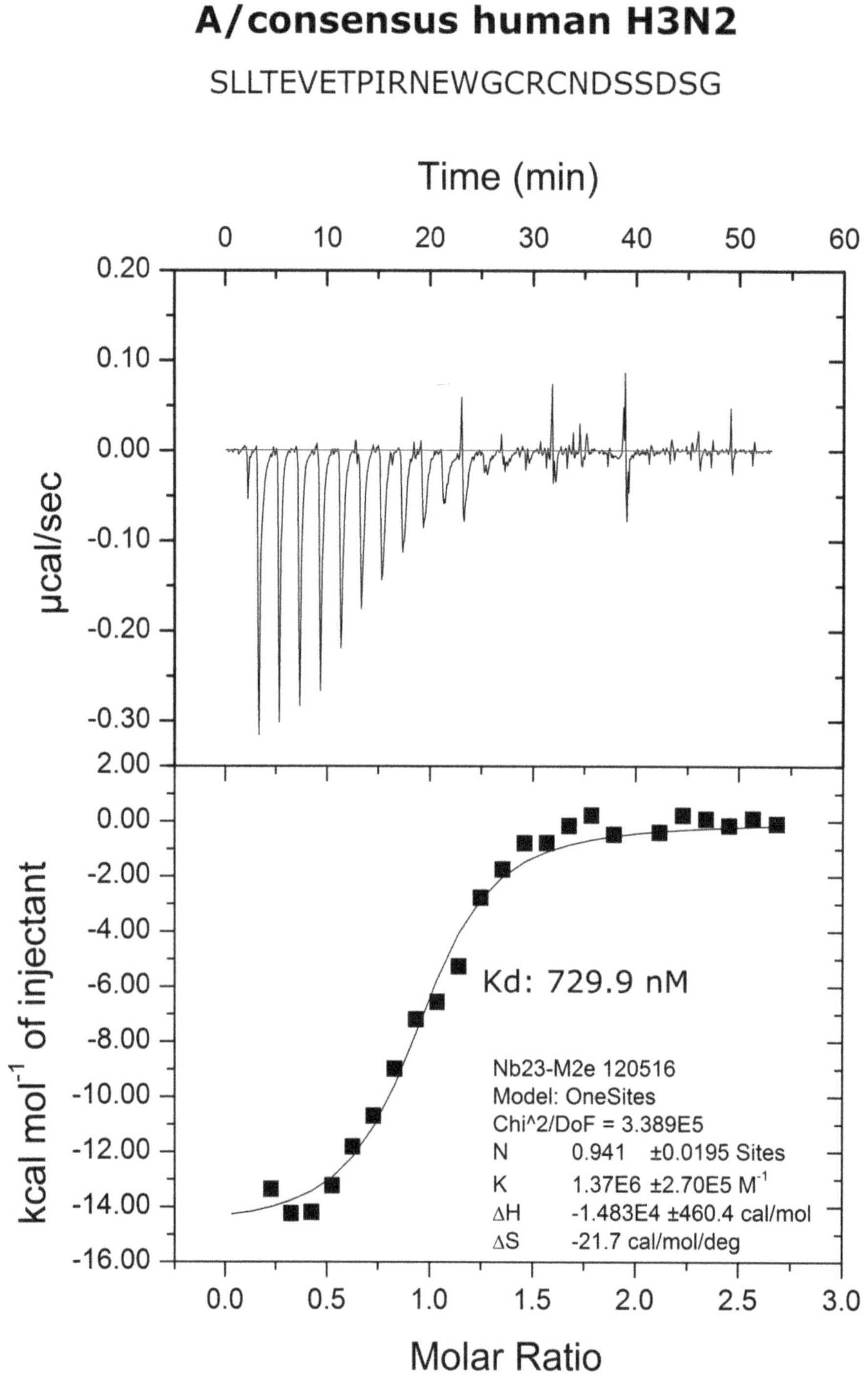

FIGURE 2 | Thermodynamic characterization of the M2e:M2e-VHH-23m interaction. Isothermal titration calorimetry of the Me peptide into M2e-VHH-23m.

FcγRs *in vitro*, by making use of a co-culture of M2-expressing cells and a set of reporter cell transfectants, which produce interleukin 2 upon the activation of a specific FcγR (**Figure 6B**) (30). As controls for FcγR activation, we used mouse M2e-specific MAb 37 (IgG1) and MAb 65 (IgG2a). In the presence of M2-expressing HEK293T cells, MAb 65 dose-dependently activated all mouse FcγRs. This is expected as mouse IgG2a antibodies can bind and activate all mouse FcγRs (16). Only mouse FcγRIIb and -RIII were activated by MAb37, again in line with the known binding specificity of mouse IgG1 antibodies for mouse FcγRs (15). In the presence of M2-expressing cells FcγRIV VHH-M2eVHH potently activated mouse FcγRIV but

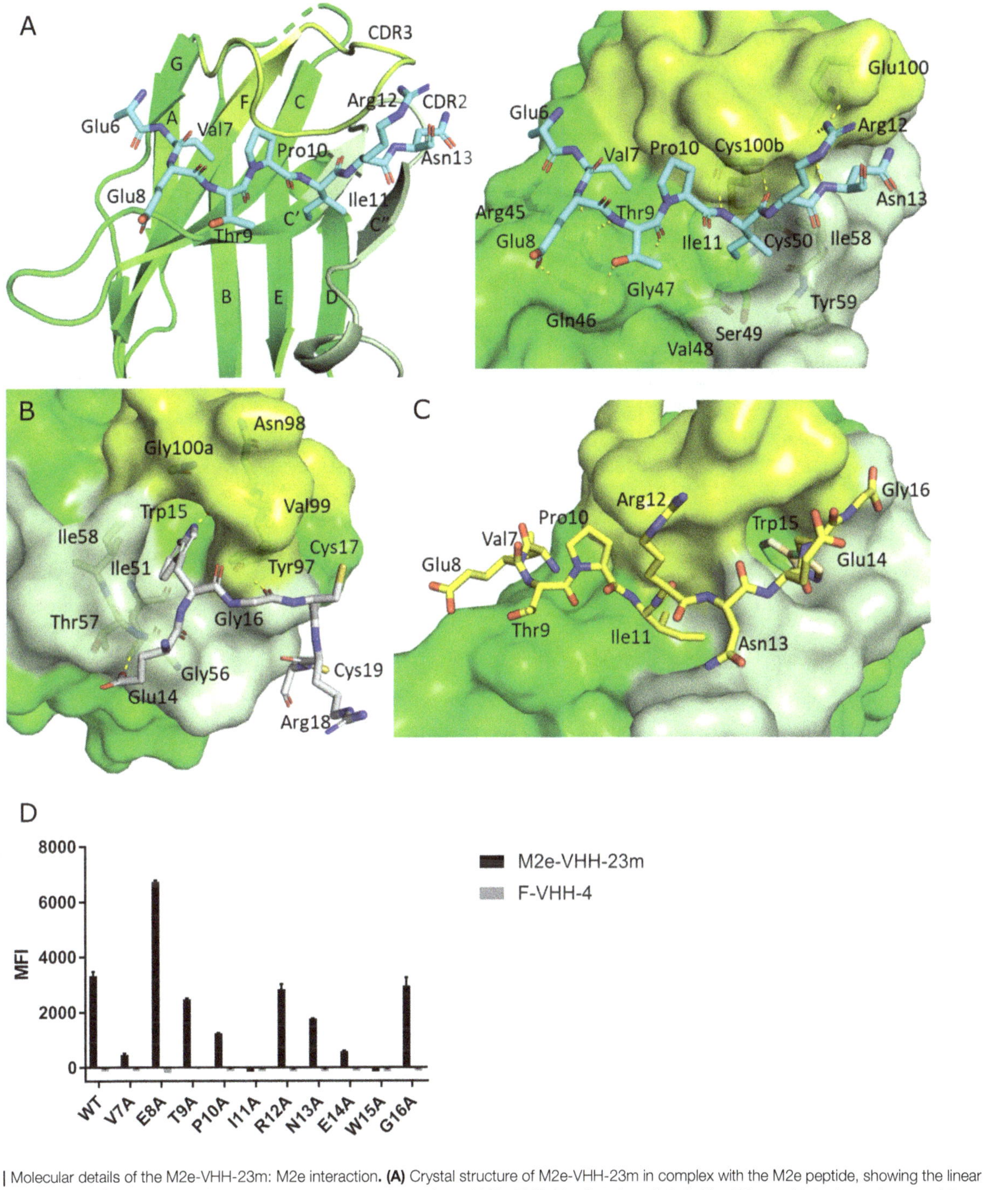

FIGURE 3 | Molecular details of the M2e-VHH-23m: M2e interaction. **(A)** Crystal structure of M2e-VHH-23m in complex with the M2e peptide, showing the linear binding epitope of M2e residues 6–13 binding to a shallow groove on the surface of M2e-VHH-23m (Interface 1). Left: The M2e peptide is shown in cyan stick representation, the M2e-VHH-23m in green cartoon representation. CDR2 and CDR3 are colored pale and lime green, respectively. Right: Details of the interactions between M2e residues 6–13 and the residues making up interface 1 on M2e-VHH-23m. **(B)** Details of the interactions between M2e residues 14–19 and the residues making up interface 2 on M2e-VHH-23m. Coloring of M2e-VHH-23m as in A, M2e shown in gray stick representation. **(C)** Docking of the M2e peptide on the crystal structure of M2e-VHH-23m confirms the ligand swapping hypothesis, showing that M2e binds an extended grove on M2e-VHH-23m comprising both Interface 1 and Interface 2. Coloring of M2e-VHH-23m as in A, M2e shown in yellow stick representation. **(D)** Binding of M2e-VHH-23m to M2e Ala scan mutants. HEK293T cells were transfected with Flag-tagged M2 wild type (WT) and M2e Ala scan mutant expression constructs and subsequently incubated with 20 μg/ml of M2e-VHH-23m or F-VHH-4. After fixation with 2% paraformaldehyde and permeabilization, binding was detected with a mouse anti-Histidine tag antibody and rabbit anti-Fag tag antibody followed by an anti-mouse IgG Alexa 647 and anti-rabbit IgG Alexa 488, respectively. The median fluorescence intensity (MFI) was calculated by subtracting the median fluorescence of binding of M2e-VHH-23m or F-VHH-4 to transfected cells from the median fluorescence of non-transfected cells bound by M2e-VHH-23m or F-VHH-4.

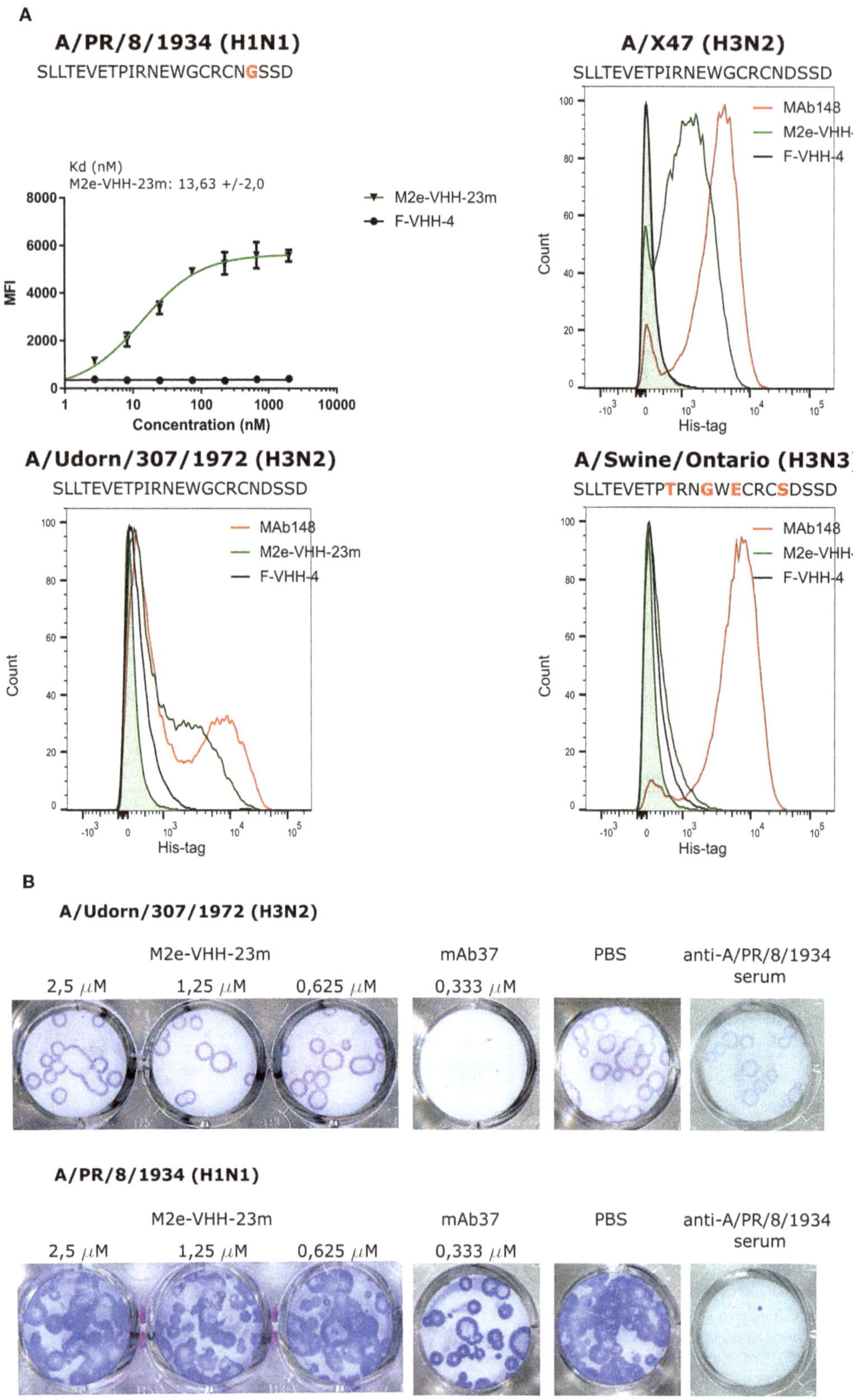

FIGURE 4 | M2e-VHH-23m bind infected cells and lacks *in vitro* antiviral activity. **(A)** HEK293T cells were infected with A/Puerto Rico/8/1934 (H1N1), A/X47 (H3N2), A/Udorn/307/1972 (H3N2) or A/Swine/Ontario (H3N3) virus. The M2e sequences of the different viruses are shown above each graph, residues that differ from the

(Continued)

FIGURE 4 | consensus human H3N2 M2e sequence are colored red. Twenty-four hours after infection, the cells were stained with 20 μg/ml M2e VHH-23m, 20 μg/ml F-VHH-4 or 10 μg/ml MAb148. The A/Puerto Rico/8/1934 (H1N1) infected cells were stained with 1/3 dilution series of M2e-VHH-23m or F-VHH-4. After fixation with 2% paraformaldehyde, infected cells were stained with goat anti-A/Puerto Rico/8/1934 serum followed by anti-goat IgG Alexa 647 and bound VHHs were detected with a mouse anti-Histidine tag antibody followed by anti-mouse IgG Alexa 488. The mean fluorescence intensity (MFI) was calculated by subtracting the median fluorescence of binding of M2e-VHH-23m or F-VHH-4 to infected cells from the median fluorescence of uninfected cells bound by M2e-VHH-23m or F-VHH-4. Data points represent averages of triplicates and error bars represent standard deviations. Results of a representative of 3 repeat experiments is depicted for the binding to the A/Puerto Rico/8/1934 (H1N1) infected cells, the dissociation constant (Kd), is the average of three independent experiments together with the standard deviation. The green shading in the histograms corresponds to the binding of M2e-VHH-23m to mock-infected HEK cells. **(B)** M2e-VHH-23m (2.5, 1.25, or 0.625 μM), 0.333 μM MAb37 or sera of mice infected with A/Puerto Rico/8/1934 (H1N1) virus were incubated with 10 to 20 plaque forming units/well of A/Udorn/307/1972 (H3N2) or A/Puerto Rico/8/1934 (H1N1) virus and then added to MDCK cells. After 1 h, the cells were overlaid with Avicel supplemented with TPCK-treated trypsin. The overlay was removed after 2 days, cells were fixed with paraformaldehyde and viral plaques were stained with convalescent mouse anti- A/Puerto Rico/8/1934 or A/Udorn/307/1972 serum followed by HRP-linked anti-mouse IgG (NXA931, GE Healthcare) and TrueBleu substrate.

not FcγRI, -III, and -IIb. None of the control VHH fusion constructs activated any of the FcγRs, indicating that specificity for both M2e and FcγRIV of the VHH fusion constructs was required. Moreover, activation of the mouse FcγRIV reporter cells by FcγRIV VHH-M2eVHH was only observed in the presence of M2 expressing target cells (**Figure S5**). Potent and dose-dependent activation of mouse FcγRIV by the FcγRIV VHH-M2e VHH fusion was also observed when A/Puerto Rico/8/1934 infected MDCK cells were used as target cells (**Figure 6C**). Finally, FcγRIIIa VHH-M2e VHH, but not FcγRIV VHH-M2eVHH, activated the human FcγRIIIa, the ortholog of mouse FcγRIV, in the presence of A/Puerto Rico/8/1934 infected targeted cells (**Figure 6D**). We conclude that the tail-to-head fusion of the FcγRIV- with the M2e-specific VHHs allows selective, M2-dependent *in vitro* activation of the mouse FcγRIV.

Intranasal Administration of Bispecific FcγRIV VHH-M2e VHH Protects Mice From a Potentially Lethal Influenza A Virus Challenge

In a final set of experiments, we explored the protective potential of FcγRIV VHH-M2e VHH *in vivo*. SPF-housed female BALB/c mice were treated intranasally with 50 μg FcγRIV VHH-M2e VHH 4 h before and 24 h after challenge with 2xLD$_{50}$ of A/X47 (H3N2) influenza virus. As controls, mice were treated with PBS, 50 μg of FcγRIIIa VHH-M2e VHH or FcγRIV VHH-F VHH. The mice that had been treated with FcγRIV VHH-M2e VHH were significantly better protected from body weight loss and lethality caused by the influenza virus infection compared, to mice that had been treated with the negative control VHH fusion constructs, which combine targeting of FcγRIIIa with M2e-specificity or targeting of RSV-F with FcγRIII-specificity (**Figure 7A**). In addition, the protection mediated by FcγRIV VHH-M2e VHH was associated with a modest but statistically significant reduction in lung viral titer (**Figure 7B**). To verify if the protection by FcγRIV VHH-M2e VHH was mediated by FcγRIV engagement, wild-type and $Fc\gamma RIV^{-/-}$ C57BL/6 mice were intranasally treated with 50 μg FcγRIV VHH-M2e VHH or FcγRIIIa VHH-M2e VHH, as negative control, 4 h before and 24 h after challenge with 2xLD$_{50}$ of A/X47 (H3N2) influenza virus. While treatment with FcγRIV VHH-M2e VHH could protect wild-type mice, $Fc\gamma RIV^{-/-}$ mice and control-treated wild-type mice did not survive the virus challenge (**Figure 7C**). Moreover, body weight loss after challenge was statistically significantly reduced in FcγRIV VHH-M2e VHH treated wild-type mice, compared to $Fc\gamma RIV^{-/-}$ mice ($p < 0.001$). Thus, selective targeting of mouse FcγRIV with the recombinant two-domain construct FcγRIV VHH-M2e VHH, can protect mice against a potentially lethal influenza A virus challenge.

DISCUSSION

Formatting of VHH fragments to develop biologicals to prevent or treat infectious diseases is a powerful and attractive approach to develop biologicals with enhanced specificity, activity, half-life and breadth of protection. Here, VHH formatting was used to test if arming of a virus surface antigen-specific VHH with an artificial and selective FcγR activation function can potentiate its activity to combat viral infections in the absence of direct virus neutralization. To explore this possibility, we focused on influenza A M2e as a viral target. This antigen is conserved among influenza A viruses and is therefore an attractive target to achieve broad protection. M2e-specific VHHs were obtained after immunization of a llama with M2e fused to a heterologous tetramerizing domain, to mimic the natural quaternary structure of M2, followed by panning on M2e peptide or cells that stably express M2. We isolated and characterized in more detail three M2e-specific VHHs. Although several M2e-specific conventional MAbs have been described in recent years, to our knowledge, these are the first reported single domain antibodies that specifically bind to M2e. Recently, a M2-specific VHH was isolated from a synthetic VHH library by Wei et al. (57), however their VHH failed to bind to M2e peptide.

We determined the crystal structure of M2e-VHH-23m in complex with a M2e peptide, that corresponds to the consensus sequence of human H1N1 viruses that circulated between 1933 and 2008, human H2N2 and H3N2 viruses. This structure revealed that the M2e antigen is bound by the VHH in an extended conformation that wraps around two main interfaces on the VHH. A first interface is a shallow groove formed by the CDR2 and CDR3 loops and the C, C', C", and F β-strands (**Figure 3A**). This interface binds the M2e region spanning residues 6–12, where Val7, Pro10 and Ile 11 bind hydrophobic patches on the VHH. In addition to three main chain interactions, the side chains of M2eGlu8 and -Thr9 each go into an H-bond interaction with the VHH. A second binding interface is found on the "back" side of the VHH, interacting with

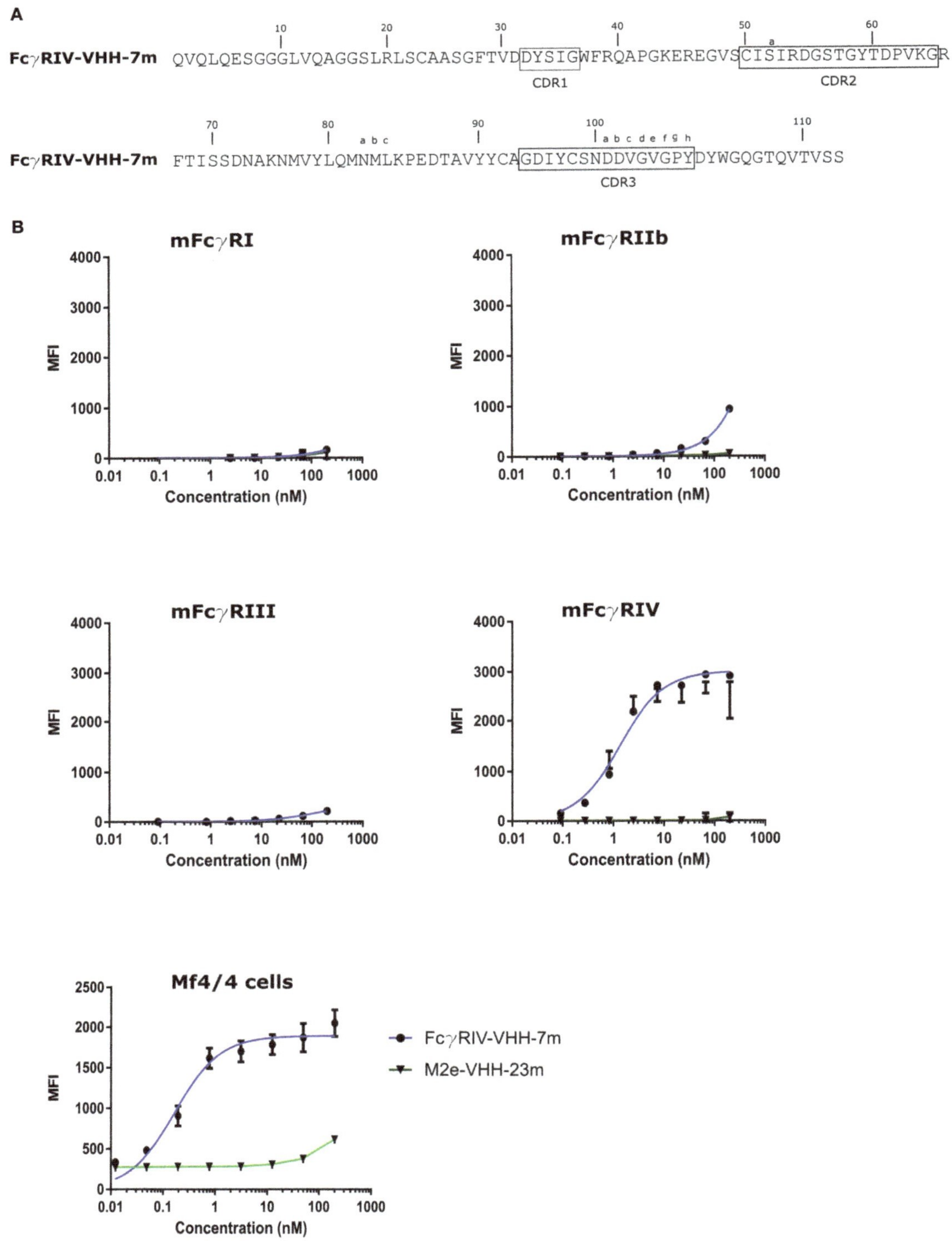

FIGURE 5 | Characterization of the isolated FcγRIV-specific VHH. **(A)** The predicted amino acid residue sequence of FcγRIV-VHH-7m, isolated after panning on recombinant mouse FcγRIV protein of a VHH library derived from a llama immunized with immature mouse dendritic cells. Above the sequences the Kabat numbering is indicated. CDR1, −2, and −3 are boxed. **(B)** Flow cytometric analysis showing binding of FcgRIV-VHH-7m and M2e-VHH-23m to HEK 293T cells transiently transfected with expression vectors coding for mouse FcγRI, FγRIIb, FcγRIII, and FcγRIV along with the common γ-chain for the activating FcγRs and a GFP expression plasmid. The lower graph depicts binding to Mf4/4 cells. The cells were incubated with fourfold serial dilution of Alexa Fluor™ 647 labeled FcγRIV-VHH-7m or M2e-VHH-23m, starting at a concentration of 0.2 μM, binding of the VHHs to the GFP positive cells was analyzed. Data points represent averages of triplicates and error bars standard deviations.

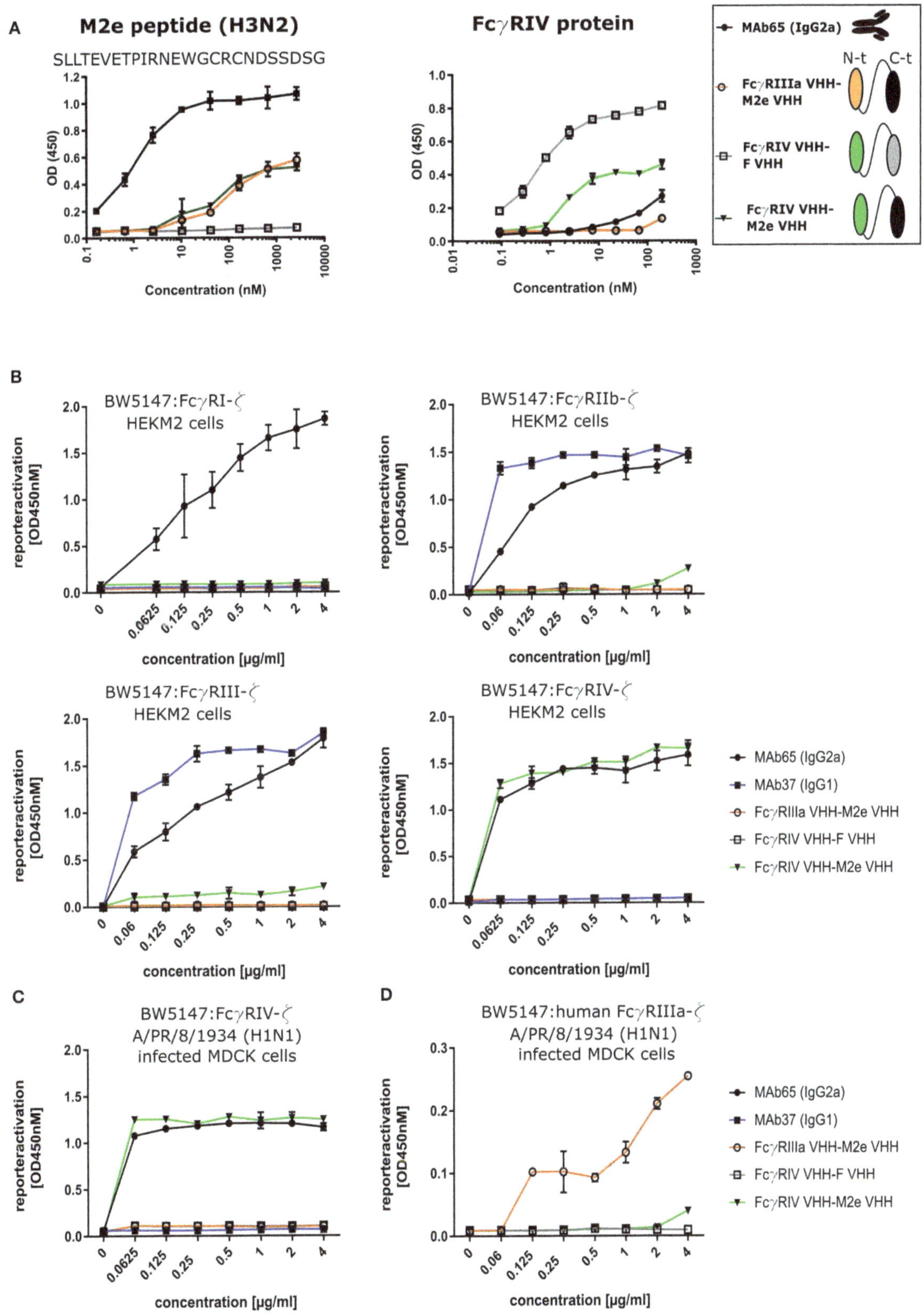

FIGURE 6 | Bispecific fusion construct of anti-mouse FcγRIV VHH with M2e-VHH-23m selectively activates FcγRIV *in vitro*. **(A)** Schematic representation of the bispecific VHHs and ELISA on human H3N2 M2e peptide and recombinant FcγRIV protein is shown on the right. Wells of microtiter plates were coated with 100 ng

(Continued)

FIGURE 6 | peptide or protein. Dilution series of the bispecific VHH fusion constructs were added to the coated plates. Binding was detected with a mouse anti-His tag MAb, followed by a secondary sheep anti-mouse IgG Ab conjugated to HRP for the peptide ELISA. In the ELISA with coated recombinant FcγRIV protein, binding was detected with a HRP-conjugated rabbit anti-camelid VHH antibody. **(B)** Serial dilutions of the bispecific VHH fusion construct or monoclonal antibodies were added to HEK293T cells stably transfected with an influenza M2 expression plasmid. Thirty minutes later, FcγR-ς BW5147 reporter cells were added to the HEK293T cells. After overnight incubation produced mIL-2 was measured in a sandwich-ELISA, which served as an indicator for the magnitude of FcγR activation. (C) MDCK cells were infected with A/Puerto Rico/8/1934 (H1N1) virus for 1 h. Unbound virus particles were washed away and serial dilutions of the bispecific VHHs or monoclonal antibodies were added and incubated for 30 min, followed by the addition of the FcγRIV-ς BW5147 reporter cells **(C)** or human FcγRIIIa-ς BW5147 reporter cells **(D)**. After overnight incubation supernatants were analyzed by an anti mIL-2 sandwich ELISA. Data points represent averages of triplicates and error bars represent standard deviations. The graphs are a representative of one out of three repeat experiments.

residues 14–19 of M2e. This interface contains a well-defined hydrophobic pocket that captures the side chain of the highly conserved Trp15. Most avian and swine influenza A viruses, and, since the 2009 pandemic, also most circulating human H1N1 viruses, have a threonine instead of an isoleucine at position 11 of M2(e). Threonine is not hydrophobic and would be incompatible to the VHH's hydrophobic pocket. This likely explains why M2e-VHH-23m fails to bind to the tested avian and swine M2e peptide variants. In contrast to Ile11, M2e-Trp15, which occupies the second hydrophobic pocket of the VHH, is strictly conserved in all known influenza A viruses. M2e Ala-scan analysis revealed that next to Ile11 and Trp15 also substitution of Val7 or Glu14 considerably impairs binding of M2e-VHH-23m. M2eVal7 is strictly conserved in all influenza A viruses and M2eGlu14 is highly conserved in human influenza A viruses. Since M2eVal7, -Ile11, -Glu14, and -Trp15 are highly conserved in all H3N2 influenza A strains, M2e-VHH-23m might have the potential to recognize the vast majority of these strains. The M2e N-terminus (SLLTEVET) is highly conserved among all influenza A viruses and is recognized by some conventional monoclonal antibodies such as MAb 148 and TCN-032. Despite employing various panning strategies using avian and swine M2e variants, we could not yet isolate a VHH that specifically binds the strictly conserved region in the M2e N-terminus.

Earlier we reported the crystal structures of M2e in complex with the Fab fragment of two different mouse monoclonal antibodies (MAb 65 and MAb 148) that recognize partially overlapping epitopes of M2e (50, 58). In these two crystal structures, M2e adopted two different conformations. The epitopes of the MAb 65 and M2e-VHH-23m are highly similar: they both span the TEVETPIRNEW fragment and in both M2eIle11 and -Trp15 are important for binding. Nevertheless, the conformation of the TEVETPIRNEW part of M2e in complex with M2e-VHH-23m is very different from that in complex with the MAb 65 (**Figure S3**). This indicates that M2e indeed has little intrinsic structure and can adopt multiple conformations dependent on the bound antibody. This flexible nature of the M2e peptide could explain why it appears to be difficult to isolate a VHH that recognizes the N-terminal part of M2e. Moreover, due to the absence of the light chain, VHHs typically bind to concave epitopes rather than to convex or protruding peptide termini (59, 60). Nevertheless a few VHHs directed against linear peptides have been described (61, 62). De Genst et al. reported on a VHH that binds to the C-terminus of the intrinsically disordered a-synuclein protein with nanomolar range affinity (61). The crystal structure revealed that this VHH binds the four C-terminal amino acids of α-synuclein by a narrow pocket formed by its CDR2 and CDR3. This suggests that it may be possible to isolate VHHs that specifically bind the highly conserved N-terminus of M2.

In this study, we also report the isolation of a FcγRIV-specific VHH from a llama that had been immunized with immature mouse dendritic cells. This VHH bound to mouse FcγRIV and showed no cross reactivity with the other FcγRs. To our knowledge, this is the first report of an FcγRIV-specific VHH. A fibronectin scaffold protein that could specifically bind to FcγRIV with high affinity has been reported (63). In addition, this scaffold protein was able to delay tumor growth in a mouse model when linked to an anti-tumor antigen-specific single-chain antibody and mouse serum albumin (to extend the half-life of the fusion construct).

The bivalent VHH comprising the FcγRIV-specific VHH and the M2e-specific VHH, could activate the mouse FcγRIV in the presence of influenza A virus infected cells. Specifically targeting only FcγRIV might be an advantage over conventional antibodies since the activation of the inhibitory FcγRIIb receptor, which dampens the immune cell activation, is circumvented this way. In this context, other strategies such as site-directed mutagenesis, bispecific antibody formats and glycan engineering have been explored to try to increase Fc binding to activating receptors and decrease the interaction with the inhibitory receptor FcγRIIb (64–67). For example, afucosylated antibodies against RSV, Ebola virus and HIV with enhanced FcγR binding showed enhanced efficacy in rodent models (67–69).

When administered 4 h before and 24 h after infection, the bispecific FcγRIV VHH-M2e VHH construct protected wild-type but not $Fc\gamma RIV^{-/-}$ mice against an otherwise lethal influenza A virus challenge. It is well documented that protection by M2e-specifc antibodies is FcγR mediated (6–9). We recently reported that wild type mice treated with an M2e-specific IgG2a showed significantly less body weight loss after infection compared with *FcγRIV-/-* mice, suggesting that FcγRIV could contribute to protection by M2e-specific IgG2a (13). Here we show that the selective activation of the mouse FcγRIV with a bispecific VHH fusion that also binds to M2e is sufficient to protect mice against a potentially lethal influenza A virus challenge. Antitumor activity has been reported for bispecific VHH fusion constructs that consist of a VHH directed against the human FcγRIIIa (the ortholog of the mouse FcγRIV), fused to either a VHH directed against carcinoembryonic antigen (CEA) or HER2 (70, 71). In the context of viral infections, it has been reported that selective engagement of human FcγRIIIa could

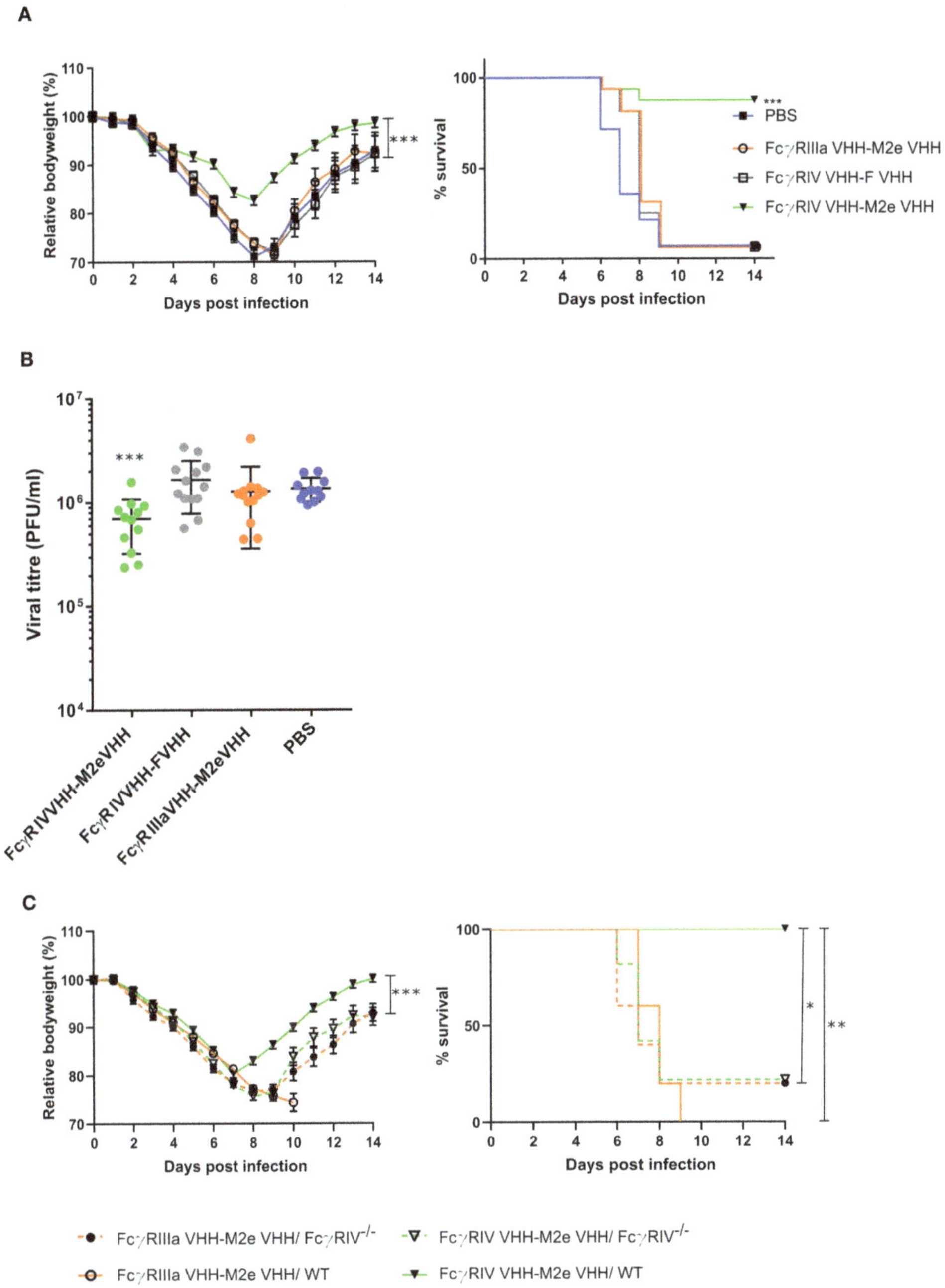

FIGURE 7 | Bispecific fusion construct of a FcγRIV- and M2e-specific VHH protects mice against a potentially lethal influenza A virus infection. **(A)** Groups of 16 (bispecific VHHs) or 14 (PBS) BALB/c mice were intranasally treated with 50 µg of the bispecific VHHs or PBS 4 h before and 24 h after challenge with $2xLD_{50}$ of A/X47 (H3N2) influenza virus. Body weight change (left) and survival (right) were monitored for 14 days. The mean relative changes in body weight together with their standard errors, are represented. The difference in body weight loss between FcγRIV VHH-M2e VHH and the negative-control groups was statistically significant (***$P < 0.001$, REML variance components analysis). The survival rate of the group receiving FcγRIV VHH-M2e VHH was significantly different from FcγRIV VHH-F VHH control treatment group (***$p < 0.001$, Log-rank test). **(B)** To determine the effect on the viral load in the lungs, groups of 13 (bispecific VHHs) or 11 (PBS) BALB/c mice received 50 µg of the bispecific VHHs or PBS 4 h before and 24 h after viral challenge with $2xLD_{50}$ of A/X47 (H3N2) influenza virus. On day 6 after infection, the lungs were harvested and the viral titer was determined by plaque assay. The viral titer of mice FcγRIV VHH-M2e VHH was significantly different compared to mice that received the FcγRIV VHH-F VHH control treatment (***$P < 0.001$, unpaired *t*-test). **(C)** Groups of 5 wild-type and *FcγRIV*$^{-/-}$ C57BL/6 mice (male and female mice) were treated with 50 µg of the bispecific VHHs 4 h before and 24 h after viral challenge with $2xLD_{50}$ of A/X47 (H3N2) influenza virus and body weight (left) and survival (right) were monitored. In the left-hand graph, data points represent means and error bars represent the standard errors of the means. Body weight changes between FcγRIV VHH-M2e VHH treated wild-type and FcγRIV$^{-/-}$ mice were significantly different (***$P < 0.001$, REML variance components analysis). The survival rate of wild-type mice that received FcγRIV VHH-M2e VHH was significantly different from wild-type mice treated with FcγRIIIa VHH-M2e VHH (**$P < 0.01$, REML variance components analysis) and FcγRIV$^{-/-}$ mice treated with FcγRIV VHH-M2e VHH and FcγRIIIa VHH-M2e VHH (*$P < 0.05$, REML variance components analysis). Data in **(A,B)** are pooled from 2 independent experiments.

mediate killing of HIV infected target cells by NK cells (72, 73). It remains to be investigated whether exchanging the mouse FcγRIV specific VHH by a human FcγRIIIa specific VHH in the bispecific fusion construct described here, would be able to protect against influenza A virus infection in the context of a human FcγR repertoire. Moreover, the M2e-specific VHH could be exchanged by a VHH direct against another (conserved) viral target antigen such as the hemagglutinin stalk domain, since FcγRs also seem to play an important role in the protection mediated by anti-stalk antibodies (74, 75).

In summary, we have demonstrated that an intranasally administered, bi-specific VHH fusion construct that selectively binds to and activates FcγRIV with one moiety and M2e as present on infected target cells can protect against influenza A virus challenge. However, the treated mice still showed substantial bodyweight loss following challenge whereas intranasal administration of a M2e-specific IgG2a monoclonal antibody largely controlled the morbidity following challenge of the mice (unpublished result). In future studies one could try to optimize the Fcγ Receptor engaging VHH-fusions by extending their lung retention, and further increasing the affinity for both the viral target and the specific FcγR. Finally, when humanized, formatted M2e-specific VHHs might provide a new treatment option in the battle against influenza A virus infections. This approach could also be of interest for other viral infections. Such VHHs might be especially well suited to prevent or treat respiratory infections because VHHs can be delivered directly to the site of infection as inhaled biotherapeutics by nebulization (27).

ETHICS STATEMENT

All mouse experiments complied with national (Belgian Law 14/08/1986 and 22/12/20333, Belgian Royal Decree 06/04/2010) and European legislation (EU Directives 2010/63/EU and 86/609EEG) on animal regulations. All experiments were approved by and performed according to the guidelines of the animal ethical committee of Ghent University (permit number LA1400091, ethical applications EC2017-66 and EC2018-12).

AUTHOR CONTRIBUTIONS

DD, BS, and XS planned the study. DD, KH, IV, WN, LV, MB, SC, and BS performed the research. DD, BS, IV, and XS wrote the manuscript with contributions from KH, WN, HR, and HH. All authors reviewed the manuscript before submission.

ACKNOWLEDGMENTS

We thank the VIB Nanobody Core facility for the llama immunizations and preparation of the VHH phage libraries. We also thank Marnik Vuylsteke for performing the statistical analysis and Geert Raes for providing the phage library of a llama immunized with immature mouse dendritic cells. We thank the beamline scientists at the i03 beamline of the Diamond Light Source synchrotron facility.

REFERENCES

1. Paules CI, Fauci AS. Influenza vaccines: good, but we can do better. *J Infect Dis.* (2019) 219:S1–4. doi: 10.1093/infdis/jiy633
2. Koszalka P, Tilmanis D, Roe M, Vijaykrishna D, Hurt AC. Baloxavir marboxil susceptibility of influenza viruses from the Asia-Pacific, 2012–2018. *Antiviral Res.* (2019) 164:91–6. doi: 10.1016/j.antiviral.2019.02.007
3. Lee N, Hurt AC. Neuraminidase inhibitor resistance in influenza: a clinical perspective. *Curr Opin Infect Dis.* (2018) 31:520–6. doi: 10.1097/QCO.0000000000000498
4. Saelens X. The role of M2e in the development of universal influenza vaccines. *J Infect Dis.* (2019) 219:S68–74. doi: 10.1093/infdis/jiz003
5. Ito T, Gorman OT, Kawaoka Y, Bean WJ, Webster RG. Evolutionary analysis of the influenza A virus M gene with comparison of the M1 and M2 proteins. *J Virol.* (1991) 65:5491–8.
6. Neirynck S, Deroo T, Saelens X, Vanlandschoot P, Jou WM, Fiers W. A universal influenza A vaccine based on the extracellular domain of the M2 protein. *Nat Med.* (1999) 5:1157–63. doi: 10.1038/13484
7. Fan J, Liang X, Horton MS, Perry HC, Citron MP, Heidecker, GJ, et al. Preclinical study of influenza virus A M2 peptide conjugate vaccines in mice, ferrets, and rhesus monkeys. *Vaccine.* (2004) 22:2993–3003. doi: 10.1016/j.vaccine.2004.02.021
8. Turley CB, Rupp RE, Johnson C, Taylor DN, Wolfson J, Tussey L, et al. Safety and immunogenicity of a recombinant M2e-flagellin influenza vaccine (STF2.4xM2e) in healthy adults. *Vaccine.* (2011) 29:5145–52. doi: 10.1016/j.vaccine.2011.05.041
9. Slepushkin VA, Katz JM, Black RA, Gamble WC, Rota PA, Cox NJ. Protection of mice against influenza A virus challenge by vaccination with baculovirus-expressed M2 protein. *Vaccine.* (1995) 13:1399–402. doi: 10.1016/0264-410X(95)92777-Y
10. Ramos EL, Mitcham JL, Koller TD, Bonavia A, Usner DW, Balaratnam G, et al. Efficacy and safety of treatment with an anti-m2e monoclonal antibody in experimental human influenza. *J Infect Dis.* (2015) 211:1038–44. doi: 10.1093/infdis/jiu539
11. Pendzialek J, Roose K, Smet A, Schepens B, Kufer P, Raum T, et al. Bispecific T cell engaging antibody constructs targeting a universally conserved part of the viral M2 ectodomain cure and prevent influenza A virus infection. *Antiviral Res.* (2017) 141:155–64. doi: 10.1016/j.antiviral.2017.02.016
12. El Bakkouri K, Descamps F, De Filette M, Smet A, Festjens E, Birkett A, et al. Universal vaccine based on ectodomain of matrix protein 2 of influenza A: Fc receptors and alveolar macrophages mediate protection. *J Immunol.* (2011) 186:1022–31. doi: 10.4049/jimmunol.0902147
13. Van den Hoecke S, Ehrhardt K, Kolpe A, El Bakkouri K, Deng L, Grootaert H, et al. Hierarchical and redundant roles of activating FcγRs in protection against influenza disease by M2e-specific IgG1 and IgG2a antibodies. *J Virol.* (2017) 91:1–13. doi: 10.1128/JVI.02500-16
14. Song A, Myojo K, Laudenslager J, Harada D, Miura T, Suzuki K, et al. Evaluation of a fully human monoclonal antibody against multiple influenza A viral strains in mice and a pandemic H1N1 strain in nonhuman primates. *Antiviral Res.* (2014) 111:60–8. doi: 10.1016/j.antiviral.2014.08.016
15. Guilliams M, Bruhns P, Saeys Y, Hammad H, Lambrecht BN. The function of Fcγ receptors in dendritic cells and macrophages. *Nat Rev Immunol.* (2014) 14:94–108. doi: 10.1038/nri3582
16. Bruhns P. Properties of mouse and human IgG receptors and their contribution to disease models. *Blood.* (2012) 119:5640–9. doi: 10.1182/blood-2012-01-380121
17. Ra C, Jouvin MH, Blank U, Kinet JP. A macrophage Fc gamma receptor and the mast cell receptor for IgE share an identical subunit. *Nature.* (1989) 341:752–4. doi: 10.1038/341752a0

18. Daëron M, Latour S, Malbec O, Espinosa E, Pina P, Pasmans S, Fridman WH. The same tyrosine-based inhibition motif, in the intracytoplasmic domain of Fc gamma RIIB, regulates negatively BCR-, TCR-, and FcR-dependent cell activation. *Immunity.* (1995) 3:635–46. doi: 10.1016/1074-7613(95)90134-5
19. Cambier JC. New nomenclature for the Reth motif (or ARH1/TAM/ARAM/YXXL). *Immunol Today.* (1995) 16:110. doi: 10.1016/0167-5699(95)80105-7
20. Nimmerjahn F, Bruhns P, Horiuchi K, Ravetch JV. FcgammaRIV: a novel FcR with distinct IgG subclass specificity. *Immunity.* (2005) 23:41–51. doi: 10.1016/j.immuni.2005.05.010
21. Hamers-Casterman C, Atarhouch T, Muyldermans S, Robinson G, Hamers C, Songa EB, et al. Naturally occurring antibodies devoid of light chains. *Nature.* (1993) 363:446–8. doi: 10.1038/363446a0
22. Wu Y, Jiang S, Ying T. Single-domain antibodies as therapeutics against human viral diseases. *Front Immunol.* (2017) 8:1802. doi: 10.3389/fimmu.2017.01802
23. De Vlieger D, Ballegeer M, Rossey I, Schepens B, Saelens X. Single-domain antibodies and their formatting to combat viral infections. *Antibodies.* (2019) 8:1. doi: 10.3390/antib8010001
24. *A Multicentre Study in Otherwise Healthy Infants and Toddlers Hospitalised For and Diagnosed With RSV Lower Respiratory Tract Infection to Evaluate the Safety, Tolerability, and Clinical Activity of ALX-0171 - Full Text View - ClinicalTrials.gov.* Available online at: https://clinicaltrials.gov/ct2/show/NCT02309320 (accessed May 17, 2019).
25. van der Linden RH, Frenken LG, de Geus B, Harmsen MM, Ruuls RC, Stok W, et al. Comparison of physical chemical properties of llama VHH antibody fragments and mouse monoclonal antibodies. *Biochim Biophys Acta.* (1999) 1431:37–46. doi: 10.1016/S0167-4838(99)00030-8
26. Dumoulin M, Conrath K, Van Meirhaeghe A, Meersman F, Heremans K, Frenken LGJ, et al. Single-domain antibody fragments with high conformational stability. *Protein Sci.* (2002) 11:500–15. doi: 10.1110/ps.34602
27. Van Heeke G, Allosery K, De Brabandere V, De Smedt T, Detalle L, de Fougerolles A. Nanobodies® as inhaled biotherapeutics for lung diseases. *Pharmacol Ther.* (2017) 169:47–56. doi: 10.1016/j.pharmthera.2016.06.012
28. De Filette M, Martens W, Roose K, Deroo T, Vervalle F, Bentahir M, et al. An influenza A vaccine based on tetrameric ectodomain of matrix protein 2. *J Biol Chem.* (2008) 283:11382–7. doi: 10.1074/jbc.M800650200
29. Desmedt M, Rottiers P, Dooms H, Fiers W, Grooten J. Macrophages induce cellular immunity by activating Th1 cell responses and suppressing Th2 cell responses. *J Immunol.* (1998) 160:5300–8.
30. Corrales-Aguilar E, Trilling M, Reinhard H, Mercé-Maldonado E, Widera M, Schaal H, et al. A novel assay for detecting virus-specific antibodies triggering activation of Fcγ receptors. *J Immunol Methods.* (2013) 387:21–35. doi: 10.1016/j.jim.2012.09.006
31. Corrales-Aguilar E, Trilling M, Hunold K, Fiedler M, Le VTK, Reinhard H, et al. Human cytomegalovirus Fcγ binding proteins gp34 and gp68 antagonize Fcγ receptors I, II and III. *PLoS Pathog.* (2014) 10:e1004131. doi: 10.1371/journal.ppat.1004131
32. Deschacht N, Groeve KD, Vincke C, Raes G, Baetselier PD, Muyldermans S. A novel promiscuous class of camelid single-domain antibody contributes to the antigen-binding repertoire. *J Immunol.* (2010) 184:5696–704. doi: 10.4049/jimmunol.0903722
33. Schoonooghe S, Kaigorodov V, Zawisza M, Dumolyn C, Haustraete J, Grooten J, et al. Efficient production of human bivalent and trivalent anti-MUC1 Fab-scFv antibodies in Pichia pastoris. *BMC Biotechnol.* (2009) 9:70. doi: 10.1186/1472-6750-9-70
34. Lin-Cereghino J, Wong WW, Xiong S, Giang W, Luong LT, Vu J, et al. Condensed protocol for competent cell preparation and transformation of the methylotrophic yeast Pichia pastoris. *BioTechniques.* (2005) 38:44–8. doi: 10.2144/05381BM04
35. McCoy AJ, Grosse-Kunstleve RW, Adams PD, Winn MD, Storoni LC, Read RJ. Phaser crystallographic software. *J Appl Crystallogr.* (2007) 40:658–74. doi: 10.1107/S0021889807021206
36. Vagin A, Teplyakov A. Molecular replacement with MOLREP. *Acta Crystallogr D Biol Crystallogr.* (2010) 66:22–5. doi: 10.1107/S0907444909042589
37. Adams PD, Afonine PV, Bunkóczi G, Chen VB, Davis IW, Echols N, et al. PHENIX: a comprehensive Python-based system for macromolecular structure solution. *Acta Crystallogr D Biol Crystallogr.* (2010) 66:213–21. doi: 10.1107/S0907444909052925
38. Emsley P, Cowtan K. Coot: model-building tools for molecular graphics. *Acta Crystallogr D Biol Crystallogr.* (2004) 60:2126–32. doi: 10.1107/S0907444904019158
39. Afonine PV, Grosse-Kunstleve RW, Echols N, Headd JJ, Moriarty NW, Mustyakimov M, et al. Towards automated crystallographic structure refinement with phenix.refine. *Acta Crystallogr D Biol Crystallogr.* (2012) 68:352–67. doi: 10.1107/S0907444912001308
40. Murshudov GN, Vagin AA, Dodson EJ. Refinement of macromolecular structures by the maximum-likelihood method. *Acta Crystallogr D Biol Crystallogr.* (1997) 53:240–55. doi: 10.1107/S0907444996012255
41. Guex N, Peitsch MC. SWISS-MODEL and the Swiss-PdbViewer: an environment for comparative protein modeling. *Electrophoresis.* (1997) 18:2714–23. doi: 10.1002/elps.1150181505
42. Hanwell MD, Curtis DE, Lonie DC, Vandermeersch T, Zurek E, Hutchison GR. Avogadro: an advanced semantic chemical editor, visualization, and analysis platform. *J Cheminform.* (2012) 4:17. doi: 10.1186/1758-2946-4-17
43. Morris GM, Huey R, Lindstrom W, Sanner MF, Belew RK, Goodsell DS, et al. AutoDock4 and AutoDockTools4: automated docking with selective receptor flexibility. *J Comput Chem.* (2009) 30:2785–91. doi: 10.1002/jcc.21256
44. Trott O, Olson AJ. AutoDock vina: improving the speed and accuracy of docking with a new scoring function, efficient optimization and multithreading. *J Comput Chem.* (2010) 31:455–61. doi: 10.1002/jcc.21334
45. Koes DR, Baumgartner MP, Camacho CJ. Lessons learned in empirical scoring with smina from the CSAR 2011 benchmarking exercise. *J Chem Inf Model.* (2013) 53:1893–904. doi: 10.1021/ci300604z
46. *PyMOL | pymol.org.* Available online at: https://pymol.org/2/ (accessed July 3, 2019).
47. Sarrion-Perdigones A, Vazquez-Vilar M, Palací J, Castelijns B, Forment J, Ziarsolo P, et al. GoldenBraid 2.0: a comprehensive DNA assembly framework for plant synthetic biology. *Plant Physiol.* (2013) 162:1618–31. doi: 10.1104/pp.113.217661
48. Behar G, Sibéril S, Groulet A, Chames P, Pugnière M, Boix C, et al. Isolation and characterization of anti-FcgammaRIII (CD16) llama single-domain antibodies that activate natural killer cells. *Protein Eng Des Sel.* (2008) 21:1–10. doi: 10.1093/protein/gzm064
49. Nimmerjahn F, Lux A, Albert H, Woigk M, Lehmann C, Dudziak D, et al. FcγRIV deletion reveals its central role for IgG2a and IgG2b activity *in vivo*. *Proc Natl Acad Sci USA.* (2010) 107:19396–401. doi: 10.1073/pnas.1014515107
50. Cho KJ, Schepens B, Seok JH, Kim S, Roose K, Lee J-H, et al. Structure of the extracellular domain of matrix protein 2 of influenza A virus in complex with a protective monoclonal antibody. *J Virol.* (2015) 89:3700–11. doi: 10.1128/JVI.02576-14
51. Kunz P, Zinner K, Mücke N, Bartoschik T, Muyldermans S, Hoheisel JD. The structural basis of nanobody unfolding reversibility and thermoresistance. *Sci Rep.* (2018) 8:7934. doi: 10.1038/s41598-018-26338-z
52. Rossey I, Gilman MSA, Kabeche SC, Sedeyn K, Wrapp D, Kanekiyo M, et al. Potent single-domain antibodies that arrest respiratory syncytial virus fusion protein in its prefusion state. *Nat Commun.* (2017) 8:14158. doi: 10.1038/ncomms14158
53. Liu Y, Eisenberg D. 3D domain swapping: as domains continue to swap. *Protein Sci.* (2002) 11:1285–99. doi: 10.1110/ps.0201402
54. Zebedee SL, Lamb RA. Influenza A virus M2 protein: monoclonal antibody restriction of virus growth and detection of M2 in virions. *J Virol.* (1988) 62:2762–72.
55. Kolpe A, Schepens B, Ye L, Staeheli P, Saelens X. Passively transferred M2e-specific monoclonal antibody reduces influenza A virus transmission in mice. *Antiviral Res.* (2018) 158:244–54. doi: 10.1016/j.antiviral.2018.08.017
56. Kolpe A, Arista-Romero M, Schepens B, Pujals S, Saelens X, Albertazzi L. Super-resolution microscopy reveals significant impact of M2e-specific monoclonal antibodies on influenza A virus filament formation at the host cell surface. *Sci Rep.* (2019) 9:4450. doi: 10.1038/s41598-019-41023-5
57. Wei G, Meng W, Guo H, Pan W, Liu J, Peng T, et al. Potent neutralization of influenza A virus by a single-domain antibody blocking M2 ion channel protein. *PLoS ONE.* (2011) 6:e28309. doi: 10.1371/journal.pone.0028309

58. Cho KJ, Schepens B, Moonens K, Deng L, Fiers W, Remaut H, et al. Crystal structure of the conserved amino terminus of the extracellular domain of matrix protein 2 of influenza A virus gripped by an antibody. *J Virol.* (2015) 90:611–5. doi: 10.1128/JVI.02105-15
59. Pírez-Schirmer M, Rossotti M, Badagian N, Leizagoyen C, Brena BM, González-Sapienza G. Comparison of three antihapten VHH selection strategies for the development of highly sensitive immunoassays for microcystins. *Anal Chem.* (2017) 89:6800–6. doi: 10.1021/acs.analchem.7b01221
60. De Genst E, Silence K, Decanniere K, Conrath K, Loris R, Kinne J, et al. Molecular basis for the preferential cleft recognition by dromedary heavy-chain antibodies. *Proc Natl Acad Sci USA.* (2006) 103:4586–91. doi: 10.1073/pnas.0505379103
61. De Genst EJ, Guilliams T, Wellens J, O'Day EM, Waudby CA, Meehan S, et al. Structure and properties of a complex of α-synuclein and a single-domain camelid antibody. *J Mol Biol.* (2010) 402:326–43. doi: 10.1016/j.jmb.2010.07.001
62. Braun MB, Traenkle B, Koch PA, Emele F, Weiss F, Poetz O, et al. Peptides in headlock – a novel high-affinity and versatile peptide-binding nanobody for proteomics and microscopy. *Sci Rep.* (2016) 6:19211. doi: 10.1038/srep19211
63. Chen TF, Li KK, Zhu EF, Opel CF, Kauke MJ, Kim H, et al. Artificial anti-tumor opsonizing proteins with fibronectin scaffolds engineered for specificity to each of the murine FcγR types. *J Mol Biol.* (2018) 430:1786–98. doi: 10.1016/j.jmb.2018.04.021
64. Shields RL, Namenuk AK, Hong K, Meng YG, Rae J, Briggs J, et al. High resolution mapping of the binding site on human IgG1 for Fc gamma RI, Fc gamma RII, Fc gamma RIII, and FcRn and design of IgG1 variants with improved binding to the Fc gamma R. *J Biol Chem.* (2001) 276:6591–604. doi: 10.1074/jbc.M009483200
65. Mori K, Iida S, Yamane-Ohnuki N, Kanda Y, Kuni-Kamochi R, Nakano R, et al. Non-fucosylated therapeutic antibodies: the next generation of therapeutic antibodies. *Cytotechnology.* (2007) 55:109–14. doi: 10.1007/s10616-007-9103-2
66. Müller D, Karle A, Meissburger B, Höfig I, Stork R, Kontermann RE. Improved pharmacokinetics of recombinant bispecific antibody molecules by fusion to human serum albumin. *J Biol Chem.* (2007) 282:12650–60. doi: 10.1074/jbc.M700820200
67. Hiatt A, Bohorova N, Bohorov O, Goodman C, Kim D, Pauly MH, et al. Glycan variants of a respiratory syncytial virus antibody with enhanced effector function and *in vivo* efficacy. *Proc Natl Acad Sci USA.* (2014) 111:5992–7. doi: 10.1073/pnas.1402458111
68. Bardhi A, Wu Y, Chen W, Li W, Zhu Z, Zheng JH, et al. Potent *in vivo* NK cell-mediated elimination of HIV-1-infected cells mobilized by a gp120-bispecific and hexavalent broadly neutralizing fusion protein. *J Virol.* (2017) 91:1–19. doi: 10.1128/JVI.00937-17
69. Zeitlin L, Pettitt J, Scully C, Bohorova N, Kim D, Pauly M, et al. Enhanced potency of a fucose-free monoclonal antibody being developed as an Ebola virus immunoprotectant. *Proc Natl Acad Sci USA.* (2011) 108:20690–4. doi: 10.1073/pnas.1108360108
70. Rozan C, Cornillon A, Pétiard C, Chartier M, Behar G, Boix C, et al. Single-domain antibody-based and linker-free bispecific antibodies targeting FcγRIII induce potent antitumor activity without recruiting regulatory T cells. *Mol Cancer Ther.* (2013) 12:1481–91. doi: 10.1158/1535-7163.MCT-12-1012
71. Turini M, Chames P, Bruhns P, Baty D, Kerfelec B. A FcγRIII-engaging bispecific antibody expands the range of HER2-expressing breast tumors eligible to antibody therapy. *Oncotarget.* (2014) 5:5304–19. doi: 10.18632/oncotarget.2093
72. Li W, Wu Y, Kong D, Yang H, Wang Y, Shao J, et al. One-domain CD4 fused to human anti-CD16 antibody domain mediates effective killing of HIV-1-infected cells. *Sci Rep.* (2017) 7:9130. doi: 10.1038/s41598-017-07966-3
73. Gleason MK, Verneris MR, Todhunter DA, Zhang B, McCullar V, Zhou SX, et al. Bispecific and trispecific killer cell engagers directly activate human NK cells through CD16 signaling and induce cytotoxicity and cytokine production. *Mol Cancer Ther.* (2012) 11:2674–84. doi: 10.1158/1535-7163.MCT-12-0692
74. DiLillo DJ, Tan GS, Palese P, Ravetch JV. Broadly neutralizing hemagglutinin stalk-specific antibodies require FcγR interactions for protection against influenza virus *in vivo*. *Nat Med.* (2014) 20:143–51. doi: 10.1038/nm.3443
75. Thulin NK, Wang TT. The role of Fc gamma receptors in broad protection against influenza viruses. *Vaccines (Basel).* (2018) 6:36. doi: 10.3390/vaccines6030036

2

The Genetics of Human Schistosomiasis Infection Intensity and Liver Disease

Estelle M. Mewamba[1†] *Oscar A. Nyangiri*[2†], *Harry A. Noyes*[3], *Moses Egesa*[4,5], *Enock Matovu*[2] *and Gustave Simo*[1*] *for the TrypanoGEN+ research group of the H3Africa consortium*

[1] *Molecular Parasitology and Entomology Unit, Faculty of Science, University of Dschang, Dschang, Cameroon,* [2] *College of Veterinary Medicine Animal Resources and Biosecurity, Makerere University, Kampala, Uganda,* [3] *Centre for Genomic Research, School of Biological Sciences, University of Liverpool, Liverpool, United Kingdom,* [4] *Medical Research Council/Uganda Virus Research Institute and London School of Hygiene & Tropical Medicine Uganda Research Unit, Entebbe, Uganda,* [5] *London School of Hygiene and Tropical Medicine, London, United Kingdom*

Correspondence:
Gustave Simo
gsimoca@yahoo.fr

† These authors have contributed equally to this work and share first authorship

Schistosomiasis remains the fourth most prevalent parasitic disease affecting over 200 million people worldwide. Control efforts have focussed on the disruption of the life cycle targeting the parasite, vector and human host. Parasite burdens are highly skewed, and the majority of eggs are shed into the environment by a minority of the infected population. Most morbidity results from hepatic fibrosis leading to portal hypertension and is not well-correlated with worm burden. Genetics as well as environmental factors may play a role in these skewed distributions and understanding the genetic risk factors for intensity of infection and morbidity may help improve control measures. In this review, we focus on how genetic factors may influence parasite load, hepatic fibrosis and portal hypertension. We found 28 studies on the genetics of human infection and 20 studies on the genetics of pathology in humans. *S. mansoni* and *S. haematobium* infection intensity have been showed to be controlled by a major quantitative trait locus *SM1*, on chromosome 5q31-q33 containing several genes involved in the T_h2 immune response, and three other loci of smaller effect on chromosomes 1, 6, and 7. The most common pathology associated with schistosomiasis is hepatic and portal vein fibroses and the *SM2* quantitative trait locus on chromosome six has been linked to intensity of fibrosis. Although there has been an emphasis on T_h2 cytokines in candidate gene studies, we found that four of the five QTL regions contain T_h17 pathway genes that have been included in schistosomiasis studies: *IL17B* and *IL12B* in *SM1*, *IL17A* and *IL17F* in 6p21-q2, *IL6R* in 1p21-q23 and *IL22RA2* in *SM2*. The T_h17 pathway is known to be involved in response to schistosome infection and hepatic fibrosis but variants in this pathway have not been tested for any effect on the regulation of these phenotypes. These should be priorities for future studies.

Keywords: schistosomiasis, fibrosis, Th17, intensity of infection, QTL, linkage

INTRODUCTION

Schistosomiasis is caused by digenic trematodes of the genus *Schistosoma* with *Schistosoma mansoni* and *Schistosoma haematobium* causing the majority of human infections. Adult parasites live in the veins around the gut and bladder and eggs are excreted in feces or urine and infect snails in fresh water. Parasite numbers are amplified in the snail intermediate host and human infective stages then emerge that can penetrate human skin when people enter the water. Schistosomiasis induces acute, severe, and chronic morbidity among those who are infected and can cause liver and bladder fibrosis and eventually bladder or colorectal cancer (1). Although exposure to water infested with the infective schistosome cercariae is the main risk factor for schistosomiasis there is considerable variation in infection intensity between people with similar exposures and schistosomiasis cases aggregate in families, some of this variation has been attributed to the genetics of the human immune response (2–4).

A review of the genetics of human susceptibility to schistosomiasis related fibrosis has been published recently (5), but there has been no review of the genetics of schistosome infection since 2008 (2).

A fundamental understanding of the genetics of schistosomiasis susceptibility and high worm load may contribute to rational design of interventions, including vaccines (6). For example, it has recently been shown that a set of 32 SNPs in 10 genes can predict susceptibility to severe hepatic disease among Brazilians with 63% sensitivity and 90% specificity (5). In the present review of the genetics of human susceptibility to schistosomiasis we focus on loci associated with egg/worm burden and hepatic fibrosis.

We therefore present an updated review of the genes and variants that have been found associated with schistosomiasis infection intensity and liver disease, together with a review of genes within QTL that could be prioritized for future analyses. We have excluded the HLA region since we have only identified one study of genes in this region since they were was last reviewed (7, 8).

Epidemiology and Treatment

The disease affects almost 240 million people, and 700 million are at risk of infection in 74 countries, the majority being in Africa, Asia and South America (9, 10). Between 3 and 56 million disability-adjusted life years (DALYs) are lost per annum and 280,000 deaths per annum have been attributed to effects of schistosomiasis (11–13). Approximately 85% of infections occur in sub-Saharan Africa and at least 90% of people requiring treatment for schistosomiasis live in Africa (14). Schistosomiasis can also be associated with chronic anemia, childhood growth stunting, protein calorie malnutrition, cognitive disability, and poor school performance (15–20).

Control of schistosomiasis has continued to rely mainly on mass drug administration (MDA) of school-aged children using the anti-schistosomal drug praziquantel (PZQ) (21, 22). Although this strategy has reduced morbidity, the impact on prevalence has been more limited, because praziquantel does not kill immature schistosomes (23, 24), coverage remains restricted and only school age children are routinely treated. Vaccines are in development but phase three trials have not been successful (25).

Immune Responses During Schistosome Infections

Immune responses to penetrating and migrating *Schistosoma* larvae (schistosomula) and maturing adults are predominantly T_h1 (26). Excretory/secretory *Schistosoma* antigens damage host barrier cells which release alarmins, activate innate cells and induce proinflammatory cytokines (IL1B, IL6, IL17, TNF, and IFNG) (27). About 6 weeks after infection, *Schistosoma* eggs are deposited in tissues (the liver and the intestine or the bladder) and trigger an expansion of T_h2 cells (28). *Schistosoma* egg antigens also directly bind receptors on antigen presenting cells inhibiting IL12 production and consequently T_h1 responses (29). T_h2 responses can also be induced independently of egg deposition as infection with single sex schistosomes induce pre-patent IL4 production by CD4 T cells (30). Schistosome specific T_h2 responses are downmodulated in long-standing infections (31) and this is associated with a development of regulatory cells producing IL10 and transforming growth factor beta (TGFB). This not only allows the parasite to survive in the host and minimize host tissue damage but also modulates host immune responses to unrelated antigens including allergens, self-antigens, and vaccines.

Schistosome egg secretions are highly antigenic (31) and typically induce polarized granulomatous T_h2 responses (32). Granulomas form around eggs lodged in tissues to protect tissue cells (33) but persistent host CD4 T_h2 cell mediated responses to parasite eggs cause fibrosis (34). The pro-fibrotic T_h2 cytokine IL13 is associated with periportal fibrosis in humans (35). Beyond T_h2 cytokine responses, intensified hepatic granulomatous inflammation in *S. mansoni* infected mice is associated with high levels of IL17 and controlled by IFNG (36). In human schistosomiasis, IL17 producing CD4 T helper cells are associated with ultrasound textural abnormalities while T regulatory cells are associated with reductions in this pathology (37).

Phenotypes

Schistosomal Fecal Egg Count and Worm Burden

Studies of the human genetics of susceptibility to schistosomiasis have focussed on two classes of phenotype; infection associated phenotypes and pathology related phenotypes. Infection associated phenotypes are usually egg counts or worm burden estimates but sometimes total IgE as a marker of the immune response (38). Eggs counts are obtained by the Kato Katz (KK) method for *S. mansoni* and by urine filtration for *S. haematobium* and worm burdens are estimated by measuring the circulating cathodic antigen (CCA) in urine or circulating anodic antigen (CAA) in plasma (39) that are produced by adult worms.

Approximately 80% of the environmental egg burden from helminths including schistosomes, derives from ~20% of the cases (40). For example 22 out of 119 Kenyan school children had developed high *S. mansoni* egg burden (>100 eggs per gram of feces) 12 months after treatment, whilst 70 children still had low (<30 epg) egg burdens (41) and this effect was not correlated with the amount of water contact. This tendency for some people to develop high infections even after treatment has been attributed to variation in genetic risk (42).

Schistosome egg burdens are also highly skewed by age with egg burdens increasing up to the age of puberty and declining thereafter (43–46). A study in Brazil found that children under 19 had egg burdens that were over ten times higher than older adults (42). The higher intensity and frequency of infections in children may be due to the slow development of immunity to schistosomes. Possibly, the antigens that are exposed by dying worms cross react with larval antigens and stimulate a protective anti-larval IgE response. The long life span of adult worms (5–15 years) means that it takes many years for children to be exposed to sufficient dying worms to develop an IgE response to the larvae (47). High anti-parasite IgE levels have been associated with resistance and high specific IgG4 has been associated with susceptibility and it has been proposed that the ratio of these two immunoglobulins controls resistance to schistosomiasis (48–51).

Schistosomiasis Associated Hepatic and Periportal Fibrosis and Portal Vein Hypertension

Although schistosomes cause a wide range of symptoms and fibrotic lesions can form around egg granulomas in many tissues, the main indicator of *S. mansoni* and *S. japonicum* pathology is hepatic fibrosis (HF) and periportal fibrosis (PPF) (52). WHO guidelines provide scoring scales for HF and PPF (53) and both scales are used as phenotypes in genetic research (54). HF and PPF is caused by extracellular matrix forming around schistosome eggs. In the hepatic portal vein this can lead to portal hypertension (PH) (55, 56), ultimately, some patients with PH die of internal bleeding, superinfections, or heart or kidney failure. *S. haematobium* is associated with bladder cancer and *S. mansoni* may be associated with hepatocellular carcinoma (57) but genetic studies of the pathology of schistosomiasis have focussed almost exclusively on hepatic and periportal fibrosis and in this review all references to pathology are to these closely related conditions unless otherwise indicated. Fibrosis can be measured by ultrasound scan, although there are concerns about the accuracy and reproducibility of ultrasound (58); additional markers and protocols for grading pathology are being developed but are not well-validated (59–61).

GENOME WIDE LINKAGE STUDIES DISCOVER SCHISTOSOMIASIS SUSCEPTIBILITY LOCI

The reviews of linkage and candidate gene studies of schistosomiasis are broken down into two sections by phenotype: (1) studies of infection status, which is usually determined by egg count in urine or feces and (2) studies of pathology which is mainly periportal fibrosis determined by ultra-sound. Relevant publications were identified by searching PubMed using the terms in **Supplementary Table 1**.

Heritability of Schistosomiasis Infection Risk

Heritability, the proportion of risk attributable to genetic variation, must be substantial to be detectable. A summary of heritability estimates for schistosomiasis are shown in **Table 1**. Studies in Brazil (62–64); Kenya (46); and China (65, 66) have each estimated similar proportions of the variance of *S. mansoni* egg count that are attributable to genetic variation, with additive heritability (*h2*) estimates of 23–31%. However, there were striking differences in the two estimates for heritability of infection with *S. japonicum* in China using variance components (VC) (0 & 58%) (**Table 1**), which have been discussed by others (2).

Linkage Studies for *Schistosoma* Egg Count

The initial study of the genetics of human schistosomiasis used segregation analysis, which determines whether the distribution of the disease on family pedigrees is consistent with the presence of a major gene (3). This study demonstrated the presence of a major gene which was subsequently named *SM1* and located on chromosome five by parametric linkage analysis (4). A major gene has alleles that cause a difference in phenotype between family members that is large enough to be able to categorize individuals as carriers or non-carriers on the basis of phenotype alone (67) and parametric linkage analysis requires estimates of the disease allele frequency and penetrance of the phenotype for the three possible genotypes.

The *SM1* quantitative trait locus (QTL) on chromosome 5 5q31-q33 for *S. mansoni* fecal egg count was the first QTL to be mapped in humans for any infectious disease (**Table 2**, **Figure 1**) (4). The great success of this study was partially attributable to the very large effect size of the *SM1* locus (66% of the variance after accounting for water contact, age and sex). This is in striking contrast to the very modest proportions of the variance explained by most loci identified by GWAS in which loci rarely explain more than 10% of the variance of the trait that is not attributable to covariates (96). Three further loci (1p22.2, 7q36 and 21q22-22-qter) had evidence of association and contained genes known to be involved in the response to schistosomes but did not achieve genome wide significance (68). A reanalysis of the same data controlling for *SM1* genotype identified additional genome wide significant loci at 1p21-q23 and 6p21-q21 (**Table 2**, **Figure 1**) (69), since the effect of these loci was small in comparison to the effect of *SM1,* they were only identifiable when using *SM1* genotype as a parameter of the model.

A further study on a Senegalese population, by the same group that conducted the original study in Brazil, confirmed an association at the *SM1* locus. However, the effect was not as strong and the association could only be demonstrated by non-parametric pedigree tests for an effect at the *SM1* locus (70). Non-parametric analysis requires no prior knowledge of the disease allele frequency or the disease penetrance of the different genotypes.

TABLE 1 | Heritability estimates for genetic component of risk of schistosomiasis in different populations.

Parasite	Phenotype	Country and district	Heritability estimate and method eg *h2*	References
S. mansoni	Egg count	Brazil, Minas Gerais	23% (*h2*)	(62)
S. mansoni	Egg count	Brazil, Minas Gerais	27% (VC)	(63)
S. mansoni	Egg count	Brazil, Bahia	31% (VC)	(64)
S. mansoni	IgE	Brazil, Bahia	59% (VC)	(64)
S. haematobium	Egg count	Kenya, Coast	9% (*h2*)	(46)
S. haematobium	Bladder morbidity	Kenya, Coast	14% (*h2*)	(46)
S. japonicum	Infection	China, Jiangxi	58% (VC)	(65)
S. japonicum	Infection	China Sichuan	0% (VC)	(66)

h2 additive heritability, VC variance components.

TABLE 2 | Loci associated with *S. mansoni* infection discovered by linkage studies.

Phenotypes	Locus name	5' Marker (Position)	3'Marker (Position)	References	Candidate genes, Tested (Untested)
Egg count	*SM1* 5q31-q33	D5S642 (128Mb)	D5S412 (158Mb)	(4, 68–70)	***IL4, IL5, IL9, IL13,*** *(IL3, CXCL14, CD14, 1IL17B, IL12B)*
Egg count	1p21-q23	D1S236 (95Mb)	D1S196 (168Mb)	(69)	*(IL6R, CRP)*
Egg count	6p21-q21	D6S271 (43Mb)	D6S283 (67Mb)	(69)	*(VEGFA, IL17A, IL17F)*
Hepatic fibrosis	*SM2* 6q22-q23	D6S1009 (137Mb)	D6S310 (142Mb)	(71)	***CTGF, IFNGR1, IL22RA2***
Egg count	7q35-q36	D7S483 (152Mb)	D7S550 (156Mb)	(69)	*(TRB, NOS3, SHH)*

*Marker positions are shown in GRCh37 co-ordinates. Candidate genes that have been found associated with the phenotype are shown in bold (**Tables 3, 4**). Other plausible candidates (See **Figure 2**) in the regions are in brackets. Genes associated with the T_h17 response are underlined. These loci are shown graphically in **Figures 1, 2**.*

Linkage Studies Identify QTL for Pathology That Are Independent of QTL for Parasite Burden

A study in Sudan found that 12% of the study population had moderate or advanced fibrosis and that half of these also had portal hypertension (97). A linkage study of four candidate gene regions in the same population identified a locus (*SM2*) on chromosome six near the interferon-gamma receptor (*IFNGR1*) associated with hepatic fibrosis (**Table 2, Figure 1**) (98). Fifty percentage of people with risk alleles at *SM2* had some continuous thickening of periportal vein branches within 19 years of coming to live within the study area. IFNG is strongly anti-fibrogenic and polymorphisms in *IFNGR1* could plausibly regulate fibrosis. No linkage was found with the *SM1* locus suggesting that control of infection and pathology were independent. The *SM2* locus at 6q22-q23 did not overlap either the HLA region on chromosome six or the 6p21-q21 region that was associated with *S. mansoni* worm burden in Brazil (69) (**Table 2, Figure 1**).

The *SM2* locus was replicated in a linkage study of 11 candidate gene regions in Egypt where 32.7% of individuals 11 years and older had significant fibrosis and rs1327475 in *IFNGR1* was significantly associated with severe PPF. In contrast to the earlier study in Sudan, this study found a weak association with the T_h2 cytokine cluster (IL4, IL13) in *SM1* (54), suggesting that worm burden does contribute to risk of pathology. There is evidence for a potentially protective role of a high IFNG response to schistosome infection, consistent with the anti-fibrogenic properties of IFNG [reviewed by Abath et al. (99)] and a SNP in *IFNG* has been associated with time to reinfection (**Table 3**) (72). Consequently, it appears that the variation in the IFNG system is involved in both the outcome of infection and pathology. Variation in *IFNGR1* has only been shown to be involved in the development of pathology but it has yet to be tested in a candidate gene study for effect on infection response.

ANNOTATION OF GENES IN QTL REGIONS

Very few genes were known in the 5 QTL regions for schistosomiasis (**Table 2**) at the time that the QTL were discovered, and we are not aware of any attempts to identify the genes that are responsible for the QTL effect. Hundreds of genes are now known in these loci, each of which could potentially regulate the phenotype and we prepared a short list of the most likely candidates in each region. In order to discover which genes in each schistosomiasis QTL region might be involved in the response to schistosomiasis we used a custom Perl script to search

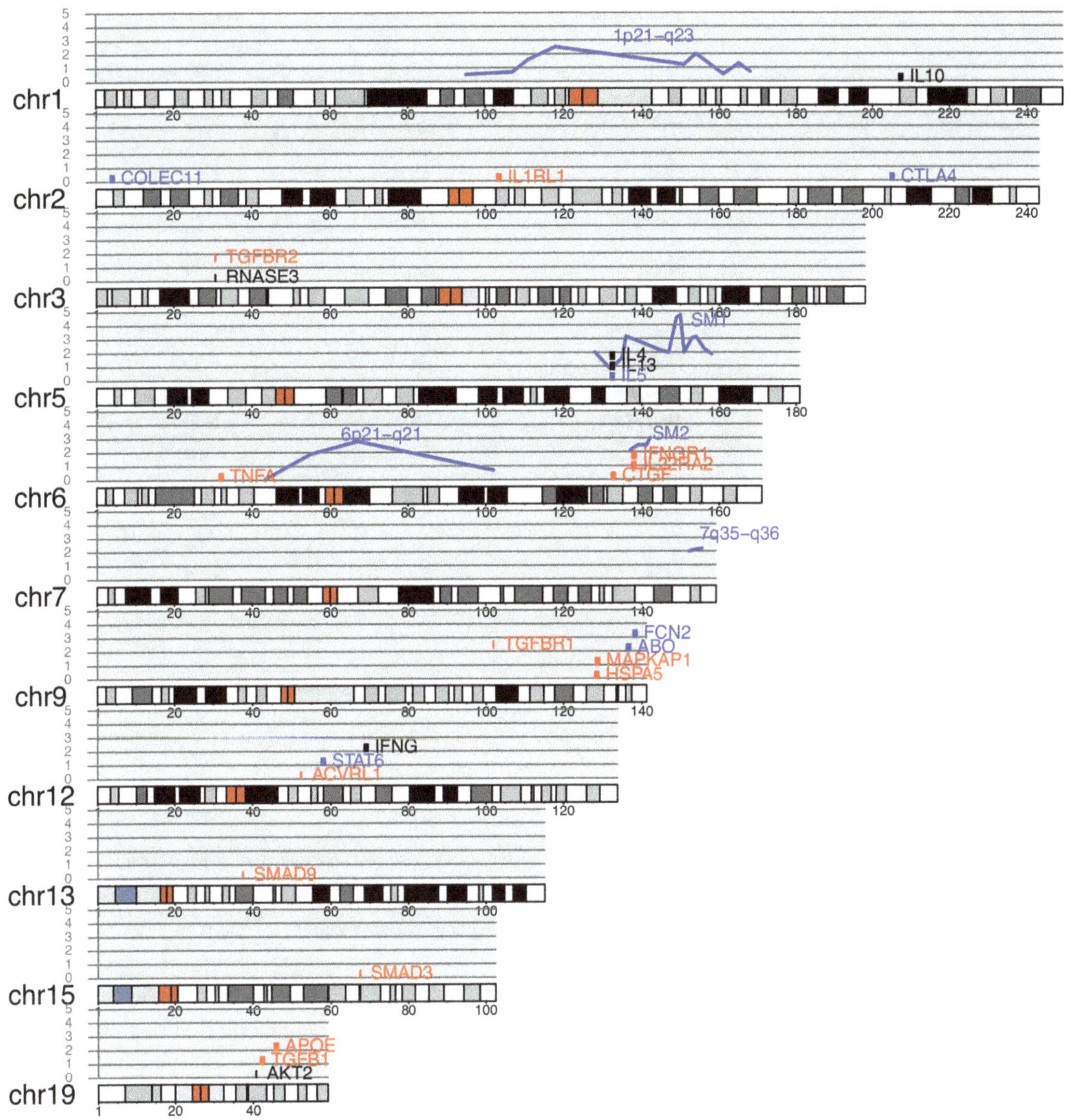

FIGURE 1 | Genes and quantitative trait loci associated with schistosomiasis plotted on a human karyotype. Blue lines indicate QTL, with reported −log *p*-value for association shown on the y axis. Genes containing SNP associated with schistosomiasis infection (**Table 3**) are shown in blue, genes associated with pathology (**Table 4**) are shown in red and genes associated with both pathology and infection are shown in black. Genes are arranged vertically on the plot for clarity and their position on the y axis is arbitrary.

PubMed with terms for schistosomiasis and each gene name and its aliases and obtained a count of the number of publications returned as detailed in **Supplementary Table 4**.

We assumed that the genes that are most likely to be the QTL genes will already have been shown to be involved in the response to schistosome infection. In order to identify these genes, we systematically searched PubMed for papers that included terms for schistosomiasis and each of the gene names in the 5 QTL regions in **Table 2** or their synonyms (**Supplementary Table 4**). The genes that have been mentioned most frequently in the abstract of a paper that also mentions schistosomiasis and that are in one of the QTL are shown in **Figure 2**, **Table 2**. A complete list of all genes that are in the QTL and that have been studied in the context of schistosomiasis is in **Supplementary Table 4**. The number of papers shown in **Figure 2** is an indicator of the genes most commonly associated with schistosomiasis in these regions. The genes with the largest literature were the T_h2 cytokine genes originally identified by Marquet (4) in *SM1* (*IL3, IL4, IL5, IL9*, and *IL13*), that each had between 17 and 511 publications associated with schistosomiasis. Only *CSF1* and *TRB*

TABLE 3 | SNP which have been found to be associated with schistosomiasis infection phenotypes in candidate gene studies.

SNP	Gene	Phenotype	Parasite	Neg refs	Pos refs
rs2430561	*IFNG*	T2R	Sm	none	(72)
rs3024495	*IL10*	FEC	Sm	None	(38)*
rs1800896	*IL10*	IgE	Sm	None	(38)
rs1800871	*IL10*	IgE	Sm	None	(38)*
rs1800872	*IL10*	IgE	Sm	None	(38)*
IL10(-1082/-819/-592)	*IL10*	UEC	Sh	(73)	(74)*
rs20541	*IL13*	FEC	Sm	(75, 76)	(77)
rs2066960	*IL13*	FEC	Sm	(78)	(77)
rs7719175	*IL13*	UEC	Sh	(73)	(79)*
rs2069743	*IL13*	UEC	Sh	(78)	(80)
rs1800925	***IL13***	**UEC, FEC, T2R**	**Sh, Sm**	**None**	**(72, 77–79)***
rs2243250	***IL4***	**UEC, T2R**	**Sh**	**(80)**	**(73), (72)***
rs2079103	*IL5*	IF	Sj	None	(75)*
rs2706399	*IL5*	IF	Sj	None	(75)*
rs3024974	*STAT6*	UEC	Sh	None	(73)*
rs324013	*STAT6*	UEC	Sh	None	(78)*
rs733618	*CTLA4*	UEC	Sh	None	(81)
rs11571316	*CTLA4*	UEC	Sh	None	(81)
rs231775	*CTLA4*	UEC	Sh	None	(81)
rs3124952	*FCN2*	UEC	Sh	None	(82)
rs17514136	*FCN2*	UEC	Sh	None	(82)
rs7567833	*COLECC11*	UEC	Sh	None	(83)
COLEC11*TCCA	*COLECC11*	UEC	Sh	None	(83)
Blood group O	*ABO*	FEC,UEC	Sh,Sm	None	(84)
rs746822072	*RNASE3*	FEC	Sm	None	(85)

*Loci that have been found associated with schistosomiasis in more than one study are shown in bold. * Loci that are not significant after Bonferroni correction. IL10 (−1082/−819/−592) = a haplotype of rs1800870, rs1800871 and rs1800872. COLEC11*TCCA is a haplotype of rs1864480 (−676T/C), rs4849953 (−472T/C), rs6714770 (−469C>G), and (−276C>T). Blood Group O is most commonly defined by genotypes at three SNP rs8176719, rs8176746(CC), rs8176747(GG). IF, Infection Frequency; T2R Time to Reinfection; UEC, Urine Egg Count; FEC, Fecal Egg Count: Sh, S. haematobium; Sm, S. mansoni; Sj, S. japonicum. "Pos refs" column contains citations for the studies that showed a significant association with phenotype and "Neg refs" column contains citations of studies that failed to show a significant association at that locus.*

(beta T cell receptor) were identified as candidate genes by the original authors in the 1p21-q23 and 7q35-q36 egg burden loci (69) and *IFNGR1* was the candidate gene that was used for the linkage study at *SM2* (98). The large literature on T_h2 cytokines and schistosomiasis is expected given the important role of this pathway in response to egg antigens and the development of pathology. The T_h2 cytokines in *SM1* are therefore credible candidate genes at this locus.

Our annotation of these QTL also revealed the presence of T_h17 related genes in four of the five QTL: *IL17B* and *IL12B* in *SM1*, *IL22RA2* in *SM2*, *IL17A* and *IL17F* in 6p21-q21 and *IL6R* in1p21-q23. Although *IL12B* (*IL12p40*) in *SM1* is primarily known as a T_h1 cytokine it is also a component of the heterodimeric IL23 cytokine which is important for T_h17 maintenance and expansion (100) and IL6 is important in T_h17 T helper cell differentiation (101). IL17 cytokines are involved in regulation of worm and egg burdens as well as the development of fibrosis and granuloma in response to eggs (102). The presence of T_h17 related cytokines in four of the five QTL suggests that variation in this system may also contribute to variation in outcome of infection in addition to that caused by variation in the T_h2 system.

CANDIDATE GENE STUDIES

Infection Status and Intensity

We have identified 28 candidate gene studies of *Schistosoma* infection or worm burden that reported associations between 24 loci in eleven candidate genes and seven different phenotypes (**Table 3**, **Supplementary Tables 2, 3**). The genes with associations were *IFNG, IL10, IL13, IL4, IL5, STAT6, CTLA4, FCN2, COLECC11, ABO,* and *RNASE3*. These genes were all chosen because their protein products were known to be involved in the response to infection. One study of *MASP2* (103) and one on *LTA* (104) only reported negative results and are not included in **Table 3**. We have not attempted any formal meta-analysis since few loci were replicated and there were important differences in study design and data reporting in the studies of loci that were replicated, making any meta-analysis hard to interpret.

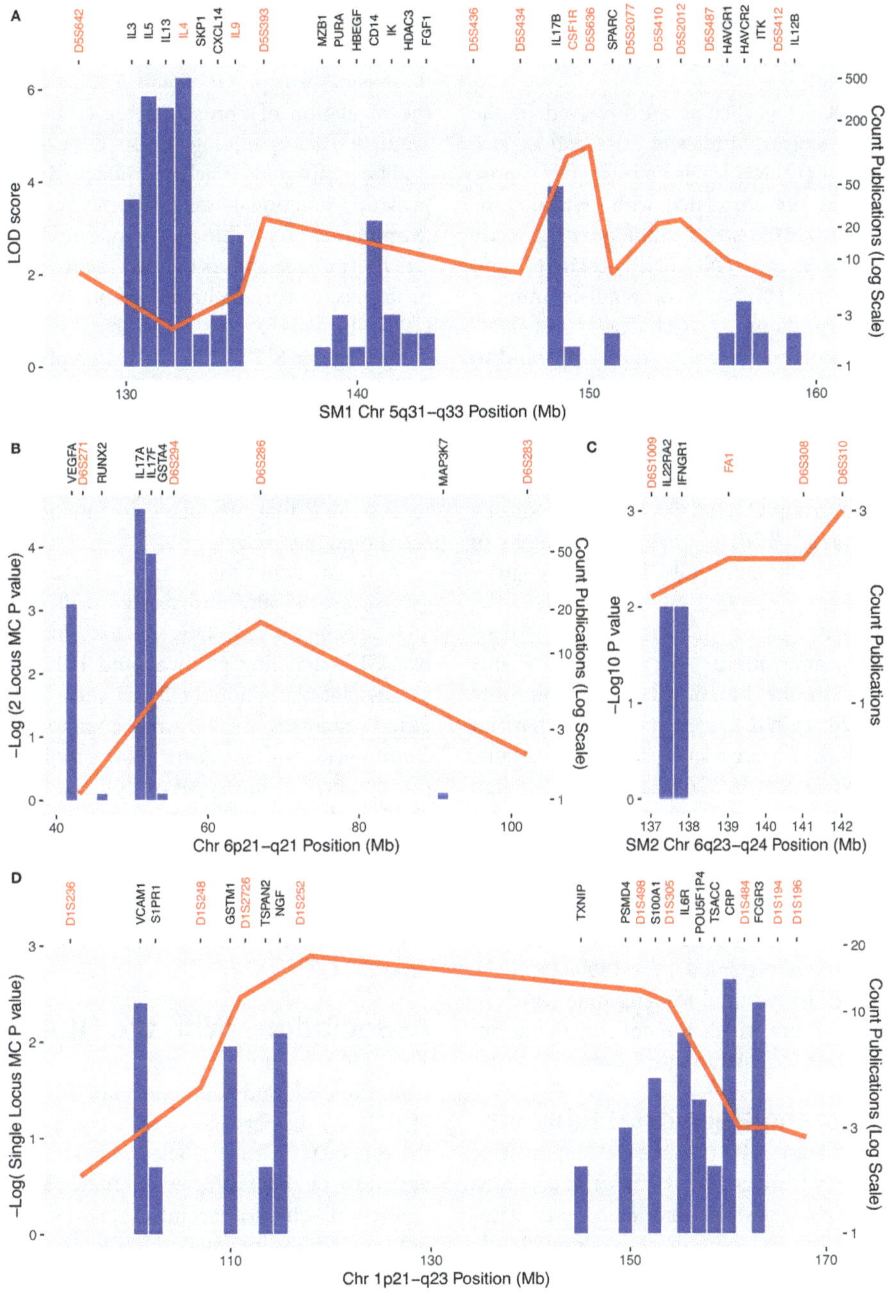

FIGURE 2 | Schistosomiasis QTL and numbers of publications mentioning each gene in each QTL regions. **(A)** *SM1* region 5q31-q33; **(B)** 6p21-q21; **(C)** *SM2* 6q23-q24; **(D)** 1p21-q23. Negative log *p*-values for associations between markers and schistosomiasis are shown on the left-hand axis. Counts of publications which mention both schistosomiasis and genes in the QTL are shown by the blue columns and on a log scale on the right-hand y axis. Markers used in mapping are shown in red on the top axis (including genes used as markers). Genes for which there was only one publication are omitted for clarity and positions of genes and markers have been adjusted by up to 1Mb for clarity. Note the cluster of T_h2 cytokine genes (*IL3, IL4, IL5, IL9, IL13*) in *SM1* with large numbers of publications between 131 and 135 Mb but low LOD scores. However, in a reanalysis of the same data using weighted pairwise correlations the peak of the QTL shifted toward this cytokine cluster (69).

Schistosome eggs induce granulomatous T_h2 responses (*IL4, IL5, IL9, IL10*, and *IL13*) (32) and antigen-specific IgG1, IgG4, and IgE (105). The *SM1* region on chromosome five identified by Marquet et al. (4) (**Figure 1**) included the prototypical T_h2 cytokines *IL4, IL5, IL9*, and *IL13*, these are strong candidates for the QTL gene(s) and SNP and all except *IL9* have been found associated with schistosomiasis in candidate gene studies (**Table 3**). *IL13* and *IL4* regulate *STAT6* expression which in turn regulates IgE class switching (106) and *STAT6* variants are also associated with schistosomiasis (**Table 3**). *IL13, IL4, IL5*, and *STAT6* are also involved in regulation of the T_h2 response to schistosomiasis (72, 75, 77–80).

T_h1 cytokines and IFNG in particular are involved in the resistance to the immature worms. Studies of mice and *ex vivo* human PBMC have shown that IFNG levels increase in response to schistosome antigens and are correlated with resistance or tolerance to infection (27, 107, 108) and a candidate gene study found an association between the *IFNG* SNP rs2430561 and time to reinfection (72). IL10 and CTLA4 downregulate immune responses in long standing infections (31). *COLECC11* and *FCN2* are involved in the innate immune response, they both bind to specific pathogen-associated molecular patterns (PAMPs) on the pathogen surface and stimulate the complement lectin cascade, thereby clearing the pathogens by opsonization (82, 83). *ABO* regulates blood group and a meta-analysis found evidence for a protective effect for blood group O (84). RNASE3 also known as eosinophil cationic protein (ECP) is a secretory protein of eosinophil granulocytes that efficiently kills the larval stage of *S. mansoni* (85).

The Ensembl Variant Effect Predictor was used to provide functional annotations for these variants (**Supplementary Table 5**). In the functional annotation only rs231775 in *CTLA4* and rs20541 in *IL13* were predicted to have an effect on function. Both of which were non-synonymous variants and were classified as risk factors by ClinVar (109), although SIFT (110), and Polyphen (111) predicted the effect of these SNP would be benign. Other SNP had no predicted effects on function, possibly because they are not functional but are linked to functional SNP nearby. However, the functional annotation cannot detect all functional variants and experimental work has shown that *IL13* expression is regulated by rs1800925 (112). Further detailed studies will be required to determine which of the SNP are truly functional and which are not functional but still potentially useful markers for risk of schistosomiasis.

Pathology: Hepatic and Periportal Fibrosis

It has been noted since at least 1974 that the development of severe fibrosis is clustered in families and is not well-correlated with intensity of infection suggesting that the mechanisms regulating infection intensity and pathology are not closely coupled (5). We found 20 studies which identified associations with schistosomiasis related pathology at 46 candidate SNP or haplotypes in 21 genes outside the HLA complex (**Table 4, Supplementary Table 2**). Few of the studies applied any multiple testing corrections and 15 out of the 43 associations would not be significant after a Bonferroni correction (**Table 4**).

There are sixteen genes for which an effect has only been reported for fibrosis and not for infection: *APOE, CCN2, HSPA5, IFNGR1, IL22RA2, MAPKAP1, IL1RL1, TNFA*, mTOR, AKT2, *TGFB1, TGFBR1, TGFBR2, ACVRL1, SMAD9*, and *SMAD3* (**Tables 3, 4**). Five genes have been associated with both fibrosis and intensity of infection (*RNASE3, IL4, IL10, IFNGI*, and *IL13*). Four genes were associated with fibrosis in more than one population: *IFNGR1, IL22RA2, CCN2*, and *MAPKAP1* (**Table 4**), the two former genes are also in the *SM2* QTL (55, 71, 86, 90, 93). Although these sixteen genes have not been tested for associations with infection status or intensity it is plausible that some of them are only associated with pathology. All of these genes except *APOE* and *IL1RL1* have been associated with the regulation of fibrosis (**Table 4**) and variation in these may regulate risk of pathology irrespective of intensity of infection.

The Ensembl Variant Effect Predictor was used to provide functional annotations for the SNP in **Table 4** (**Supplementary Table 5**). Two non-synonymous SNP in *APOE* (rs7412 and rs429358) were predicted by ClinVar to be a risk factor, pathogenic and involved in drug response (109), the rs7412 SNP was also predicted to be deleterious or damaging by SIFT (110) and Polyphen (111). A non-coding SNP in *LTA* (rs1800629) was predicted to be involved in drug response by ClinVar (109) and a non-coding SNP (rs1800872) in *IL10* was predicted to be risk factor by ClinVar. Other SNP in **Table 4** did not have functional annotations, and many may be marker SNP that are linked to functional variants rather than functional themselves.

A recent study found that just 32 SNPs could predict who gets severe hepatic fibrosis in Brazil with 63% sensitivity and 90% specificity (5). This review emphasized the importance of TGFB signaling pathway and IL22. TGFB is also involved in the differentiation of T_h17 cells (113), and together with SMAD regulates T_h17 in response to another worm infection *Echinococus multilocularis* (114) providing further justification for systematic investigation of the role of variants in the T_h17 pathway in differences in response to infection. IL22 and IL17 are co-expressed by T_h17 CD4+ T cells and polymorphisms have been associated with hepatic fibrosis in the *IL22* receptor *IL22RA2* (5, 90). IL22 also has protective effects on the intestinal epithelium against toxic bacterial products (5).

Associations With the HLA Region

The HLA region is associated with response to many communicable and non-communicable diseases. The importance of CD4+ T helper cells in the response to schistosomiasis, and the role of HLA class II alleles in recruiting these, suggests that variation in the HLA region may play an important role in control of schistosome infections. However, associations were not found in this region in the whole genome linkage scans either for worm burden or pathology (4, 68, 71).

Two reviews reported 17 and 18 studies, respectively, of associations of HLA markers with schistosomiasis induced PPF (7, 8), but surprisingly we could not find any studies of HLA genes and worm burden (**Table 3, Supplementary Table 3**). We have found only one study of genes in the HLA region and schistosomiasis that has been published in the 9 years since those reviews. A SNP in Major histocompatibility complex class I chain-related A (*MICA*) was associated with liver fibrosis in a Han Chinese population (76).

It has been emphasized that the problems of extensive linkage disequilibrium within the HLA region, the small sizes of the studies reviewed, the allelic diversity and large variations in allele frequencies between populations mean that these studies may not replicate in different populations and need further confirmation

TABLE 4 | SNP which have been found to be associated with schistosomiasis pathology related phenotypes in candidate gene studies.

SNP	Gene	Phenotype	Species	Not associated	Associated	References
rs1327475	*IFNGR1*	HF	Sm	NA	Egypt	(54)
rs2243250[§]	*IL4*	HF	Sm	NA	Egypt	(54)
rs1056854	*TGFB1*	HF	Sm	NA	Egypt*	(54)
rs373880612	*IFNG*	PPF, HF, PH	Sm	NA	Sudan*	(55)
rs1861494	*IFNG*	PPF, HF, PH	Sm	NA	Sudan*	(55)
IFN-gR1 6q22-q23	*IFNGR1*	HF, PH	Sm	NA	Sudan	(71)
rs3037970	*CCN2(CTGF)*	HF, PH	Sj Sm	China Sudan Brazil	China	(71)
rs1257705	*CCN2(CTGF)*	HF, PH	Sj Sm	Sudan Brazil China	China*	(86)
rs2151532	*CCN2(CTGF)*	HF, PH	Sj Sm	China Egypt	China*	(54, 86)
rs9402373	*CCN2(CTGF)*	HF, PH	Sj Sm	NA	2 China* Sudan Brazil*	(86)
rs9399005	*CCN2(CTGF)*	HF, PH	Sj	China	China*	(86)
rs6918698	*CCN2(CTGF)*	HF, PH	Sj Sm	China Sudan	China* Brazil*	(86)
rs1931002	*CCN2(CTGF)*	HF, PH	Sj	China	China	(86)
rs12526196	*CCN2(CTGF)*	HF, PH	Sj Sm	Sudan Brazil	2 China*	(86)
rs1800925C-rs20541A[§]	*IL13*	HF, PH	Sj	NA	China	(87)
rs1800925[§]	*IL13*	HF PH	Sj	NA	China*	(87)
rs12712135	*ST2 (IL1RL1)*	IL1RL1	Sj Sm	NA	China Brazil	(88)
rs1420101	*ST2 (IL1RL1)*	IL1RL1	Sj Sm	NA	China Brazil	(88)
rs6543119	*ST2 (IL1RL1)*	IL1RL1	Sj Sm	NA	China Brazil	(88)
rs7412, rs429358 APOE3	*APOE*	TC, LDL	Sm	Brazil	NA	(89)
rs6570136	*IL22RA2*	HF, PH	Sj Sm	NA	China Brazil* Sudan*	(90)
rs7774663	*IL22RA2*	HF, PH	Sj Sm	China	Sudan Brazil*	(90)
rs2064501	*IL22RA2*	HF, PH, IL22	Sj Sm	NA	China* Brazil* Sudan*	(90)
rs11154915	*IL22RA2*	HF, PH, IL22	Sj Sm	China Brazil	Sudan*	(90)
rs7749054	*IL22RA2*	HF, PH, IL22 level	Sj Sm	China Sudan	Brazil*	(90)
rs1800870	*IL10*	PPF	Sm	NA	Brazil	(91)
IL10 (-1082/-819/-592)[§]	*IL10*	PPF	Sm	NA	Brazil	(91)
rs1800629	*TNFA*	PPF, TNFA	Sm	NA	Brazil	(92)
rs10118570	*MAPKAP1*	HF, infection	Sj	NA	2 China	(93)
rs391957	*HSPA5*	HF, infection	Sj	NA	China	(93)
rs17025963 rs185882198 rs71093915	*TGFBR2*	HF	Sm	NA	Brazil	(5)

(Continued)

TABLE 4 | Continued

SNP	Gene	Phenotype	Species	Not associated	Associated	References
rs1690215 rs56368010	*ACVRL1(ALK1)*	HF	Sm	NA	Brazil	(5)
rs114046193 rs12345675	*TGFbR1 (ALK5)*	HF	Sm	NA	Brazil	(5)
rs138079455 rs10555873 rs77414361	*SMAD9*	HF	Sm	NA	Brazil	(5)
rs12913547 rs12914140 rs12439500	*SMAD3*	HF	Sm	NA	Brazil	(5)
rs746822072	*RNASE3 (ECP)*	HF	Sm	NA	Uganda	(85)
rs1800629	*TNFA*	PPF regression after treatment	Sm	NA	Brazil	(94)
rs2295080	*mTOR*	HF, infection	Sj	NA	China	(95)
rs7254617	*AKT2*	HF, infection	Sj	NA	China*	(95)

*Loci that have been found associated with schistosomiasis in more than one population are shown in bold. *Loci that are not significant after Bonferroni correction. §SNP which are also associated with infection (**Table 3**). Studies of classical HLA loci have been excluded since they have been fully reviewed elsewhere (7, 8). Sh, S. haematobium; Sm, S. mansoni; Sj, S. japonicum. The "Associated" column shows the locations of studies where a significant association has been found and the "Not Associated" column shows the location of studies that failed to show a significant association. PPF Periportal Fibrosis; PH Portal Hypertension; PT Portal thickness, including portal vein diameter and portal vein branch point thickness, HF Hepatic Fibrosis; AHSD Advanced HepatoSplenic Disease, TC Total Cholesterol, HDL High Density Lipoprotein, TNFA Median levels TNFA higher in patients with PPF, IL22 level of IL22 in plasma, IL1RL1 level of soluble IL1RL1 in plasma. IL-10 (−1082/−819/−592) represents a haplotype of rs1800870, rs1800871, and rs1800872. NA, Not applicable.*

from larger studies (7). However, some alleles of HLA class II loci DQA1, DQB1 and DRB1 and HLA class I HLA-A and HLA-B were associated with PPF in a meta-analysis that combined evidence from 2 to 3 studies for each allele evaluated (8) and these associations may be robust.

DISCUSSION

Replication of Candidate Gene Studies for Infection

Few of the candidate gene studies shown in **Tables 3, 4** applied correction for testing multiple SNPs and the 32 associations that would not remain significant after such a correction are indicated by asterisks. The lack of Bonferroni corrections suggests that some of these studies will not replicate and, for some of these loci, there are studies that have not replicated the association (**Tables 3, 4**), although this is often when using a different phenotype. Notably, half of these studies that did not replicate an association were at loci that were significant after a Bonferroni correction.

There are many instances of failures to replicate candidate gene studies. One review found that only 6 out of 166 associations replicated in more than 75% of studies, although 97 of the 166 associations (58%) were reproduced in at least one study (115). Failure to replicate can be due to the initial observation being due to random variation in allele frequencies between test and control samples (a type one error). However, genuine associations can fail to replicate because of linkage between the marker SNP and the functional SNP varying between populations, small study sizes, variable penetrance, population variation at modifier loci, (occult) population stratification within study populations or differences in allele frequencies between populations leading to type two errors. In addition, it is also possible for different SNP in the same gene to be most important in regulating a response in different populations or individuals (116). Therefore, most of these observations should be considered provisional until adequately powered meta-analyses can be conducted.

Associations with infection were replicated at two SNP (*IL13* rs1800925; *IL4* rs2243250), and both of these SNP and also the *IL10* (−1082/−819/−592) haplotype were also found to be associated with pathology (**Tables 3, 4**), despite the studies using different phenotypes and in one case different parasite species. The *IL13* rs1800925 SNP was associated with schistosomiasis in four infection related studies and one pathology study and all studies that included this SNP found an association with it, despite the association not being significant after a Bonferroni correction in any of these studies. The high level of replication at this SNP suggests that these associations may be robust despite the lack of significance in individual studies. Functional data also supports a role for rs1800925, which is in the promoter of *IL13,* and is associated with increased expression of IL13 from stimulated cells *in vitro* (112). Since IL13 regulates IgE levels via STAT6 (106), there is a plausible mechanism for a role for this SNP in response to infection, increasing the confidence that it is a genuine association. Although *IL4* expression is also associated with IgE levels, the rs2243250 SNP is not (117), so its impact on intensity of infection must be via some other mechanism.

The Th17 Pathway Has Been Neglected in Schistosomiasis Association Studies

Since the Th2 pathway is the dominant response to helminth infections and is the main pathway for response to egg antigens

(28, 30), genes in this pathway have been well-represented in association studies (**Tables 3, 4**) and these have confirmed the importance of variation in this pathway for outcome of infection. However, the Th1 and Th17 pathways are also important, particularly in the early stages of the infection (26, 29, 36, 37). Variants in *IL17F* and *IL17RA* have been found associated with cerebral malaria (118) and similar variation may contribute to the outcome of schistosome infection. Our annotation of QTL, with the genes that have published associations with schistosomiasis, revealed an excess of Th17 pathway genes in these QTL (**Figures 1, 2**). There have been no association studies to test candidate gene hypothesis for three out of the five QTL (**Table 2**) and there are Th17 genes in four of the five QTL (underlined in **Table 2**), which could be priorities for future association studies.

It is possible that variation in other Th17 pathway genes outside of the QTL also contribute to variation in response to infection. A KEGG pathway diagram of Th17 cell differentiation and a list of 108 genes in this pathway is shown in **Supplementary Table 6.** We have obtained a list of the 1,742,019 SNP in these genes from dbSNP and kept the 1,052 SNP that were predicted to be "pathogenic" by ClinVar, irrespective of minor allele frequency (**Supplementary Table 7**). We also kept SNP with minor allele frequency > 5% and that had any of the following functional classifications: splice acceptor variant, stop gained, initiator codon variant, stop lost, splice donor variant, missense variant, terminator codon variant, frameshift variant. This left a list of 2,701 SNP in the Th17 pathway which are most likely to have an effect on function and that could be priorities for further testing (**Supplementary Table 7**).

Which Are the Optimal Study Designs to Discover Susceptibility Loci?

Approaches for discovering susceptibility loci for parasitic infections have been reviewed previously (119). The major approaches are association studies in unrelated individuals and linkage studies within families, the merits of which have been evaluated by Abel and Dessein (120). We noted in this review that family based designs were the first to discover QTL loci in schistosomiasis (4), and these were followed up with considerable success by candidate gene studies in these QTL. Schistosomiasis affected communities are frequently geographical clusters of related individuals where case control studies can be confounded by cryptic relatedness. In contrast family-based association studies exploit this relatedness by estimating disequilibrium in transmission of alleles within families.

Schistosomiasis is also an excellent setting for family-based linkage studies of infection intensity because children are the most heavily infected; therefore, parents are often available for genotyping to create complete families, unlike adult onset diseases. However, it is more difficult to collect full families for complications of chronic schistosomiasis such as fibrosis that affect adults. Whole genome linkage studies have only been undertaken on two populations, one in Brazil and one in Senegal, further studies to identify loci regulating intensity of infection in additional populations should be undertaken and could enlarge our understanding of the mechanisms of response to infection. It has already been shown that 32 SNP can be used to identify those at highest risk of developing pathology after *S. mansoni* infection (5). If the 20% of the people that shed 80% of the eggs could also be identified they could be targeted for regular treatment which could dramatically reduce the number of eggs in the environment and the pressure of infection on the whole community.

CONCLUSION

Despite the remarkable success of the early linkage studies that identified major QTL loci, no further whole genome scans for association have been conducted and the QTL genes underlying these loci have not been definitively identified. All subsequent studies have been candidate gene linkage and association studies focussing on genes within the QTL regions *SM1*, *SM2*, and the T_h2 pathway that are hypothesized to play a role in schistosomiasis progression. No candidate gene studies have attempted to identify QTL genes in three of the QTL for *S. mansoni* egg count (**Table 2**). This review has presented evidence that the T_h17 pathway has been overlooked in studies of the genetics of schistosomiasis and should be prioritized in future investigations of susceptibility genes.

The rapid development of genotyping technologies makes large scale genomic studies easier than ever, provided that well-characterized samples can be obtained. The studies of Dessein et al. (86) on populations from China, Sudan and Brazil have demonstrated the value of replicating analyses in multiple populations and similar replication is needed for other candidate SNP and genes.

AUTHOR CONTRIBUTIONS

GS and EMa conceived the review. EMe and ON wrote the draft and collected all the relevant literature. HN significantly reviewed the draft and analyzed QTL data. ME contributed to the draft and revised the manuscript. All authors read and approved the final manuscript.

ACKNOWLEDGMENTS

The authors are grateful to Alison Elliott of the London School of Hygiene and Tropical Medicine for helpful discussions and reviewing the manuscript.

THE TRYPANOGEN+ RESEARCH GROUP OF THE H3AFRICA CONSORTIUM

Membership of the TrypanoGEN+ research group is available at http://www.trypanogen.net/.

SUPPLEMENTARY MATERIAL

Supplementary Table 1 | Search strategy: Summary of PubMed search strategy.

Supplementary Table 2 | All included references: Papers included in the review.

Supplementary Table 3 | Details of Refs Populations, study design, phenotypes, and effects from studies.

Supplementary Table 4 | Genes in QTL. List of genes in QTL regions with lists of publications associated with each gene and schistosomiasis.

Supplementary Table 5 | VEP SNP Annotations. Functional annotation of SNP from candidate genes studies with the Ensembl Variant Effect predictor.

Supplementary Table 6 | Th17 genes. List of Genes in Th17 pathway with KEGG pathway diagram.

Supplementary Table 7 | Th17 SNP. List of potentially function SNP in genes in the Th17 pathway.

REFERENCES

1. Ismail HAHA, Hong ST, Babiker ATEB, Hassan RMAE, Sulaiman MAZ, Jeong HG, et al. Prevalence, risk factors, and clinical manifestations of schistosomiasis among school children in the White Nile River basin, Sudan. *Parasites Vectors.* (2014) 7:478. doi: 10.1186/s13071-014-0478-6
2. Bethony JM, Quinnell RJ. Genetic epidemiology of human schistosomiasis in Brazil. *Acta Trop.* (2008) 108:166–174. doi: 10.1016/j.actatropica.2007.11.008
3. Abel L, Demenais F, Prata A, Souza AE, Dessein A. Evidence for the segregation of a major gene in human susceptibility/resistance to infection by *Schistosoma mansoni*. *Am J Hum Genet.* (1991) 48:959–70.
4. Marquet S, Abel L, Hillaire D, Dessein H, Kalil J, Feingold J, et al. Genetic localization of a locus controlling the intensity of infection by *Schistosoma mansoni* on chromosome 5q31-q33. *Nat Genet.* (1996) 14:181–4. doi: 10.1038/ng1096-181
5. Dessein H, Duflot N, Romano A, Opio C, Pereira V, Mola C, et al. Genetic algorithms identify individuals with high risk of severe liver disease caused by schistosomes. *Hum Genet.* (2020) 139:821–31. doi: 10.1007/s00439-020-02160-4
6. Alsallaq RA, Gurarie D, Ndeffo Mbah M, Galvani A, King C. Quantitative assessment of the impact of partially protective anti-schistosomiasis vaccines. *PLoS Negl Trop Dis.* (2017) 11:e0005544. doi: 10.1371/journal.pntd.0005544
7. Blackwell JM, Jamieson SE, Burgner D. HLA and infectious diseases. *CMR.* (2009) 22:370–85. doi: 10.1128/CMR.00048-08
8. Huy NT, Hamada M, Kikuchi M, Lan NTP, Yasunami M, Zamora J, et al. Association of HLA and post-schistosomal hepatic disorder: a systematic review and meta-analysis. *Parasitol Int.* (2011) 60:347–56. doi: 10.1016/j.parint.2011.05.008
9. Colley DG, Bustinduy AL, Secor WE, King CH. Human schistosomiasis. *Lancet.* (2014) 383:2253–64. doi: 10.1016/S0140-6736(13)61949-2
10. Hotez PJ, Kamath A. Neglected tropical diseases in sub-saharan Africa: review of their prevalence, distribution, and disease burden. *PLoS Negl Trop Dis.* (2009) 3:e412. doi: 10.1371/journal.pntd.0000412
11. Steinmann P, Keiser J, Bos R, Tanner M, Utzinger J. Schistosomiasis and water resources development: systematic review, meta-analysis, and estimates of people at risk. *Lancet Infect Dis.* (2006) 6:411–25. doi: 10.1016/S1473-3099(06)70521-7
12. Murray CJL, Vos T, Lozano R, Naghavi M, Flaxman AD, Michaud C, et al. Disability-adjusted life years (DALYs) for 291 diseases and injuries in 21 regions, 1990-2010: a systematic analysis for the Global Burden of Disease Study 2010. *Lancet.* (2012) 380:2197–223. doi: 10.1016/S0140-6736(12)61690-0
13. van der Werf MJ, de Vlas SJ, Brooker S, Looman CWN, Nagelkerke NJD, Habbema JDF, et al. Quantification of clinical morbidity associated with schistosome infection in sub-Saharan Africa. *Acta Trop.* (2003) 86:125–39. doi: 10.1016/S0001-706X(03)00029-9
14. Gbalégba NGC, Silué KD, Ba O, Ba H, Tian-Bi NTY, Yapi GY, et al. Prevalence and seasonal transmission of *Schistosoma haematobium* infection among school-aged children in Kaedi town, southern Mauritania. *Parasites Vectors.* (2017) 10:353. doi: 10.1186/s13071-017-2284-4
15. Ezeamama AE, Friedman JF, Acosta LP, Bellinger DC, Langdon GC, Manalo DL, et al. Helminth infection and cognitive impairment among filipino children. *Am J Trop Med Hyg.* (2005) 72:540–8. doi: 10.4269/ajtmh.2005.72.540
16. Ezeamama AE, Bustinduy AL, Nkwata AK, Martinez L, Pabalan N, Boivin MJ, et al. Cognitive deficits and educational loss in children with schistosome infection—a systematic review and meta-analysis. *PLoS Negl Trop Dis.* (2018) 12:e0005524. doi: 10.1371/journal.pntd.0005524
17. Friedman JF, Kanzaria HK, McGarvey ST. Human schistosomiasis and anemia: the relationship and potential mechanisms. *Trends Parasitol.* (2005) 21:386–92. doi: 10.1016/j.pt.2005.06.006
18. King CH, Dangerfield-Cha M. The unacknowledged impact of chronic schistosomiasis. *Chronic Illn.* (2008) 4:65–79. doi: 10.1177/1742395307084407
19. King CH, Dickman K, Tisch DJ. Reassessment of the cost of chronic helmintic infection: a meta-analysis of disability-related outcomes in endemic schistosomiasis. *Lancet.* (2005) 365:1561–9. doi: 10.1016/S0140-6736(05)66457-4
20. Koukounari A, Gabrielli AF, Toure S, Bosque-Oliva E, Zhang Y, Sellin B, et al. *Schistosoma haematobium* infection and morbidity before and after large-scale administration of praziquantel in Burkina Faso. *J Infect Dis.* (2007) 196:659–69. doi: 10.1086/520515
21. Utzinger J, Raso G, Brooker S, De Savigny D, Tanner M, Ornbjerg N, et al. Schistosomiasis and neglected tropical diseases: towards integrated and sustainable control and a word of caution. *Parasitology.* (2009) 136:1859–74. doi: 10.1017/S0031182009991600
22. Evan Secor W. Water-based interventions for schistosomiasis control. *Pathogens Global Health.* (2014) 108:246–54. doi: 10.1179/2047773214Y.0000000149
23. Ross AGP, Olveda RM, Li Y. An audacious goal: the elimination of schistosomiasis in our lifetime through mass drug administration. *Lancet.* (2015) 385:2220–1. doi: 10.1016/S0140-6736(14)61417-3
24. Gray DJ, McManus DP, Li Y, Williams GM, Bergquist R, Ross AG. Schistosomiasis elimination: lessons from the past guide the future. *Lancet Infect Dis.* (2010) 10:733–6. doi: 10.1016/S1473-3099(10)70099-2
25. Riveau G, Schacht AM, Dompnier JP, Deplanque D, Seck M, Waucquier N, et al. Safety and efficacy of the rSh28GST urinary schistosomiasis vaccine: a phase 3 randomized, controlled trial in Senegalese children. *PLoS Negl Trop Dis.* (2018) 12:e0006968. doi: 10.1371/journal.pntd.0006968
26. Egesa M, Lubyayi L, Tukahebwa EM, Bagaya BS, Chalmers IW, Wilson S, et al. *Schistosoma mansoni* schistosomula antigens induce Th1/Pro-inflammatory cytokine responses. *Parasite Immunol.* (2018) 40:e12592. doi: 10.1111/pim.12592
27. Perrigoue JG, Marshall FA, Artis D. On the hunt for helminths: innate immune cells in the recognition and response to helminth parasites. *Cellular Microbiology.* (2008) 10:1757–1764. doi: 10.1111/j.1462-5822.2008.01174.x
28. Grzych JM, Pearce E, Cheever A, Caulada ZA, Caspar P, Heiny S, et al. Egg deposition is the major stimulus for the production of Th2 cytokines in murine schistosomiasis mansoni. *J Immunol.* (1991) 146:1322–7.
29. Pearce EJ, M Kane C, Sun JJ, Taylor J, McKee AS, Cervi L. Th2 response polarization during infection with the helminth parasite *Schistosoma mansoni*. *Immunol Rev.* (2004) 201:117–26. doi: 10.1111/j.0105-2896.2004.00187.x
30. de Oliveira Fraga LA, Torrero MN, Tocheva AS, Mitre E, Davies SJ. Induction of type 2 responses by schistosome worms during prepatent infection. *J Infect Dis.* (2010) 201:464–72. doi: 10.1086/649841
31. Joseph S, Jones FM, Kimani G, Mwatha JK, Kamau T, Kazibwe F, et al. Cytokine production in whole blood cultures from a fishing community in an area of high endemicity for *Schistosoma mansoni* in Uganda: the differential effect of parasite worm and egg antigens. *IAI.* (2004) 72:728–34. doi: 10.1128/IAI.72.2.728-734.2004
32. Everts B, Perona-Wright G, Smits HH, Hokke CH, van der Ham AJ, Fitzsimmons CM, et al. Omega-1, a glycoprotein secreted by *Schistosoma mansoni* eggs, drives Th2 responses. *J Exp Med.* (2009) 206:1673–80. doi: 10.1084/jem.20082460

33. Kaplan MH, Whitfield JR, Boros DL. Th2 Cells are required for the *schistosoma mansoni* egg-induced granulomatous response. *J Immunol.* (1998) 160:1850–6.
34. Dunne DW, Lucas S, Bickle Q, Pearson S, Madgwick L, Bain J, et al. Identification and partial purification of an antigen (ω1 from *Schistosoma mansoni* eggs which is putatively hepatotoxic in T-cell deprived mice. *Trans R Soc Trop Med Hyg.* (1981) 75:54–71. doi: 10.1016/0035-9203(81)90013-4
35. Alves Oliveira LF, Moreno EC, Gazzinelli G, Martins-Filho OA, Silveira AMS, Gazzinelli A, et al. Cytokine production associated with periportal fibrosis during chronic schistosomiasis mansoni in humans. *Infect Immun.* (2006) 74:1215–21. doi: 10.1128/IAI.74.2.1215-1221.2006
36. Rutitzky LI, Stadecker MJ. Exacerbated egg-induced immunopathology in murine Schistosoma mansoni infection is primarily mediated by IL-17 and restrained by IFN-γ. *Eur J Immunol.* (2011) 41:2677–87. doi: 10.1002/eji.201041327
37. Mbow M, Larkin BM, Meurs L, Wammes LJ, de Jong SE, Labuda LA, et al. T-Helper 17 cells are associated with pathology in human schistosomiasis. *J Infect Dis.* (2013) 207:186–95. doi: 10.1093/infdis/jis654
38. Grant AV, Araujo MI, Ponte EV, Oliveira RR, Cruz AA, Barnes KC, et al. Polymorphisms in IL10 are associated with total Immunoglobulin E levels and *Schistosoma mansoni* infection intensity in a Brazilian population. *Genes Immun.* (2011) 12:46–50. doi: 10.1038/gene.2010.50
39. Corstjens PLAM, De Dood CJ, Kornelis D, Tjon Kon Fat EM, Wilson RA, Kariuki TM, et al. Tools for diagnosis, monitoring and screening of *Schistosoma* infections utilizing lateral-flow based assays and upconverting phosphor labels. *Parasitology.* (2014) 141:1841–55. doi: 10.1017/S0031182014000626
40. Woolhouse MEJ, Dye C, Etard JF, Smith T, Charlwood JD, Garnett GP, et al. Heterogeneities in the transmission of infectious agents: implications for the design of control programs. *PNAS.* (1997) 94:338–42. doi: 10.1073/pnas.94.1.338
41. Butterworth AE, Capron M, Cordingley JS, Dalton PR, Dunne DW, Kariuki HC, et al. Immunity after treatment of human *Schistosomiasis mansoni*. II. Identification of resistant individuals, and analysis of their immune responses. *Trans R Soc Trop Med Hyg.* (1985) 79:393–408. doi: 10.1016/0035-9203(85)90391-8
42. Abel L, Demenais F, Prata A, Souza AE, Dessein A. Evidence for the segregation of a major gene in human susceptibility/resistance to infection by *Schistosoma mansoni*. *Am J Hum Genet.* (1991) 48:959–70.
43. Wilkins HA, Goll PH, Marshall TF, Moore PJ. Dynamics of *Schistosoma haematobium* infection in a Gambian community. III. Acquisition and loss of infection. *Trans R Soc Trop Med Hyg.* (1984) 78:227–32. doi: 10.1016/0035-9203(84)90283-9
44. Bradley DJ, McCullough FS. Egg output stability and the epidemiology of *Schistosoma haematobium*. II. An analysis of the epidemiology of endemic S. haematobium. *Trans R Soc Trop Med Hyg.* (1973) 67:491–500. doi: 10.1016/0035-9203(73)90080-1
45. Warren KS. Regulation of the prevalence and intensity of schistosomiasis in man: immunology or ecology? *J Infect Dis.* (1973) 127:595–609. doi: 10.1093/infdis/127.5.595
46. King CH, Kariuki HC, Kadzo H, Koech DK, Magak P, Ouma JH, et al. Low heritable component of risk for infection intensity and infection-associated disease in urinary schistosomiasis among Wadigo village populations in Coast province, Kenya. *Am J Trop Med Hyg.* (2004) 70:57–62. doi: 10.4269/ajtmh.2004.70.57
47. Fitzsimmons CM, Jones FM, Pinot de Moira A, Protasio AV, Khalife J, Dickinson HA, et al. Progressive cross-reactivity in IgE responses: an explanation for the slow development of human immunity to schistosomiasis? *Infect Immun.* (2012) 80:4264–70. doi: 10.1128/IAI.00641-12
48. Demeure CE, Rihet P, Abel L, Ouattara M, Bourgois A, Dessein AJ. Resistance to *Schistosoma mansoni* in humans: influence of the IgE/IgG4 Balance and IgG2 in immunity to reinfection after chemotherapy. *J Infect Dis.* (1993) 168:1000–8. doi: 10.1093/infdis/168.4.1000
49. Figueiredo JP, Oliveira RR, Cardoso LS, Barnes KC, Grant AV, Carvalho EM, et al. Adult worm-specific IgE/IgG4 balance is associated with low infection levels of *Schistosoma mansoni* in an endemic area. *Parasite Immunol.* (2012) 34:604–10. doi: 10.1111/pim.12001
50. Hagan P, Dunn D, Simpson G, Wilkins HA. Human IgE, IgG4 and resistance to reinfection with *Schistosoma haematobium*. (1991) 349:3. doi: 10.1038/349243a0
51. Ndombi EM, Abudho B, Kittur N, Carter JM, Korir H, Riner DK, et al. Effect of four rounds of annual school-wide mass praziquantel treatment for *Schistosoma mansoni* control on schistosome-specific immune responses. *Parasite Immunol.* (2018) 40:e12530. doi: 10.1111/pim.12530
52. McManus DP, Dunne DW, Sacko M, Utzinger J, Vennervald BJ, Zhou XN. Schistosomiasis. *Nat Rev Dis Primers.* (2018) 4:13. doi: 10.1038/s41572-018-0013-8
53. Richter,J, Hatz,C, Campagne,G, Bequist,N, Jenkins,J. *Ultrasound in Schistosomiasis. A Practical Guide to the Standardized Use of Ultrasonography for the Assessment of Schistosomiasis-Related Morbidity.* Niamey: WHO. (2000).
54. Blanton RE, Salam EA, Ehsan A, King CH, Goddard KA. Schistosomal hepatic fibrosis and the interferon gamma receptor: a linkage analysis using single-nucleotide polymorphic markers. *Eur J Hum Genet.* (2005) 13:660–8. doi: 10.1038/sj.ejhg.5201388
55. Chevillard C, Moukoko CE, Elwali N-EMA, Bream JH, Kouriba B, Argiro L, et al. IFN-gamma polymorphisms (IFN-gamma +2109 and IFN-gamma +3810) are associated with severe hepatic fibrosis in human hepatic schistosomiasis (*Schistosoma mansoni*). *J Immunol.* (2003) 171:5596–601. doi: 10.4049/jimmunol.171.10.5596
56. Hirayama K, Chen H, Kikuchi M, Yin T, Gu X, Liu J, et al. HLA-DR-DQ alleles and HLA-DP alleles are independently associated with susceptibility to different stages of post-schistosomal hepatic fibrosis in the Chinese population. *Tissue Antigens.* (1999) 53:269–74. doi: 10.1034/j.1399-0039.1999.530307.x
57. Palumbo E. Association between schistosomiasis and cancer: a review. *Infect Dis Clin Pract.* (2007) 15:145–8. doi: 10.1097/01.idc.0000269904.90155.ce
58. Asztely MS, Eriksson B, Gabone RM, Nilsson L Å. Is ultrasonography useful for population studies on schistosomiasis mansoni? An evaluation based on a survey on a population from Kome Island, Tanzania. *Acta Radiol Open.* (2016) 5:2058460116686392. doi: 10.1177/2058460116686392
59. Barreto AVMS, Alecrim VM, Medeiros TB de, Domingues ALC, Lopes EP, Martins JRM, et al. New index for the diagnosis of liver fibrosis in *Schistosomiasis mansoni*. *Arq Gastroenterol.* (2017) 54:51–6. doi: 10.1590/s0004-2803.2017v54n1-10
60. Olveda DU, Inobaya M, Olveda RM, Vinluan ML, Ng S-K, Weerakoon K, et al. Diagnosing schistosomiasis-induced liver morbidity: implications for global control. *Int J Infect Dis.* (2017) 54:138–44. doi: 10.1016/j.ijid.2016.10.024
61. Pereira TA, Syn WK, Pereira FEL, Lambertucci JR, Secor WE, Diehl AM. Serum osteopontin is a biomarker of severe fibrosis and portal hypertension in human and murine *Schistosomiasis mansoni*. *Int J Parasitol.* (2016) 46:829–32. doi: 10.1016/j.ijpara.2016.08.004
62. Pullan RL, Bethony JM, Geiger SM, Correa-Oliveira R, Brooker S, Quinnell RJ. Human helminth co-infection: no evidence of common genetic control of hookworm and *Schistosoma mansoni* infection intensity in a Brazilian community. *Int J Parasitol.* (2010) 40:299–306. doi: 10.1016/j.ijpara.2009.08.002
63. Gazzinelli A, Coelho L, Alves-Fraga L, Soares-Filho B, Williams-Blangero S, Bethony J, et al. Additive host genetic factors influence fecal egg excretion rates during *Schistosoma mansoni* infection in a rural area in Brazil. *Am J Med Hyg.* (2002) 67:336–43. doi: 10.4269/ajtmh.2002.67.336
64. Grant A, Araujo MI, Ponte EV, Oliveira RR, Cruz AA, Barnes KC, et al. High heritability but uncertain mode of inheritance for total serum IgE level and *Schistosoma mansoni* infection intensity in a Schistosomiasis-Endemic Brazilian Population. *J Infect Dis.* (2008) 198:1227–36. doi: 10.1086/591946
65. Ellis MK, McManus DP. Familial aggregation of human helminth infection in the Poyang lake area of China with a focus on genetic susceptibility to schistosomiasis japonica and associated markers of disease. *Parasitology.* (2009) 136:699–712. doi: 10.1017/S003118200900612X
66. Spear RC, Zhong B, Kouch J, Seto EYW, Hubbard A. Genetic and household risk factors for *Schistosoma japonicum* infection in the

presence of larger scale environmental differences in the mountainous transmission areas of China. *Am J Trop Med Hyg.* (2005) 73:1145–50. doi: 10.4269/ajtmh.2005.73.1145
67. King, R.C, Stransfield, W.D. *Dictionary of Genetics*. Oxford: Oxford University Press. (1998).
68. Marquet S, Abel L, Hillaire D, Dessein A. Full results of the genome-wide scan which localises a locus controlling the intensity of infection by *Schistosoma mansoni* on chromosome 5q31-q33. *Eur J Hum Genet.* (1999) 7:88–97. doi: 10.1038/sj.ejhg.5200243
69. Zinn-Justin A, Marquet S, Hillaire D, Dessein A, Abel L. Genome search for additional human loci controlling infection levels by *Schistosoma mansoni*. *Am J Trop Med Hyg.* (2001) 65:754–8. doi: 10.4269/ajtmh.2001.65.754
70. Müller-Myhsok B, Stelma FF, Guissé-Sow F, Muntau B, Thye T, Burchard GD, et al. Further evidence suggesting the presence of a locus, on human chromosome 5q31-q33, influencing the intensity of infection with Schistosoma mansoni. *Am J Hum Genet.* (1997) 61:452–4. doi: 10.1086/524851
71. Dessein AJ, Hillaire D, Elwali NE, Marquet S, Mohamed-Ali Q, Mirghani A, et al. Severe Hepatic Fibrosis in *Schistosoma mansoni* Infection Is Controlled by a Major Locus That Is Closely Linked to the Interferon-Gamma Receptor Gene. *Am J Hum Genet.* (1999) 65:709–21. doi: 10.1086/302526
72. Gatlin MR, Black CL, Mwinzi PN, Secor WE, Karanja DM, Colley DG. Association of the gene polymorphisms IFN-gamma +874, IL-13−1055 and IL-4−590 with patterns of reinfection with Schistosoma mansoni. *PLoS Negl Trop Dis.* (2009) 3:e375. doi: 10.1371/journal.pntd.0000375
73. Adedokun SA, Seamans BN, Cox NT, Liou G, Akindele AA, Li Y, et al. Interleukin-4 and STAT6 promoter polymorphisms but not interleukin-10 or 13 are essential for schistosomiasis and associated disease burden among Nigerian children. *Infect Genetics Evol.* (2018) 65:28–34. doi: 10.1016/j.meegid.2018.07.012
74. Adedoja A, Hoan NX, Tong H van, Adukpo S, Tijani DB, Akanbi AA, et al. Differential contribution of interleukin-10 promoter variants in malaria and schistosomiasis mono- and co-infections among Nigerian children. *Trop Med Int Health.* (2018) 23:45–52. doi: 10.1111/tmi.13007
75. Ellis MK, Zhao ZZ, Chen HG, Montgomery GW, Li YS, McManus DP. Analysis of the 5q31 33 locus shows an association between single nucleotide polymorphism variants in the IL-5 gene and symptomatic infection with the human blood fluke, *Schistosoma japonicum*. *J Immunol.* (2007) 179:8366–71. doi: 10.4049/jimmunol.179.12.8366
76. Gong Z, Luo Q-Z, Lin L, Su Y-P, Peng H-B, Du K, et al. Association of MICA gene polymorphisms with liver fibrosis in schistosomiasis patients in the Dongting Lake region. *Braz J Med Biol Res.* (2012) 45:222–9. doi: 10.1590/S0100-879X2012007500024
77. Grant AV, Araujo MI, Ponte EV, Oliveira RR, Gao P, Cruz AA, et al. Functional polymorphisms in IL13 are protective against high *Schistosoma mansoni* infection intensity in a Brazilian population. *PLoS ONE.* (2012) 7:e35863. doi: 10.1371/journal.pone.0035863
78. He H, Isnard A, Kouriba B, Cabantous S, Dessein A, Doumbo O, et al. A STAT6 gene polymorphism is associated with high infection levels in urinary schistosomiasis. *Genes Immun.* (2008) 9:195–206. doi: 10.1038/gene.2008.2
79. Isnard A, Kouriba B, Doumbo O, Chevillard C. Association of rs7719175, located in the IL13 gene promoter, with *Schistosoma haematobium* infection levels and identification of a susceptibility haplotype. *Genes Immun.* (2011) 12:31–9. doi: 10.1038/gene.2010.43
80. Kouriba B, Chevillard C, Bream JH, Argiro L, Dessein H, Arnaud V, et al. Analysis of the 5q31-q33 Locus Shows an Association between IL13-1055C/T IL-13-591A/G Polymorphisms and *Schistosoma haematobium* Infections. *J Immunol.* (2005) 174:6274–81. doi: 10.4049/jimmunol.174.10.6274
81. Idris ZM, Yazdanbakhsh M, Adegnika AA, Lell B, Issifou S, Noordin R. A pilot study on Cytotoxic T Lymphocyte-4 gene polymorphisms in urinary schistosomiasis. *Genetic Testing Mol Biomarkers.* (2012) 16:488–92. doi: 10.1089/gtmb.2011.0209
82. Ouf EA, Ojurongbe O, Akindele AA, Sina-Agbaje OR, Van Tong H, Adeyeba AO, et al. Ficolin-2 Levels and FCN2 genetic polymorphisms as a susceptibility factor in schistosomiasis. *J InfectDis.* (2012) 206:562–70. doi: 10.1093/infdis/jis396
83. Antony JS, Ojurongbe O, Kremsner PG, Velavan TP. Lectin complement protein collectin 11 (CL-K1) and susceptibility to urinary schistosomiasis. *PLoS Negl Trop Dis.* (2015) 9:e0003647. doi: 10.1371/journal.pntd.0003647
84. Tiongco RE, Paragas NA, Dominguez MJ, Lasta SL, Pandac JK, Pineda-Cortel MR. ABO blood group antigens may be associated with increased susceptibility to schistosomiasis: a systematic review and meta-analysis. *J Helminthol.* (2018) 94:e21. doi: 10.1017/S0022149X18001116
85. Eriksson J, Reimert CM, Kabatereine NB, Kazibwe F, Ireri E, Kadzo H, et al. The 434(G>C) polymorphism within the coding sequence of Eosinophil Cationic Protein (ECP) correlates with the natural course of *Schistosoma mansoni* infection. *Int J Parasitol.* (2007) 37:1359–66. doi: 10.1016/j.ijpara.2007.04.001
86. Dessein A, Chevillard C, Arnaud V, Hou X, Hamdoun AA, Dessein H, et al. Variants of CTGF are associated with hepatic fibrosis in Chinese, Sudanese, and Brazilians infected with schistosomes. *J Exp Med.* (2009) 206:2321–8. doi: 10.1084/jem.20090383
87. Long X, Chen Q, Zhao J, Rafaels N, Mathias P, Liang H, et al. An IL-13 promoter polymorphism associated with liver fibrosis in patients with *Schistosoma japonicum*. *PLoS ONE.* (2015) 10:e0135360. doi: 10.1371/journal.pone.0135360
88. Long X, Daya M, Zhao J, Rafaels N, Liang H, Potee J, et al. The role of ST2 and ST2 genetic variants in schistosomiasis. *J Allergy Clin Immunol.* (2017) 140:1416–22.e6. doi: 10.1016/j.jaci.2016.12.969
89. Martins da Fonseca CS, Pimenta Filho AA, dos Santos BS, da Silva CA, Domingues ALC, Owen JS, et al. Human plasma lipid modulation in schistosomiasis mansoni depends on apolipoprotein E polymorphism. *PLoS ONE.* (2014) 9:e101964. doi: 10.1371/journal.pone.0101964
90. Sertorio M, Hou X, Carmo RF, Dessein H, Cabantous S, Abdelwahed M, et al. IL-22 and IL-22 binding protein (IL-22BP) regulate fibrosis and cirrhosis in hepatitis C virus and schistosome infections. *Hepatology.* (2015) 61:1321–31. doi: 10.1002/hep.27629
91. Silva PCV, Gomes AV, de Souza TKG, Coêlho MRCD, Cahu GG de OM, Muniz MTC, et al. Association of SNP (-G1082A) IL-10 with increase in severity of periportal fibrosis in Schistosomiasis, in the Northeast of Brazil. *Genetic Testing Mol Biomarkers.* (2014) 18:646–52. doi: 10.1089/gtmb.2014.0098
92. Silva PCV, Gomes AV, de Britto LRPB, de Lima ELS, da Silva JL, Montenegro SML, et al. Influence of a TNF-α Polymorphism on the severity of schistosomiasis periportal fibrosis in the Northeast of Brazil. *Genet Test Mol Biomarkers.* (2017) 21:658–62. doi: 10.1089/gtmb.2017.0133
93. Zhu X, Zhang J, Fan W, Gong Y, Yan J, Yuan Z, et al. MAPKAP1 rs10118570 polymorphism is associated with anti-infection and anti-hepatic fibrogenesis in schistosomiasis japonica. *PLoS ONE.* (2014) 9:e105995. doi: 10.1371/journal.pone.0105995
94. Oliveira JB, Silva PCV, Vasconcelos LM, Gomes AV, Coêlho MRCD, Cahu GGOM, et al. Influence of polymorphism (-G308A) TNF-α on the periportal fibrosis regression of schistosomiasis after specific treatment. *Genet Test Mol Biomarkers.* (2015) 19:598–603. doi: 10.1089/gtmb.2015.0091
95. Xiao Q, Yu H, Zhu X. The associations of hub gene polymorphisms in PI3K/AKT/mTOR pathway and Schistosomiasis Japonica infection and hepatic fibrosis. *Infect Genet Evol.* (2020) 85:104423. doi: 10.1016/j.meegid.2020.104423
96. Manolio TA, Collins FS, Cox NJ, Goldstein DB, Hindorff LA, Hunter DJ, et al. Finding the missing heritability of complex diseases. *Nature.* (2009) 461:747–53. doi: 10.1038/nature08494
97. Mohamed-Ali Q, Elwali NE, Abdelhameed AA, Mergani A, Rahoud S, Elagib KE, et al. Susceptibility to periportal (Symmers) fibrosis in human *Schistosoma mansoni* infections: evidence that intensity and duration of infection, gender, and inherited factors are critical in disease progression. *J Infect Dis.* (1999) 180:1298–306. doi: 10.1086/314999
98. Dessein AJ, Marquet S, Henri S, El Wali NE, Hillaire D, Rodrigues V, et al. Infection and disease in human *Schistosoma mansoni* are under distinct major gene control. *Microbes Infect.* (1999) 1:561–7. doi: 10.1016/S1286-4579(99)80096-3
99. Abath FGC, Morais CNL, Montenegro CEL, Wynn TA, Montenegro SML. Immunopathogenic mechanisms in schistosomiasis: what can be learnt from human studies? *Trends Parasitol.* (2006) 22:85–91. doi: 10.1016/j.pt.2005.12.004

100. Schön MP, Erpenbeck L. The Interleukin-23/Interleukin-17 axis links adaptive and innate immunity in psoriasis. *Front Immunol.* (2018) 9:1323. doi: 10.3389/fimmu.2018.01323
101. Kimura A, Kishimoto T. IL-6: Regulator of Treg/Th17 balance. *Eur J Immunol.* (2010) 40:1830–5. doi: 10.1002/eji.201040391
102. Wen X, He L, Chi Y, Zhou S, Hoellwarth J, Zhang C, et al. Dynamics of Th17 cells and their role in *Schistosoma japonicum* infection in C57BL/6 Mice. *PLoS Neglected Trop Dis.* (2011) 5:e1399. doi: 10.1371/journal.pntd.0001399
103. Ojurongbe O, Antony JS, Tong HV, Meyer CG, Akindele AA, Sina-Agbaje OR, et al. Low MBL-associated serine protease 2 (MASP-2) levels correlate with urogenital schistosomiasis in Nigerian children. *Trop Med Int Health.* (2015) 20:1311–9. doi: 10.1111/tmi.12551
104. Elsammak MY, Al-Sharkaweey RM, Ragab MS, Amin GM, Kandil MH. In Egyptians, a mutation in the lymphotoxin-alpha gene may increase susceptibility to hepatitis C virus but not that to schistosomal infection. *Ann Trop Med Parasitol.* (2008) 102:709–16. doi: 10.1179/136485908X337599
105. Nutman TB. Looking beyond the induction of Th2 responses to explain immunomodulation by helminths. *Parasite Immunol.* (2015) 37:304–13. doi: 10.1111/pim.12194
106. Goenka S, Kaplan MH. Transcriptional regulation by STAT6. *Immunol Res.* (2011) 50:87–96. doi: 10.1007/s12026-011-8205-2
107. Brito CF, Caldas IR, Filho C, Correa-Oliveira R, Oliveira SC. CD4+ T cells of schistosomiasis naturally resistant individuals living in an endemic area produce interferon-γ and tumour necrosis factor-α in response to the recombinant 14kda *Schistosoma mansoni* fatty acid-binding protein. *Scand J Immunol.* (2000) 51:595–601. doi: 10.1046/j.1365-3083.2000.00710.x
108. Fonseca CT, Oliveira SC, Alves CC. Eliminating schistosomes through vaccination: what are the best immune weapons? *Front Immunol.* (2015) 6:1–8. doi: 10.3389/fimmu.2015.00095
109. Landrum MJ, Lee JM, Benson M, Brown GR, Chao C, Chitipiralla S, et al. ClinVar: improving access to variant interpretations and supporting evidence. *Nucleic Acids Res.* (2018) 46:D1062–7. doi: 10.1093/nar/gkx1153
110. Sim N-L, Kumar P, Hu J, Henikoff S, Schneider G, Ng PC. SIFT web server: predicting effects of amino acid substitutions on proteins. *Nucleic Acids Res.* (2012) 40:W452–7. doi: 10.1093/nar/gks539
111. Adzhubei IA, Schmidt S, Peshkin L, Ramensky VE, Gerasimova A, Bork P, et al. A method and server for predicting damaging missense mutations. *Nat Methods.* (2010) 7:248–249. doi: 10.1038/nmeth0410-248
112. van der Pouw Kraan T, van Veen A, Boeije L, van Tuyl S, de Groot E, Stapel S, et al. An IL-13 promoter polymorphism associated with increased risk of allergic asthma. *Genes Immun.* (1999) 1:61–65. doi: 10.1038/sj.gene.63 63630
113. Patel DD, Kuchroo VK. Th17 cell pathway in human immunity: lessons from genetics and therapeutic interventions. *Immunity.* (2015) 43:1040–51. doi: 10.1016/j.immuni.2015.12.003
114. Pang N, Zhang F, Ma X, Zhu Y, Zhao H, Xin Y, et al. TGF-β/Smad signaling pathway regulates Th17/Treg balance during Echinococcus multilocularis infection. *Int Immunopharmacol.* (2014) 20:248–57. doi: 10.1016/j.intimp.2014.02.038
115. Hirschhorn JN, Lohmueller K, Byrne E, Hirschhorn K. A comprehensive review of genetic association studies. *Genet Med.* (2002) 4:45–61. doi: 10.1097/00125817-200203000-00002
116. McClellan J, King M-C. Genetic heterogeneity in human disease. *Cell.* (2010) 141:210–7. doi: 10.1016/j.cell.2010.03.032
117. Choi WA, Kang MJ, Kim YJ, Seo JH, Kim HY, Kwon JW, et al. Gene-gene interactions between candidate gene polymorphisms are associated with total IgE levels in Korean Children with Asthma. *J Asthma.* (2012) 49:243–52. doi: 10.3109/02770903.2012.660294
118. Marquet S, Conte I, Poudiougou B, Argiro L, Cabantous S, Dessein H, et al. The IL17F and IL17RA genetic variants increase risk of cerebral malaria in two African Populations. *Infect Immunity.* (2016) 84:590–7. doi: 10.1128/IAI.00671-15
119. Campino S, Kwiatkowski D, Dessein A. Mendelian and complex genetics of susceptibility and resistance to parasitic infections. *Semin Immunol.* (2006) 18:411–22. doi: 10.1016/j.smim.2006.07.011
120. Abel L, Dessein AJ. Genetic epidemiology of infectious diseases in humans: design of population-based studies. *Emerging Infect Dis.* (1998) 4:593–603. doi: 10.3201/eid0404.9 80409

3

Enhanced Delivery of Rituximab into Brain and Lymph Nodes Using Timed-Release Nanocapsules in Non-Human Primates

Meng Qin[1,2], *Lan Wang*[1,2], *Di Wu*[3], *Christopher K. Williams*[4], *Duo Xu*[3], *Emiko Kranz*[2,5], *Qi Guo*[2,6], *Jiaoqiong Guan*[7], *Harry V. Vinters*[4], *YooJin Lee*[1,2], *Yiming Xie*[1,2], *Yun Luo*[8], *Guibo Sun*[8], *Xiaobo Sun*[8], *Zhanlong He*[7], *Yunfeng Lu*[3], *Masakazu Kamata*[2,5*†], *Jing Wen*[1,2*] and *Irvin S. Y. Chen*[1,2*]

[1] Department of Microbiology, Immunology and Molecular Genetics, David Geffen School of Medicine at University of California, Los Angeles, Los Angeles, CA, United States, [2] UCLA AIDS Institute, Los Angeles, CA, United States, [3] Department of Chemical and Biomolecular Engineering, School of Engineering, UCLA, Los Angeles, CA, United States, [4] Departments of Pathology & Laboratory Medicine (Neuropathology) and Neurology, David Geffen School of Medicine at UCLA, Los Angeles, CA, United States, [5] Division of Hematology-Oncology, David Geffen School of Medicine at UCLA, Los Angeles, CA, United States, [6] School of Nursing, UCLA, Los Angeles, CA, United States, [7] Institute of Medical Biology, Peking Union Medical College, Chinese Academy of Medical Sciences, Kunming, China, [8] Institute of Medicinal Plant Development, Peking Union Medical College, Chinese Academy of Medical Sciences, Beijing, China

***Correspondence:**
Masakazu Kamata
masa3k@uab.edu
Jing Wen
wjjulia@ucla.edu
Irvin S. Y. Chen
syuchen@mednet.ucla.edu

†Present address:
Masakazu Kamata,
Department of Microbiology,
University of Alabama at Birmingham,
Birmingham, AL, United States

Tumor metastasis into the central nervous system (CNS) and lymph nodes (LNs) is a major obstacle for effective therapies. Therapeutic monoclonal antibodies (mAb) have revolutionized tumor treatment; however, their efficacy for treating metastatic tumors-particularly, CNS and LN metastases-is poor due to inefficient penetration into the CNS and LNs following intravenous injection. We recently reported an effective delivery of mAb to the CNS by encapsulating the anti-CD20 mAb rituximab (RTX) within a thin shell of polymer that contains the analogs of choline and acetylcholine receptors. This encapsulated RTX, denoted as n-RTX, eliminated lymphoma cells systemically in a xenografted humanized mouse model using an immunodeficient mouse as a recipient of human hematopoietic stem/progenitor cells and fetal thymus more effectively than native RTX; importantly, n-RTX showed notable anti-tumor effect on CNS metastases which is unable to show by native RTX. As an important step toward future clinical translation of this technology, we further analyzed the properties of n-RTX in immunocompetent animals, rats, and non-human primates (NHPs). Our results show that a single intravenous injection of n-RTX resulted in 10-fold greater levels in the CNS and 2-3-fold greater levels in the LNs of RTX, respectively, than the injection of native RTX in both rats and NHPs. In addition, we demonstrate the enhanced delivery and efficient B-cell depletion in lymphoid organs of NHPs with n-RTX. Moreover, detailed hematological analysis and liver enzyme activity tests indicate n-RTX treatment is safe in NHPs. As this nanocapsule platform can be universally applied to other therapeutic mAbs, it holds great promise for extending mAb therapy to poorly accessible body compartments.

Keywords: monoclonal antibody, central nervous system delivery, LNs delivery, non-human primate, nanocapsules

INTRODUCTION

Therapeutic monoclonal antibodies (mAbs) such as rituximab (RTX, anti-CD20 for B-cell lymphomas) and trastuzumab (anti-HER2 for breast cancer) have revolutionized treatment for various types of cancers. However, their benefit in treating metastasized tumors of the central nervous system (CNS) or through lymphatic vessels into lymph nodes (LNs) (1, 2), is transient and limited, increasing life expectancy by only a few months. A major mechanism that renders metastasis more resistant to mAb treatment than primary tumors is limited antibody delivery into the CNS and lymphatic vessels (3, 4). Intraventricular or intrathecal administration of mAbs allows for bypass of the blood-brain barrier (BBB), resulting in relative effectiveness of antibody therapy in treating brain tumor metastases (5, 6); however, neurotoxicity and rapid efflux are known to hinder mAb application for brain tumor treatment (7). Subcutaneous administration of mAb targeting metastatic tumors shows the advantages of entering lymphatic vessels and binding to metastases in lymph nodes (LNs) (8). However, the restriction to regional nodes, toxicity at injection sites, and limited reach to organs without lymphatic vessels are major obstacles to using subcutaneous administration of mAb in treating systemic metastases (9). Therefore, a systemic intravenous injection route is the ideal means for administration of mAb treatment against metastatic tumors.

To improve BBB penetration for mAb delivery to the brain, modifications with various chemicals or biological components, such as lipidation or molecular targeting ligands, have been attempted (10, 11). Another strategy uses colloidal carriers such as liposomes, micelles, and nanoparticles, which transport cargos across the BBB by endocytosis and/or transcytosis (12–14). Improved therapeutic efficacy of these approaches has been demonstrated in rodents with brain tumors, Alzheimer's disease, acute ischemic stroke, and Parkinson's disease (15–17); however, non-specific tissue accumulation—including in liver, spleen, and kidney—is known to mediate acute toxicity and further decrease the effective amount of mAbs in the CNS (18). Moreover, none of those approaches achieved improvement of both LN and brain delivery at the same time.

Our nanotechnology platform utilizes "nanocapsules" which form a thin polymer shell that encapsulates individual macromolecules, protein, RNA, or DNA inside and protects them from the physiological environment (19–27). The shell is formed by *in situ* polymerization of monomers and stabilized by environmentally-responsive crosslinkers; cargoes can be released only through cleavage of these crosslinkers. We tailored these nanocapsules for CNS delivery with zwitterionic properties imbued by polymer shells composed of 2-methacryloyloxyethyl phosphorylcholine (MPC), which is clinically approved for use in coatings on implanted medical devices. MPC renders the polymer shells of nanocapsules highly biocompatible and efficacious due to low protein adsorption, improved circulation times, and minimal immunogenicity (28, 29). Moreover, such nanocapsules can effectively penetrate the BBB and deliver encapsulated macromolecules to the CNS via nicotinic acetylcholine receptors and choline transporters (30). This technology has demonstrated efficacy for neural regeneration in mice with spinal cord injuries (31) and antibody therapies for primary brain tumors (32) in mice.

Rituximab (RTX), a chimeric anti-CD20 monoclonal antibody, is used for treatment of B-cell malignancies such as non-Hodgkin's lymphomas (NHL) as well as chronic lymphocytic leukemia (CLL) (33). RTX administration contributes significant advancements toward systemic CD20+ NHL control, but treatment of primary and relapsed CNS lymphomas is inefficient due to poor penetration through the BBB (4). We recently demonstrated clearance of human B-cell tumors with brain metastases in xenograft humanized NOD-SCID-IL2receptor γ^{null} (NSG) mouse models by RTX nanocapsules (n-RTX) (34). Though these results are promising, further studies are limited by the challenge in collecting successive samples of cerebrospinal fluid (CSF) from the same mouse for analysis; moreover, the delivery into LNs, which are highly atrophic, cannot be confirmed in NSG mice. To address these limitations, we designed studies of n-RTX in both rats and non-human primates (NHPs) to further investigate delivery and biodistribution in both lymphatic tissues and CNS, and B-cell ablation in NHPs. Following a single IV dose of n-RTX, encapsulated RTX is released and maintained in blood for weeks resulting in effective B-cell ablation in blood and lymphatic tissues of NHPs. Importantly, we show significantly improved RTX delivery to the CNS and lymph nodes with no notable adverse effects.

RESULTS

Formulation of Nanocapsules With Hydrolysable Crosslinkers to Release mAbs

A formulation of nanocapsules with timed-release capabilities *in vivo* was synthesized based on previously published nanocapsules (19). We screened and selected two crosslinkers to sustain release at physiological conditions *in vivo*: hydrolysable crosslinker—poly (lactide-co-glycolide)-b-poly(ethylene glycol)-b-poly(lactide-co-glycolide) (PLA-PEG-PLA) and non-hydrolysable crosslinker—glycerol dimethacrylate (GDMA), which degrade rapidly and slowly, respectively, at physiological pH conditions. The ratios between and GDMA impact the release kinetics. With a higher PLA-PEG-PLA ratio, the crosslinkers will degrade in a shorter time. As the crosslinkers degrade, the shells of nanocapsules will loosen, swell, and dissociate resulting in the release of encapsulated mAbs. As shown in **Figure 1A**, nanocapsules encapsulating mAbs are synthesized through the following processes: first, the zwitterionic monomer (MPC) and two crosslinkers, PLA-PEG-PLA and GDMA, are enriched around the surface of the mAb (in this case, RTX) through hydrogen bonding (Step 1). Subsequent polymerization in an aqueous solution at 4°C wraps each molecule with a thin shell of polymer through *in situ* free-radical polymerization (Step 2). Finally, crosslinkers stabilize the polymer structure and release mAbs upon hydrolysis (Step 3). Transmission

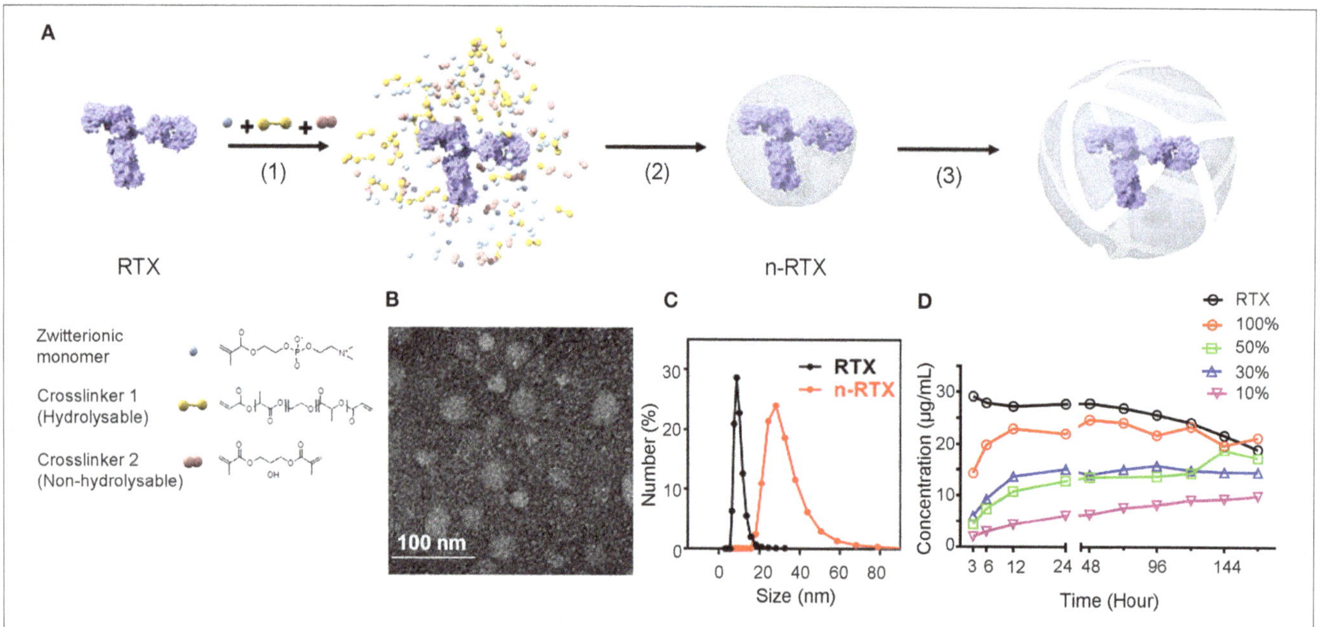

FIGURE 1 | Developing timed-release nanocapsules of RTX. **(A)** Scheme of the synthesis of and release by timed-release RTX nanocapsules (n-RTX) by (1) enriching zwitterionic monomer (MPC), hydrolysable crosslinker 1 (PLA-PEG-PLA) and non-hydrolysable crosslinker 2 (GDMA) around a RTX molecule, (2) *in-situ* polymerization of the monomer and crosslinkers forming a thin shell of polymer around an RTX molecule, and (3) releasing RTX when polymer shells are degraded under physiological condition. **(B)** Transmission Electron Microscopy image of n-RTX. **(C)** Size distribution of n-RTX measured by dynamic light scattering measurement. **(D)** Nanocapsules with mixed hydrolysable crosslinkers achieve timed release of RTX in rhesus macaque plasma. The nanocapsules synthesized with mixed PLA-PEG-PLA and GDMA crosslinkers at different ratios. Release kinetics of n-RTX with 100, 50, 30, 10, and 0% of PLA-PEG-PLA were tested. Thirty micrograms of nanocapsules were incubated in 1 mL of rhesus macaque plasma at 37°C. The concentration of released RTX was determined by ELISA.

electron microscopy (TEM) and dynamic light scattering (DLS) measurements show that these nanocapsules form a spherical morphology of 20–30 nm encasing mAb molecules inside (**Figures 1B,C**). Dependent on the ratios between PLA-PEG-PLA and GDMA, nanocapsules release RTX at different rates when incubated in rhesus macaque plasma *in vitro* (**Figure 1D**). The RTX concentration was detected by enzyme-linked immunosorbent assay (ELISA) using anti-RTX (anti-idiotype) antibody, which can only detect the free RTX released from nanocapsules since nanocapsules shields the epitopes of encapsulated antibodies by the polymer shells. The n-RTX with 50 and 30% PLA-PEG-PLA crosslinkers showed an intermediate level of release over 6 days. We already demonstrated improved CNS delivery of n-RTX with 50% PLA nanocapsules in mice in our published work (35), so the same formulation for following *in vivo* studies in rats and NHPs was used. We also demonstrated that improvement of CNS delivery with this nanocapsules formulation is applicable to other therapeutic mAbs. To prove this point, we tested Herceptin (anti-Her2) for breast cancer; similarly to n-RTX, Herceptin nanocapsules (n-Hercepin) show increased delivery to the CNS (**Figure S1**).

Improved Delivery to CNS and LNs of Rats by RTX Nanocapsules

We demonstrated the improved delivery to CNS and LNs by n-RTX using rats where greater amounts of CSF facilitate serial sampling within the same animals and mature LN formation enables clear visualization and detection in the lymphatic system. Native RTX and n-RTX, normalized with of the same amount of RTX for a single IV dose, showed comparable RTX level in plasma (**Figure 2A**). Whereas, native RTX in CSF was <0.1% of plasma levels, RTX released from n-RTX was 1%, and was maintained this level to days 14 and 21 when native antibody was barely detectable at day 4 (**Figure 2B**). At the endpoint, RTX levels in brain tissue were consistent with the CSF results; higher levels of RTX were observed in the n-RTX treated animals (**Figure 2C**). These results provide proof of concept for improved antibody delivery in the CNS compared to the native form. Improved levels of RTX from n-RTX are also observed in lymphatic-tissues, which include organs such as spleen, LNs in different locations, and three sections of the small intestine (**Figure 2C**). Tissue imaging shows clear biodistribution of fluorescently labeled native RTX and n-RTX on day 1 post-injection (**Figure 2D**). Compared to native RTX, n-RTX shows an improved distribution in lymphatic-tissues containing organs including LNs and spleen and, importantly, reduced accumulation in lung, liver, and kidney—major organs involved with clearance of recombinant antibodies. The decreased accumulation in lung, liver, and kidney is due to the superior anti-fouling property of n-RTX, which decrease the uptake by immune surveillance cells. The difference in biodistribution between RTX and n-RTX is further confirmed by quantifying the relative fluorescence units of the fluorescence label from each organ (**Figure 2E**).

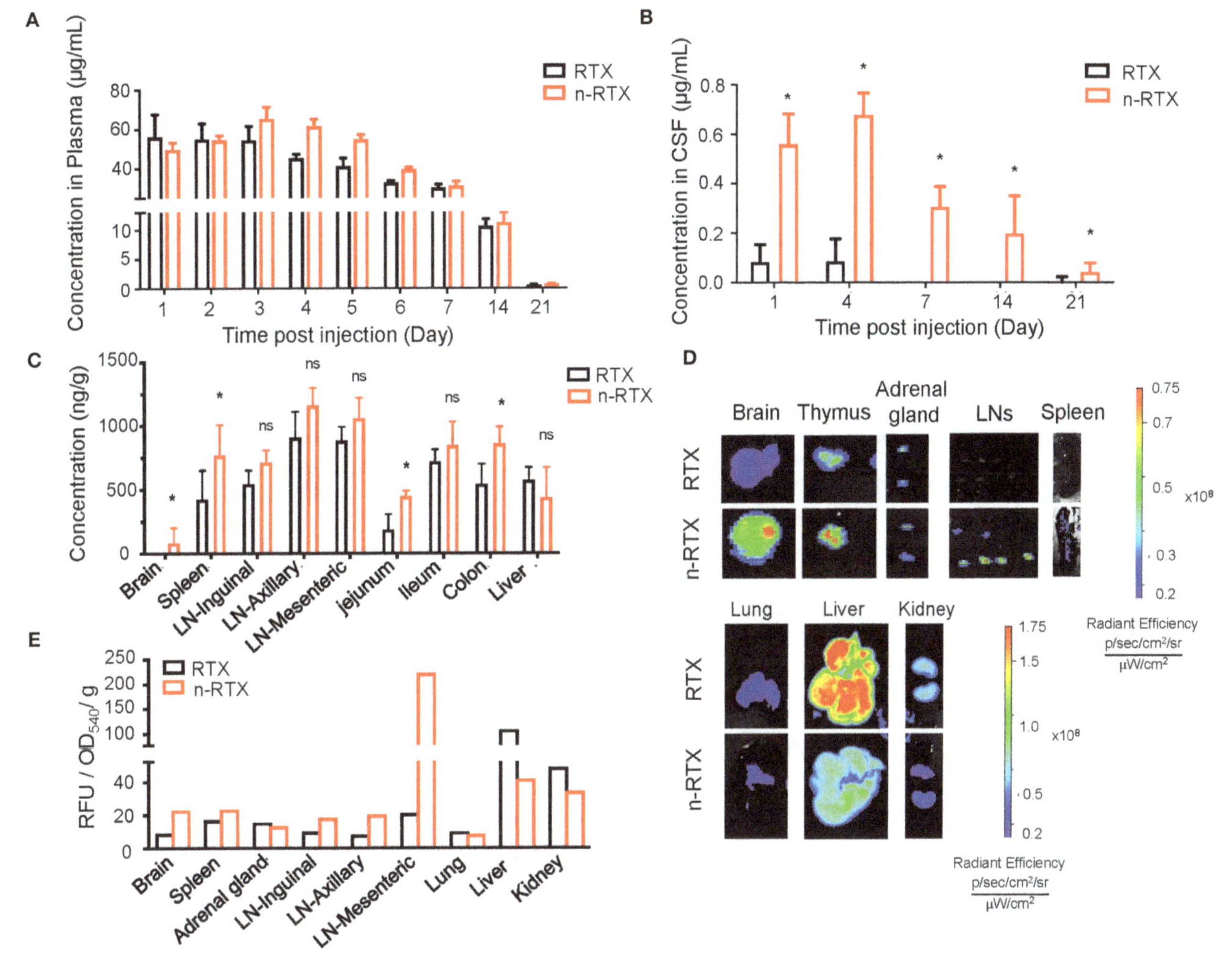

FIGURE 2 | Nanocapsulation of RTX improves levels of its tissue penetration, including CNS, in rats. A single dose (5 mg/kg) of native RTX or n-RTX was administered in rats through IV (intravenous) injection ($n = 3$). **(A–C)** The concentrations of free RTX in plasma **(A)** on Days 1, 2, 3, 4, 5, 6, 7, 14, and 21 and CSF **(B)** on Days 1, 4, 7, 14, and 21 were determined by ELISA. **(C)** Tissues, including LNs at three different locations, jejunum, ileum, colon, spleen, liver, and brain, were harvest at necropsy after perfusion on Day 22. Tissues were homogenized in PBS (1 mg tissue in 100 μl PBS), and tested by ELISA for RTX concentrations. A higher single dose (15 mg/kg) of fluorescent labeled native RTX or n-RTX was administered in rats through IV injection ($n = 1$) and monitored on IVIS *in vivo* imaging **(D,E)**. Organs were isolated and monitored by IVIS imaging on Day7 after injection. **(E)** Signal intensity from free RTX in each organ was quantified by software Living Image. Data were generated from $n = 3$ rats. Data are shown as means ± s.d. of biological triplicate. Statistical significance between native and nanocapsules was determined by one-tailed Mann–Whitney–Wilcoxon test. *Significant, $p < 0.1$; ns, not significant.

Enhanced Delivery of RTX Nanocapsules to the Brain of Rhesus Macaques

As an essential step toward future clinical translation of nanocapsules, we further analyzed the properties of n-RTX in non-human primates (NHPs). The study design is summarized in **Figure 3**. Four rhesus macaques were intravenously infused with a single dose (5 mg/kg, normalized for the RTX amount) of native RTX or n-RTX and processed for necropsy on Day 21 (Group I, #12025 and #13029) or Day 63 (Group II, #12069 and 12019). Blood samples were collected on Days 1, 3, 5, and 7 in the first week, and every 7 days after that (**Figure 3**, Stars). CSF sample collection started before infusion as a baseline (**Figure 3**, Day-12), on Day 3 post-infusion, and continued every 7 days until Day 21 for Group I; for Group II, CSF collection was initiated on Day 1 post-infusion and continued every week until Day 63. Lymph node (LN) biopsies were performed on Days 3 and 14 in Group I and on Days 3, 17, 28, and 42 in Group II (**Figure 3**, Double triangles). Eight tissues, including brain, thymus, lung, liver, spleen, kidney, intestine, and LNs, were harvested at necropsy following perfusion. LNs from different locations (inguinal LN, axillary LN, and mesenteric LN), and three pieces (3 × 3 cm) from each of other tissues were collected and used for ELISA assays. Brain and LN samples were also used for immunohistochemical (IHC) analysis.

We successfully demonstrated the enhanced CNS delivery of n-RTX in rhesus macaques (**Figure 4**). The levels of RTX released from n-RTX in rhesus macaque plasma was slightly lower on Day 1 compared to that of native RTX, probably due to the controlled

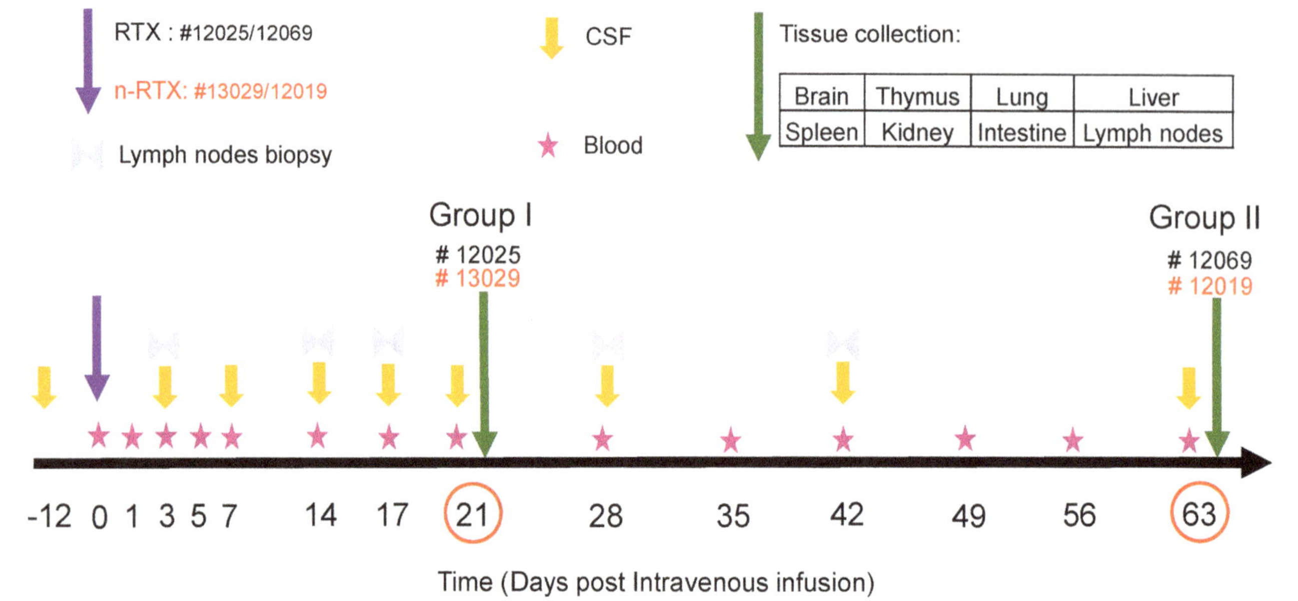

FIGURE 3 | Experimental schedule of RTX brain delivery in non-human primates. Four rhesus macaques were administered with a single 5 mg/kg dose of native RTX (Monkey ID #12025 and #12069) and n-RTX (Monkey ID #13029 and 12019) via IV infusion. Peripheral blood, CSF, and Inguinal lymph nodes were collected as scheduled. Other tissues were harvested at necropsy on Days 21 or 63 after perfusion.

RTX release from n-RTX in plasma (**Figure 4A**). The plasma level remained stable for 1 week, followed by a gradual decreased over time. Two animals treated with n-RTX (#13029 and 12019) showed 5- and 2.5-fold greater levels of free RTX in the CSF compared to those in native RTX-treated animals (#12025 and 12069), respectively, within the first week (**Figure 4B**). Native RTX fell below detection limits by Day 14, whereas free RTX released from n-RTX persisted until Day 21 in both groups. RTX concentration in the tissue homogenates was also assessed by ELISA (**Figure 4C**). In Group I, the animal treated with n-RTX (#13029) showed significantly higher levels of RTX in all tissues than that treated with native RTX (#12025) in all tissues. A similar trend was confirmed with animals in Group II, but the difference between those two treatments was less significant. Five regions of the brain, including the frontal, parietal, temporal occipital lobes, as well as cerebellum, were homogenized separately for ELISA. RTX was only detectable in Group I. RTX released from n-RTX was observed at approximately 4-fold levels in all brain regions than that in the brain tissues from the RTX-treated animal (**Figure 4D**).

Liver toxicity is a major concern for use of nanomedicines *in vivo* (35). Thus, liver damage is the one of the indexes of nanomedicine safety. In order to show that this nanocapsule platform improves brain delivery efficiency of therapeutic antibodies through systemic injection without inducing liver toxicity, three liver enzymes indicating acute liver toxicity were closely measured over the course of experiments: alanine aminotransferase (ALT), aspartate aminotransferase (AST), and alkaline phosphatase (ALP) (**Figure 5A**). As we confirmed in mice previously (34), no notable differences exist in levels between animals treated with RTX or n-RTX. Neither a complete liver function assay including serum globulin (GLB), indirect bilirubin (IBIL), gamma-glutamyl transferase (γ-GT), total protein (TP), and albumin (ALB), nor a blood chemistry test for white blood cell (WBC) count, lymphocyte count, monocyte count, neutrophil count, hemoglobin (HGB), hematocrit (HCT), and platelet counts (PLT), showed major differences between those animals (**Figure S2**). We have hereby concluded that n-RTX increases antibody delivery into the CNS by 4–10-fold with no detectable level of acute systemic toxicity.

We further showed no potential neurotoxicity caused by n-RTX treatment. Two well-known neurotoxicity markers were used in this test: glial fibrillary acidic protein (GFAP), of which levels increase with reactive gliosis (36), and ionized calcium-binding adapter molecule (IBA-1), of which levels increase upon mediating neuroinflammation (37). Compared to native RTX-treated animals, brain tissues of n-RTX treated animals showed normal morphology and no elevated expressions of those two markers (**Figures 5B,C**).

Comparison of Effector Activity Mediated by Native RTX and n-RTX

Lastly, we observed comparable B cell depletion by RTX and n-RTX in peripheral blood of NHPs. CD20 can be internalized by the binding of RTX (38, 39), so single staining for cell surface CD20 may underestimate total B cell levels. To more accurately measure B cell levels, we stained cells with both CD19 and CD20 antibodies. To minimize CD20 epitope masking by RTX, we used the CD20 antibody clone L26, which recognizes different epitope on rhesus CD20 molecules not blocked by RTX (40). Analysis by single staining for CD19+ showed similar results to double staining for CD19+/CD20+ cells (data not shown).

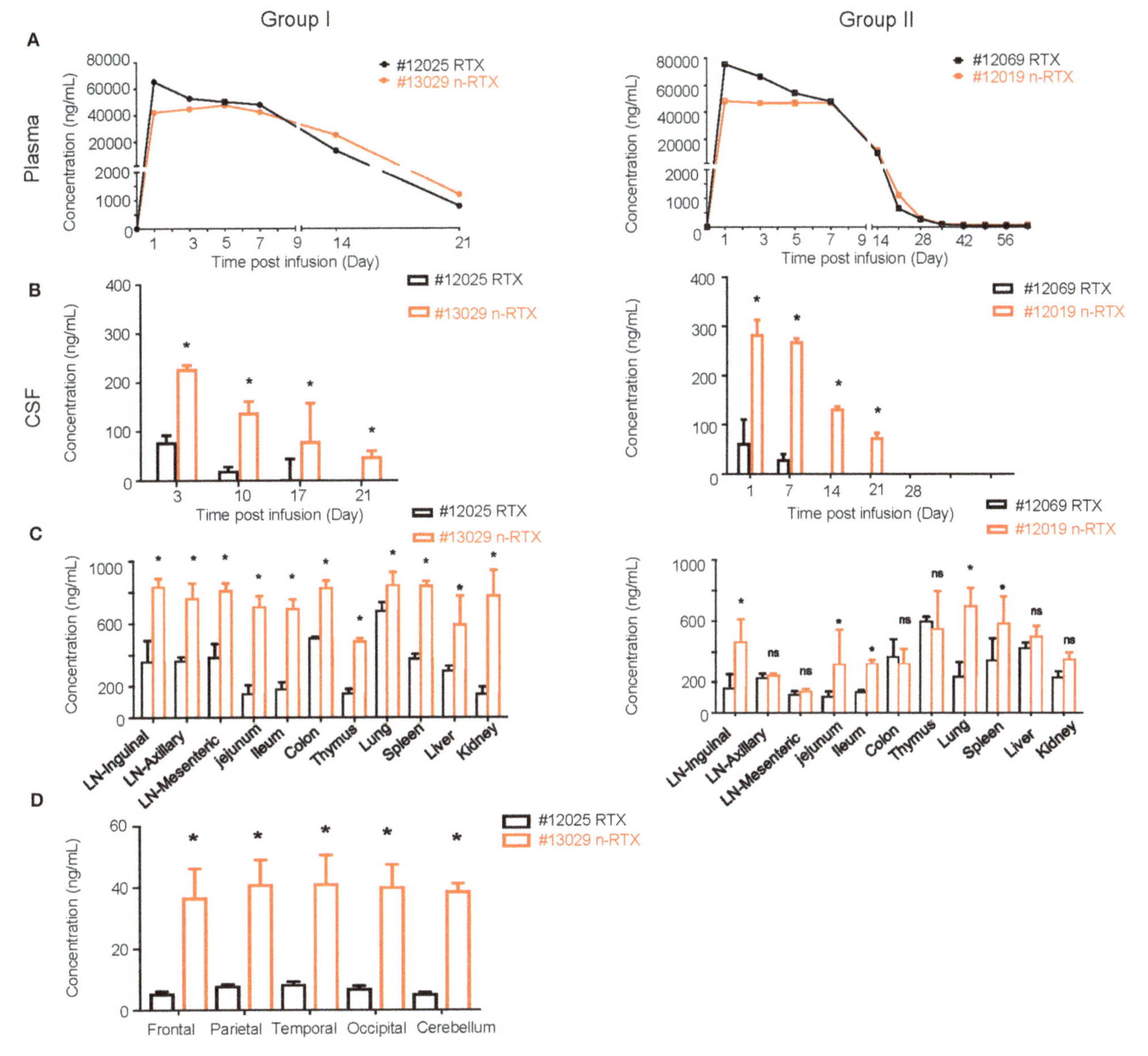

FIGURE 4 | Nanocapsulation of RTX improves levels of its tissue penetration in non-human primates. A single dose (5 mg/kg) of native RTX or n-RTX was administered in rhesus macaques through IV infusion **(A,B)**. The concentrations of free RTX in plasma **(A)** and CSF **(B)** were determined by ELISA. **(C)** At the endpoint of Group I (Day 21) and Group II (Day 63), LNs at three different locations, jejunum, ileum, colon, thymus, lung, spleen, liver, kidney, and brain were harvest after perfusion. Whole LNs and three pieces (3 × 3 cm) of other tissues were homogenized in PBS (1 mg tissue in 100 μl PBS) for ELISA test. **(D)** Five different regions of the brain (frontal, parietal, temporal occipital lobes, and cerebellum) were homogenized in PBS (1 mg tissue in 100 μl PBS) for ELISA test. Data are shown as means ± s.d. of biological triplicate. Statistical significance between native and nanocapsules was determined by one-tailed Mann–Whitney–Wilcoxon test. *Significant, $p < 0.1$, ns, not significant.

CD19+/CD20+ B cell levels dropped ~80–90% within the first 7 days after treatment by both RTX and n-RTX (**Figure 6A**). Aside from the expected drop in B cells, the numbers of total WBCs, neutrophils, lymphocytes, and monocytes were relatively stable (**Figure S3**), indicating B-cell specific depletion by RTX in both forms. Levels of total CD3+ cells, CD3+/CD4+ T cells, and CD3+/CD8+ T cells were also stable over the course of treatment (**Figures 6B–D**).

To assess the specificity of depletion and accessibility to B cells in lymphoid tissues, we analyzed levels of B-cell depletion in LNs at three different localities: axillary, mesenteric and inguinal, by IHC analysis. Antibodies for CD20+, CD3+, and Bcl-6 were included to distinguish three different types of cells, B cells, T cells, and T follicular helper cells (**Figure 7A**). By further quantitative analysis of IHC staining results, CD20+ B cells showed a lower density in all three LNs of animals treated with n-RTX compared to that of native RTX on Day 21 (**Figure 7B**). Ratios of B cell against T cell (B/T ratio) detected by flow cytometry in inguinal LN indicated that n-RTX mediated prolonged B cell depletion over the course of treatment compared

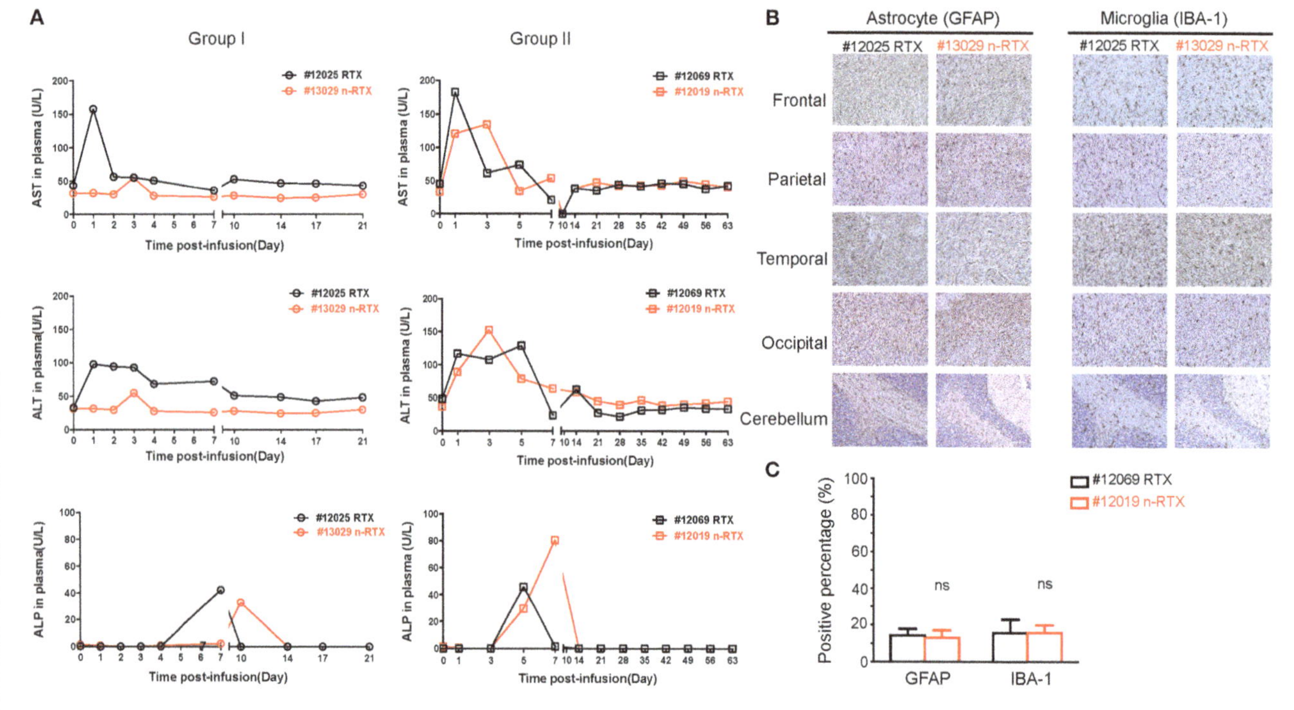

FIGURE 5 | RTX nanocapsules do not mediate notable levels of acute toxicity in the liver and brain. **(A)** Rhesus macaques were administrated with a single dose (5 mg/kg) of native RTX or n-RTX. Plasma samples were collected as scheduled and served for measuring levels of aspartate transaminase (AST), alanine transaminase (ALT), and alkaline phosphatase (ALP) by ELISA. **(B)** Brain tissues obtained from five different parts were fixed by 4% paraformaldehyde and processed for IHC analysis. Representative images of immunohistochemical staining for GFAP (astrocyte marker) and IBA-1 (microglial marker) were shown. Scale bar = 100 μm. **(C)** A positive pixel count in images (4 mm^2) from five different brain parts was quantified using Aperio ScanScope slide scanner. Positive pixel calculation for GFAP used the following variables: hue width = 0.371 and color saturation threshold = 9.7e-002. Positive pixel calculation for IBA-1 used the following variables: hue width = 0.5 and color saturation threshold = 4.0e-007. % positivity was calculated by total number of positive pixels divided by the total number of pixels. Data are shown as means ± s.d. of biological triplicate. Statistical significance, compared with the native RTX group, was determined by one-tailed *t*-test with Welch's correction. ns, not significant.

to native RTX (**Figure S4**). In contrast, no significant difference in levels of CD3+ T cells was confirmed between LNs treated with native RTX or n-RTX. The level of Bcl-6 expression in LNs, a marker of germinal center B cells and T follicular helper cells, showed no difference between two animals.

DISCUSSION

We utilized a platform wherein single mAbs are encapsulated within a thin polymer shell, called a "nanocapsule," to improve delivery of anti-tumor antibodies to the brain. Formulations were modified to utilize neutral polymers with zwitterionic properties (MPC polymers) and crosslinkers that hold the shell together which are later gradually hydrolyzed for timed release of mAb in a suitable microenvironment. This successful nanocapsule design sustains RTX in circulation, allows penetration into the brain, reaches deep tissues including LNs, and releases RTX in a controlled fashion. Our results detail the first test of a zwitterionic nanocarrier—nanocapsule—for therapeutic mAb delivery in NHPs. Importantly, the data clearly show efficient and prolonged delivery of RTX into both the CNS and LNs by a single dose of intravenous injection with no notable acute liver toxicity nor neurotoxicities.

Therapeutic mAbs are effective for treating several tumors; however, their performance is limited in the treatment of metastases in CNS and LNs, where the physical barriers are considered as one of the major obstacles to achieve effective mAbs delivery. Although subcutaneous administration is considered as an effective route for LN delivery through the absorption by lymphatic capillaries, the delivery into the lymphatic system is delayed due to the limitation of the absorption rate (41, 42). Moreover, the brain delivery of mAbs through subcutaneous administration is challenging due to the low concentration of mAbs in plasma. Therefore, intravenous injection is still a commonly used administration route for mAb therapy. However, achieving a high plasma concentration is insufficient for treatment of brain cancers due to poor delivery through the BBB. While multiple strategies have been attempted to facilitate greater antibody penetration through the BBB, the potential risks outweigh most benefits. One approach is to disrupt the tight junctions, allowing for passage, however, this approach raises safety concerns for the brain environment (43). Other approaches are the modification and engineering of mAbs to improve brain delivery; attaching charged or lipophilic moieties to mAbs to enhance absorptive-mediated transport, but those modifications are known to result in unexpected biodistribution, low sustainability, and insufficient

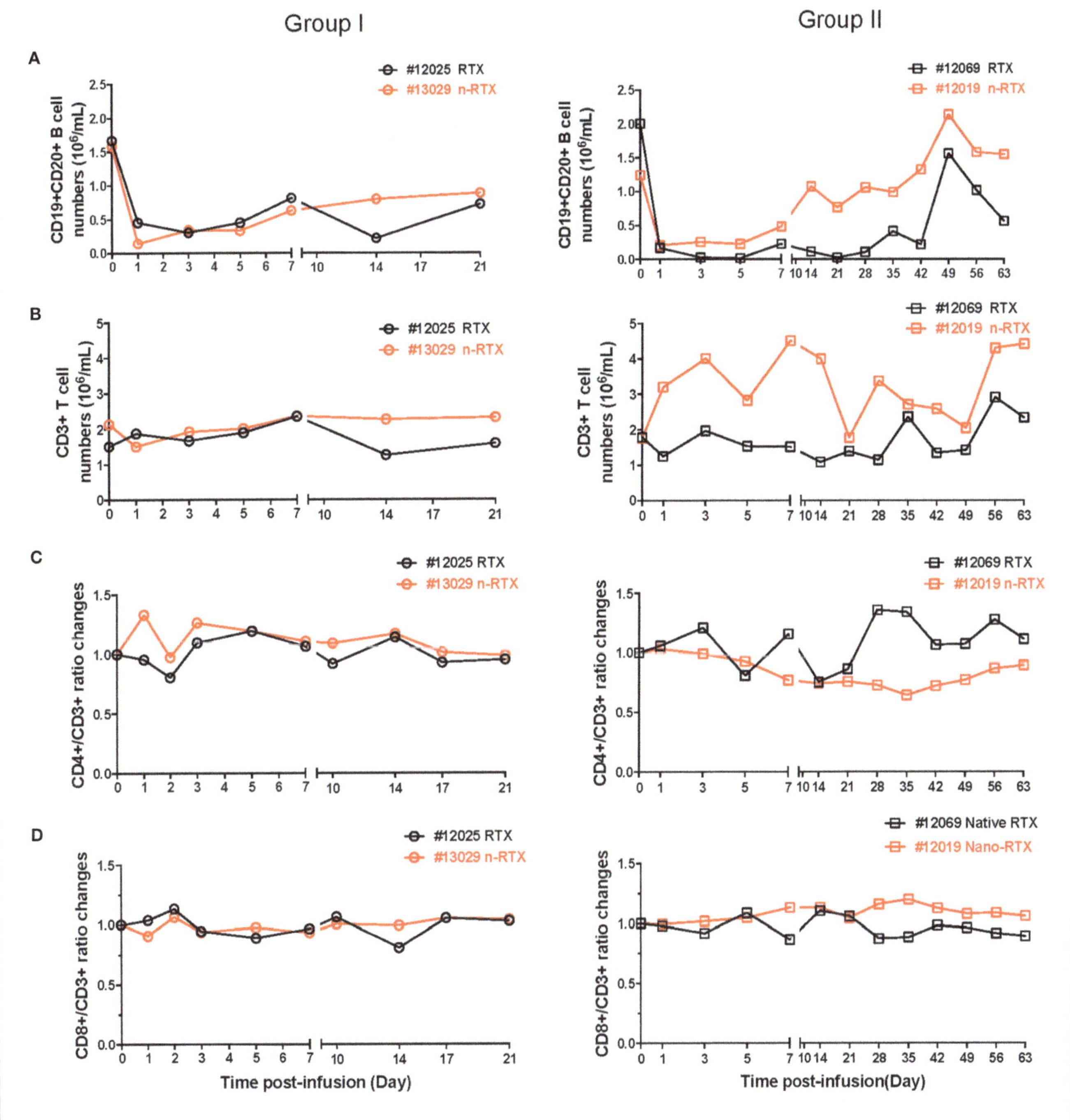

FIGURE 6 | Both native and nanocapsulated RTXs mediate similar levels of peripheral blood B cell depletion in rhesus macaques. Whole blood was collected as scheduled and processed for monitoring immunophenotyping by flow cytometry. **(A)** CD19+CD20+ B cells, **(B)** CD3+ total T cells, **(C)** CD4+T cells, and **(D)** CD8+T cells. **(A,B)** CD19+CD20 B cells and CD3+ T cells were showed by absolute numbers per 1 mL of blood. **(C,D)** The percentages of CD4+ T cells and CD8+ T cells in CD3+ T cells were normalized over baseline.

efficacy (44, 45). mAbs have also been encapsulated or conjugated with nanoparticles or liposomes to induce receptor-mediated transcytosis on the BBB (46, 47), but the efficacy, safety, and stability in NHPs are still unknown. Thus, despite decades of effort, effective delivery of mAbs to the both LNs and the CNS remains challenging.

We used the nanocapsule platform to achieve systemic delivery of RTX into both the CNS and LNs in both rodents and NHPs with single intravenous injection. The choline and acetylcholine analogous structures on the MPC polymer chains of nanocapsules, which can induce transcytosis through the BBB via nicotinic acetylcholine receptors and choline transporters,

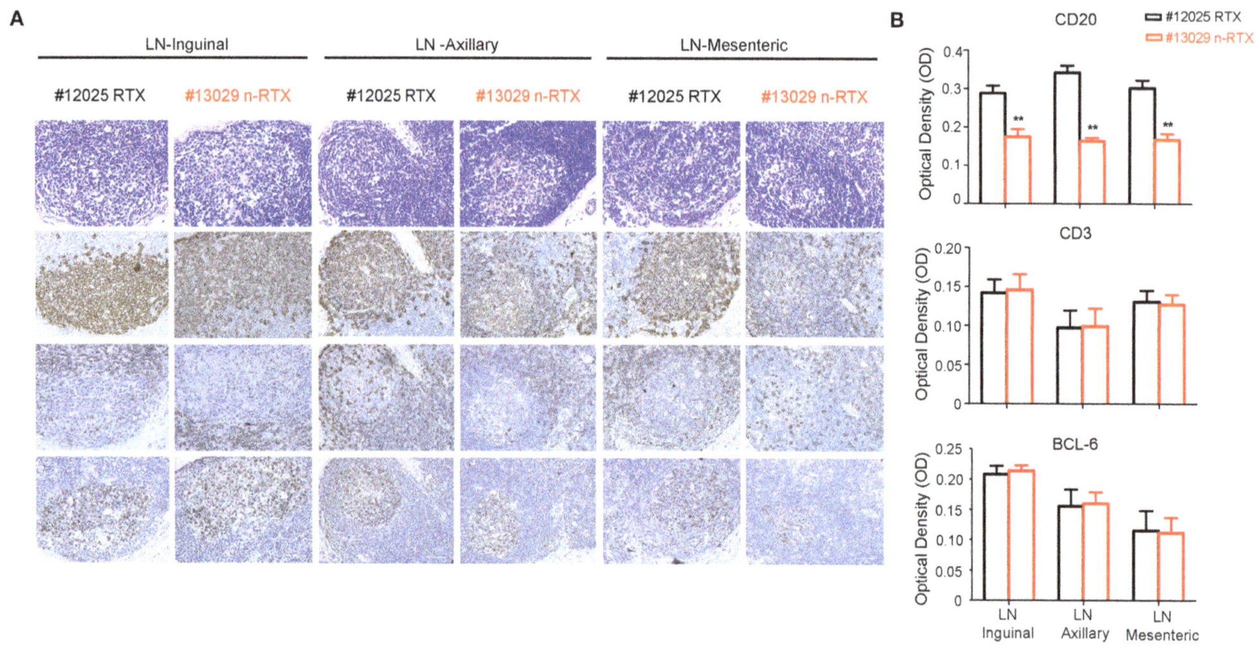

FIGURE 7 | Nanocapsulated RTX mediates superior B-cell depletion in LNs of rhesus macaques. LNs from three different locations (inguinal, axillary, and mesenteric) were collected at necropsy on Day 21 from Group I rhesus macaques with a single dose (5 mg/kg) of native RTX or n-RTX via IV and processed for immunohistochemical (IHC) analyses. **(A)** H&E (top) and IHC staining of CD20 (B cell, second), CD3 (T cell, third), and Bcl-6 (Germinal center, bottom) were performed on serial sections. Panels from left to right show the expression level in axillary, mesentery, and inguinal LNs, respectively. Scale bar = 50 μm. **(B)** 6.8 × 5 cm of each CD20 and CD3 positive staining ($n = 7$), and 3.4 × 4.2 cm of Bcl-6 ($n = 4$) were randomly selected and gray pixel values were measured by Image J software. Each bar indicates the mean inverse gray value ± standard deviation (mean ± SD). One-tailed t-test with Welch's correction was used for the statistical analysis. $^{**}p < 0.01$. H&E, hematoxylin and eosin stain.

play an important role to accomplish CNS penetration (30). In NHPs treated with nanoencapsulated RTX, levels of RTX in the CSF were 100 to 300 ng/mL over 14 days, which are 4–10-fold greater than that observed for native RTX in the CSF. It indicates that our nanocapsule platform achieved higher brain delivery compared to animals treated with native RTX. Moreover, similar to animals treated with native RTX, those treated with nanocapsules exhibited no notable blood, liver, or neuronal toxicities. These studies were conducted in immune competent rats and outbred NHP more closely modeling human therapy than in our previous studies utilizing immunodeficient mice. While these levels of RTX in the CNS were sufficient to clear xenografted B cell lymphomas in the immunodeficient mice, it is unclear whether these levels are high enough to have therapeutic efficacy in humans. Our results on biodistribution and safety profiles provide a rationale for further assessing efficacy and safety in human clinical studies.

CONCLUSION

Our studies suggest a non-invasive facile solution suitable for human application to address this critical issue of poor anti-cancer mAb deliverance to both LNs and the CNS. To date, similar results are obtained with one additional clinically approved anti-cancer mAb, anti-Her2 (Herceptin), as well as other non-therapeutic mAbs such as anti-CD4 (OKT4) (unpublished data). The platform is highly versatile, with biodistribution and pharmacokinetics being readily adjustable by rational choice of chemical formulation of the polymer shell. In addition to timed-release functionality via hydrolysis of crosslinkers under physiological pH conditions, mAb release can be further controlled by crosslinkers sensitive to environmental factors such as endosomal low pH and proteases (21). Our study supports the translation of therapy from animals to human clinical studies. Further enhancements of the platform may produce therapeutic delivery options for other diseases requiring mAbs delivery into the CNS and/or LNs.

MATERIALS AND METHODS

Materials

All chemicals were purchased from Sigma-Aldrich (St. Louis, MO, USA) unless otherwise noted. All cell culture reagents were purchased from ThermoFisher Scientific (Waltham, MA) unless otherwise noted. Hydrolysable crosslinker Poly(DL-lactide)-b-Poly(ethylene glycol)-b-Poly(DL-lactide)-diacrylate triblock (PLA-PEG-PLA) was purchased from PolySciTech Akina, Inc. (West Lafeyette, IN). Capture antibody for ELISA against rituximab was purchased from Bio-Rad Laboratories (HCA0620, Hercules, CA). Anti-CD19, anti-CD20, anti-CD3, anti-CD4, and anti-CD8 for flow cytometry were purchased from BioLegend, Inc (San Diego, CA, USA). Antibodies for

IHC staining were purchased from different vendors, identifying separately in Immunohistochemistry section. Rituximab, RITUXAN (Genentech, Inc.) was purchased from the UCLA hospital pharmacy.

Synthesis of Nanocapsules

The mAbs (RTX and Herceptin) were encapsulated via *in-situ* polymerization technology. The mAb solution (2.2 mg/mL in PBS) was mixed with MPC as monomer (40% m/v in PBS) and AI102 (PLA-PEG-PLA, 10% m/v in PBS) as well as glycerol dimethacrylate (GDMA, 10% m/v in DMSO) as degradable crosslinkers. Then the polymerization was initiated by adding ammonium persulfate (APS, 10% m/v in PBS) and N, N, N′, N′-tetramethylethylenediamine (TEMED) solution. Synthesized nanocapsules were dialyzed against PBS and purified by passing through a hydrophobic interaction column (Phenyl-Sepharose 4BCL). Since the nanocapsules possess a super-hydrophilic surface, their binding affinity to the column is much weaker than the native mAb. Thus, encapsulated protein will be eluted out with a high salt concentration buffer (10xPBS), whereas the native mAb binds on the column. Purification is confirmed by DLS and ELISA to show no free mAbs. Detailed parameters of the synthesis are provided in the **Table S1**.

Transmission Electron Microscopy (TEM) and Dynamic Light Scattering (DLS) Measurements of the Nanocapsules

The nanocapsule solution (0.2 mg/mL) 10 μL was dropped onto a carbon-coated copper grid. After 45 s incubation, excess amount of the samples was removed. The samples are stained with 1% phosphotungstic acid (PTA) at pH 7.0 after being rinsed with distilled water for three times. To investigate the size and zeta potential of the nanocapsules, DLS measurements were taken under the concentration of 0.5 mg/mL.

Pharmacokinetics and Bio-Distribution Studies

Four male rhesus macaques were single administered with 5 mg/kg of RTX and n-RTX via intravenous infusion in 30 mL sterile saline through femoral vein. 2–3 mL peripheral blood was collected in EDTA anticoagulant tubes and centrifuged at 5000 rpm/min for 2 min, the plasma was separated and freeze down in −80°C for further purposes. 300–500 μL CSF with no apparent blood contamination continually collected through 3–4th lumbar spine by 1 mL syringe and frozen in −80°C for ELISA test. All animals were anesthetized with an intraperitoneal injection of FFM mix (2.5 mg Fluanisone, 0.105 mg Fentanylcitrate, and 1.25 mg Midozalam HCl/kg in distilled water). On Days 21 and 64 post-injection, animals were euthanized; tissues were removed following heart perfusion with ice-cold saline and fixed in 4% paraformaldehyde for further analyses.

Flow Cytometry

Five hundred microliters peripheral blood was used for staining following the plasma separation. Cells was rinsed by cold PBS (pH7.4) once, counted, and then suspended in FACS buffer (2% FBS/PBS), followed by blocking with 2 μL Human Trustain FcX (BioLegend, US) at room temperature for 10 min. Following the staining of dead cells with LIVE/DEAD Fixable Violet Dead cell staining kit, cells were incubated with PerCP-CY5.5-conjugated mouse anti-human CD3, FITC-conjugated mouse anti-human CD8, BV605-conjugated mouse anti-human CD4, PE-conjugated mouse anti-human CD19, APC-CY7-conjugated mouse anti-human CD20 in dark at 4°C for 30 min. Cells were then rinsed with PBS for two times and fixed by 2% paraformaldehyde in PBS. Expression levels were assessed by BD LSRFortessa™ (BD Biosciences, Inc.), and analyzed with FlowJo (FlowJo, LLC).

Preparation of Fluorescence Labeled RTX

Rhodamine-B-labeled RTX was prepared by following the protocol provided by the manufacturer of fluorescence dyes. Fluorescent dyes, Rhodamine-B (RhB), were first dissolved in anhydrous DMSO to get 10 mg/mL stock solution, respectively. Then 50 μL of dye solutions were added gradually into 2 mL enzyme solutions (10 mg protein/mL, pH = 8.2, sodium carbonate, 100 mM). The reactions were carried out overnight at 4°C. Labeled RTX were then dialyzed against phosphate buffer (20 mM, pH = 7), condensed by centrifugal filtration (MWCO = 10 kDa) and stored at 4°C for further use. The concentration and dye/mAb ratio (D/P) were determined by the extinction coefficients of 2,101,000 M^{-1} cm^{-1} at 280 nm (RTX) and 108,000 M^{-1} cm^{-1} at 555 nm (RhB).

Tissue Imaging

The bioluminescence imaging of organs was performed with IVIS Spectrum imager (PerkinElmer, Waltham, MA). Rats were injected through IV with 15 mg/kg of fluorescent labeled native RTX or n-RTX and scarified at Day 7 post-injection. The tissue images present the total photon flux *per second* within each organ with rainbow color scales. To further quantifiably compare the fluorescent intensity, and the fluorescent intensity from tissue homogenates was quantified as Relative Fluorescence Unit (RFU) per g.

Immunohistochemistry

Axillary, mesenteric, and inguinal lymph nodes, frontal, parietal, temporal, occipital lobes, and cerebellum, were collected separately and fixed in formaldehyde. Four micrometers thickness section were cut serially post paraffin embedding. For staining, slides were first heated at 60°C for 1 h, then deparaffinized in xylene twice and rehydrated in an ethanol gradient. For antigen retrieval, LNs and brain lobes were treated with citrate buffer (Vector Laboratories and Biocare Medical, respectively) for 25 min at 100°C and for 50 min in pressure cooker post ddH_2O rinse, respectively. Sections were incubated with BLOXALL endogenous peroxidase (Vector Laboratories) and alkaline phosphatase blocking solution (Vector Laboratories) for 10 min at room temperature, followed with PBST (0.1% Tween-20) wash and serum blocking at room temperature for 1 h. Primary mouse anti-human CD20 (1:200, clone L26, Santa Cruz Biotechnology), which recognizes different epitopes on rhesus CD20 molecules not covered by RTX to minimize CD20 epitope masking by rituximab, rabbit anti-human CD3 (1:100, cloneSP7, Invitrogen), and mouse anti-human Bcl-6 (1:100, cloneD8, Santa Cruz Biotechnology), were incubated overnight at 4°C, separately. Rabbit anti-human glia fibrillary acidic protein (GFAP) (1:200, Biocare Medical), mouse anti-human ionized calcium-binding adapter molecule 1 (IBA-1) (1:100, clone 20A12.1, Millipore) were separately used to identify astrocyte and microglia, respectively in brain lobes. After rinsed in PBST, the slides were incubated with ImmPRESS HRP universal secondary antibody at room temperature for 30 min. Followed with PBST wash, 3,3′-diaminobenzidine (DAB) staining, nucleus counterstaining, graded ethanol dehydration, xylene clear, the sections were covered with mounting medium (Thermo Fisher). Images were captured by inverted microscope (DMi1, Leica), brown staining was considered as positive signal, otherwise was considered as negative. Slides of lymph nodes were analyzed with Image J (NIH); slides of brain lobes were scanned by Aperio ScanScope slide scanner by 4 × 4 grid (20×).

For analysis of lymph nodes, 6.8 × 5 cm of each 40 magnified CD20 and CD3 positive staining ($n = 7$) and 3.4 × 4.2 cm of Bcl6 ($n = 4$), was randomly selected and their optical density (OD) numbers were calculated with the following formula: OD = log (max intensity/Mean intensity), where max intensity = 255 for 8-bit images. Brain slides were performed with the Aperio Positive Pixel Count v9 algorithm. Positive pixel calculation for GFAP used the following variables: hue width = 0.371 and color saturation threshold = 9.7e-002. Positive pixel calculation for IBA-1 used the following variables: hue width = 0.5 and color saturation threshold = 4.0e-007. Positivity was calculated by total number of positive pixels divided by the total number of pixels. The value was then multiplied by 100 to give a percentage for positive pixels. Total area analyzed for both GFAP and IBA is 4 mm^2. One-way ANOVA from SPSS software (IBM) was used for the analysis of statistical significance ($^{**}P < 0.01$), the inversed gray value of positive stained tissue was showed in histogram (mean ± SD).

MAb Detection by Enzyme-Linked Immunosorbent Assays (ELISA)

The concentration of RTX in animal body fluids and tissue homogenates was measured by ELISA against RTX. RTX levels were measured by ELISA using a monoclonal antibody (HCA062, clone#AbD02844, Bio-Rad, Hercules, CA), which specifically recognizes the idiotypic determinants of RTX. The 96-well plates were coated with 1 µg/mL of anti-RTX antibody (diluted in sodium carbonate-bicarbonate buffer), followed by blocking with 1% BSA/PBS for 2 h at room temperature. Diluted samples of RTX in PBST from 0 to 500 ng/mL were then added and incubated for 1 h at room temperature to obtain calibration curves. Animal body fluids and tissue homogenates containing encapsulated RTX in non-degradable nanocapsules were treated with 100 mM sodium acetate buffer (pH 5.4) at 4°C overnight and used for ELISA measurement. Released RTX from hydrolysable nanocapsules was directly measured with animal body fluids and tissue homogenates. All animal samples were added and incubated for an additional hour at room temperature. After washing with PBST for five times, peroxidase-conjugated anti-human Fc antibody was added and incubated for a further hour at room temperature. The substrate 3,3′,5,5′-Tetramethylbenzidine (TMB) solution was added and incubated until the appropriate color developed. The reaction was stopped and absorbance at 450 nm was measured with a plate reader (FLUOstar OPTIMA).

Animal Care and Ethics Statements

All research involving animals was conducted according to relevant national and international guidelines. Male SD rats (weighting 180–220 g, 6–8 weeks old) were provided by the Experimental Animal Center of Medical Department of Peking University. All interventions and animal care procedures were performed in accordance with the Guidelines and Policies for Anima l Surgery provided by our collaborator institute (Chinese Academy of Medical Sciences & Peking Union Medical College, Beijing, China) and were approved by the Institutional Animal Use and Care Committee. The rats were maintained in a temperature-controlled facility (temperature: 22 ± 1°C, humidity: 60%) with a 14 h light/10 h dark photoperiod and free access to food and water. Male rhesus macaques (weighing 4.8–5.2 kg, 4–5 years old) were purchased from the Medical Primate Research Center of the Institute of Medical Biology, Chinese Academy of Medical Sciences, and housed and bred according to the guidelines. The experimental protocols were reviewed and approved by the Yunnan Province Experimental Animal Management Association (SYXK-YN 2010-0009) and the Experimental Animal Ethic Committee of the Institute, which complied with the humane regulations of replacement, refinement, and reduction.

ETHICS STATEMENT

The animal study was reviewed and approved by 1. Institutional Animal Use and Care Committee, Chinese Academy of Medical Sciences and Peking Union Medical College, Beijing, China. 2. Yunnan Province Experimental Animal Management Association (SYXK-YN 2010-0009) and the Experimental Animal Ethic Committee of the Institute.

AUTHOR CONTRIBUTIONS

MQ, MK, and JW designed studies. MQ, LW, DW, CW, DX, QG, JG, EK, YLuo, YLee, and YX performed experiments. HV, GS, XS, ZH, YLu, MK, JW, and IC discussed and interpreted data. MQ, JW, MK, and IC wrote the paper.

ACKNOWLEDGMENTS

We thank Kathy Situ for editing the manuscript, Rina Lee-Cha for providing editorial assistance.

REFERENCES

1. Stacker SA, Achen MG, Jussila L, Baldwin ME, Alitalo K. Lymphangiogenesis and cancer metastasis. *Nat Rev Cancer.* (2002) 2:573–83. doi: 10.1038/nrc863
2. Tobler NE, Detmar M. Tumor and lymph node lymphangiogenesis–impact on cancer metastasis. *J Leukoc Biol.* (2006) 80:691–6. doi: 10.1189/jlb.1105653
3. Muldoon L, Soussain C, Jahnke K, Johanson C, Siegal T, Smith Q, et al. Chemotherapy delivery issues in central nervous system malignancy: a reality check. *J Clin Oncol.* (2007) 25:2295–305. doi: 10.1200/JCO.2006.09.9861
4. Rubenstein JL, Combs D, Rosenberg J, Levy A, McDermott M, Damon L, et al. Rituximab therapy for CNS lymphomas: targeting the leptomeningeal compartment. *Blood.* (2003) 101:466–8. doi: 10.1182/blood-2002-06-1636
5. Owonikoko T, Arbiser J, Zelnak A, Shu H, Shim H, Robin A, et al. Current approaches to the treatment of metastatic brain tumours. *Nat Rev Clin Oncol.* (2014) 11:203–22. doi: 10.1038/nrclinonc.2014.25
6. Komori M, Lin Y, Cortese I, Blake A, Ohayon J, Cherup J, et al. Insufficient disease inhibition by intrathecal rituximab in progressive multiple sclerosis. *Ann Clin Transl Neurol.* (2016) 3:166–79. doi: 10.1002/acn3.293
7. Groothuis D. The blood-brain and blood-tumor barriers: a review of strategies for increasing drug delivery. *Neuro Oncol.* (2000) 2:45–59. doi: 10.1093/neuonc/2.1.45
8. Weinstein JN, Steller MA, Keenan AM, Covell DG, Key ME, Sieber SM, et al. Monoclonal antibodies in the lymphatics: selective delivery to lymph node metastases of a solid tumor. *Science.* (1983) 222:423–6. doi: 10.1126/science.6623082
9. Weinstein JN, Parker RJ, Holton OD 3rd, Keenan AM, Covell DG, Black CD, et al. Lymphatic delivery of monoclonal antibodies: potential for detection and treatment of lymph node metastases. *Cancer Invest.* (1985) 3:85–95. doi: 10.3109/07357908509040610
10. Chacko A, Li C, Pryma D, Brem S, Coukos G, Muzykantov V. Targeted delivery of antibody-based therapeutic and imaging agents to CNS tumors: crossing the blood-brain barrier divide. *Expert Opin Drug Deliv.* (2013) 10:907–26. doi: 10.1517/17425247.2013.808184
11. Georgieva JV, Hoekstra D, Zuhorn IS. Smuggling drugs into the brain: an overview of ligands targeting transcytosis for drug delivery across the blood-brain barrier. *Pharmaceutics.* (2014) 6:557–83. doi: 10.3390/pharmaceutics6040557
12. Yang H. Nanoparticle-mediated brain-specific drug delivery, imaging, and diagnosis. *Pharmaceutical Res.* (2010) 27:1759–71. doi: 10.1007/s11095-010-0141-7
13. Zara G, Cavalli R, Fundaro A, Bargoni A, Caputo O, Gasco M. Pharmacokinetics of doxorubicin incorporated in solid lipid nanospheres (SLN). *Pharmacol Res.* (1999) 40:281–6. doi: 10.1006/phrs.1999.0509
14. Costantino L, Tosi G, Ruozi B, Bondioli L, Vandelli MA, Forni F. Chapter 3 - Colloidal systems for CNS drug delivery. *Progr Brain Res.* (2009) 180:35–69. doi: 10.1016/S0079-6123(08)80003-9
15. Garcion E, Lamprecht A, Heurtault B, Paillard A, Aubert-Pouessel A, Denizot B, et al. A new generation of anticancer, drug-loaded, colloidal vectors reverses multidrug resistance in glioma and reduces tumor progression in rats. *Mol Cancer Ther.* (2006) 5:1710–22. doi: 10.1158/1535-7163.MCT-06-0289
16. Lu C, Zhao Y, Wong H, Cai J, Peng L, Tian X. Current approaches to enhance CNS delivery of drugs across the brain barriers. *Int J Nanomed.* (2014) 9:2241–57. doi: 10.2147/IJN.S61288
17. Wong H, Wu X, Bendayan R. Nanotechnological advances for the delivery of CNS therapeutics. *Adv Drug Deliv Rev.* (2012) 64:686–700. doi: 10.1016/j.addr.2011.10.007
18. Scott A, Wolchok J, Old L. Antibody therapy of cancer. *Nat Rev Cancer.* (2012) 12:278–87. doi: 10.1038/nrc3236
19. Liang S, Liu Y, Jin X, Liu G, Wen J, Zhang LL, et al. Phosphorylcholine polymer nanocapsules prolong the circulation time and reduce the immunogenicity of therapeutic proteins. *Nano Res.* (2016) 9:1022–31. doi: 10.1007/s12274-016-0991-3
20. Yan M, Du J, Gu Z, Liang M, Hu Y, Zhang W, et al. A novel intracellular protein delivery platform based on single-protein nanocapsules. *Nat Nanotechnol.* (2010) 5:48–53. doi: 10.1038/nnano.2009.341
21. Wen J, Anderson SM, Du J, Yan M, Wang J, Shen M, et al. Controlled protein delivery based on enzyme-responsive nanocapsules. *Adv Mater.* (2011) 23:4549–53. doi: 10.1002/adma.201101771
22. Wen J, Yan M, Liu Y, Li J, Xie Y, Lu Y, et al. Specific elimination of latently HIV-1 infected cells using HIV-1 protease-sensitive toxin nanocapsules. *PLoS ONE.* (2016) 11:e0151572. doi: 10.1371/journal.pone.0151572
23. Tian H, Du J, Wen J, Liu Y, Montgomery SR, Scott TP, et al. Growth-factor nanocapsules that enable tunable controlled release for bone regeneration. *ACS Nano.* (2016) 10:7362–9. doi: 10.1021/acsnano.5b07950
24. Liu C, Wen J, Meng Y, Zhang K, Zhu J, Ren Y, et al. Efficient delivery of therapeutic miRNA nanocapsules for tumor suppression. *Adv Mater.* (2015) 27:292–7. doi: 10.1002/adma.201403387
25. Liu Y, Du JJ, Yan M, Lau MY, Hu J, Han H, et al. Biomimetic enzyme nanocomplexes and their use as antidotes and preventive measures for alcohol intoxication. *Nat Nanotechnol.* (2013) 8:187–92. doi: 10.1038/nnano.2012.264
26. Gu Z, Yan M, Hu B, Joo KI, Biswas A, Huang Y, et al. Protein nanocapsule weaved with enzymatically degradable polymeric network. *Nano Lett.* (2009) 9:4533–8. doi: 10.1021/nl902935b
27. Yan M, Wen J, Liang M, Lu YF, Kamata M, Chen ISY. Modulation of gene expression by polymer nanocapsule delivery of DNA cassettes encoding small RNAs. *PLoS ONE.* (2015) 10:e127986. doi: 10.1371/journal.pone.0127986
28. Chen S, Li L, Zhao C, Zheng J. Surface hydration: principles and applications toward low-fouling/nonfouling biomaterials. *Polymer.* (2010) 51:5283–93. doi: 10.1016/j.polymer.2010.08.022
29. Young G, Bowers R, Hall B, Port M. Six month clinical evaluation of a biomimetic hydrogel contact lens. *CLAO J.* (1997) 23:226–36.
30. Wu D, Qin M, Xu D, Wang L, Liu C, Ren J, et al. A bioinspired platform for effective delivery of protein therapeutics to the central nervous system. *Adv Mater.* (2019) 31:e1807557. doi: 10.1002/adma.201970127
31. Xu D, Wu D, Qin M, Nih LR, Liu C, Cao Z, et al. Efficient Delivery of nerve growth factors to the central nervous system for neural regeneration. *Adv Mater.* (2019) 31:e1900727. doi: 10.1002/adma.201900727
32. Han L, Liu C, Qi H, Zhou J, Wen J, Wu D, et al. Systemic delivery of monoclonal antibodies to the central nervous system for brain tumor therapy. *Adv Mater.* (2019) 31:e1805697. doi: 10.1002/adma.201805697
33. Rezvani AR, Maloney DG. Rituximab resistance. *Best Pract Res Cl Ha.* (2011) 24:203–16. doi: 10.1016/j.beha.2011.02.009
34. Wen J, Wu D, Qin M, Liu C, Wang L, Xu D, et al. Sustained delivery and molecular targeting of a therapeutic monoclonal antibody to metastases in the central nervous system of mice. *Nat Biomed Eng.* (2019) 3:706–16. doi: 10.1038/s41551-019-0434-z
35. Shi J, Kantoff P, Wooster R, Farokhzad O. Cancer nanomedicine: progress, challenges and opportunities. *Nat Rev Cancer.* (2017) 17:20–37. doi: 10.1038/nrc.2016.108
36. Eng LF, Ghirnikar RS. GFAP and astrogliosis. *Brain Pathol.* (1994) 4:229–37. doi: 10.1111/j.1750-3639.1994.tb00838.x
37. Ito D, Imai Y, Ohsawa K, Nakajima K, Fukuuchi Y, Kohsaka S. Microglia-specific localisation of a novel calcium binding protein, Iba1. *Brain Res Mol Brain Res.* (1998) 57:1–9. doi: 10.1016/S0169-328X(98)00040-0
38. Lim SH, Vaughan AT, Ashton-Key M, Williams EL, Dixon SV, Chan HT, et al. Fc gamma receptor IIb on target B cells promotes rituximab internalization and reduces clinical efficacy. *Blood.* (2011) 118:2530–40. doi: 10.1182/blood-2011-01-330357
39. Boross P, Leusen JH. Mechanisms of action of CD20 antibodies. *Am J Cancer Res.* (2012) 2:676–90.
40. Mason DY, Comans-Bitter WM, Cordell JL, Verhoeven MA, van Dongen JJ. Antibody L26 recognizes an intracellular epitope on the B-cell-associated CD20 antigen. *Am J Pathol.* (1990) 136:1215–22.
41. McLennan DN, Porter CJ, Charman SA. Subcutaneous drug delivery and the role of the lymphatics. *Drug Discov Today Technol.* (2005) 2:89–96. doi: 10.1016/j.ddtec.2005.05.006
42. Richter WF, Jacobsen B. Subcutaneous absorption of biotherapeutics: knowns and unknowns. *Drug Metab Dispos.* (2014) 42:1881–9. doi: 10.1124/dmd.114.059238
43. Carman AJ, Mills JH, Krenz A, Kim DG, Bynoe MS. Adenosine receptor signaling modulates permeability of the blood-brain barrier. *J Neurosci.* (2011) 31:13272–80. doi: 10.1523/JNEUROSCI.3337-11.2011
44. Triguero D, Buciak JB, Yang J, Pardridge WM. Blood-brain barrier transport of cationized immunoglobulin G: enhanced delivery compared to native

protein. *Proc Natl Acad Sci USA*. (1989) 86:4761–5. doi: 10.1073/pnas.86.12.4761

45. Yesilyurt V, Ramireddy R, Azagarsamy MA, Thayumanavan S. Accessing lipophilic ligands in dendrimer-based amphiphilic supramolecular assemblies for protein-induced disassembly. *Chemistry*. (2012) 18:223–9. doi: 10.1002/chem.201102727
46. Barar J, Rafi MA, Pourseif MM, Omidi Y. Blood-brain barrier transport machineries and targeted therapy of brain diseases. *Bioimpacts*. (2016) 6:225–48. doi: 10.15171/bi.2016.30
47. Tang X, Sun J, Ge T, Zhang K, Gui Q, Zhang S, et al. PEGylated liposomes as delivery systems for Gambogenic acid: characterization and *in vitro/in vivo* evaluation. *Colloids Surf B Biointerfaces*. (2018) 172:26–36. doi: 10.1016/j.colsurfb.2018.08.022

4

Combining Host Genetics and Functional Analysis to Depict Inflammasome Contribution in Tuberculosis Susceptibility and Outcome in Endemic Areas

Dhêmerson Souza De Lima [1], Caio C. B. Bomfim [2], Vinícius N. C. Leal [1], Edione C. Reis [1], Jaíne L. S. Soares [1], Fernanda P. Fernandes [1], Eduardo P. Amaral [2], Flavio V. Loures [3], Mauricio M. Ogusku [4], Maria R. D'Imperio Lima [2], Aya Sadahiro [5] and Alessandra Pontillo [1]*

[1] Laboratório de Imunogenética, Departamento de Imunologia, Instituto de Ciências Biomédicas, Universidade de São Paulo, São Paulo, Brazil, [2] Laboratório de Imunologia das Doenças Infecciosas, Departamento de Imunologia, Instituto de Ciências Biomédicas, Universidade de São Paulo, São Paulo, Brazil, [3] Instituto de Ciência e Tecnologia, Universidade Federal de São Paulo, São José dos Campos, Brazil, [4] Laboratório de Micobacteriologia, Instituto Nacional de Pesquisas da Amazônia, Manaus, Brazil, [5] Departamento de Parasitologia, Universidade Federal do Amazonas, Manaus, Brazil

***Correspondence:**
Alessandra Pontillo
alepontillo@usp.br

The interplay between *M. tuberculosis* (Mtb) and humans is multifactorial. The susceptibility/resistance profile and the establishment of clinical tuberculosis (TB) still remains elusive. The gain-of-function variant rs10754558 in the *NLRP3* gene (found in 30% of the world population) confers protection against the development of TB, indicating a prominent role played by NLRP3 inflammasome against Mtb. Through genotype-guided assays and various Mtb strains (BCG, H37Rv, Beijing-1471, MP287/03), we demonstrate that Mtb strains activate inflammasome according to the NLRP3/IL-1ß or NLRC4/IL18 preferential axis. *NLRP3* and *NLRC4* genetic variants contribute to the presentation of TB. For the first time, we have shown that loss-of-function variants in *NLRC4* significantly contribute to the development of extra-pulmonary TB. The analysis of inflammasome activation in a cohort of TB patients and their "household contacts" (CNT) revealed that plasma IL-1ß/IFN-α ratio lets us distinguish patients from Mtb-exposed-but-healthy individuals from an endemic region. Moreover, NLRP3 inflammasome seemed "exhausted" in TB patients compared to CNT, indicating a more efficient activation of inflammasome in resistant individuals. These findings suggest that inflammasome genetics as well as virulence-dependent level of inflammasome activation contribute to the onset of a susceptible/resistant profile among Mtb-exposed individuals.

Keywords: tuberculosis, inflammasome, genetics, NLRP3, Nlrc4

INTRODUCTION

Tuberculosis (TB) is caused by a *Mycobacterium tuberculosis* (Mtb) infection. Only 5–10% of Mtb-infected individuals develop active TB and, in the majority of cases, the bacteria is either eliminated or remains in a latent state (1, 2). The cross-talk among host, pathogen and environment determines the outcome of an infection (3).

Host innate immune genes have been recently taken into account to explain how the first host/pathogen contact could shape one's subsequent response to Mtb (resistance vs. susceptibility). After accessing the host airways, Mtb is phagocyted by alveolar macrophages which initiate an innate immune response that leads to pathogen eradication, with the occasional contribution of an adaptive cell-mediated response (mainly driven by interferon (IFN)-γ) (4). Alternatively, a chronic inflammatory process begins with Mtb persistance in the lung and that may result in tissue damage through the formation of granulomas and lung fibrosis. In more severe infections, a dramatic lung parenchyma destruction occurs (5, 6). As such, the host innate immune response and further tissue inflammation could either be beneficial or detrimental in the fight against Mtb, possibly due to a delicate balance among several mediators.

Recently, Mayer Barber et al. showed that the plasma level of interleukin (IL)-1ß, type I IFN (IFN-I) and prostaglandin (PG)-E2—among several other inflammatory mediators—characterized the clinical presentation (severe vs. mild) of Mtb infections in TB patients (7), suggesting that a fine-tune regulation of innate immune response is crucial for TB outcomes.

Inflammasome is a cytosolic multi-protein complex that mediates the maturation and release of IL-1β and IL-18 (8). Pathogen- or damage-associated molecular patterns (PAMPs and DAMPs, respectively) activate the inflammasome through a group of cytosolic pathogen recognition receptors (PRRs), including NLRP1, NLRP3, NLRC4, NAIP, AIM2, and pyrin (8, 9). During infection, pathogens carry or inject PAMPs into cell cytosol and/or induce damage and break into the host homeostasis through the release of DAMPs. These are detected by inflammasome sensors, which in turn can recruit the adaptor molecule ASC and the effector molecule caspase-1, which is responsible for the maturation of IL-1ß and IL-18. Moreover, caspase-1 can mediate the cleavage of the pore-forming protein gasdermin D, leading to pro-inflammatory active cell death called pyroptosis (8).

Inflammasome activation constitutes a very efficient and rapid mechanism for host defense against pathogens. In this case, the inflammation is triggered either by leukocyte recruitment, *via* IL-1ß and IL-18 or by the destruction of the pathogen *niche* and inflammation amplification through pyroptosis. However, pathogen-induced response may be excessive with inflammasome-mediated tissue damage or, on the other hand, pathogens may evade host detection and/or inflammasome activation itself (9).

In murine bone marrow-derived macrophages, Mtb activates inflammasome through NLRP3 (10, 11) and mice lacking NLRP3 showed a reduced IL-1β production in response to an Mtb infection (12), suggesting that this sensor is crucial to trigger an animal response to this bacteria.

Besides being one of the most studied inflammasome sensors, researchers still have not completely demonstrated how NLRP3 is activated, as it responds to several PAMPs and DAMP, such as bacterial lipopolysaccharide (LPS), bacterial secretion systems, bacterial toxins, viral proteins, nucleic acids, increased extracellular concentration of ATP and alarmins (released by dead cells), organic and inorganic crystal or fibers (i.e., uric acid, cholesterol, ß-amyloid). Scientific evidence indicate that PAMPs and DAMPs activate NLRP3 through the induction of cytosolic alterations, such as K+ efflux, mediated by membrane pore-forming toxins or the binding of extracellular ATP to the purinergic receptor P2X7; or even in the case of damage in cell organelles (mitochondria or lysosome) with the consequent release of their contents, including reactive oxygen species, mitochondrial DNA or lysosomal cathepsins (8). As NLRP3 can be activated by such a plethora of signals, it is strongly regulated at several levels, including transcription and post-transcriptional events, including the feed-back mechanism induced by nitric oxide (NO), interferons and PGE2 (13–15).

Intriguingly, Mtb not only induces NLRP3 inflammasome activation but also the production of NO and IFN-I in mice (16). Accordingly, Wasserman et al. have shown that in THP-1, the human monocytic cell line, Mtb H37Rv triggers both NLRP3 and AIM2 inflammasome activation and IFN-1 production, most likely as an escape mechanism (17). In TB patients, the relative balance between the serum level of IL-1ß, IFN-I, and PGE-2 allows for classification according to disease severity (7). Altogether, these findings suggest that correct NLRP3 inflammasome activation can certainly contribute to bacterial clearance.

We previously reported the protective gain-of-function effect of a Single Nucleotide Variant (SNV) in the *NLRP3* 3'UTR region (rs10754558; found in about 30% of the world population) against the development of pulmonary TB (18). This led us to hypothesize genes coding factors taking part in the inflammasome assembling and function, which directly influences the IL-1ß and/or IL-18 production, could affect the outcome of an Mtb infection, therefore determining either the susceptibility and/or the prognosis for a TB patients.

In this study, we proposed a model of host/pathogen interplay including host inflammasome genetics, Mtb aggressiveness and inflammasome response rate, to evaluate the relative contribution of each parameter in individual TB susceptibility and outcome.

MATERIALS AND METHODS

Cohort for Cellular Assays

Three groups of adult volunteers were recruited for the *in vitro* study: healthy donors (HD) from TB non-endemic area, TB patients and their household contacts from TB endemic area. Thirty unrelated healthy volunteers from the metropolitan area of São Paulo (SP, Brazil) were recruited at the Blood Bank of "Oswaldo Cruz" hospital. Twenty-seven unrelated adults recently diagnosed with active pulmonary TB were recruited at the Reference Centre for Sanitary Pneumology "Cardoso Fontes" (Manaus, AM, Brazil). Twenty-seven unrelated adults in daily contact with TB patients ("household contacts") but without TB symptoms and negative for Mtb detection tests were included in the study as Mtb-exposed TB negative individuals. Diagnosis of active pulmonary TB is based on the evaluation of clinical symptoms together with Mtb detection tests: sputum smears analyses (19, 20) and/or GeneXpert MTB/RIF tests (*Cepheid*). Main characteristics of the volunteers recruited for the study are presented in **Table 1.**

Cohort for Genotyping Study

Genomic DNA from 352 unrelated TB patients and 288 healthy adults (without clinical signs or symptoms of TB) from the Brazilian State of Amazonas (not indigenous people from the Amazon forest) was used for the genetic association study. Diagnosis of TB is based on the evaluation of clinical symptoms together with Mtb detection tests, as above mentioned. Main characteristics of this cohort are presented in **Table 2**.

Mycobacterial Culture Conditions and Preparation for Cell Infection

Non-virulent Bacillus Calmette-Guerin (BCG), common virulent H37Rv and hyper-virulent Beijing 1471 (Bj) and MP287/03 (MP) mycobacterium strains were used in this study. *M. tuberculosis* H37Rv and Beijing 1471, *M. bovis strains* Bacillus Calmette-Guerin and MP287/03 were sourced from the laboratory of Professor Maria Regina D'Imperio Lima (Department of Immunology, Institute of Biomedical Sciences, University of São Paulo). Mtb were grown at 37°C, either in 7H9 medium (*Difco*) supplemented with 10% albumin-dextrose-catalase (ADC, *Middlebrook*) or on 7H10 agar plates supplemented with 10% oleic acid-albumin-dextrose-catalase (OADC, *Middlebrook*). Bacteria were grown to the exponential phase (optical density at 600 nm, OD_{600}, of 0.1), washed once in a 7H9 medium, and resuspended in 7H9 to an OD_{600}, of 1—equivalent to 2 x 10^8 bacilli/ml for BCG, 1 x10^7 bacilli/mL for H37Rv and Bj, 2 x 10^7 for MP. The required volume for Mtb bacterial suspension was then added to the cell culture medium for infection of human monocyte-derived macrophages (MDM) at a multiplicity of infection (MOI) of 0.033. This MOI was selected after pilot experiments as the minimum MOI capable of activating IL-1ß production in MDM. We avoided using a higher MOI in an attempt to mimic natural infection in humans (21). For colony formation unit (CFU) assays, infected MDM were lysed and serial dilutions were plated in a complete agar medium. After 21 days, bacterial growth in MDM was evaluated by CFU counting.

TABLE 1 | Characteristics of the individuals recruited for the cellular assays.

Characteristics	HD (*n* = 30)	TB (*n* = 27)	CNT (*n* = 27)
State of origin	SP	AM	AM
Age, years (Mean ± SD)	45 ± 13	51 ± 11	52 ± 12
Male/Female, *n* (%)	14/16 (46.7/54.3)	16/11 (59/41)	11/16 (41/59)
BCG vaccinated, *n* (%)	30 (100)	27 (100)	27 (100)
TST+, *n* (%)	0	5 (18.6)	3 (11.1)
IGRA+, *n* (%)	n.d.	12 (44.4)	13 (48.1)
Mtb detection test +, *n* (%)	n.d.	27 (100)	0
Mtb detection test in sputum smear +, *n* (%)	n.d.	13 (50)	0

State of origin in Brazil, mean age, gender distribution and BCG vaccination are reported for the three groups of studied individuals: healthy donors (HD; n = 30), TB patients (TB; n = 27) and contacts (CNT; n = 27). Positive results for TST test, IGRA, Mtb detection test as well as s Mtb detection test in the sputum smear were indicated for the TB patients and contacts.

SP, São Paulo State; AM, Amazonas State; n: number of individuals; SD, standard deviation; %, percentage; BCG, Bacillus Calmette Guerin; TST, Tuberculin Skin Test or Mantoux test; IGRA, Interferon Gamma Release Assay; Mtb, Mycobacterium tuberculosis.

TABLE 2 | General characteristics of the TB cohort for genotyping study.

Characteristics	TB (*n* = 288)	ETB (*n* = 64)	HD (*n* = 288)
Gender			
Male, *n* (%)	193 (67.0%)	30 (47.0%)	155 (46.4%)
Female, *n* (%)	95 (33.0%)	34 (53.0%)	133 (53.6%)
Mean age ± SD	38.2 ± 13.2	33.0 ± 13.02	35.8 ± 12.0
BCG-vaccinated			
Yes, *n* (%)	212 (73.6%)	55 (86.0%)	180 (62.5%)
No, *n* (%)	25 (8.70%)	9 (14.0%)	36 (12.5%)
Data not available, *n* (%)	51 (17.7%)		72 (25.0%)

Mean age, gender distribution and BCG vaccination are reported for the three groups of studied individuals from the Brazilian State of Amazonas: healthy donors (HD; n = 288), pulmonary TB (TB; n = 288) and extra-pulmonary (ETB; n = 64).

MDM Generation and *in-vitro* Infection

Peripheral blood mononuclear cells (PBMC) were isolated from donor blood using the Ficoll-Paque® density gradient centrifugation (*GE Healthcare, Biosciences*). Monocytes were separated from total PBMC by plastic adherence and cultivated at 0.4 × 10^6 cells/mL in RPMI-1640 (*Gibco, ThermoFisher Scientific*), supplemented with 10% fetal bovine serum (FBS; *Gibco*) and 25 ng/mL monocyte colony stimulating factor (M-CSF; *PreproTech*) for 5 days at 37°C in 5% CO_2 atmosphere to obtain MDM. Monocytes-to-MDM differentiation was confirmed by flow cytometry analyses of the CD14 and CD68 surface markers (**Supplementary File 1**). MDM were infected with H37Rv, Bj, MP, and BCG strains at MOI 0.033 for 3 h, washed, and then cultivated for 24 h. In some experiments. MDM were treated with 10 μM parthenolide (PTD; *Sigma-Adrich*), a general inhibitor of inflamamsome (22); or 10 μM MCC-950 (*InvivoGen*), a specific inhibitor of NLRP3 (23); or 10 μM CA074-Me (CA074; *Merck*), an inhibitor of intracellular cathepsin B; or 10 μM of cytocalasin-D (Cyt-D; *Sigma-Aldrich*), an inhibitor of actin polymerization which impairs phagocytosis. PTD, MCC-950, and Ca074 were added to MDM cultures for 1 h prior to bacterial infection. Cyt-D was added to MDM cultures during *in vitro* infection. In some experiments, 1 mM ATP (*Sigma-Aldrich*) was added at the end of treatment for another 15 min. The treatment with 1 μg/mL LPS (*E. coli* strain O111:B4; *Sigma-Aldrich*) for 24 h and 1 mM ATP for another 15 min were used as positive control for NLRP3 inflammasome activation (24, 25). For CFU assays, 10 ng/mL of recombinant human IL-1ß (rh-IL-1ß; *Peptotech*) or 10 μM PTD were added to the culture. Inflammasome activation was analyzed by IL-1ß and IL-18 release in the culture supernatants, 'cleaved/activated caspase-1 and "speck" formation.

Cytokines Quantification

IL-1ß, IL-18, IFN-ß, and TNF levels in serum and culture supernatants were measured using commercial

ELISA Kits (*Biolegend, R&D Systems*) according to the manufacturer's instructions.

Caspase-1 Activity Assay

The detection of caspase-1 activity in MDM FAM-FLICA® Caspase-1 Assay Kit (*Immunochemistry Technologies*) and flow cytometry, according to the manufacturer's instructions. Briefly, 2 x 10^5 MDM were stimulated according to the above-mentioned protocol, and then incubated with the fluorescent inhibitor probe FAM-YVAD-FMK for 1 h at 37°C, 5% CO_2. The samples were then washed, incubated with Live/Dead Fixable Cell Stain Kit (*Thermo Fisher Scientific*), and analyzed by flow cytometry. The caspase-1 activity was expressed as percentage of FAM-FLICA positive (+) live cells.

Cell Cytotoxicity

Cell cytotoxicity was assessed by the quantification of Lactate dehydrogenase (LDH) release in supernatants using the LDH Cytotoxicity Assay Kit (*ThermoFisher Scientific*), according to the manufacturer's protocol. The cytotoxicity is expressed as percentage of LDH release relative to the positive control (Triton).

"Specks" Formation

Inflammasome complex assembly was evaluated by the detection of "specks" formation using immunofluorescence microscopy. MDM were fixed and permeabilized with Cytofix/Cytoperm reagent (*BD Biosciences*) for 30 min at 37°C and 5% CO_2 and incubated with primary antibody for NLRP3 (1:100 mouse anti-human NLRP3, *Abram*) and/or NLRC4 (1:200 rabbit anti-human NLRC4; *Biolegend*) overnight at room temperature. Fluorescent secondary antibodies (Alexa 488-conjugated goat-anti-mouse IgG1, or Alexa 647-conjugated goat-anti-rabbit IgG1; *Thermofisher Scientific)* were then added for 1 h. 4',6-Diamidine-2'-phenylindole dihydrochloride (DAPI; *Sigma-Aldrich*) was used for nuclear counterstaining. Image acquisition was performed at the microscope facility at the Laboratory of Cellular Biology from the Butantan Institute (São Paulo, SP, Brazil) using a DMi8 confocal laser scanning microscope equipped with a digital camera DFC310 FX (Leica). The counting of NLRP3+ and NLRC4+ *specks* in MDM was performed manually by observing speck formation within the cells in 10 fields (26).

Inflammasome' Genes Expression Analysis

Total RNA was isolated from 0.4 × 10^6 MDM using the RNAqueous-Micro kit (*Ambion, Thermo Fisher Scientific*), according to the manufacturer's protocol, and quantified using Nanodrop N-1000 (*Agilent*). Total RNA was converted into cDNA using Superscript III RT kit and random primers (*Invitrogen, Thermo Fisher Scientific*). *NLRP3* (*Hs00366465*), *NLRC4* (*Hs00368367*), *IL1B* (hs01555410), and *IL18 (Hs01038788)* genes were amplified using TaqMan® gene-specific assays (*Applied Biosystems, Thermo Fisher Scientific*) and qPCR on the QuantStudio 3.0 Real-Time PCR equipment (*Applied Biosystems*). The QuantStudio 3.0 software was used to obtain cycle threshold values (Ct) for relative gene expression analysis according to the Fold Change (FC) method (27). Raw expression data (Ct) were normalized with the expression of the house-keeping gene glyceraldehyde-3-phosphate dehydrogenase/*GAPDH* (*Hs02758991; TaqMan® assay*) (ΔCt), and the FC was calculated comparing stimulated and unstimulated (UN) conditions ($FC=2^{--\Delta\Delta Ct}$; $\Delta\Delta Ct = \Delta Ct_{stimulated} - \Delta Ct_{UN}$). Alternatively, basal (constitutive) gene expression was calculated as $2^{-\Delta Ct}$.

SNVs Genotyping

NLRP3 rs10754558 C>G and *NLRC4* rs479333 G>C single nucleotide variants were selected based on their known functional effect, and elevated minor allele frequency (MAF) in the general population (0.30 and 0.49 respectively, from *www.ensembl.org*). *NLRP3* rs10754558 is a 3'UTR variant previously associated with increased *NLRP3* mRNA stability and supposed augmented inflammasome activation (28). *NLRC4* rs479333 is an intronic polymorphism which negatively affects *NLRC4* expression (29) and serum IL-18 level (30). They were genotyped in the TB cohort with TaqMan®-type allele-specific commercial assays (*Applied Biosystems*) and qPCR on the QuantStudio 3.0 Real-Time PCR equipment. The QuantStudio 3.0 software was used for allelic discrimination.

Data Analysis

All data were collected and analyzed from at least three independent experiments. A normality test was applied to the data, and a parametric or non-parametric analysis was used accordingly to compare two or more data sets, as specified for each graph. The level of significance was $p < 0.05$. Calculations were performed using the statistical software package GraphPad Prism (v8.01). Genotyping data were analyzed through multivariate analysis according to the general linear model (GLM) using the package SNPassoc and R-project. Bonferroni correction for multiple comparisons (2 SNVs) required a $p < 0.025$ (0.05/2).

RESULTS

M. tuberculosis Induces Inflammasome Activation and IL-1ß Production Plays a Major Role in Bacterial Restriction *in vitro* as Well as *in vivo*

Mtb triggers NLRP3 inflammasome in mice (10–12), as well as in some *in-vitro* models of human macrophages (17, 31, 32); however, the multiplicity of infection (MOI) implied is always high (1–10 or more) compared to what expected during natural infection (<<1) (21).

Considering this, we first investigated whether the common virulent reference strain Mtb H37Rv activates the inflammasome at a physiologic MOI. For this, we measured cytokine production and caspase-1 activation at a MOI of 0.033 in Mtb-infected monocyte-derived macrophages (MDM).

At this MOI, H37Rv was also able to induce a significant release of inflammasome cytokines IL-1ß (**Figure 1A**) and IL-18

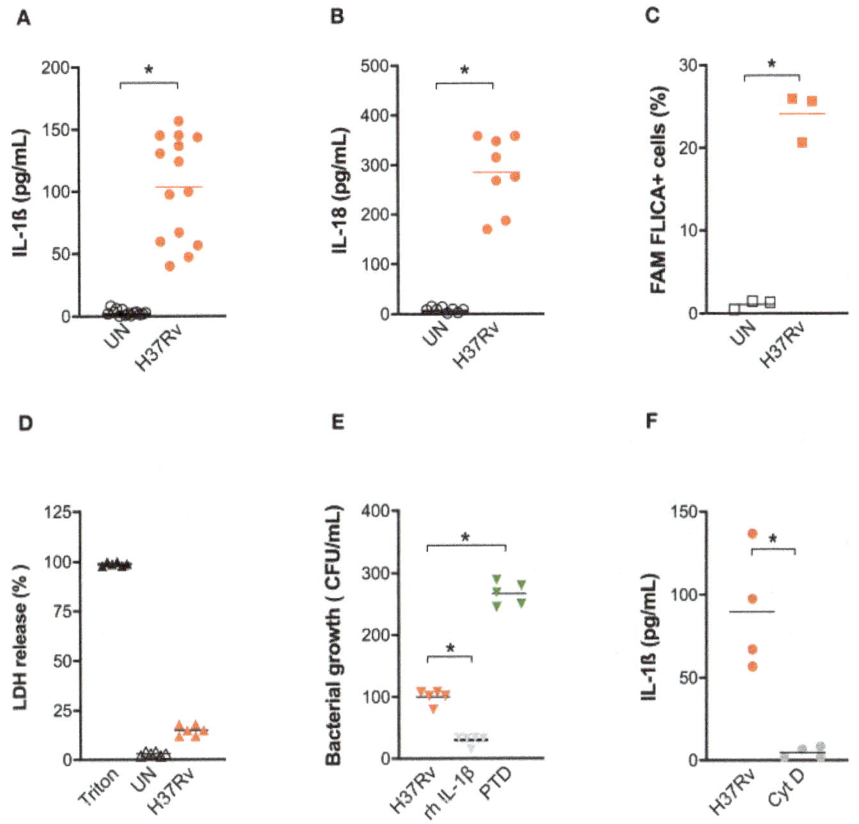

FIGURE 1 | *M. tuberculosis* strain H37Rv induces inflammasome activation in human MDM and IL-1ß production plays a major role in bacterial restriction. The healthy donors' monocyte-derived macrophages (MDM; $n = 14$) were challenged with the *M. tuberculosis* (Mtb) strain H37Rv (MOI: 0.033) for 3 h, then washed and cultured for 24 h. The release of IL-1ß ($n = 14$) **(A)** and IL-18 ($n = 8$) **(B)** was measured in culture supernatants of untreated (UN) and infected (H37Rv) MDM. Cells were harvested for an analysis of caspase-1 activity by a FAM-FLICA® assay and flow cytometry from three independent experiments. The percentage of FAM-FLICA+ cells was reported for H37Rv-infected (H37Rv) and untreated (UN) MDM **(C)**. Lactate Dehydrogenase (LDH) liberation was measured in culture supernatants in three independent experiments. Data are expressed as a percentage in respect to the positive control (Triton, 100% cell lysis) **(D)**. The healthy donors' MDM ($n = 5$) were infected with Mtb H37Rv (MOI: 0.033) for 3 h in the presence of exogenous recombinant human IL-1ß (rh-IL-1ß) or parthenolide (PTD; 10 μM), then lysed. Serial dilutions were plated in a complete agar medium. Bacterial growth was evaluated after 21 days by counting colony formation units (CFU) **(E)**. The healthy donors' MDM ($n = 4$) were infected with Mtb H37Rv (MOI: 0.033) for 3 h in the presence of cytochalasin D (Cyt D; 10 μM), then washed and cultured for 24 h. The release of IL-1ß was measured at the end of incubation in infected MDM (H37Rv) and infected MDM in the presence of a phagocytosis inhibitor (Cyt D) **(F)**. Individual data are reported with their mean. The Mann–Whitney test was used to compare treated and untreated groups **(A–C,F)**. The Kruskall–Wallis test followed by a Bonferroni post-test were used to compare H37Rv, rh-IL-1ß, and PTD groups **(E)**. Differences with a $p < 0.05$ were considered statistically significant (*).

(**Figure 1B**) from MDM, which was accompanied by the increase of caspase-1 cleavage (**Figure 1C**) but not by a significant release of LDH (**Figure 1D**), suggesting the induction of the canonical pathway of inflammasome activation, but without high rates of pyroptosis.

Little is known about a possible function of IL-18 against mycobacteria, while IL-1ß plays a role in macrophages phagocytosis (33) Therefore, we performed a bacterial growth assay in Mtb-infected MDM in the presence of exogenous recombinant IL-1ß or pre-treated with the inflammasome inhibitor parthenolide (PTD). H37Rv bacterial growth was significantly inhibited by IL-1ß (70.2% CFU inhibition). At the same time, a significant increase of Mtb growth was observed when PTD was added to cultures (160% CFU increase) (**Figure 1E**). H37Rv-driven inflammasome activation seems to be direct, as the inhibition of mycobacterial phagocytosis completely abolished IL-1ß production (**Figure 1F**).

These data emphasize that the activation of inflammasome and IL-1β production are mandatory for Mtb containment.

NLRP3 Contributes to Inflammasome Activation by the *Mtb* Common Virulence Strain H37Rv in Human MDM

As our previous results pointed out the protective role of a gain-of-function genetic variant in *NLRP3* (rs10754558) (18), and given the central role of this receptor in the mouse model of Mtb infection as well (10–12), we next asked whether the observed activation of inflammasome complex by Mtb H37Rv in MDM could be dependent on NLRP3. The formation of *specks* indicates the activation of inflammasome and also allows for the visualization of a mounted complex platform, including the activated sensor (26). Thus, we subsequently replicated MDM infection with Mtb H37Rv to confirm NLRP3 participation in inflammasome responses. To do so, cells were stained using specific antibodies and samples analyzed at the end of infection assay under a fluorescence microscope. A significant increase of NLRP3+ specks were detected in Mtb-infected MDM compared to untreated cells (**Figures 2A,B**).

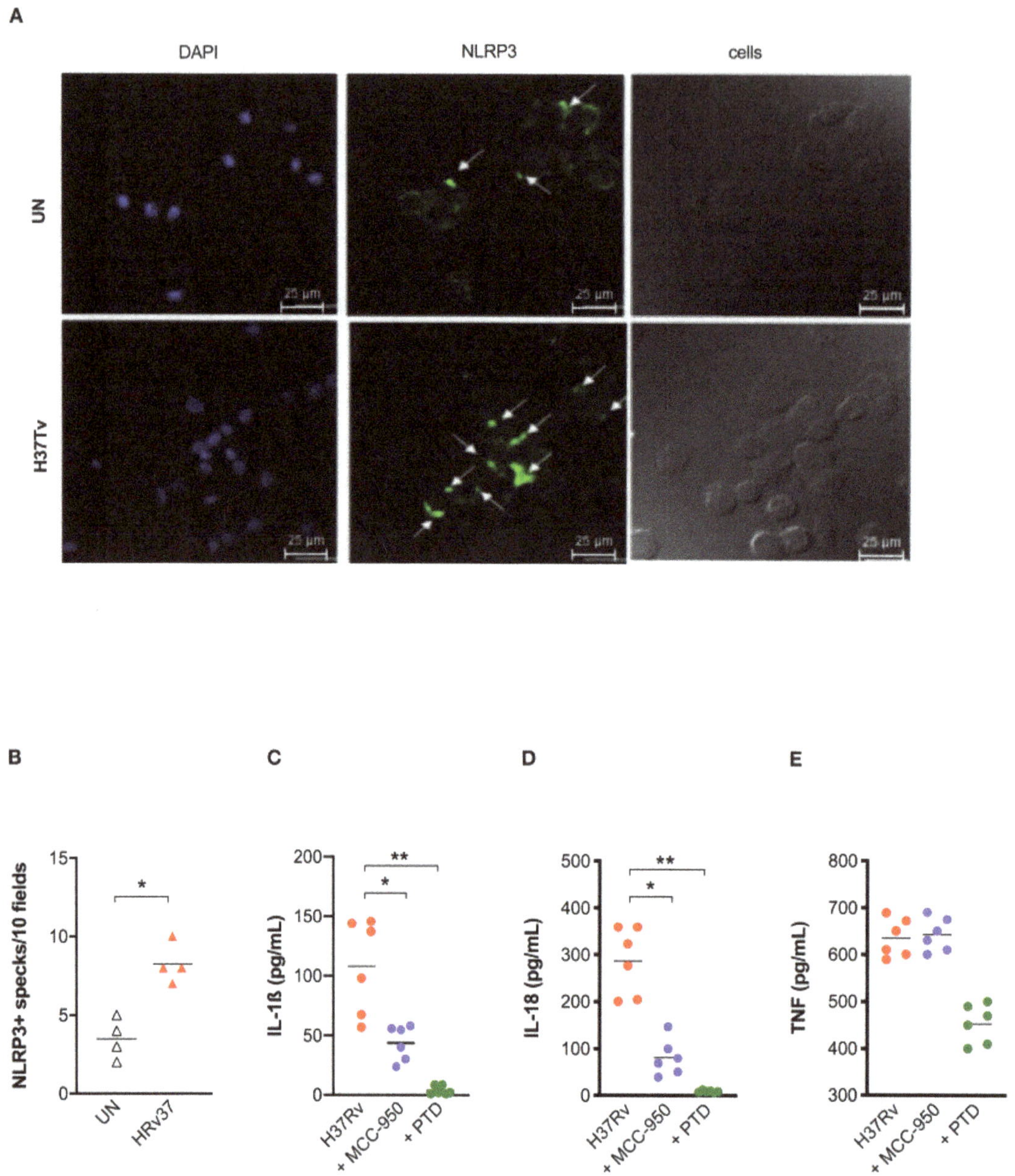

FIGURE 2 | NLRP3 contributes to inflammasome activation by *Mtb* H37Rv in human MDM. The healthy donors' monocyte-derived macrophages (MDM; $n = 4$) were cultivated (0.08×10^6) in 16-well chamber slides (*Thermo Fisher Scientific*), challenged with *M. tuberculosis* (Mtb) H37Rv (MOI: 0.033) for 3 h, then washed and cultured for 24 h. Mouse anti-human NLRP3 and a fluorescent secondary antibody (Alexa 488-conjugated goat-anti-mouse IgG1) were used to label NLRP3. DAPI was used to counterstain the nuclei. NLRP3+ speck formation in untreated (UN) and infected MDM (H37Rv) was analyzed using fluorescence microscopy. A representative experiment was reported. Arrows indicated NLRP3+ specks. **(A)**. The number of NLRP3+ specks was manually counted for each independent experiment **(B)**. The healthy donors' monocyte-derived macrophages (MDM; $n = 6$) were treated with 10 µM MCC-950 or 10 µM parthenolide (PTD) 1 h before infection with *M. tuberculosis* H37Rv (MOI: 0.033) for 3 h, then washed and cultured for 24 h. The release of IL-1ß **(C)**, IL-18 **(D)**, and TNF **(E)** was measured in culture supernatants. Individual data are reported with their mean. The Mann-Whitney test was used to compare treated and untreated groups **(B)**. The Kruskall-Wallis test followed by a Bonferroni post-test were used to compare H37Rv, MCC-950 and PTD groups **(C–E)**. Differences with a $p < 0.05$ were considered statistically significant (*). $^{**}p < 0.001$.

Next, we applied another approach, based on the use of known chemical inhibitors, to confirm NLRP3 involvement in the response. IL-1ß and IL-18 release was measured in Mtb infected-MDM and pre-treated with the NLRP3 inhibitor MCC-950 (10 μM) (23). As a positive control of inhibition, we also pre-treated MDM with the general inflammasome inhibitor parthenolide (PTD; 10 μM) (22). As expected, PTD entirely abolished cytokines production, while MCC-950 significantly reduced, but not completely abrogated, the release of IL-1ß (**Figure 2C**) and IL-18 (**Figure 2D**) in infected-MDM (48.7 and 71.7% inhibition, respectively). The secretion of a non-inflammasome-dependent pro-inflammatory cytokine, TNF, was not significantly affected by the use of inhibitors (**Figure 2E**).

Altogether, these findings corroborate previous data about the importance of NLRP3 in macrophage' response against virulent Mtb (10–12, 17, 31, 32), including at physiologic condition of infection (MOI: 0.033), and support the protective effect observed for *NLRP3* rs10754558 against the development of active pulmonary TB (18).

TB Patients Present an Impaired NLRP3 Response and IL-1ß Release

In order to better understand the relative contribution of inflammasome activation and IL-1ß release in Mtb infection *in vivo*, we analyzed IL-1ß, IL-18, IFN-α, and TNF levels in the plasma of patients recently diagnosed with active pulmonary TB (TB) and their "household contacts" (CNT) from an endemic TB area (Brazilian State of Amazonas). A group of healthy donors from a non-endemic area (São Paulo, SP, Brazil) was also included. All cytokines, with the exception of IL-18, were up-regulated in TB and CNT individuals with respect to HD (**Figures 3A–D**). Of note, a significant difference was observed in the plasma level of IL-1ß (**Figure 3A**) and IFN-α (**Figure 3C**) between the TB and the CNT groups. The IL-1ß concentration is significantly lower in the TB than in the CNT samples, while the IFN-α level increased in the TB compared to the CNT sample (**Figures 3A,C**).

These results emphasize that the TB patients presented an imbalance between IL-1ß and IFN-α, as suggested from animal models and *in-vitro* assays (17). These results also show that "household contacts" from endemic areas are characterized by a different plasma cytokine profile compared to TB patients or to the general population from non-endemic TB areas. In part, our findings also correspond with Mayer-Barber et al. (7), even if the unbalance was described specifically for severe TB vs. mild form of the disease in that study.

When we performed a canonical correlation between plasma IL-1ß levels and sputum positivity for Mtb, we observed that the IL-1ß level inversely correlated with the Mtb positive sputum, leading us to clearly separate the CNT and TB groups (**Figure 3E**). This once more confirms that the production of IL-1ß is an important contributing factor for Mtb infection control, and that this response could be measured systemically.

Next, taking in account the role of NLRP3 in the IL-1ß release by Mtb-infected MDM and the fact that IFN-I is a known inhibitor of NLRP3 (31), we questioned whether the imbalance between IL-1ß and IFN-α, observed in the plasma of TB patients could be related to an impairment of NLRP3 inflammasome.

In an attempt to respond to this tricky question, we first compared the constitutive expression of *NLRP3*, *CASP1*, *IL1B*, and *IL18* in MDM from the TB patients, their household contacts (CNT) and heathy donors from a non-endemic region (HD); however, no significant difference resulted among the groups (**Figure 3F**).

We then treated MDM with 1 μg/mL of LPS for 24 h—with or without the further addition of 1 mM ATP for 15 min—and compared the IL-1ß release among the TB, CNT and HD groups. In cells with normal NLRP3, the addition of ATP significantly increased the LPS-induced release of IL-1ß (24). As expected, ATP boosted IL-1ß release in LPS-treated MDM from HD, and intriguingly also from CNT; however, it did not significantly affect the cytokine release in LPS-treated MDM from TB patients (**Figure 3G**).

This unresponsiveness of MDM seems to be, at least in part, due to the poor induction of *NLRP3* and *IL1B* expression in TB-treated cells, compared to MDM from HD or CNT (**Figure 3H**). This condition could be a consequence of high IFN-α production, which possibly prevents NLRP3 inflammasome response (13).

Altogether, these results demonstrate that recently diagnosed TB patients present defective NLRP3 inflammasome and IL-1ß release and, conversely, increased IFN-α production, which can be at least in part responsible for NLRP3 inhibition. Moreover, for the first time to our knowledge, we showed that exposed but healthy subjects ("household contacts") display an inflammasome response similar to non-exposed healthy donors, allowing us to hypothesize that "Mtb-resistant" individuals may have an IL-1ß production that is better able to counteract IFN-I induction by mycobacteria.

Inhibition of Cathepsin Activity Abolished IL-1ß and IL-18 Release Suggesting the Contribution of NLRC4 in Inflammasome Activation by Mtb H37Rv

Among typical NLRP3 activation pathways, P2X7-mediaded K+ efflux and lysosomal cathepsins release have been reported as possible mechanisms for an inflammasome activation by mycobacteria (11, 34). To investigate the contribution of these two mechanisms in our model, exogenous ATP (1 mM) or Ca074-Me (10 μg/mL) were added for 15 min after or 1 h before Mtb infection, respectively. As a positive control for NLRP3 activation, MDM were also stimulated with 1 μg/mL of LPS for 24 h with or without 1 mM ATP for another 15 min (24).

Exogenous ATP did not significantly alter inflammasome cytokine production in H37Rv-treated MDM, or in LPS-treated ones (**Figures 4A,B**), suggesting that, at least in this model, ATP did not amplify mycobacterial stimulation as previously observed in mice (34). On the other hand, the inhibitor of lysosomal cathepsin activity Ca074-Me completely abolished IL-1ß and IL-18 release (96.7 and 97% of inhibition, respectively) (**Figures 4A,B**), reinforcing previous findings about the role of lysosomal cathepsins release in inflammasome activation by mycobacteria (11).

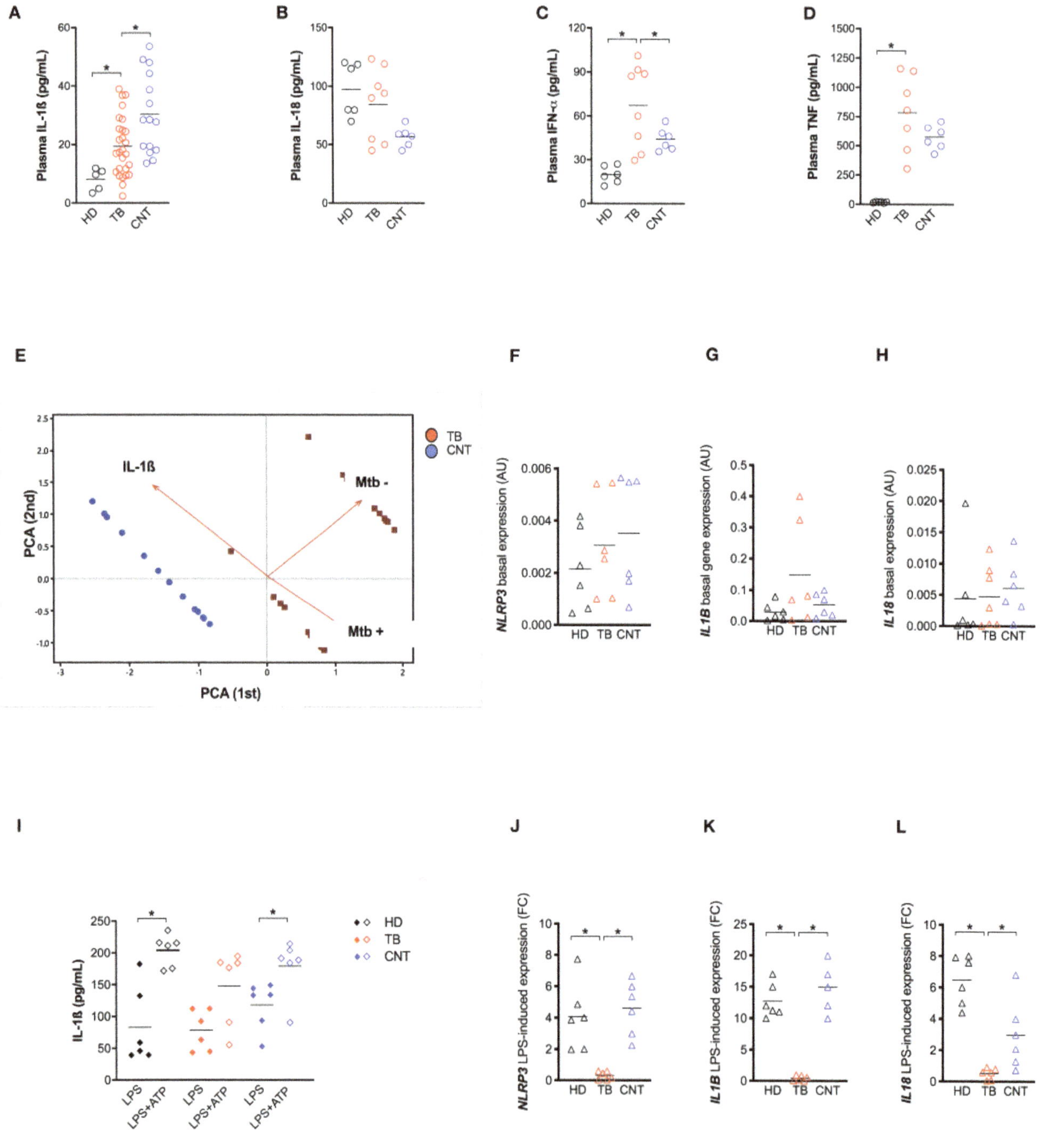

FIGURE 3 | TB patients present an impaired NLRP3 inflammasome response. IL-1ß **(A)** level were measured in plasma from recently diagnosed untreated TB patients (TB; $n = 27$) and some of their "household contacts" (CNT; $n = 15$) from an endemic TB area (Manaus, metropolitan region, AM) and from healthy donors in a non-endemic area (São Paulo metropolitan region, SP) (HD; $n = 5$). IL-18 **(B)**, IFN-a **(C)**, and TNF **(D)** dosage was executed in a group of samples (HD, $n = 6$; TB, $n = 8$; CNT, $n = 6$). **(E)** A Principal Components (PC) analysis was executed including the plasma level of IL-1ß, a mycobacteria count in a sputum analysis and a diagnosis of TB (TB or CNT). Monocyte-derived macrophages (MDM) were isolated from HD ($n = 6$), TB patients ($n = 6$), and CNT ($n = 6$) and challenged with 1 μg/mL of LPS for 24 h (LPS), or 1 μg/mL of LPS for 24 h plus 1 mM of ATP for another 15 min (LPS+ATP). Cells were lysed for RNA isolation and expression analysis. The release of IL-1ß was measured in culture supernatants. **(F–H)** Basal expression of *NLRP3, IL1B*, and *IL18* genes were analyzed in untreated MDM using gene-specific Taqman® assays and qPCR. Row target gene expression was normalized by the expression of the *GAPDH* house-keeping gene (ΔCt). Relative expression was calculated as $2^{-\Delta Ct}$. Data are expressed as arbitrary units (AU). **(I)** IL-1ß was measured in culture supernatants of treated MDM. **(J–L)** LPS-induced expression of *NLRP3, IL1B*, and *IL18* genes were analyzed in treated MDM using gene-specific Taqman® assays and qPCR. Row target gene expression was normalized by the expression of *GAPDH* house-keeping gene (ΔCt). Modulation of gene expression was calculated as Fold Change ($FC = 2^{--\Delta\Delta C}$) in respect to untreated (UN) cells. Individual data are reported with their mean. The Mann–Whitney test was used to compare two groups. The Kruskall–Wallis test followed by a Bonferroni post-test were used to compare more than two groups. Differences with a $p < 0.05$ were considered statistically significant (*).

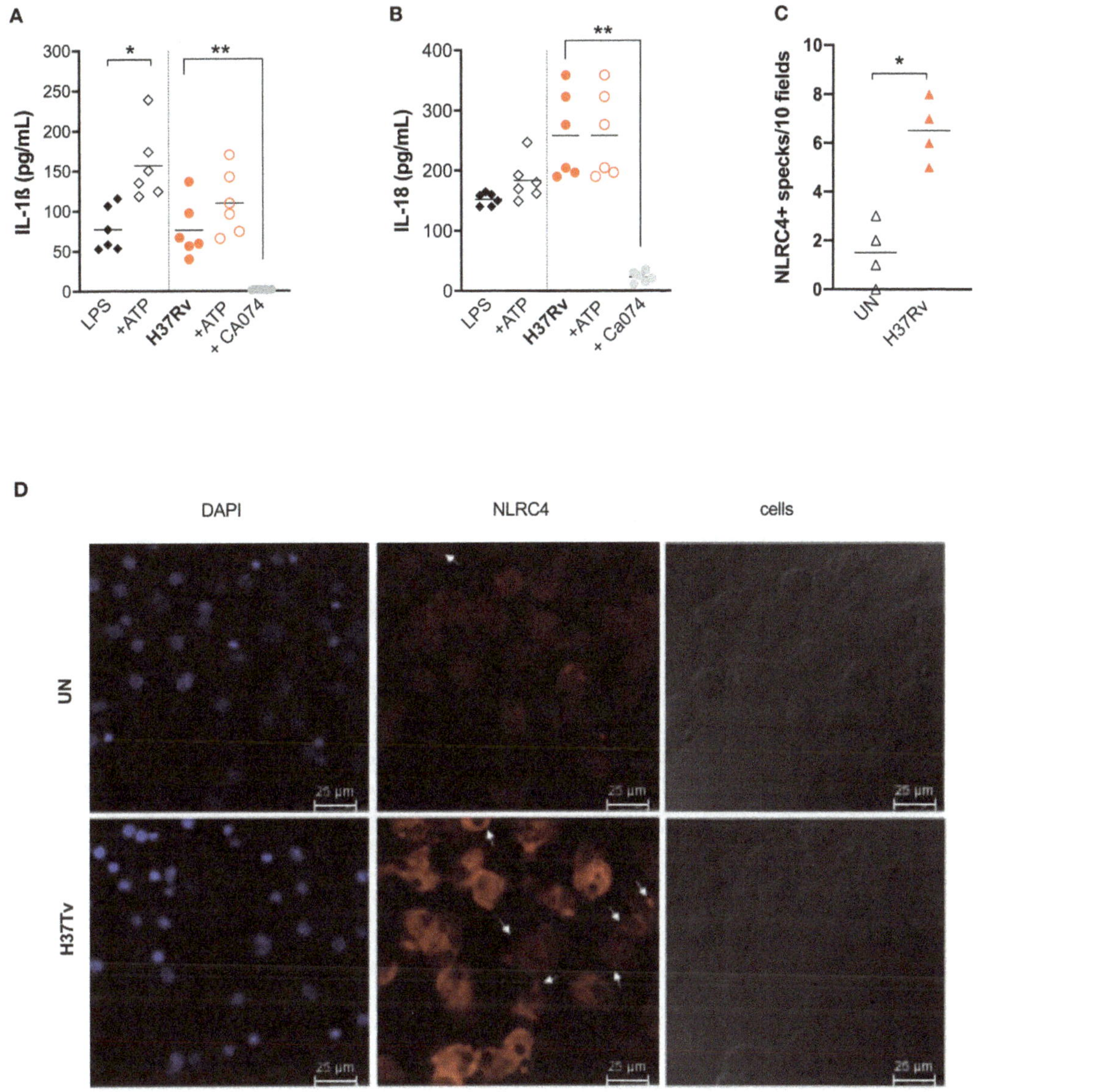

FIGURE 4 | Cathepsins activity is the major mechanism for inflammasome activation by *M. tuberculosis* H37Rv in human MDM, triggering NLRP3 and NLRC4. The healthy donors' monocyte-derived macrophages (MDM; $n = 6$) were treated or not with Ca074-Me (Ca074; 10 μM) before the infection with *M. tuberculosis* H37Rv (MOI: 0.033) for 3 h, then washed and cultured for 24 h. ATP (1 mM) was eventually added for another 15 min in H37Rv-infected MDM. The stimulation of MDM using LPS (1 μg/mL) for 24 h with or without ATP (1 mM) was included as a positive control for NLRP3 inflammasome activation. The release of IL-1ß **(A)** and IL-18 **(B)** was measured in culture supernatants. Healthy donors' monocyte-derived macrophages (MDM; $n = 4$) were cultivated (0.08×10^6) in 16-well chamber slides (*Thermo Fisher Scientific*), challenged with *M. tuberculosis* H37Rv (MOI: 0.033) for 3 h, then washed and cultured for 24 h. Rabbit anti-human NLRC4 and fluorescent secondary antibody (Alexa 647-conjugated goat-anti-rabbit IgG1) were used to label NLRC4. DAPI was used to counterstain the nuclei. NLRC4+ speck formation in untreated (UN) and infected MDM (H37Rv) was analyzed using fluorescence microscopy. The number of NLRPC+ specks was manually counted for each independent experiment **(C)**. A representative experiment was reported. Arrows indicated NLRC4+ specks. **(D)** Individual data are reported with their mean. The Kruskall–Wallis test followed by a Bonferroni post-test were used to compare more than two groups **(A,B)**. The Mann–Whitney test was used to compare treated and untreated groups **(C)**. Differences with a $p < 0.05$ were considered statistically significant (*). **$p < 0.001$.

Taking into account the discrepancy between the only partial reduction in inflammasome activation by MCC-950 (**Figures 2A,B**), the complete inhibition by Ca074-Me (**Figures 4A,B**), and the fact that cathepsin release activates another complex receptor, the NLRC4 (35), we hypothesized that this molecule could also be involved in the macrophage response to Mtb. To visualize the NLRC4 participation in inflammasome activation, we once again performed MDM infection with Mtb H37Rv assays and stained the specks using specific antibodies. Samples were observed under a fluorescence microscope. A significant increase in the number of NLRC4+ specks was observed in Mtb-infected MDM compared to untreated cells (**Figures 4C,D**).

These findings show that lysosomal cathepsins represent the main pathway for NLRP3 triggering by H37Rv, and maybe also for NLRC4, a receptor which is poorly investigated in TB and pulmonary diseases.

Genetic Variants in *NLRP3* and *NLRC4* Genes Distinctively Affect the Host Response to *M. tuberculosis* Infection and Outcome

Once confirming the central role exerted by NLRP3 in the inflammasome activation and host response against virulent Mtb, we next investigated the contribution of the TB protective *NLRP3* variant rs10754558 (18) on this response.

For this purpose, IL-1ß and IL-18 release from Mtb-challenged HD MDM was compared in carriers and non-carriers of the variant. As expected, individuals carrying the gain-of-function rs10754558 C>G variant in homozygosis (G/G) produced more IL-1ß when stimulated with the Mtb H37Rv than non-carriers (**Figure 5A**), confirming that NLRP3 is a crucial inflammasome sensor for Mtb. Moreover, in the presence of high levels of NLRP3 (28), macrophages respond to Mtb processing a larger amount of IL-1ß. Intriguingly, the IL-18 release in Mtb-treated HD MDM was not significantly affected by this SNV (**Figure 5B**). Then we performed the genotype-guided analysis with plasma cytokines levels in TB patients TB patients carrying rs10754558 G/G displayed an increased level of IL-1ß compared to non-carriers (**Figure 5C**), emphasizing that the effect of the NLRP3 gain-of-function variant against Mtb is detectable also *in vivo*. The SNV did not affect the inflammasome-dependent cytokine TNF (**Supplementary File 2A**).

In our previous genotyping analysis (18), we did not include the *NLRC4* gene. At that time, genetic association studies did not refer to *NLRC4* as an important locus for Mtb infection. Only recently, it was reported that *NLRC4* SNVs may affect the outcome of TB in chronically infected HIV patients (36). As our *in vitro* results indicate the participation of NLRC4 in

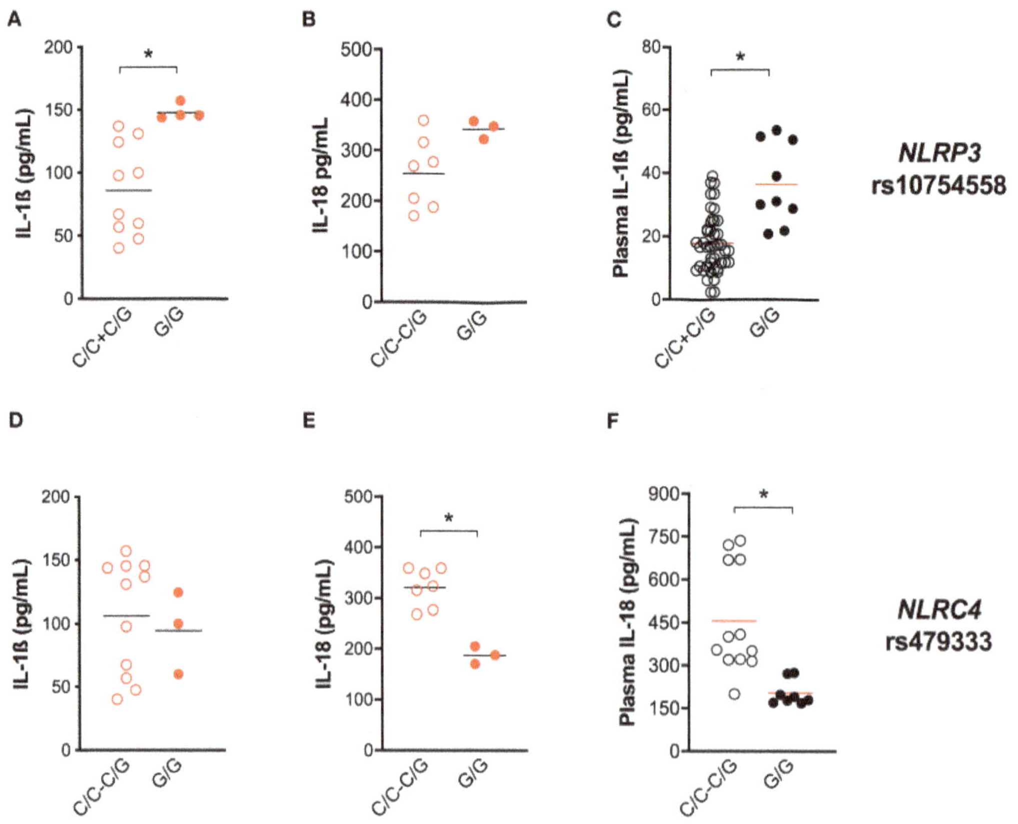

FIGURE 5 | Genetic variants in *NLRP3* and *NLRC4* genes affect host response to *M. tuberculosis*. The healthy donors' monocyte-derived macrophages (MDM; $n = 14$) were treated with *M. tuberculosis* H37Rv (MOI: 0.033) for 3 h, then washed and cultured for 24 h. The IL-1ß and IL-18 level was measured in culture supernatants at the end of experiment ($n = 14$ and 8, respectively), and in the plasma of TB patients ($n = 27$ and 20, respectively). *NLRP3* rs10754558 and *NLRC4* rs479333 SNVs were genotyped in the genomic DNA of healthy donors and TB patients. IL-1ß and IL-18 release data were then grouped by individual *NLRP3* rs10754558 genotype into homozygotes for the minor G allele (G/G) and the others (C/C+C/G), according to a recessive model of inheritance for the minor allele **(A–C)**; or by individual *NLRC4* rs479333 genotype into homozygotes for the minor C allele (C/C) and the others (G/G+G/C) according to a recessive model of inheritance for the minor allele **(D–F)**. Individual data are reported with their mean. The Mann–Whitney test was used to compare the groups. Differences with a $p < 0.05$ were considered statistically significant (*).

inflammasome activation by virulent Mtb (**Figure 4**), we selected a known functional variant in *NLRC4* (rs479333 G>C; found in 45% of the general population) and performed a genotype-guided analysis. The loss-of-function rs479333 variant did not affect IL-1ß in our *in-vitro* model of infection (**Figure 5D**), but was associated with a lower level of IL-18 both *in vitro* (**Figure 5E**) and *in vivo* (TB patients' plasma) (**Figure 5F**). The SNV did not affect the inflammasome-independent cytokine TNF (**Supplementary File 2B**).

These findings functionally demonstrate the effect of *NLRP3* rs10754558 SNV on TB protection (18), emphasizing the key role of NLRP3 in the first contact host/mycobacteria. Moreover, they suggest that *NLRC4* genetics may also affect Mtb/host interplay, even if in a different way.

Trying to assess whether *NLRC4 rs479333* can represent a susceptibility factor for TB, we performed an association study in a case/control cohort of TB. A multivariate analysis was first executed comparing *NLRC4 rs479333* and *NLRP3* rs10754558 distribution between TB patients and healthy donors. Then, to detect the possible effect on clinical presentation, we compared SNVs distribution in TB patients with pulmonary and with extra-pulmonary forms. The results are presented in **Table 3**.

As we have previously shown (18), *NLRP3* rs10754558 represents a protective factor against TB susceptibility, being more frequent in controls (G/G: 0.13) than in patients (0.04). On the other side, and for the first time to our knowledge, we observed that the loss-of-function variants in *NLRC4* (rs479333), which did not affect susceptibility to TB *per se* ($p_{adj} = 0.658$), results significantly less frequent in patients with the more severe form of infection (extra-pulmonary TB) compared to pulmonary TB, according to a dominant model of inheritance for the minor C allele (G/C+C/C: 0.40 vs. 0.61) (**Table 3**).

This genetic approach was not only useful for supporting the previously published association of the *NLRP3* rs10754558 variant with Mtb infection (18), but also for revealing that *NLRC4* could be another genetic factor important for the outcome of infection. It is interesting to emphasize that the two studied SNVs (rs10754558 and rs479333) principally affect one or the other inflammasome cytokine in Mtb-infected MDM (IL-1ß and IL-18, respectively), suggesting the distinct contribution of the mediators in TB.

Mtb Strains of Different Virulence and the Host's Genetic Background Shape NLRP3 Inflammasome Response to Mycobacteria

As the development of active TB is the complex outcome of several factors, including genetics, environment and pathogen biology (3), the next step was to evaluate the impact of Mtb phenotype on the inflammasome activation together with the host's genetic background. For this purpose, and considering the emergence of TB patients with a severe presentation caused by hyper-virulent strains (37, 38), MDM were challenged with different strains of mycobacteria: BCG and MP287/03 (MP) non-virulent and hyper-virulent strains from *M bovis* respectively; and the hyper-virulent strain Beijing-1471 (Bj) from *M. tuberculosis*. IL-1ß and IL-18 release was compared with the common virulent strain H37Rv, also from *M. tuberculosis*.

H37Rv and Bj strains induced a similar amount of IL-1ß, but higher than MP, providing to be a poor IL-1ß producer. BCG was the major inductor of IL-1ß, leading to about a 3-fold increase in cytokine compared to H37Rv or Bj (**Figure 6A**). This difference among BCG, H37Rv, and Bj was not as important in the case of IL-18 production, even if BCG tends to induce a higher amount of cytokine, especially when compared to H37Rv (**Figure 6B**). MP was able to induce significant IL-18 release compared to untreated MDM, even if in a lower amount compared to other strains (**Figure 6B**). Of note, the production of TNF was similar in all conditions (**Figure 6C**), as well as the LDH release (**Figure 6D**).

To depict the relative contribution of NLRP3 in sensing distinct Mtb strains, we performed assays in the presence of the NLRP3 specific inhibitor MCC-950 or the general inhibitor PTD. MCC-950 inhibited about half of IL-1ß and IL-18 production in H37Rv-, Bj-, and BCG-treated -MDM. Due to the low production of IL-18 induced by MP the inhibition rate observed for MCC-950 was not statistically significant ($p = 0.08$) (**Figures 6E,F**). As expected, PTD completely abolished IL-1ß and IL-18 production in all the conditions (**Figures 6E,F**).

The pattern of IL-1ß and IL-18 release by MDM was distinct depending on the Mtb strain, and these differences may be related to the different ability of Mtb strains to induce inflammasome genes expression (**Figure 6G**). In terms of cytokine production, BCG promotes the highest expression of

TABLE 3 | Association results for SNVs in inflammasome-encoding genes in the TB cohort from the Brazilian State of Amazonas.

Gene SNV ID	Effect	Genotypes	HD (*n* = 288)	TB (*n* = 352)	p_{adj} OR_{adj} (95%CI)	PTB (*n* = 288)	ETB (*n* = 64)	p_{adj} OR_{adj} (95%CI)
NLRP3 rs10754558	GoF	C/C	0.52	0.65	**0.003**	0.68	0.62	0.475
		C/G	0.35	0.31	0.16	0.27	0.34	0.96
		G/G	0.13	0.04	(1.02–1.29)	0.05	0.04	(0.64–3.56)
NLRC4 rs479333	LoF	G/G	0.66	0.49	0.658	0.39	0.60	**0.0006**
		C/G	0.20	0.31	0.78	0.39	0.23	0.20
		C/C	0.14	0.20	(0.25–2.43)	0.22	0.17	(1.92–13.16)

Gene symbol, variant identification number (SNV ID), genotypes frequencies for patients with active pulmonary TB (PTB) extra-pulmonary (ETB) and healthy donors (HD), GLM p-value (p), odds ratio (OR) and 95% confidence interval (CI) are reported adjusted for sex and age (p_{adj}, OR_{adj}). Statistically significant results after Bonferroni correction are indicated in bold characters.

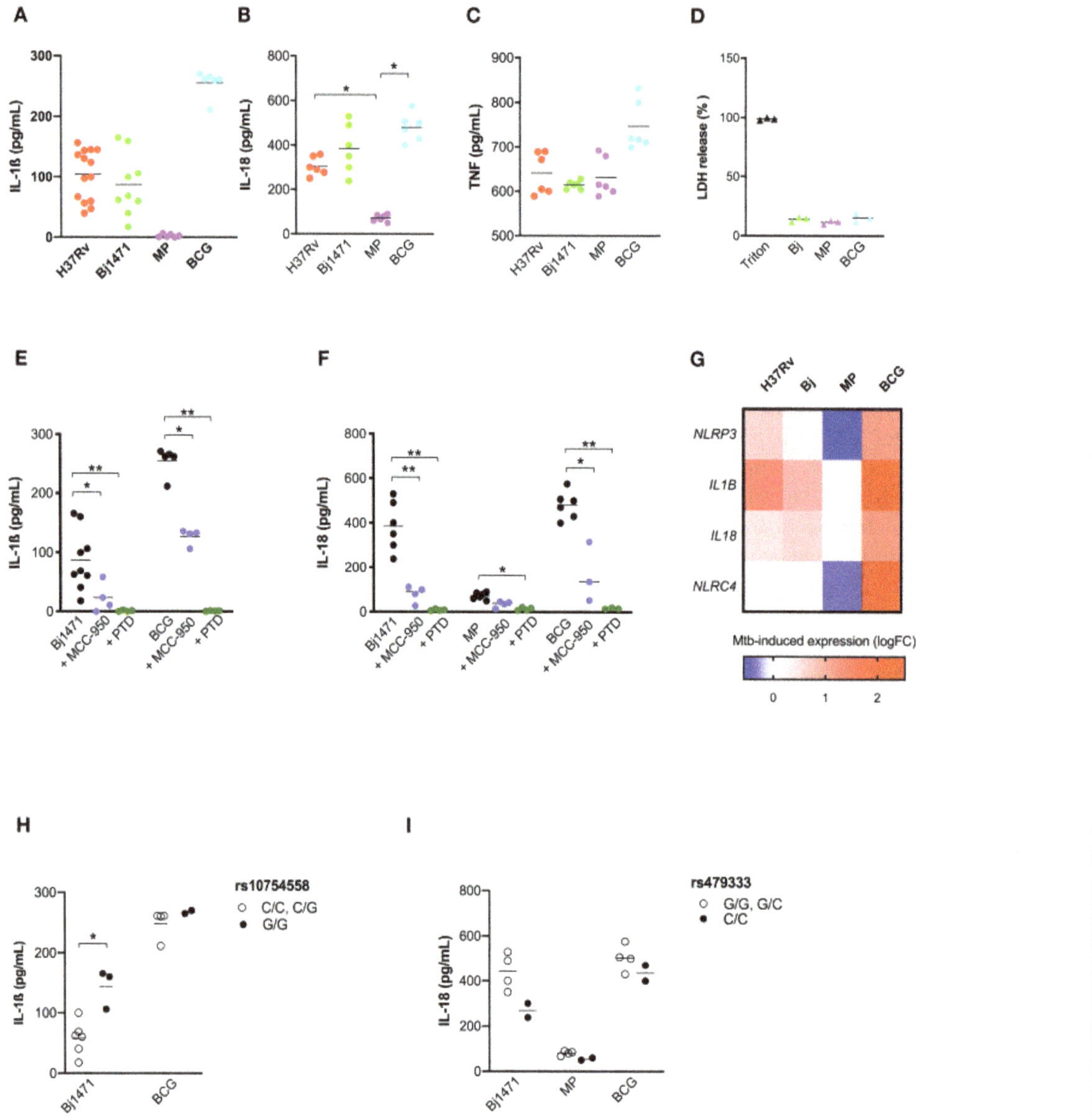

FIGURE 6 | Mtb strains of different virulence and host genetic background shaped the inflammasome response to mycobacteria. The healthy donors' monocyte-derived macrophages (MDM) were treated with 10 μM MCC-950 or 10 μM parthenolide (PTD) 1 h before infection with *M. tuberculosis* (MOI: 0.033) H37Rv ($n = 14$), Beijin-1470 (Bj-1470; $n = 9$), MP287/03 (MP; $n = 6$) and *Bacillus Calmette Guerin* (BCG; $n = 6$) for 3 h, then washed and cultured for 24 h. The release of IL-1β **(A)**, IL-18 **(B)**, TNF **(C),** and LDH **(D)** was measured in culture supernatants. Dosage for IL-1β was executed for all samples, while for IL-18 and TNF in six samples, for LDH in three sample. Cytokines and LDH release were compared among different Mtb strains. Cells were lysed for RNA isolation and gene expression analysis. *NLRP3* rs10754558 and *NLRC4* rs479333 SNVs were genotyped in the genomic DNA of healthy donors. The effect of MCC-950 and PTD on inflammasome activation in infected MDM was analyzed by the meaning of IL-1β **(E)** and IL-18 **(F)** release. Mtb-induced expression of *NLRP3, NLRC4, IL1B,* and *IL18* genes in H37Rv-, Bj-1470-, MP- and BCG-infected MDM was calculated as $2^{-\Delta\Delta Ct}$ (fold-change, FC) and reported as $\log_2$FC in a heat-map graph **(G).** IL-1β release data were grouped by individual *NLRP3* rs10754558 genotype into homozygotes for the minor G allele (G/G) and the others (C/C+C/G), according to a recessive model of inheritance for the minor allele **(H)**. IL-18 release data were grouped by *NLRC4* rs479333 genotype into homozygotes for the minor C allele (C/C) and the others (G/G+G/C) according to a recessive model of inheritance for the minor allele **(I)**. Individual data are reported with their mean. The Kruskall-Wallis test followed by a Bonferroni post-test were used to compare groups **(A–F)**. The Mann-Whitney test was used to compare two groups **(H,I)**. Differences with a $p < 0.05$ were considered statistically significant (*). **$p < 0.001$.

the 4 analyzed genes (*NLRP3, NLRC4, IL1B*, and *IL18*), and MP the lowest.

Finally, to assess the contribution of host genetics on the inflammasome activation toward different Mtb strains, we performed genotype-guided assays for the two functional variants *NLRP3* rs10754558, and *NLRC4* rs479333. Despite the limited number of tested samples ($n = 12$), MDM from donors carrying the gain-of-function *NLRP3* variant (G/G) responded to Beijin-1470 and BCG strains, producing a higher level of IL-1ß compared to MDM from non-carriers (C/C+C/G) (**Figure 6H**).

At the same time, and contrary to what was observed for H37Rv-treated MDM, the loss-of-function variant *NLRC4* rs479333 did not significantly affect IL-18 release in MDM challenged with BCG. Beijin-1470 or MP287/03 (**Figure 6I**).

This last set of experiments demonstrated that different strains of Mtb display a unique capacity to induce inflammasome activation at a rather physiologic condition (MOI: 0.033) with virulence (non-virulent more than virulent) playing a greater role than the type of bacteria (*M.bovis* BCG more than *M.bovis* MP287/03; *M. tuberculosis* H37Rv similar to *M. tuberculosis* Beijin-1470). Moreover, we showed that host genetics may affect the inflamamsome activation rate toward different Mtb strains, especially for *NLRP3* rs10754558 SNV—once again corroborating the important role of inflammasome genetics in individual responses to mycobacteria.

DISCUSSION

Extensive efforts have been made to better understand the mechanisms involved in Mtb/host interactions and how this complex interplay may determine resistance vs. susceptibility to Mtb and the development of TB. Innate immunity and first-line immune responses, including inflammasome and related cytokines, have recently been taken into account as important determinants in TB outcomes. Notwithstanding, our knowledge of the mechanisms underlying progression of Mtb infections and the development of the active disease in humans is not yet fully understood, in part due to the lack of appropriate models of study, and also due to the difficulty of interpreting complex genetics, immunologic, and microbiologic interactions.

Starting from our previous genetic data (18), we designed a study for the contemporary evaluation of how inflammasome genetics and Mtb phenotype affect inflammasome activation in primary human monocytes-derived macrophages, in turn contributing to individual responses to Mtb and/or to Mtb-susceptibility vs. resistance establishment.

Our findings show that the common virulent strain H37Rv induces NLRP3 inflammasome activation (but not pyroptosis) in human macrophages and that IL-1ß is mandatory for bacterial containment (**Figures 1, 2**). These findings corroborate previous studies in murine and human macrophages (10–12, 17, 31, 32); however, it is important to mention that in those studies, the MOI level was very high (10 or higher), while we decided to infect cells with an MOI level that was as physiologic as possible (0.033). This protective response can be modulated by host genetics, as macrophages from individuals carrying the gain-of-function rs10754558 in *NLRP3* produce significantly more IL-1ß than non-carriers (**Figure 5A**), as well as by the type of Mtb strain, as non-virulent BCG strains trigger a large amount of cytokine while the hyper-virulent MP287/03 none at all (**Figure 6A**). These data support the protective effect observed for *NLRP3* rs10754558 against the development of active pulmonary TB (18).

Trying to better understand how the host/mycobacteria interplay acts *in vivo*, we analyzed the plasma levels of inflammasome cytokines, IFN-α and TNF in a group of recently diagnosed TB patients (before treatment) and their "household contacts"—representing a group of exposed but healthy subjects. As expected, responder individuals ("household contacts") presented a higher level of IL-1ß, suggesting that their inflammasome is functioning well (**Figure 3**). On the contrary, susceptible individuals (TB patients) were characterized by an imbalance between IL-1ß and IFN-α, a known inhibitor of NLRP3 inflammasome (13). This concept of fine tuning between innate immune mediators was previously proposed by Mayer-Barber et al. (7), referring to the severity of the TB presentation; however, our study demonstrates that a "good" inflammasome activation is determinant for Mtb resistance in exposed population such as endemic TB areas. Intriguingly, TB patients also appeared to be less prone to an efficient response against PAMPs/DAMPs, as suggested by impaired NLRP3 activation by common stimuli (**Figure 3**). A similar impairment of NLRP3 was first reported in the dendritic cells of HIV patients (39), which are also characterized by elevated IFN-I levels, emphasizing a common inhibitory mechanism mediated by the antiviral mediator. Wassermann and colleagues aptly demonstrated that Mtb evolved some strategies to by-pass inflammasome activation, one being to activate pathways leading to IFN production (17).

According to Amaral et al. (11), H37Rv also activates the inflammasome in human macrophages through lysosomal damage and cathepsins release, as demonstrated by the complete inhibition of cytokine release by Ca074-Me (**Figures 4A,B**). However, the discrepancy between the dramatic effect of Ca074-Me and only partial inhibition obtained with the NLRP3 specific inhibitor MCC-950 (23) led us to hypothesize the contribution of another pathway for inflammasome activation. Besides NLRP3, other inflammasome receptors, such as the NLRC4, have been shown to contribute to the host's response to intracellular bacteria (9). Differently from NLRP3, NLRC4 can either directly recognizes bacterial patterns, such as flagellin (40), or be activated by lysosomal cathepsins release, at least in mice (35). The role of NLRC4 in TB remains elusive because it has been poorly investigated in TB and pulmonary diseases. Microscopic visualization of inflammasome aggregates ("specks"), allowed us to observe NLRC4 in the mounted complex, suggesting that it can contribute to macrophages response against Mtb; however, further investigation will be needed to better depict the role of this molecule in TB pathogenesis.

Through a genetic approach and genotype-guided assay, for the first time to our knowledge, we found a significant association between NLRC4 and the outcome of TB in an endemic area. The loss-of-function variant rs479333 in the *NLRC4* gene (minor allele frequency, 49%; from ensembl.org) was less frequent in patients with extra-pulmonary TB than in patients with pulmonary disease (**Table 3**). This SNV, previously associated to reduced *NLRC4* transcription (29) and diminished plasma level of IL-18 (30), was associated with a lower release of IL-18

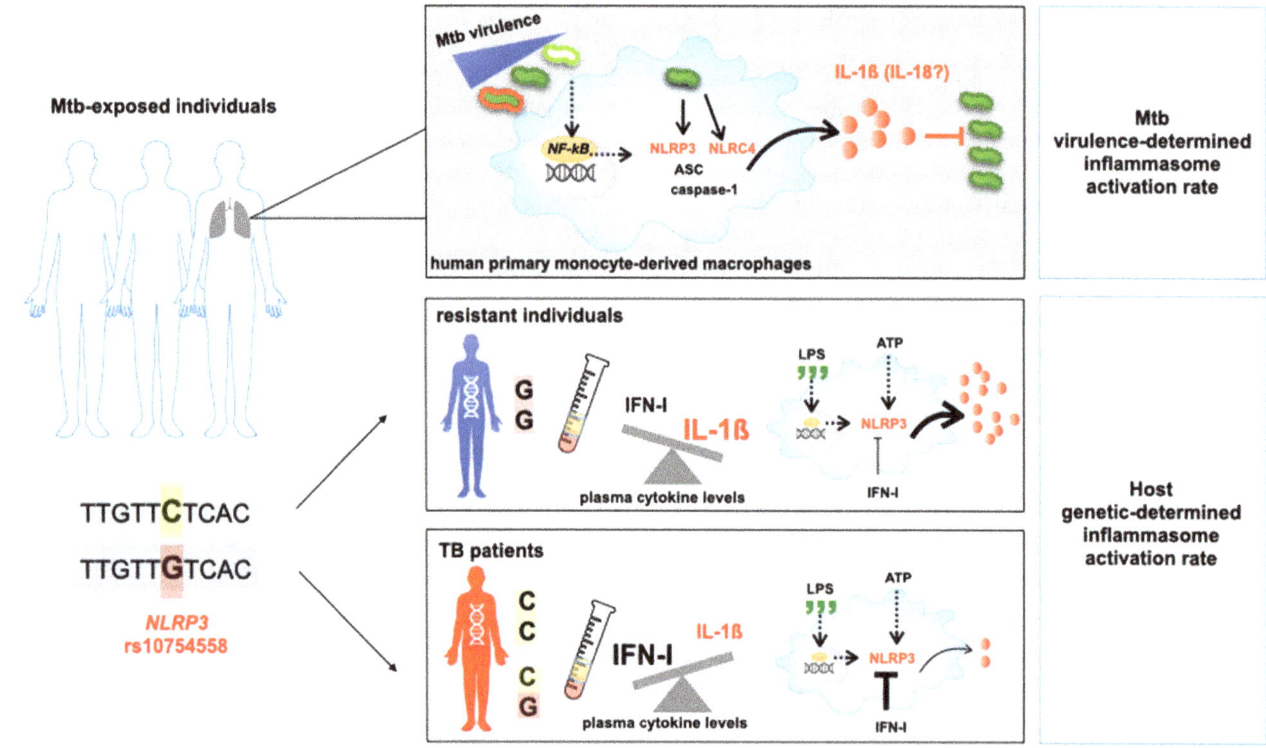

FIGURE 7 | Host genetic background and *M.tuberculosis* (Mtb) determine the outcome of TB. Schematic representation of the main results of this study.

in H37Rv-challenged MDM as well as the plasma level of the cytokine (**Figures 5E,F**), reinforcing its loss-of-function effect at both local and systemic levels.

We would like to emphasize that our data reveal two situations in Mtb/host interplay: one characterized by the preferential NLRP3/IL-1ß axis and another by NLRC4/IL18 axis. The first exerts a central role in first host/pathogen contact and in mycobacterial containment while the other is apparently more important in the outcome of Mtb infection. As we know, IL-1ß and IL-18 assume distinct roles within immune response. While IL-1ß is mainly involved in endothelium and phagocytes activation, IL-18 is involved in epithelium homeostasis and CD4+ T lymphocytes polarization toward Th1 IFN-γ-producer cells.

Considering the importance of IFN-γ-producer cells in typical TB granuloma formation, we therefore hypothesize that individuals with a defective NLRC4/IL18 axis are not able to effectively contain mycobacteria within granulomas, leading to eventual extra-pulmonary dissemination. Accordingly, at least in HIV-infected patients, the expression of *NLRC4* significantly increased in the blood of individuals with a more severe form of TB (41). Moreover, it is interesting to remember that loss-of-function SNVs in *NLRC4* have been found in HIV patents with severe TB (36) and in patients with cystic fibrosis affected by severe lung infections (42), reinforcing the important and poorly investigated role of NLRC4 in lung immunity and pulmonary diseases.

Mtb strains induce inflammasome activation in a "virulence-dependent" way. The non-virulent strain BCG promotes a dramatic inflammasome activation compared to common virulent (H37R) and rare hyper-virulent (Beijing 1471, MP287/03) strains, suggesting that Mtb virulence evolved together with some mechanism of inflammasome escape (17), and corroborating once more the importance of inflammasome activation in the immune response against Mtb.

Of note, the pattern of IL-1ß and IL-18 release is not identical in Mtb-challenged MDM (**Figure 6**), being IL-18 levels higher than IL-1ß for all tested strains. Moreover, IL-1ß production appears to be more virulence-dependent than IL-18. These findings suggest that Mtb could activate several and distinct inflammasome pathways (i.e., NLRP3/IL-1ß or NLRC4/IL-18 axis) compared to a unique PAMP, such as LPS, and these pathways could alternatively process IL-1ß or IL-18, as previously proposed (8, 9). The different level of inflammasome activation in response to distinct Mtb strains has also been observed in the murine model of infection, showing that MP287/03 is a poor inducer of IL-1ß both *in vivo* and *in vitro* compared to H37Rv or Beijing; IL-18 was not, however, evaluated in these models (34).

Masters et al. (43) proposed that the difference in the level of inflammasome activation by distinct Mtb strains is due to the virulence factor *Zmp1*. Interestingly, this group has also noted that MP287/03, which does not express *Zmp1*, activates inflammasome through NLRC4. In our assays, MP287/03 induced IL-18 but not IL-1ß. However, this Mtb strain is not able to trigger NLRC4, nor NLRP3 expression (**Figure 6**). Consequently, we cannot conclude whether Mtb strains which preferentially induce IL-18 do so through NLRC4. Nevertheless, taking into account the long co-evolution period of Mtb and humans, it would not be surprising that several inflammasome sensors could contribute to mycobacterial defense, as it was demonstrated for NLRP3 and AIM2 (17).

In conclusion, for the first time, our findings show the intricate interaction among inflammasome genetics, Mtb virulence and the resultant inflammasome activation profile at the local (*in vitro* model) as well at the systemic (plasma) level. According to our hypothesis, during the first host/pathogen contact, the Mtb activates a strong inflammasome response in term of IL-1ß as well as IL-18, especially for non-virulent strain BCG and the common virulent one, H37Rv. This response is mediated by the NLRP3/IL-1ß axis in a cathepsin-dependent way, and the gain-of-function variant in NLRP3 contributes to the elevated production of IL-1ß, which in turn is specifically responsible for bacterial containment.

In-vitro assays and genetic association data support the involvement of the NLRC4/IL18 pathway in individual responses to mycobacteria and determine the outcome of an Mtb infection as well as TB severity. These original findings highlight that the same pathogen could activate inflammasome-dependent cleavages of cytokine pro-forms based on events that are not yet fully understood, such as a bacterial strain (i.e., MP287/03), distinct steps of the disease (i.e., first host/pathogen contact, or response to the pathogen in an individual with an established infection), or even based on an individual's genetic background (**Figure 7**).

ETHICS STATEMENT

This study was approved by the Human Research Ethics Committee of the Institute of Biomedical Sciences (ICB) of the University of São Paulo (USP) (CEPSH reference number: 51780715.8.0000.5467) and the Institute of Biological Sciences (ICB) of the Federal University of Amazonas (UFAM) (reference number: 57978916.3.0000.5020). All human participants provided written informed consent and all clinical investigations were conducted according to the principles expressed in the Declaration of Helsinki. The patients/participants provided their written informed consent to participate in this study.

AUTHOR CONTRIBUTIONS

DS and AP: conceived, designed experiments, wrote the article, and conducted statistical analyse. AS and MO: selected and collected TB patients and household contacts. MO: performed microbiologic analysis. DS and CB: performed MDM experiments. EA and CB: standardized *Mycobacterial* culture and infection. DS and VL: performed the immunofluorescence experiments. ER: performed flow-cytometry experiments. FF and JS: executed ELISA, performed RNA isolation, and gene expression analyse. DS, AP, FL, MO, AS, and ML: discussed the results. All authors contributed to the article and approved the submitted version.

ACKNOWLEDGMENTS

We are very grateful to the Oswaldo Cruz Hospital Blood Bank Service (São Paulo, SP, Brazil) and to the Reference Center for Sanitary Pneumology Clínica Cardoso Fontes (Manaus, AM, Brazil) for the recruitment of healthy donors and TB patients and their household contacts, respectively. We would like to thank Professor Mario Hiroyuki Hirata (Departamento de Análises Clínicas e Toxicológicas, Universidade de São Paulo/USP), Professor Niels Olsen Saraiva Câmara (Departamento de Imunologia, Instituto de Ciências Biomédicas/ICB, USP). Dr. Telma Miyuki Oshiro (Laboratório de Investigação Médica-56, Faculdade de Medicina, USP), Professor Karina Ramalho Bortoluci (Laboratório de Imunologia Molecular, Universidade Federal de São Paulo/UNIFESP), Dr. Eliana Faquin de Lima Mauro e Alexsander Seixas de Souza (Instituto Butantan, São Paulo), Prof. Aya Sadahiro' group (ICB, Universidade Federal do Amazonas/UFAM).

REFERENCES

1. Bellamy R. Genetics and pulmonary medicine. 3. Genetic susceptibility to tuberculosis in human populations. *Thorax.* (1998) 53:588–93. doi: 10.1136/thx.53.7.588
2. Forrellad MA, Klepp LI, Gioffré A, Sabio y García J, Morbidoni HR, de la Paz Santangelo M, et al. Virulence factors of the *Mycobacterium tuberculosis* complex. *Virulence.* (2013) 4:3–66. doi: 10.4161/viru.22329
3. O'Garra A, Redford PS, McNab FW, Bloom CI, Wilkinson RJ, Berry MP. The immune response in tuberculosis. *Annu Rev Immunol.* (2013) 31:475–527. doi: 10.1146/annurev-immunol-032712-095939
4. Cooper AM. Cell-mediated immune responses in tuberculosis. *Annu Rev Immunol.* (2009) 27:393–422. doi: 10.1146/annurev.immunol.021908.132703
5. Collins AC, Cai H, Li T, Franco LH, Li XD, Nair VR, et al. Cyclic GMP-AMP Synthase Is an Innate Immune DNA Sensor for *Mycobacterium tuberculosis.* *Cell Host Microbe.* (2015) 17:820–8. doi: 10.1016/j.chom.2015.05.005
6. Watson RO, Manzanillo PS, Cox JS. Extracellular *M. tuberculosis* DNA targets bacteria for autophagy by activating the host DNA-sensing pathway. *Cell.* (2012) 150:803–15. doi: 10.1016/j.cell.2012.06.040
7. Mayer-Barber KD, Andrade BB, Oland SD, Amaral EP, Barber DL, Gonzales J, et al. Host-directed therapy of tuberculosis based on interleukin-1 and type I interferon crosstalk. *Nature.* (2014) 511:99–103. doi: 10.1038/nature13489
8. Mathur A, Hayward JA, Man SM. Molecular mechanisms of inflammasome signaling. *J Leukoc Biol.* (2018) 103:233–57.
9. Hayward JA, Mathur A, Ngo C, Man SM. Cytosolic recognition of microbes and pathogens: inflammasomes in action. *Microbiol Mol Biol Rev.* (2018) 82:e00015-18. doi: 10.1128/MMBR.00015-18
10. Jamwal SV, Mehrotra P, Singh A, Siddiqui Z, Basu A, Rao KV. Mycobacterial escape from macrophage phagosomes to the cytoplasm represents an alternate adaptation mechanism. *Sci Rep.* (2016) 6:23089. doi: 10.1038/srep23089
11. Amaral EP, Riteau N, Moayeri M, Maier N, Mayer-Barber KD, Pereira RM, et al. Lysosomal cathepsin release is required for NLRP3-inflammasome activation by *Mycobacterium tuberculosis* in infected macrophages. *Front Immunol.* (2018) 9:1427. doi: 10.3389/fimmu.2018.01427
12. Mishra BB, Moura-Alves P, Sonawane A, Hacohen N, Griffiths G, Moita LF, et al. *Mycobacterium tuberculosis* protein ESAT-6 is a potent activator of the NLRP3/ASC inflammasome. *Cell Microbiol.* (2010) 12:1046–63. doi: 10.1111/j.1462-5822.2010.01450.x

13. Guarda G, Braun M, Staehli F, Tardivel A, Mattmann C, Förster I, et al. Type I interferon inhibits interleukin-1 production and inflammasome activation. *Immunity.* (2011) 34:213–23. doi: 10.1016/j.immuni.2011.02.006
14. Sokolowska M, Chen LY, Liu Y, Martinez-Anton A, Qi HY, Logun C, et al. Prostaglandin E2 inhibits NLRP3 inflammasome activation through EP4 Receptor and intracellular cyclic AMP in Human Macrophages. *J Immunol.* (2015) 194:5472–87. doi: 10.4049/jimmunol.1401343
15. Latz E, Xiao TS, Stutz A. Activation and regulation of the inflammasomes. *Nat Rev Immunol.* (2013) 13:397–411. doi: 10.1038/nri3452
16. Briken V, Ahlbrand SE, Shah S. *Mycobacterium tuberculosis* and the host cell inflammasome: a complex relationship. *Front Cell Inform Microb.* (2013) 3:62. doi: 10.3389/fcimb.2013.00062
17. Wassermann R, Gulen MF, Sala C, Perin SG, Lou Y, Rybniker J, et al. *Mycobacterium tuberculosis* differentially activates cGAS- and inflammasome-dependent intracellular immune responses through ESX-1. *Cell Host Microbe.* (2015) 17:799–810. doi: 10.1016/j.chom.2015.05.003
18. Souza de Lima D, Ogusku MM, Sadahiro A, Pontillo A. Inflammasome genetics contributes to the development and control of active pulmonary tuberculosis. *Infect Genet Evol.* (2016) 41:240–4. doi: 10.1016/j.meegid.2016.04.015
19. Salem JI, Marója MD, Carvalho FF, Lima MO, Litaiff LR, Cardoso MS, et al. Valor relativo do exame direto, após concentração e por cultivo de escarro no diagnóstico bacteriológico da tuberculose pulmonar no Amazonas. *J.Pneumol.* (1990) 16:133–6. Available online at: https://pesquisa.bvsalud.org/portal/resource/pt/lil-94374
20. Salem JI, Carvalho CM, Ogusku MM, Maia R, Ruffino-Neto A. PKO - Alternative method for isolating mycobacteria from sputum. *Acta Amazonica.* (2007) 37:419–24. doi: 10.1590/S0044-59672007000300013
21. Kaufmann SH. How can immunology contribute to the control of tuberculosis? *Nat Rev Immunol.* (2001) 1:20–30. doi: 10.1038/35095558
22. Juliana C, Fernandes-Alnemri T, Wu J, Datta P, Solorzano L, Yu JW, et al. Anti-inflammatory compounds parthenolide and Bay 11-7082 are direct inhibitors of the inflammasome. *J Biol Chem.* (2010) 285:9792–802. doi: 10.1074/jbc.M109.082305
23. Coll RC, Robertson AA, Chae JJ, Higgins SC, Muñoz-Planillo R, Inserra MC, et al. A small-molecule inhibitor of the NLRP3 inflammasome for the treatment of inflammatory diseases. *Nat Med.* (2015) 21:248–55. doi: 10.1038/nm.3806
24. Gattorno M, Tassi S, Carta S, Delfino L, Ferlito F, Pelagatti MA, et al. Pattern of interleukin-1beta secretion in response to lipopolysaccharide and ATP before and after interleukin-1 blockade in patients with CIAS1 mutations. *Arthritis Rheum.* (2007) 56:3138–48. doi: 10.1002/art.22842
25. Mariathasan S, Weiss DS, Newton K, McBride J, O'Rourke K, Roose-Girma M, et al. Cryopyrin activates the inflammasome in response to toxins and ATP. *Nature.* (2006) 440:228–32. doi: 10.1038/nature04515
26. Stutz A, Horvath GL, Monks BG, LatzE. ASC speck formation as a readout for inflammasome activation. *Methods Mol Biol.* (2013) 1040:91–101. doi: 10.1007/978-1-62703-523-1_8
27. Schmittgen TD, Livak KJ. Analyzing real-time PCR data by the comparative C(T) method. *Nat Protoc.* (2008) 3:1101–8. doi: 10.1038/nprot.2008.73
28. Hitomi Y1, Ebisawa M, Tomikawa M, Imai T, Komata T, Hirota T, et al. Associations of functional NLRP3 polymorphisms with susceptibility to food-induced anaphylaxis and aspirin-induced asthma. *J Allergy Clin Immunol.* (2009) 124:779–85.e6. doi: 10.1016/j.jaci.2009.07.044
29. Zeller T, Haase T, Müller C, Riess H, Lau D, Zeller S, et al. Molecular characterization of the NLRC4 expression in relation to interleukin-18 levels. *Circ Cardiovasc Genet.* (2015) 8:717–26. doi: 10.1161/CIRCGENETICS.115.001079
30. Matteini AM, Li J, Lange EM, Tanaka T, Lange LA, Tracy RP, et al. Novel gene variants predict serum levels of the cytokines IL-18 and IL-1ra in older adults. *Cytokine.* (2014) 65:10–6. doi: 10.1016/j.cyto.2013.10.002
31. Welin A, Eklund D, Stendahl O, Lerm M. Human Macrophages Infected With a High Burden of ESAT-6-expressing *M. tuberculosis* Undergo caspase-1- And Cathepsin B-independent Necrosis. *Plos ONE.* (2011) 6:e20302. doi: 10.1371/journal.pone.0020302
32. Eklund D1, Welin A, Andersson H, Verma D, Söderkvist P, Stendahl O, et al. Human gene variants linked to enhanced NLRP3 activity limit intramacrophage growth of Mycobacterium tuberculosis. *J Infect Dis.* (2014) 1:209:749–53. doi: 10.1093/infdis/jit572
33. Schenk M, Fabri M, Krutzik SR, Lee DJ, Vu DM, Sieling PA, et al. Interleukin-1β triggers the differentiation of macrophages with enhanced capacity to present mycobacterial antigen to T cells. *Immunology.* (2014) 141:174–80. doi: 10.1111/imm.12167
34. Amaral EP, Ribeiro SC, Lanes VR, Almeida FM, de Andrade MR, Bomfim CC, et al. Pulmonary infection with hypervirulent mycobacteria reveals a crucial role for the P2X7 receptor in aggressive forms of tuberculosis. *PLoS Pathog.* (2014) 10:e1004188. doi: 10.1371/journal.ppat.1004188
35. Lage SL, Buzzo CL, Amaral EP, Matteucci KC, Massis LM, Icimoto MY, et al. Cytosolic flagellin-induced lysosomal pathway regulates inflammasome-dependent and -independent macrophage responses. *Proc Natl Acad Sci USA.* (2013) 110:E3321–30. doi: 10.1073/pnas.1305316110
36. Ravimohan S, Maenetje P, Auld SC, Ncube I, Mlotshwa M, Chase W, et al. A Common NLRC4 gene variant associates with inflammation and pulmonary function in human immunodeficiency virus and tuberculosis. *Clin Infect Dis.* (2019) 22:ciz898. doi: 10.1093/cid/ciz898
37. Lasunskaia E1, Ribeiro SC, Manicheva O, Gomes LL, Suffys PN, Mokrousov I, et al. Emerging multidrug resistant *Mycobacterium tuberculosis* strains of the Beijing genotype circulating in Russia express a pattern of biological properties associated with enhanced virulence. *Microbes Infect.* (2010) 12:467–75. doi: 10.1016/j.micinf.2010.02.008
38. Rocha VC, de Figueiredo SC, Rosales CA, de Hildebrand e Grisi Filho JH, Keid LB, Soares RM, et al. Molecular discrimination of *Mycobacterium bovis* in São Paulo, Brazil. *Vector Borne Zoonotic Dis.* (2013) 13:17–21. doi: 10.1089/vbz.2012.1035
39. Pontillo A, Silva LT, Oshiro TM, Finazzo C, Crovella S, Duarte AJ. HIV-1 induces NALP3-inflammasome expression and interleukin-1β secretion in dendritic cells from healthy individuals but not from HIV-positive patients. *AIDS.* (2012) 26:11–8. doi: 10.1097/QAD.0b013e32834d697f
40. Zhao Y, Yang J, Shi J, Gong YN, Lu Q, Xu H, et al. The NLRC4 inflammasome receptors for bacterial flagellin and type III secretion apparatus. *Nature.* (2011) 477:596–600. doi: 10.1038/nature10510
41. Gebremicael G, Kassa D, Quinten E, Alemayehu Y, Gebreegziaxier A, Belay Y, et al. Host gene expression kinetics during treatment of tuberculosis in HIV-coinfected individuals is independent of highly active antiretroviral therapy. *J Infect Dis.* (2018) 218:1833–46. doi: 10.1093/infdis/jiy404
42. Iannitti RG, Napolioni V, Oikonomou V, De Luca A, Galosi C, Pariano M, et al. IL-1 receptor antagonist ameliorates inflammasome-dependent inflammation in murine and human cystic fibrosis. *Nat Commun.* (2016) 7:10791. doi: 10.1038/ncomms10791
43. Master SS, Rampini SK, Davis AS, Keller C, Ehlers S, Springer B, et al. Mycobacterium tuberculosis prevents inflammasome activation. *Cell Host Microbe.* (2008) 3:224–32. doi: 10.1016/j.chom.2008.03.003

5

The Use of Both Therapeutic and Prophylactic Vaccines in the Therapy of Papillomavirus Disease

Anna Rosa Garbuglia[1*]*, Daniele Lapa*[1]*, Catia Sias*[1]*, Maria Rosaria Capobianchi*[1] *and Paola Del Porto*[2]

[1] *Laboratory of Virology, "Lazzaro Spallanzani" National Institute for Infectious Diseases, IRCCS, Rome, Italy,* [2] *Department of Biology and Biotechnology "C. Darwin," Sapienza University, Rome, Italy*

***Correspondence:**
Anna Rosa Garbuglia
argarbuglia@iol.it

Human papillomavirus (HPV) is the most common sexually transmitted virus. The high-risk HPV types (i.e., HPV16, 18, 31, 33, 35, 39, 45, 51, 52, 56, 58, 59) are considered to be the main etiological agents of genital tract cancers, such as cervical, vulvar, vaginal, penile, and anal cancers, and of a subset of head and neck cancers. Three prophylactic HPV vaccines are available that are bivalent (vs. HPV16, 18), tetravalent (vs. HPV6, 11, 16, 18), and non-avalent (vs. HPV6, 11, 16, 18, 31, 33,45, 52, 58). All of these vaccines are based on recombinant DNA technology, and they are prepared from the purified L1 protein that self-assembles to form the HPV type-specific empty shells (i.e., virus-like particles). These vaccines are highly immunogenic and induce specific antibodies. Therapeutic vaccines differ from prophylactic vaccines, as they are designed to generate cell-mediated immunity against transformed cells, rather than neutralizing antibodies. Among the HPV proteins, the E6 and E7 oncoproteins are considered almost ideal as targets for immunotherapy of cervical cancer, as they are essential for the onset and evolution of malignancy and are constitutively expressed in both premalignant and invasive lesions. Several strategies have been investigated for HPV therapeutic vaccines designed to enhance $CD4^+$ and $CD8^+$ T-cell responses, including genetic vaccines (i.e., DNA/ RNA/virus/ bacterial), and protein-based, peptide-based or dendritic-cell-based vaccines. However, no vaccine has yet been licensed for therapeutic use. Several studies have suggested that administration of prophylactic vaccines immediately after surgical treatment of CIN2 cervical lesions can be considered as an adjuvant to prevent reactivation or reinfection, and other studies have described the relevance of prophylactic vaccines in the management of genital warts. This review summarizes the leading features of therapeutic vaccines, which mainly target the early oncoproteins E6 and E7, and prophylactic vaccines, which are based on the L1 capsid protein. Through an analysis of the specific immunogenic properties of these two types of vaccines, we discuss why and how prophylactic vaccines can be effective in the treatment of HPV-related lesions and relapse.

Keywords: human papillomavirus, immune response, cancer, prophylactic vaccine, therapeutic vaccine

INTRODUCTION

Despite the introduction of prophylactic vaccines, the incidence of human papillomavirus (HPV)-related tumors remains high (1), particularly in developing countries of the sub-Saharan region. The current HPV prophylactic vaccines have indications for use in women up to the age of 45 years, but they are predominantly administered to adolescent of 9–15 years. As most cancers develop decades after an initial HPV infection, the impact of this vaccination program will be seen in the long-term. Therefore, setting-up a therapeutic vaccine that can provide results similar to surgical treatment or chemotherapy represents a challenge for the eradication of HPV-induced tumors. However, therapeutic vaccines are not yet available for clinical practice.

Several studies have suggested that administration of HPV prophylactic vaccines after surgical treatment of high-grade cervical intraepithelial neoplasia (CIN2-3) can be considered as an adjuvant to prevent HPV reactivation or reinfection. The relevance of prophylactic vaccines has also been demonstrated in the management of genital warts, although clinical studies have not delivered univocal results to date.

In this review, the HPV-related tumors and the life cycle of HPV are described, to better understand the characteristics of the different viral proteins that are targeted by prophylactic and therapeutic vaccines. Then, we summarize the leading features of prophylactic and therapeutic vaccines that target the L1 and E6, E7 oncoproteins, respectively. Finally, through an analysis of the specific immunogenic properties of these two types of vaccines, we discuss how prophylactic vaccines can be effective for the treatment of HPV-related lesions, and for prevention of HPV-related relapse.

HPV PREVALENCE

Human papillomavirus is the main agent of sexually transmitted diseases, and it can cause cancer in different anatomical districts with different prevalences (2). The highest proportion of HPV attribution as responsible for a cancer is for the cervix, where >99% of specimens are HPV-positive. In 2012, HPV-invasive cervical cancers reached >500,000 cases, which resulted in ~250,000 deaths around the world[1]. HPV-related cancers are differently distributed across genders: among women, 8.6% of cancers are linked to HPV infections, while in men, <1% of cancers are attributable to HPV[2,3]. Differences are also observed in the geographic distributions of invasive cervical cancers: more than 85% occur in developing countries, where cervical screening programs and HPV vaccination campaigns are rarely available[4] (3, 4). HPV infection in a cervical site is frequently asymptomatic, and >90% of these resolve within 2 years without medical intervention (5), apparently through rapid immune clearance. However, the protective power of natural anti-HPV antibodies and the duration of immunity after infection are not fully understood. Also, only 50–60% of women show detectable anti-HPV antibodies after infection (6).

There are 15 high-risk (HR)-HPV genotypes that can lead to cancers of the cervix, anus, penis, vagina, vulva, and oropharynx (i.e., HPV16, 18, 3, 33, 35, 39, 45, 51, 52, 56, 58, 68, 73, 82) (7). The relevance of HPV to each of these individual cancers is now considered.

Cervical Cancer

Overall, 90% of cervical cancers are attributed to HR-HPV types. HPV16 and HPV18 are the most prevalent in invasive cervical cancer, where they account for 62.5 and 15.7% of cases, respectively (8). HPV-associated cancers include cervical squamous cell carcinoma (70%), cervical adenocarcinoma (25%), and mixed histology tumors (7)[5]. An immunocompromised status represents a risk factor for cervical dysplasia, as well as for latent reactivation of HPV at genital sites. Patients with human immunodeficiency virus (HIV) infection have a 5-fold greater risk of acquiring HPV-associated cervical cancer than those without HIV infection. Precancerous (squamous) intraepithelial lesions are categorized as low-grade (LSIL) and high-grade (HSIL) (9).

Anal Cancer

Anal intraepithelial neoplasia (AIN1-3) represents the precursor of invasive anal cancers, where 65% are cervical squamous cell carcinomas. For both sexes, 88–94% of these cancerous lesions are positive for HPV DNA, with HPV16 as the most commonly detected (~87% of HPV-positive tumors), while only 9% of these anal cancers harbors HR-HPV18[6].

Annually, about 18,000 women are diagnosed with anal cancer worldwide, and this cancer is more frequent in women than in men (10). Furthermore, anal cancer incidence is increasing, which appears to be due to changes in sexual risk factors for HPV transmission (11). Persistent anal HPV infection is the major cause of anal cancer[7] (12). Women with a history of cervical cancer and cervical intraepithelial neoplasia grade 3 (HSIL) are also at increased risk of anal cancer. Cervical HR-HPV–positivity is associated with anal HR-HPV prevalence. In a study carried out by Lin, anal HR-HPV prevalence was significantly higher in cervical HR-HPV–positive women (43%) vs. cervical HR-HPV–negative women (9%) (13). These associations were even stronger for HPV16-positivity: in cervical HPV16-positive women, anal HPV16 prevalence was 41%, while in the HPV16-negative cervical group, anal HPV16 prevalence was 2%.

In men, the risk of anal cancer development is strictly related to sexual behavior and HIV immune status (14).

Penile Cancer

Approximately 50% of penile cancers can be attributed to HPV infections, although HPV also infects healthy subjects without progressing to neoplasia. In a British study carried out among 43 couples, 69% of the men were HPV-positive in the uro-genital tract (15). Another study in the USA showed similar high levels of

[1]https://gco.iarc.fr/
[2]https://publications.iarc.fr/108
[3]https://monographs.iarc.fr/wp-content/uploads/2018/06/mono100B-11.pdf
[4]http://globocan.iarc.fr/old/FactSheets/cancers/cervix-new.asp

[5]https://seer.cancer.gov/archive/csr/1975_2004/
[6]https://monographs.iarc.fr/wp-content/uploads/2018/06/mono90.pdf
[7]https://monographs.iarc.fr/wp-content/uploads/2018/06/mono100B.pdf

HPV prevalence, with 65.5% of the men HPV-positive: 51.2% of them harbored at least one typed HPV, and 14.3% of them were positive for an unclassified HPV infection (16). HPV clearance is observed in 75% of cases within 1 year (17). HPV-positivity is greater in penile intraepithelial neoplasia (PIN 1,2,3), which is considered the precursor of penile cancer, and in basaloid histological neoplasia (range, 75–80%) than in invasive cervical squamous cell carcinoma (range, 30–60%). HPV16 and HPV18 are the HPV types that are most frequently associated with all types of penile cancers[2].

Vulvar Cancer

It is estimated that 40–50% of vulvar cancers are associated with HPV. Overall, vulvar cancers represented 3% of gynecologic cancers in 2002 (18), and 60% of were observed in developed countries (18, 19)[8]. Vulvar intraepithelial neoplasia (VIN) is considered a precursor of vulvar squamous cell carcinoma, which represents >90% of vulvar cancers (20). The World Health Organization recognizes a three-grade system of VIN (i.e., VIN1-3), and VIN3 is considered as a precursor of invasive vulvar cancer. However, until recently, VIN2-3 had been considered as HSIL, and VIN1 (or LSIL) is no longer used, as there is misclassification of these low-grade lesions: these are often actually condilomata acuminata with transient HPV infection, or an inflammatory status of the vulva (21). VIN can be caused by two distinct etiological agents: HPV, which is linked to the usual form of VIN (uVIN), and differentiated VIN (dVIN) is associated with lichen sclerosus (22, 23). Generally, uVIN is common among young women, while dVIN is frequently seen for post-menopausal women. In VIN3/HSIL lesions, HPV16 had been detected in >91% of cases (24).

Vaginal Cancer

Cancer of the vagina is rare, and it accounts for only 2% of gynecological neoplasia. Nevertheless, from 2000 to 2015 there was an increase in vaginal cancer, which corresponded to 0.4% of vulvar carcinomas in the USA[9]. Vaginal intraepithelial neoplasia (VAIN) is considered a pre-malignant lesion. Previously, a three-tiered classified was used (VAIN1-3) according to epithelial involvement. In 2014, the World Health Organization revised this classification by substituting VAIN2-3 with HSIL, and VAIN1 with LSIL (25). About 82% of high-grade lesions (i.e., vaginal intraepithelial lesions, VAIN3, HSIL) and 91% of invasive vaginal carcinomas test positive for HPV DNA and/or HPV antibodies. HPV16 is the most prevalent HPV type in HSIL and vaginal cancers[2] (26–29).

Head and Neck Cancer

The most common head and neck cancers are squamous cell carcinomas (HNC) and they include neoplasia of the oral cavity, tongue, tonsils, oropharynx, hypopharynx, and larynx. The HR-HPV types most frequently detected in head and neck cancers are HPV16, followed by HPV18[2] (30, 31). Head and neck cancers are frequent in southern-central Asia (32); however, an increase in head and neck cancer incidence has been seen over recent years in developed countries (33) and among Caucasian men (34). Tonsillectomies can increase the overall survival rates of patients with diagnosis of tonsil carcinoma (35), but it does not influence the overall risk of oropharyngeal cancer (36).

A reduction in HPV-positive oropharyngeal cancer is observed in people with a specific genetic locus in the human leukocyte antigen region (HLA-DRB1*1301-HLA-DQA1*0103-HLA-DQB1*0603) (37). This protective effect might involve increased immune targeting of HPV-infected cells through the major histocompatibility complex haplotype binding to HPV peptides, resulting in a strong $CD4^+$ T-cell response (38).

Respiratory Papillomatosis

Different annual incidences of respiratory papillomatosis have been reported in different countries. For example, in Denmark, similar incidence has been reported in children (juvenile onset) (3.6/100,000 children) and in adults (3.9/100,000 adults) (38), while in the USA the annual respiratory papillomatosis incidence is 3-fold higher in children than in adults (4.6 vs. 3.9/100,000 children/adults) (39).

HPV6 and HPV11 are the main genotypes detected in respiratory papillomatosis. As spontaneous regression is rarely observed, surgical treatment is necessary to prevent progression of the lesions. Moreover, recurrence of papillomatosis is often observed, and retreatment is needed in most cases, which comes at a high economic burden (40). Although no structured trials have been carried out to date, HPV vaccine administration prior to the onset of sexual behavior might have a positive impact on prevention of respiratory papillomatosis in adulthood.

Genital Warts

Human papillomavirus infection can not only cause cancer, but also benign genital warts. These are very diffuse in the young and in adults, with prevalence from 4 to 11% (41–43). Treatment of genital warts includes therapies with imiquimod and podophyllotoxin, or surgical procedures, or cryotherapy and tricloroacetic acid. These medical interventions represent high costs for both private insurance (44) and health systems (45).

Condylomas were classically considered a benign lesion, with the exception of Buscke-Lowenstein tumors. This large tumor can undergo local invasion and can transform into anal cervical squamous cell carcinoma (46).

VIRAL CHARACTERISTICS AND IMMUNE RESPONSES

Life Cycle of HPV

Human papillomaviruses are non-enveloped icosahedral viruses that consist of 72 capsomers and are 55 nm in diameter. The viral genome is a circular double stranded DNA of ~8,000 bp in length.

According to the time-regulated expression of proteins during the viral cycle, three functional genome regions can be distinguished: (i) the early region that encodes the E1, E2, E4, E5, E6, E7, E8 viral proteins that have regulatory functions in infected epithelial cells; (ii) the late region that encodes the two

[8] https://www.ncbi.nlm.nih.gov/books/NBK12354/

[9] http://www.seer.cancer.gov

viral capsid proteins L1 and L2; and (iii) the long control regions (also known as upstream regulatory regions) that contain *cis*-acting regulatory sequences that are involved in the control of viral replication and post-transcriptional phases (**Figure 1**).

Different viral proteins are expressed in different layers of the epithelium. The early proteins are expressed in basal epithelial cells, while the late proteins are expressed in the granular layer that includes more differentiated cells, and from where the virus is assembled and released. E1 is an ATPase helicase that is involved with E2 in viral replication and transcription regulation. The E1 and E2 complex interacts with the long control region ori site, which is considered to be the origin of HPV DNA replication (47–53). In the initial phase of infection, the HPV DNA genome is in the episomal form. It shows low amplification activity and there are ~100 copies/cell (54). E2 ensures episomal maintenance of the HPV genome through interactions with other cellular factors. For example, Bromo-domain protein 4 (BRD4) is a mitotic chromosome-associated protein that is a critical binding partner for E2 for this activity (55). BRD4 and E2 co-localize on condensed mitotic chromosomes, and mediate episome segregation (55). E2 also regulates transcription of the E6 and E7 oncoproteins, the expression of which depends on an early promoter. E1 to E4 are encoded by a spliced RNA, and along with E5, they are translated under early promoter control in undifferentiated cells, and they appear to facilitate efficient productive replication in differentiating cells (56, 57).

E6 and E7 are small proteins of about 150 and 100 amino acids, respectively. The E6 oncoprotein acts through its PDZ-binding motif, which promotes its interactions with PDZ domains in multidomain proteins, to alter their functionality. These PDZ domains are present in many multidomain proteins that regulate key steps in the cellular processes of apoptosis, adhesion, and polarity (37–43, 58). E6 also impairs the activity of the p53 protein, which prevents DNA damage accumulation through induction of DNA repair, cell-cycle arrest, or apoptosis, which leads to transformation of HPV chronically infected cells.

The main targets of E7 are the pRB, p107, and p130 proteins, which are components of a complex that can repress the E2F transcription factor (59, 60). When E7 interacts with pRB, p107, and p130, it induces their degradation, and so E2F is free to activate genes such as cyclins A and E, to promote transition from G1 to S-phase of the cell cycle (61). The productive viral cycle also includes the synthesis of the late proteins L1 and L2 in the suprabasal epithelial cell layers, and this step is characterized by a change in mRNA splicing (62, 63). Icosahedral virions are composed of 360 L1 proteins that are organized in pentamers, each of which is associated with one monomer of L2. The productive life cycle is completed when the virions self-assemble, after packaging of the amplified HPV DNA genome, with the viral particles then shed from the epithelial cell layers (64).

Natural Immune Response

The immune response has an important role in clearing most HPV infections, although sometime the virus cannot be eliminated and can persist for several years, which represents a risk factor for neoplasia development (65). HPV-associated neoplastic progression is linked to dysregulated expression of the early viral genes. Specifically, increased expression of the E6 and E7 proteins in the basal epithelium leads to increased cell-cycle entry and loss of differentiation across the epithelium. The main cause of dysregulated HPV gene expression is integration of the viral genome into the host chromosomes (66). HPV DNA integrates randomly into the host DNA. During this process, the viral DNA can often be broken at any position within the E1-E2 region, with the loss of E2 function, and the consequent overexpression of E6 and E7 that promotes cellular transformation (67–69). However, a proportion of cervical cancers are associated with episomal DNA only. In such cases, the E2 open reading frame integrity is maintained, and this protein is expressed throughout the progression of the malignancy.

In natural infections, both humoral- and cell-mediated immune responses are induced. Genital infection with oncogenic HPV is common, but only a minority of infected patients develop epithelial lesions or cancer (70). Spontaneous clearance of an established infection is likely to be mediated by the cellular immune responses. Indeed, strong Th1 $CD4^+$ T-cell responses that are specific for HPV16 E6, E7, and E2 have been frequently detected in peripheral blood mononuclear cells of healthy individuals (71). In contrast, responses against HPV16 E6, E7, and E2 have rarely been detected in patients with HPV16-positive genital lesions or antigen-specific proliferative responses that show a non-inflammatory cytokine profile (72, 73).

Similarly, effective HPV18-specific T-cell responses are only seen in healthy controls, and not in HPV18-positive patients (74). For the role of $CD8^+$ T-cells in disease regression, a comparison of $CD8^+$ T-cell responses to E6 and E7 using enzyme-linked immunospot assays in individuals with incident or prevalent HPV 16 or 18 infections did not show any significant difference in the frequency of positivity between these two patient groups (33 vs. 40%) (75). At variance with this, in CIN2/3 lesions, more $CD8^+$ T-cells were seen for the epidermis of tissues that went on to regress (76). Also, large numbers of intraepithelial $CD8^+$ tumor-infiltrating lymphocytes have been associated with an absence of lymph-node metastases in patients with large early stage cervical cancer (76). Taken together, these findings indicate that the development of high-risk HPV-positive cervical cancer is associated with failure of HPV-specific T-cell responses.

The humoral immune response to HPV infection is mainly directed against conformational epitopes in the variable regions of the major coat protein L1 (77). This develops slowly, and is usually weak. Indeed, seroconversion appears to occur 6–18 months after infection, and type-specific antibodies to L1 are detected in 60–70% of women who acquire HPV infection (6, 78). HPV-seroprevalence is considerably lower in men than women, and it has been suggested that HPV-seropositive women might have higher antibody levels than HPV-seropositive men (79).

IgG and IgA are the most abundant isotypes in sera from natural infections. Other HPV antigens (e.g., E1, E2, E6, L2) do not commonly induce antibody responses in patients with acute or persistent HPV infections.

Studies that have investigated whether naturally acquired HPV antibodies can protect against subsequent HPV infections

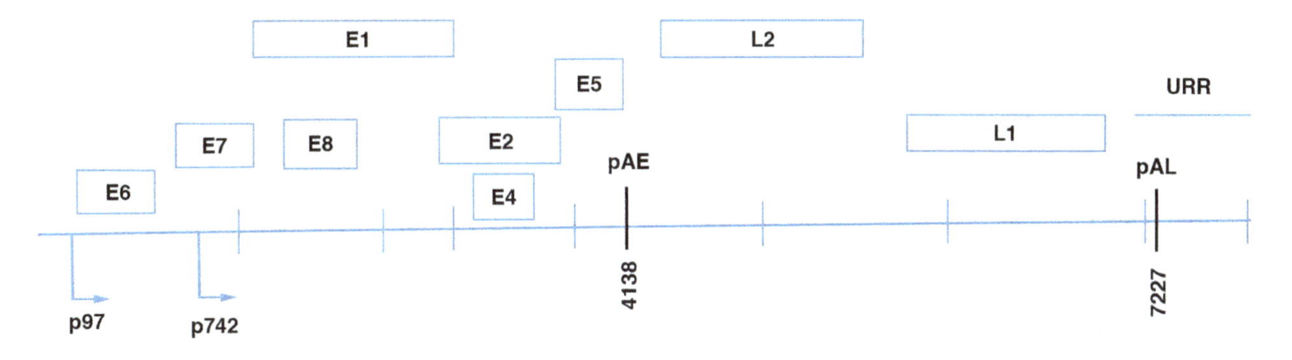

FIGURE 1 | Linear diagram of HPV16 genome showing the eight open reading frames (ORFs), the early (pAE), and the late (pAL) polyadenilation sites; p97, promoter of E6 and E7 viral oncoproteins; p670, promoter of the late proteins.

have reported mixed results (80–82). More recently a systematic review and meta-analysis that included >24,000 individuals showed that natural HPV antibodies provide protection against subsequent type-specific genital HPV infections in females. However, given that the antibody titers in natural immunity are considerably lower than those observed with vaccination, and that antibody responses are preferentially induced in women and are not induced in all infected individuals, it is likely that protection through the development of natural immunity is inferior to protection obtained from HPV vaccination (83).

HPV VACCINES

Prophylactic Vaccines

Three prophylactic vaccines for prevention of HPV infection are available at present: a bivalent vaccine against HPV16 and HPV18 (Cervarix) that was approved in 2007; a tetravalent vaccine against HPV6, 11, 16, and 18 (Gardasil) that was approved in 2006; and a nonavalent vaccine against HPV6, 11, 18, 31, 33, 45, 52, 58 (Gardasil 9) that was approved in 2016. However, the non-avalent vaccine is the only HPV vaccine that is currently available in the USA, and it was approved for males and females from 9 to 45 years by the US Food and Drug Administration in late 2018.

Initially, the administration of the HPV vaccines was in three doses, with the more recent change to a two-dose schedule driven by evaluation of girls aged 9–13 years who had received either two or three doses. The antibody responses of the young women (aged 16–26 years) who had followed a two-dose schedule were similar to those who received all three doses (84). Therefore, in 2016, the Advisory Committee on Immunization Practice declared that there was only the need for two doses of vaccine for those under 15 years of age. However, for females who start the vaccination between 15 and 45 years old, a three-dose schedule is recommended (at 0, 1–2, and 6 months) (84, 85)[10]. Also immunocompromised patients should follow the three-dose schedule regardless of sex and age at vaccination (86).

[10]https://www.cdc.gov/hpv/dowloads/9vhpv-guidance.pdf

All three of these vaccines use recombinant DNA technology and are prepared from the purified L1 protein, which self-assembles to form HPV type-specific empty shells (virus-like particles; VLPs). Only intact VLPs can generate protective antibodies, which supports the evidence that conformational epitopes of L1 are required to generate neutralizing antibodies (87).

The evidence that HPV VLP vaccines protect against high viral challenges through induction of neutralizing anti-L1 antibodies was obtained in preclinical studies in animals, which thus provided the strong rationale for development of VLP-based vaccines. In particular, in a canine model of experimentally induced oral papillomas, it was demonstrated that dogs vaccinated with the major capsid protein, L1, of canine oral papillomavirus developed antibodies against canine oral papillomavirus and became completely resistant to the viral challenge (88). Similarly, vaccination of rabbits with L1 VLPs protected them against papillomas induced by cottontail rabbit papillomavirus (89). In addition, in both of these animal models, passive transfer of immune serum protected the dogs and rabbits against the canine oral papillomavirus and cottontail rabbit papillomavirus challenges, respectively.

In humans, analysis of vaccine-induced antibody responses measured by several methods has demonstrated that almost 100% of vaccinated individuals generate a strong type-restricted serum antibody response to L1 VLP. These methods have included conventional enzyme-linked immunosorbent assays, competitive radioimmunoassays, competitive Luminex-based immunoassays, and pseudovirion-based neutralization assays.

Initial and follow-up studies that assessed the immunogenicity of the HPV 16/18 AS04-adjuvant vaccine in 15- to 25-year-old women showed that after vaccination, anti-HPV16 and anti-HPV18 total IgG antibodies peaked at month 7, reached a plateau between months 18 and 24, and remained constant for up to 76 months (90). Measurement of the neutralizing antibodies using pseudovirion-based neutralization assays confirmed high levels of functional antibodies as well. Then evaluation of long-term immunogenicity of the HPV16/18 vaccine in the serum of 15- to 55-year-old females revealed that the seropositivity for anti-HPV16 remained high in all of the age groups 10 years after the first vaccination. For anti-HPV18, there were more seropositive females in the 15- to 25-year-old group (99.2%) than for the 26- to 45-year-olds (93.7%) and 46- to 55-year-olds (83.8%) (90). In these studies, the anti-HPV16 and anti-HPV18 titers remained above natural infection levels in all of the age groups, and more interestingly, they were predicted to persist for more than 30 years after vaccination (91).

Comparisons of the immunogenicities of the HPV16/18 and HPV6/11/16/18 vaccines in healthy women aged 18–45 years revealed that 7 months after vaccination, the serum neutralizing antibody responses elicited by the bivalent vaccine were significantly higher than those for the HPV6/11/16/18 vaccine. The differences in these responses for HPV16 and HPV18 were maintained at month 24, and also up to month 60 in women aged 18–45 years.

Antibody titers induced by vaccination are higher than those produced by natural infection[11]. Responses to HPV vaccination is weakly influenced by gender, with higher seroconversion in males than females (99 vs. 93%), and by age, with higher antibody titers in women aged 9–15 years (92, 93). The FUTURE I trial demonstrated that the efficacy of the tetravalent HPV vaccine was 100% against condyloma in HPV-naïve women, and 70% (vaginal condyloma) to 78% (vulvar condyloma) in the overall population. The efficacy of the non-avalent vaccine is comparable to that of the tetravalent vaccine against condyloma (94). Prophylactic HPV vaccines show excellent protection against high-grade CIN (i.e., CIN2, CIN3) and adenocarcinoma *in situ* for HR-HPV-naïve women. In particular, the non-avalent vaccine showed the highest efficacy for prevention of onset of CIN1 (relative risk reduction, 98.9%), CIN2 (97.1%), and CIN3 (100%) neoplasia (95).

Data for vaccine prevention against AIN are more limited. In the Guanacaste study, the tetravalent HPV vaccine prevented HPV16/18 infection in anal anatomic sites in 84% of women who were HPV-seronegative at baseline (96). Palefsky reported 77.5% prevention of AIN among HPV-naïve men aged 16–26 years who had sex with men (MSM) (97). The tetravalent vaccine also protects heterosexual naïve men from both anogenital HPV infections and HPV lesions, with an efficacy against infections and associated lesions of >90% (98). Also a Finnish randomized trial reported significant reduction of genital HPV infections in men following HPV16/18 vaccine administration (99).

For oropharyngeal cancer prevention, a risk reduction of 93.3% for precursor lesions of HPV-induced oral cancer was reported for the Guanacaste study (96). However, further studies are needed to demonstrate the efficacy of these vaccines on oropharyngeal cancer development.

Therapeutic Vaccines

The therapeutic vaccines differ from the prophylactic vaccines as they are aimed at the generation of cell-mediated immunity, rather than neutralizing antibodies. Although prophylactic vaccines can prevent HPV infections in 100% of cases, and precancerous cervical lesions (i.e., CIN) caused by the HPV genotypes included in the vaccine, HPV-related lesions remain a public problem worldwide for several reasons: (i) only 8% of low and middle income countries have introduced HPV vaccination programs[12]; (ii) HPV types that are not included in vaccines might be responsible for cancers (100); (iii) the cost of requirements for a cold chain and the absence of sanitary infrastructure limits HPV vaccine deployment in developing countries; and (iv) HPV vaccines are recommended for young women (9–26 years old), and as women older than 26 years are not vaccinated, they can develop cancers. It is also estimated that the impact of HPV vaccination on cancer incidence might not be appreciated for at least 20 years from any mass vaccination.

TABLE 1 | Conventional treatment of HPV-related cancers.

Cancer HPV related lesion	Conventional treatment
High-grade CIN	1. Loop electrosurgical excision procedure. 2. Cold knife. 3. Cone biopsy. 4. Electrofulgaration. 5. Cold-coagulation. 6. Cryotherapy.
Cervical cancer	1. Conization. 2. Radical hysterectomy. 3. Chemotherapy.
Vulvar intraepithelial neoplasia (VIN) and vulvar cancer	1. Surgical excision. 2. Topical agents (imiquimod). 3. Photodynamic therapy.
AIN and anal cancer	1. Ablative. 2. Chemotherapy (5-fluoracil, imiquimod, cidofovir).
PeIN and penile cancer	1. Surgical treatment. 2. Cisplatinum-based regimen.

CIN, cervical intraepithelial neoplasia; AIN, anal intraepithelial neoplasia; PeIN, penile intraepithelial neoplasia.

Currently, the treatment of high-grade disease (CIN2-3) includes electrosurgical excision of the transformation zone, with carbon dioxide lasers or knives used to perform conization, where the entire transformation zone is removed (101, 102) (**Table 1**). Incomplete excision, however, can occur, and HPV transformed cells can remain, which will facilitate recurrent neoplasia. Hence, there is the need for a therapeutic vaccine that can fully eliminate malignant cells.

The aim of a therapeutic vaccine against HPV is to induce *in-vivo* virus-specific T-cell responses against established HPV infections and lesions. For therapeutic vaccination to deliver unequivocal clinical benefits, improvements must be achieved at two levels: by maximizing the induction of T-cell responses with optimal amplitude, specificity and effector profile; and by ensuring that vaccine-induced T-cells can reach the tumor site and perform their functions without restraint (103).

Among the HPV proteins, the E6 and E7 oncoproteins are considered to be almost ideal targets for immunotherapy of cervical cancer, as these proteins are essential for the onset and

[11]http://www.rho.org/files/WHO_HPV_tech_info_nocover_2007.pdf

[12]https://apps.who.int/iris/bitstream/handle/10665/251810/WER9148.pdf; jsessionid=12D591BAA8A2E02CEB5223020DFC3526?sequence=1

evolution of malignancy, and are constitutively expressed in both premalignant and invasive lesions, while being absent in healthy cells (104). E6 and E7 have therefore been included in most therapeutic vaccines developed to date. Usually, a DNA sequence that encodes a fusion protein of E6 and E7 is inserted into a vector, and mutations are introduced into the regions that are responsible for the E6 interactions with p53, and the E7 interactions with pRB, to reduce their oncogenic power. The E1 and E2 viral proteins are also attractive candidates for therapeutic vaccines that target early viral infections, as they are highly expressed before viral genome integration (105).

Several strategies have been investigated for HPV therapeutic vaccines designed to enhance $CD4^{+}$ and $CD8^{+}$ T-cell responses, including genetic vaccines (e.g., DNA/ RNA/ virus/ bacterial), and protein-based, peptide-based or dendritic-cell-based vaccines. Among the bacterial vectors, live attenuated *Listeria monocytogenes* has been used to generate a promising HPV therapeutic vaccine. *L. monocytogenes* is considered a potent vaccine vector because it enters professional antigen-presenting cells and induces antigen-presenting cell maturation, and strong innate and adaptive immunity (106). In addition, *L. monocytogenes* grows very efficiently *in vitro* and lacks lipopolysaccharides, which are a major toxicity factor with Gram-negative bacteria (104). The safety of a recombinant live attenuated *L. monocytogenes* secreting E7 as a fusion protein joined to non-hemolytic listeriolysin O (*Lm*-LLO-E7) was demonstrated in a phase I clinical study that was conducted with 15 patients with late-stage metastatic cervical cancer (107). Evaluation of the efficacy of *Lm*-LLO-E7 (also known as ADXS11-001) in a prospective phase II clinical trial as second-line and third line for patients with recurrent metastatic cervical cancer showed that 12-month overall survival was 38%, which exceeded the historical overall survival of such patients, of 25%. A phase III clinical trial of *Lm*-LLO-E7 for high-grade cervical cancer is being conducted at the time of writing (see NCT02853604).

Encouraging data have also been obtained in clinical studies that have tested DNA-based vaccines. DNA vaccination consists of direct introduction into tissues of a plasmid that contains the DNA sequence that encodes the antigen(s) against which an immune response is sought. This relies on *in-situ* production of the antigen(s) as a result of the transfection of antigen-presenting cells and non-antigen-presenting cells, with the presentation of the expressed antigen(s) by both MHC class I and class II molecules. Furthermore, this results in activation of all three arms of the adaptive immune response (i.e., helper T cells, cytotoxic T cells, antibodies).

However, although DNA vaccines have been shown to induce balanced $CD4^{+}$ and $CD8^{+}$ T cells as well as humoral immune responses in small animal models, clinical data from multiple studies have demonstrated that they induce poor T-cell responses (108).

Many strategies to facilitate antigen processing and presentation, and also antigen delivery, have been adopted to ameliorate the immunogenicity of DNA vaccines against HPV (109–111).

A phase I study was carried out using the DNA vaccine VGX-3100 that consists of a mixture of two plasmids that encode the optimized consensus of the E6 and E7 genes of HPV genotypes 16 and 18. These were delivered via intramuscular injection, followed by electroporation, with 18 patients who had been previously treated for cervical intraepithelial neoplasia (CIN2/3). This study showed that 78% of the patients developed CD8+ T-cell responses, and 100% showed antibody positivity to at least two vaccine antigens (112). Notably, the peripheral blood T-cell responses elicited by VGX-3100 were an order of magnitude greater than naturally occurring responses, and a log unit greater than those previously reported for HPV therapeutic vaccines (112).

In 2015, the efficacy, safety, and immunogenicity of VGX-3100 was assessed in a phase II clinical trial in patients with CIN2/3. In the per-protocol analysis, 30.6% of the placebo recipients and 49.5% of the VGX-3100 recipients showed histological regression. Concomitant histopathological regression and viral clearance occurred in 14.3% of placebo recipients compared with 40.2% of vaccinated recipients (113). *Post-hoc* immunological analysis here demonstrated that VGX-3100 elicited significantly increased frequency of T-cell responses against HPV16/18 E6 and E7, and that the magnitude of the T-cell response against E6 was associated with clinical outcome. Humoral immune responses were also lower in placebo recipients than in VGX-3100 recipients, and the antibody responses against HPV16, HPV18, and E7 were significantly higher in the patients who had concomitant histopathological regression and viral clearance, compared to those who did not (113). A phase III clinical trial of VGX-3100 for women with CIN was initiated in 2017, and it is expected to end in 2021 (see NCT03185013).

Viral vectors including adenoviruses, adeno-associated viruses, alphaviruses, and vaccinia viruses (e.g., modified vaccinia Ankara virus; MVA) can be used to express the E2, E6, and E7 oncoproteins, and they can stimulate $CD4^{+}$ and $CD8^{+}$ T-cell responses. A MVA vector was used to produce the Tipapkinogen Sovacivec vaccine, which includes three exogenous genes that encode the human cytokine interleukin-2, and non-oncogenic E6 and E7. This vaccinia virus can induce interferon-α production and express HPV16 E6 and E7, which are presented by dendritic cells to activate naïve T cells in lymph nodes. At a follow-up of 2.5 years, compared to the placebo cohort at 10% viral clearance, the administration of Tipapkinogen Sovacivec vaccine provided complete resolution for 24% of patients with CIN2/3, irrespective of their HR-HPV baseline infection (i.e., HPV16, 18, 31, 33, 35, 39, 45, 52, 56, 58, 59, or 68). However, despite this significantly improved HPV viral clearance with this vaccine, it has still not been licensed for clinical use because of the modest efficacy (104).

Finally, a vaccine designed on recombinant MVA that contained the bovine papillomavirus E2 protein (MVA E2) was used to treat HPV-induced ano-genital intraepithelial lesions. A phase III study showed that 90% of female patients had complete elimination of lesions after treatment with MVA E2, with 100% seen for men. All of these patients treated with MVA E2 developed antibodies against the MVA E2 vaccine and generated a specific cytotoxic response against the papilloma-transformed cells (114).

Interestingly, novel vaccination strategies aimed to maximize systemic as well as genital resident memory T cell responses to treat sexually transmitted infections and human papilloma virus neoplasia are being developed. In this context several studies have investigated the effect of either the topical delivery of host and pathogen derived immunomodulatory molecules or the delivery route of immunization in the induction of cervicovaginal long lived CD8+ T cell responses (115).

HPV PROPHYLACTIC VACCINES USED AS THERAPEUTIC VACCINES

The treatment of premalignant lesions (CIN2,3) by LLEP or conization sometimes fails to prevent lesion recurrence (116–118). This is often linked to incomplete excision of transformation zone consciously carried out by gynecologists. In fact, evidence shows that large excision of the cervix can compromise cervix integrity and can cause adverse neonatal outcome with preterm risk (119, 120). Moreover, recurrence risk is greater in presence of HR HPV infection (116, 121).

A systematic review of studies of the treatment of high-grade lesions (HSIL/ CIN2-3) reported that a median of 28% of the women remained positive for oncogenic HPV types 3 months after treatment. A decrease in this HPV persistence was seen during follow-up, as it fell to 21% after 6 months (102). Also, higher risks for the development of cervical and vaginal neoplasia have been reported for women who had previously been treated for CIN3, in comparison to the general female population, with this higher risk persisting for 20–25 years, and possibly longer (122). The risk of cervical cancer after treatment also increases with age. A large study with long-term follow-up for women treated for CIN3 reported standard incidence and mortality ratios (i.e., treated vs. placebo) for cervical and vaginal cancers of 10.58 and 7.60, respectively, for women aged 60–69 years, and 2.03 and 1.52, respectively, for women aged 30–39 years (123). Also, women who had previously reported CIN3 lesions showed greater probability of developing other HPV-related neoplasia of the genital tract (e.g., vaginal, vulvar, anal) or the oropharyngeal district (124).

As no vaccine has yet been licensed for therapeutic use, the prophylactic vaccines have been tested in several trials to determine their effectiveness for prevention of HPV disease recurrence or reinfection after CIN2-3 treatment. The recurrence for MSM who undergo treatment for high-grade anal intraepithelial neoplasia (HGAIN) is particularly high, as 50% show recurrence within 1 year (123). This makes it essential to find a treatment that can reduce the development of high-grade lesions in treated patients. In 2011, the effectiveness of the tetravalent HPV vaccine for the prevention of recurrent HGAIN was evaluated in HIV-negative, self-identified MSM with a history of biopsy-proven and treated HGAIN. In the 340.4 person-years of follow-up, 30.7% of the non-vaccinated patients developed recurrent HGAIN, compared to 13.6% of the vaccinated patients. Among these patients who were infected with HR-HPV types, the tetravalent vaccine was associated with significantly decreased risk of recurrent HGAIN at 2 years from study entry (hazard ratio, 0.47). To explain the partial effectiveness of the tetravalent vaccine in this study, it was speculated that some of these patients might have developed diseases that were related to the HPV genotypes not covered by the tetravalent vaccine or to multiple HPV infections. Further, some HGAIN might not have been identified and treated before the vaccinations, or the viral integration into the host genome had already occurred. Unfortunately, these aspects were not investigated.

In 2013, Kang et al. investigated the effectiveness of the tetravalent HPV vaccine to prevent recurrence of CIN2-3 in patients with high-grade CIN treated by the loop electrosurgical excision procedure (125). Recurrence was seen for 7.2% of the non-vaccinated patients and by 2.5% of the vaccinated patients. In patients infected with HPV16 and/or HPV18, 8.5% of the non-vaccinated patients and 2.5% of the vaccinated patients developed recurrent disease related to these HPV types. Although encouraging, these data indicate that the prophylactic HPV vaccine had weak activity against such HPV16/18-related high-grade lesions. Recently, a prospective clinical project, the SPERANZA study, was carried out to determine the effectiveness of the tetravalent vaccine for reduction of the risk of clinical relapse in women treated for CIN2 (126). Overall, 344 women were included in the study, and 6.4% of the non-vaccinated women showed clinical disease recurrence, while for the vaccinated women, there was only 1.2% recurrence. Vaccination here was associated with significantly reduced risk of subsequent HPV-related high-grade CIN after cervical surgery, at 81.2%. For the non-vaccinated women, the recurrent clinical disease was attributed to HPV11, 16, 18, 31, 33, 45, 53, 82, while for the vaccinated women, the two cases of clinical disease recurrence were associated with HPV33 and HPV82. In this study, about 40% of the patients enrolled were >36 years old, although neither the age range nor the age of women with recurrent clinical disease were reported, and thus it cannot be determined if the efficacy of the tetravalent HPV vaccine was influenced by the age of the patients at the time of their vaccination. At variance with this, a study by Hildesheim et al. included 1,711 women with carcinogenic human HPV infection and 311 women who received loop electrosurgical excision for cervical precancer. Here, there was no evidence that HPV16/18 vaccination alters the fate of an HPV infection present at the time of vaccination, or the rates of cervical infections and lesions after loop electrosurgical excision. For these HPV16/18 infections, in the cohort of women with HPV infection but without precancer, the efficacy of clearance was 5.4%, with progression to CIN1 seen for 15.5%, and to CIN2, for 0.3%. Moreover, after the loop electrosurgical excision, the vaccination had no significant effects on HPV16/18 infections and/or HPV16/18-associated cytological and histological lesions (127).

The data obtained on the efficacy of the tetravalent HPV vaccine for the prevention of anal condylomas are, however, more encouraging (128). Three hundred and thirteen MSM (mean age, 42 years) were enrolled for a median of 981 days. During the follow-up, condyloma developed in 18.8% of non-vaccinated patients, and in 8.6% of vaccinated patients. Moreover, several clinical studies have demonstrated activity for HPV vaccination in the treatment of genital warts (129–131).

Altogether, these data suggest that there is possibility that prophylactic vaccines reduce the risk of HSIL recurrence in previously infected patients, although the exact protective mechanisms in infected individuals is not understood. The high risk of recurring infections is consistent with either auto-inoculation across anatomic sites or new inoculation or episodic reactivation of latent infection. As HPV vaccines prevent infection by induction of L1-specific antibodies that block viral entry, and L1 is not generally expressed during the oncogenic process, it is expected that these vaccines will be effective in the prevention of auto-inoculation or new infections.

The greater effectiveness obtained with prophylactic vaccines in the prevention and regression of genital warts might be related to the integration state of the HPV genome. In genital warts, the virus is not generally integrated into the host genome, and therefore viral particles are produced. In this case, the prophylactic vaccines that block viral entry through induction of L1-specific antibodies can prevent reinfections, which will favor the elimination of the virus. Conversely, in high-grade lesions, the virus genome is often integrated into the host genome, and infected cells do not express L1 and do not produce viral particles. Thus, as transformed cells are frequently in the basal layer of the derma, they will not be recognized by vaccine-induced antibodies, which are ineffective in the control of the disease course.

Furthermore, there are some cases in the treatment of HPV-related cancers where the use of prophylactic vaccines might not be recommended:

(1) Anal and cervical cancers that are not attributable to the HPV types that are included in the non-avalent HPV vaccine. Several studies have demonstrated that half of the HPV infections in MSM are caused by HPV types that are not included in the non-avalent HPV vaccine (132, 133) (**Table 2**). Here, over 2 years of observation, only about 30% of HIV-positive MSM had incidents of HR-HPV infections that were covered by the non-avalent vaccine (134). This situation can be also observed for women (**Table 2**).

(2) HPV DNA-negative cervical tumors. Over recent decades, several studies have reported that some cervical cancers are HPV-negative (135–139). Often, HPV DNA negativity is due to the sensitivity of the methods used in the HPV DNA detection, and so samples that have tested as HPV-negative might show as HPV-positive when retested with more sensitive assays (e.g., nested PCR) (136). The Cancer Genome and Molecular Characterization of Cervical Cancer Study used next-generation sequencing to characterize primary cervical cancers, and it established that 5% of the specimens were HPV-negative. This subset of HPV DNA-negative cancers is mainly observed among adenocarcinoma cancers, and predominantly in gastric-type adenocarcinomas. The pattern of immunostaining of gastric-type adenocarcinomas shows strong and diffuse positivity for MUC-6 and HIK1083 antibodies, which recognize epitopes of gastric pyloric glycoproteins, although they are p16 negative, which is a cell-cycle regulatory protein (140). Gastric-type adenocarcinomas have significantly higher rates of recurrence and mortality than HPV-positive cancers (141, 142). Furthermore, progression and regression of gastric-type adenocarcinomas are independent of HPV infection, and thus HPV vaccine administration here would be inappropriate.

TABLE 2 | Detail of cervical and anal samples from HIV positive patients with squamous intraepithelial lesions and HPV DNA negative or positive for HPV types that are not included in nonavalent vaccine.

		N. of cases (%) Pt HPV- 9v Neg	N. of cases (%) Pt HPV DNA Neg
Cervical samples	LSIL ($n = 231$)	72 (31.2)	70 (30.3)
	HSIL ($n = 55$)	17 (30.9)	6 (10.9)
Anal samples	AIN 1 ($n = 18$)	9 (50)	3 (16.7)
	AIN 2 ($n = 7$)	5 (71.4)	0
	AIN 3 ($n = 1$)	1	0

Pt, patient; LSIL, Low Grade Squamous Intraepithelial Lesion; HSIL, High Grade Squamous Intraepithelial Lesion; AIN, Anal intraepithelial neoplasia; 9v, nonavalent vaccine. These data are partially presented in CME event "Novità nel campo dell'infezione da HPV," Rome, 20th June 2018 INMI L Spallanzani IRCCS.

CONCLUSIONS

The data reported in this review highlight the significant efforts that have been carried out to set-up therapeutic vaccines against HPV-related malignancies. Although several approaches to produce an effective vaccine have been attempted, including the use of proteins, synthetic peptides, and viral proteins expressed in different vectors, and although some of the data appear encouraging, no therapeutic vaccines have been licensed in clinical practice yet. Recently, prophylactic vaccines have been used for treatment of recurrent forms or reinfections in subjects who have previously undergone surgical resection. However, the trials here have offered conflicting results, and vaccination did not guarantee 100% effectiveness. This is probably due to a residual burden of transformed cells that can persist after the surgical treatment, and that are not targeted by the humoral L1-specific immune response induced by the prophylactic vaccines. Although it cannot be excluded that the therapeutic potential of prophylactic vaccines could be improved by using different adjuvants or route of immunization, an additional limit in using prophylactic vaccines for therapeutic purposes is seen by the evidence that the non-avalent vaccine does not include all of the HR-HPV types. As the real extent of protection given by the non-avalent vaccine against other HPV types is not known, its use in the treatment of tumors related to these other HR-HPV types is questionable. Furthermore, for endometrial adenocarcinomas, such as gastric-type adenocarcinomas, which are HPV DNA-negative, careful virological and histological diagnosis must be made before administration of HPV prophylactic vaccines to treat HPV recurrence or reinfection.

REFERENCES

1. Ferlay J, Colombet M, Soerjomataram I, Mathers C, Parkin DM, Piñeros M, et al. Estimating the global cancer incidence and mortality in 2018: GLOBOCAN sources and methods. *Int J Cancer.* (2019) 144:1941–53. doi: 10.1002/ijc.31937
2. Plummer M, de Martel C, Vignat J, Ferlay J, Bray F, Franceschi S. Global burden of cancers attributable to infections in 2012: a synthetic analysis. *Lancet Glob Health.* (2016) 4:e609–16. doi: 10.1016/S2214-109X(16)30143-7
3. Crosbie EJ, Einstein MH, Franceschi S, Kitchener HC. Human papillomavirus and cervical cancer. *Lancet.* (2013) 382:889–99. doi: 10.1016/S0140-6736(13)60022-7
4. Vaccarella S, Franceschi S, Engholm G, Lönnberg S, Khan S, Bray F. 50 years of screening in the Nordic countries: quantifying the effects on cervical cancer incidence. *Br J Cancer.* (2014) 111:965–9. doi: 10.1038/bjc.2014.362
5. Moscicki AB, Schiffman M, Kjaer S, Villa LL. Chapter 5: updating the natural history of HPV and anogenital cancer. *Vaccine.* (2006) 24 (Suppl. 3):S3/42–51. doi: 10.1016/j.vaccine.2006.06.018
6. Carter JJ, Koutsky LA, Hughes JP, Lee SK, Kuypers J, Kiviat N, et al. Comparison of human papillomavirus types 16, 18, and 6 capsid antibody responses following incident infection. *J Infect Dis.* (2000) 181:1911–9. doi: 10.1086/315498
7. Cutts FT, Franceschi S, Goldie S, Castellsague X, de Sanjose S, Garnett G, et al. Human papillomavirus and HPV vaccines: a review. *Bull World Health Organ.* (2007) 85:719–26. doi: 10.2471/BLT.06.038414
8. Guan P, Howell-Jones R, Li N, Bruni L, de Sanjosé S, Franceschi S, et al. Human papillomavirus types in 115,789 HPV-positive women: a meta-analysis from cervical infection to cancer. *Int J Cancer.* (2012) 131:2349–59. doi: 10.1002/ijc.27485
9. Nayar R, Solomon D. Second edition of 'wfhe Bethesda System for reporting cervical cytology' - atlas, website, and Bethesda interobserver reproducibility project. *Cytojournal.* (2004)1:4. doi: 10.1007/978-1-4612-2042-8
10. de Martel C, Plummer M, Vignat J, Franceschi S. Worldwide burden of cancer attributable to HPV by site, country and HPV type. *Int J Cancer.* (2017) 141:664–70. doi: 10.1002/ijc.30716
11. Daling JR, Madeleine MM, Johnson LG, Schwartz SM, Shera KA, Wurscher MA, et al. Human papillomavirus, smoking, and sexual practices in the etiology of anal cancer. *Cancer.* (2004) 101:270–80. doi: 10.1002/cncr.20365
12. Lin C, Franceschi S, Clifford GM. Human papillomavirus types from infection to cancer in the anus, according to sex and HIV status: a systematic review and meta-analysis. *Lancet Infect Dis.* (2018) 18:198–206. doi: 10.1016/S1473-3099(17)30653-9
13. Lin C, Slama J, Gonzalez P, Goodman MT, Xia N, Kreimer AR, et al. Cervical determinants of anal HPV infection and high-grade anal lesions in women: a collaborative pooled analysis. *Lancet Infect Dis.* (2019) 19:880–91. doi: 10.1016/S1473-3099(19)30164-1
14. Garbuglia AR, Gentile M, Del Nonno F, Lorenzini P, Lapa D, Lupi F, et al. An anal cancer screening program for MSM in Italy: prevalence of multiple HPV types and vaccine-targeted infections. *J Clin Virol.* (2015) 72:49–54. doi: 10.1016/j.jcv.2015.09.001
15. Dunne EF, Nielson CM, Stone KM, Markowitz LE, Giuliano AR. Prevalence of HPV infection among men: a systematic review of the literature. *J Infect Dis.* (2006) 194:1044–57. doi: 10.1086/507432
16. Nielson CM, Flores R, Harris RB, Abrahamsen M, Papenfuss MR, Dunne EF, et al. Human papillomavirus prevalence and type distribution in male anogenital sites and semen. *Cancer Epidemiol Biomarkers Prev.* (2007) 16:1107–14. doi: 10.1158/1055-9965.EPI-06-0997

AUTHOR CONTRIBUTIONS

AG and PD wrote the original version and edited versions. MC edited versions. DL and CS prepared figures and tables.

17. Nielson CM, Harris RB, Dunne EF, Abrahamsen M, Papenfuss MR, Flores R, et al. Risk factors for anogenital human papillomavirus infection in men. *J Infect Dis.* (2007) 196:1137–45. doi: 10.1086/521632
18. Giuliano AR, Tortolero-Luna G, Ferrer E, Burchell AN, de Sanjose S, Kjaer SK, et al. Epidemiology of human papillomavirus infection in men, cancers other than cervical and benign conditions. *Vaccine.* (2008) 26 (Suppl. 10):K17–28. doi: 10.1016/j.vaccine.2008.06.021
19. Sankaranarayanan R, Ferlay J. Worldwide burden of gynaecological cancer: the size of the problem. *Best Pract Res Clin Obstet Gynaecol.* (2006) 20:207–25. doi: 10.1016/j.bpobgyn.2005.10.007
20. de Sanjosé S, Alemany L, Ordi J, Tous S, Alejo M, Bigby SM, et al. Worldwide human papillomavirus genotype attribution in over 2000 cases of intraepithelial and invasive lesions of the vulva. *Eur J Cancer.* (2013) 49:3450–61. doi: 10.1016/j.ejca.2013.06.033
21. Hoang LN, Park KJ, Soslow RA, Murali R. Squamous precursor lesions of the vulva: current classification and diagnostic challenges. *Pathology.* (2016) 48:291–302. doi: 10.1016/j.pathol.2016.02.015
22. Bornstein J, Bogliatto F, Haefner HK, Stockdale CK, Preti M, Bohl TG, et al. The 2015 International society for the study of vulvovaginal disease (ISSVD) terminology of vulvar squamous intraepithelial lesions. *J Low Genit Tract Dis.* (2016) 20:11–4. doi: 10.1097/LGT.0000000000000169
23. van der Avoort IA, Shirango H, Hoevenaars BM, Grefte JM, de Hullu JA, de Wilde PC, et al. Vulvar squamous cell carcinoma is a multifactorial disease following two separate and independent pathways. *Int J Gynecol Pathol.* (2006) 25:22–9. doi: 10.1097/01.pgp.0000177646.38266.6a
24. Srodon M, Stoler MH, Baber GB, Kurman RJ. The distribution of low and high-risk HPV types in vulvar and vaginal intraepithelial neoplasia (VIN and VaIN). *Am J Surg Pathol.* (2006) 30:1513–8. doi: 10.1097/01.pas.0000213291.96401.48
25. Reich O, Regauer S, Marth C, Schmidt D, Horn LC, Dannecker C, et al. Precancerous lesions of the cervix, vulva and vagina according to the 2014 WHO classification of tumors of the female genital tract. *Geburtshilfe Frauenheilkd.* (2015) 75:1018–20. doi: 10.1055/s-0035-1558052
26. Hildesheim A, Han CL, Brinton LA, Kurman RJ, Schiller JT. Human papillomavirus type 16 and risk of preinvasive and invasive vulvar cancer: results from a seroepidemiological case-control study. *Obstet Gynecol.* (1997) 90:748–54. doi: 10.1016/S0029-7844(97)00467-5
27. Daling JR, Madeleine MM, Schwartz SM, Shera KA, Carter JJ, McKnight B, et al. A population-based study of squamous cell vaginal cancer: HPV and cofactors. *Gynecol Oncol.* (2002) 84:263–70. doi: 10.1006/gyno.2001.6502
28. Carter JJ, Madeleine MM, Shera K, Schwartz SM, Cushing-Haugen KL, Wipf GC, et al. Human papillomavirus 16 and 18 L1 serology compared across anogenital cancer sites. *Cancer Res.* (2001) 61:1934–40.
29. Lamos C, Mihaljevic C, Aulmann S, Bruckner T, Domschke C, Wallwiener M, et al. Detection of human papillomavirus infection in patients with vaginal intraepithelial neoplasia. *PLoS ONE.* (2016) 11:e0167386. doi: 10.1371/journal.pone.0167386
30. Parkin DM, Bray F. Chapter 2: The burden of HPV-related cancers. *Vaccine.* (2006) 24 (Suppl. 3):S3/11–25. doi: 10.1016/j.vaccine.2006.05.111
31. Kreimer AR, Clifford GM, Boyle P, Franceschi S. Human papillomavirus types in head and neck squamous cell carcinomas worldwide: a systematic review. *Cancer Epidemiol Biomarkers Prev.* (2005) 14:467–75. doi: 10.1158/1055-9965.EPI-04-0551
32. Pintos J, Black MJ, Sadeghi N, Ghadirian P, Zeitouni AG, Viscidi RP, et al. Human papillomavirus infection and oral cancer: a case-control study in Montreal, Canada. *Oral Oncol.* (2008) 44:242–50. doi: 10.1016/j.oraloncology.2007.02.005
33. Bosch FX, Broker TR, Forman D, Moscicki AB, Gillison ML, Doorbar J, et al. Comprehensive control of human papillomavirus

infections and related diseases. *Vaccine.* (2013) 31 (Suppl. 7):H1–31. doi: 10.1016/j.vaccine.2013.07.026

34. Herrero R, Quint W, Hildesheim A, Gonzalez P, Struijk L, Katki HA, et al. Reduced prevalence of oral human papillomavirus (HPV) 4 years after bivalent HPV vaccination in a randomized clinical trial in Costa Rica. *PLoS ONE.* (2013) 8:e68329. doi: 10.1371/journal.pone.0068329
35. Vokes EE, Agrawal N, Seiwert TY. HPV-associated head and neck cancer. *J Natl Cancer Inst.* (2015) 107:djv344. doi: 10.1093/jnci/djv344
36. Fakhry C, Andersen KK, Christensen J, Agrawal N, Eisele DW. The impact of tonsillectomy upon the risk of oropharyngeal carcinoma diagnosis and prognosis in the danish cancer registry. *Cancer Prev Res.* (2015) 8:583–9. doi: 10.1158/1940-6207.CAPR-15-0101
37. Lesseur C, Diergaarde B, Olshan AF, Wünsch-Filho V, Ness AR, Liu G, et al. Genome-wide association analyses identify new susceptibility loci for oral cavity and pharyngeal cancer. *Nat Genet.* (2016) 48:1544–50. doi: 10.1038/ng.3685
38. Bomholt A. Juvenile laryngeal papillomatosis. an epidemiological study from the Copenhagen region. *Acta Otolaryngol.* (1988) 105:367–71. doi: 10.3109/00016488809097020
39. Dickens P, Srivastava G, Loke SL, Larkin S. Human papillomavirus 6, 11, and 16 in laryngeal papillomas. *J Pathol.* (1991) 165:243–6. doi: 10.1002/path.1711650308
40. Derkay CS, Darrow DH. Recurrent respiratory papillomatosis. *Ann Otol Rhinol Laryngol.* (2006) 115:1–11. doi: 10.1177/000348940611500101
41. Fenton KA, Korovessis C, Johnson AM, McCadden A, McManus S, Wellings K, et al. Sexual behaviour in Britain: reported sexually transmitted infections and prevalent genital Chlamydia trachomatis infection. *Lancet.* (2001) 358:1851–4. doi: 10.1016/S0140-6736(01)06886-6
42. Grulich AE, de Visser RO, Smith AM, Rissel CE, Richters J. Sex in Australia: knowledge about sexually transmissible infections and blood-borne viruses in a representative sample of adults. *Aust N Z J Public Health.* (2003) 27:230–3. doi: 10.1111/j.1467-842X.2003.tb00813.x
43. Kjaer SK, Tran TN, Sparen P, Tryggvadottir L, Munk C, Dasbach E, et al. The burden of genital warts: a study of nearly 70,000 women from the general female population in the 4 Nordic countries. *J Infect Dis.* (2007) 196:1447–54. doi: 10.1086/522863
44. Insinga RP, Dasbach EJ, Myers ER. The health and economic burden of genital warts in a set of private health plans in the United States. *Clin Infect Dis.* (2003) 36:1397–403. doi: 10.1086/375074
45. Insinga RP, Dasbach EJ, Elbasha EH. Assessing the annual economic burden of preventing and treating anogenital human papillomavirus-related disease in the US: analytic framework and review of the literature. *Pharmacoeconomics.* (2005) 23:1107–22. doi: 10.2165/00019053-200523110-00004
46. Albuquerque A, Sarmento J, Rios E, Macedo G. Gastrointestinal: anal buschke loewenstein tumor. *J Gastroenterol Hepatol.* (2012) 27:1537. doi: 10.1111/j.1440-1746.2012.07204.x
47. Kasukawa H, Howley PM, Benson JD. A fifteen-amino-acid peptide inhibits human papillomavirus E1-E2 interaction and human papillomavirus DNA replication *in vitro*. *J Virol.* (1998) 72:8166–73. doi: 10.1128/JVI.72.10.8166-8173.1998
48. Stanley MA, Browne HM, Appleby M, Minson AC. Properties of a non-tumorigenic human cervical keratinocyte cell line. *Int J Cancer.* (1989) 43:672–6. doi: 10.1002/ijc.2910430422
49. Bedell MA, Hudson JB, Golub TR, Turyk ME, Hosken M, Wilbanks GD, et al. Amplification of human papillomavirus genomes *in vitro* is dependent on epithelial differentiation. *J Virol.* (1991) 65:2254–60. doi: 10.1128/JVI.65.5.2254-2260.1991
50. Parish JL, Bean AM, Park RB, Androphy EJ. ChlR1 is required for loading papillomavirus E2 onto mitotic chromosomes and viral genome maintenance. *Mol Cell.* (2006) 24:867–76. doi: 10.1016/j.molcel.2006.11.005
51. McBride AA. Replication and partitioning of papillomavirus genomes. *Adv Virus Res.* (2008) 72:155–205. doi: 10.1016/S0065-3527(08)00404-1
52. Van Tine BA, Dao LD, Wu SY, Sonbuchner TM, Lin BY, Zou N, et al. Human papillomavirus (HPV) origin-binding protein associates with mitotic spindles to enable viral DNA partitioning. *Proc Natl Acad Sci USA.* (2004) 101:4030–5. doi: 10.1073/pnas.0306848101
53. Bergvall M, Melendy T, Archambault J. The E1 proteins. *Virology.* (2013) 445:35–56. doi: 10.1016/j.virol.2013.07.020
54. Groves IJ, Coleman N. Pathogenesis of human papillomavirus-associated mucosal disease. *J Pathol.* (2015) 235:527–38. doi: 10.1002/path.4496
55. You J, Srinivasan V, Denis GV, Harrington WJ Jr, Ballestas ME, Kaye KM, et al. Kaposi's sarcoma-associated herpesvirus latency-associated nuclear antigen interacts with bromodomain protein Brd4 on host mitotic chromosomes. *J Virol.* (2006) 80:8909–19. doi: 10.1128/JVI.00502-06
56. Egawa N, Wang Q, Griffin HM, Murakami I, Jackson D, Mahmood R, et al. HPV16 and 18 genome amplification show different E4-dependence, with 16E4 enhancing E1 nuclear accumulation and replicative efficiency via its cell cycle arrest and kinase activation functions. *PLoS Pathog.* (2017) 13:e1006282. doi: 10.1371/journal.ppat.1006282
57. Hladik F, Liu H, Speelmon E, Livingston-Rosanoff D, Wilson S, Sakchalathorn P, et al. Combined effect of CCR5-Delta32 heterozygosity and the CCR5 promoter polymorphism−2459 A/G on CCR5 expression and resistance to human immunodeficiency virus type 1 transmission. *J Virol.* (2005) 79:11677–84. doi: 10.1128/JVI.79.18.11677-11684.2005
58. Suarez I, Trave G. Structural insights in multifunctional papillomavirus oncoproteins. *Viruses.* (2018) 10:37. doi: 10.3390/v10010037
59. Huh K, Zhou X, Hayakawa H, Cho JY, Libermann TA, Jin J, et al. Human papillomavirus type 16 E7 oncoprotein associates with the cullin 2 ubiquitin ligase complex, which contributes to degradation of the retinoblastoma tumor suppressor. *J Virol.* (2007) 81:9737–47. doi: 10.1128/JVI.00881-07
60. Zhang B, Chen W, Roman A. The E7 proteins of low- and high-risk human papillomaviruses share the ability to target the pRB family member p130 for degradation. *Proc Natl Acad Sci USA.* (2006) 103:437–42. doi: 10.1073/pnas.0510012103
61. Moody CA, Laimins LA. Human papillomavirus oncoproteins: pathways to transformation. *Nat Rev Cancer.* (2010) 10:550–60. doi: 10.1038/nrc2886
62. Bernard HU. Regulatory elements in the viral genome. *Virology.* (2013) 445:197–204. doi: 10.1016/j.virol.2013.04.035
63. Schwartz S. Papillomavirus transcripts and post-transcriptional regulation. *Virology.* (2013) 445:187–96. doi: 10.1016/j.virol.2013.04.034
64. Johansson C, Schwartz S. Regulation of human papillomavirus gene expression by splicing and polyadenylation. *Nat Rev Microbiol.* (2013) 11:239–51. doi: 10.1038/nrmicro2984
65. zur Hausen H. Papillomavirus infections–a major cause of human cancers. *Biochim Biophys Acta.* (1996) 1288:F55–78. doi: 10.1016/0304-419X(96)00020-0
66. Pett M, Coleman N. Integration of high-risk human papillomavirus: a key event in cervical carcinogenesis? *J Pathol.* (2007) 212:356–67. doi: 10.1002/path.2192
67. Stanley M. Immunobiology of HPV and HPV vaccines. *Gynecol Oncol.* (2008) 109 (Suppl. 2):S15–21. doi: 10.1016/j.ygyno.2008.02.003
68. Liaw KL, Hildesheim A, Burk RD, Gravitt P, Wacholder S, Manos MM, et al. A prospective study of human papillomavirus (HPV) type 16 DNA detection by polymerase chain reaction and its association with acquisition and persistence of other HPV types. *J Infect Dis.* (2001) 183:8–15. doi: 10.1086/317638
69. Woodman CB, Collins S, Winter H, Bailey A, Ellis J, Prior P, et al. Natural history of cervical human papillomavirus infection in young women: a longitudinal cohort study. *Lancet.* (2001) 357:1831–6. doi: 10.1016/S0140-6736(00)04956-4
70. van der Burg SH, de Jong A, Welters MJ, Offringa R, Melief CJ. The status of HPV16-specific T-cell reactivity in health and disease as a guide to HPV vaccine development. *Virus Res.* (2002) 89:275–84. doi: 10.1016/S0168-1702(02)00196-X
71. de Jong A, van Poelgeest MI, van der Hulst JM, Drijfhout JW, Fleuren GJ, Melief CJ, et al. Human papillomavirus type 16-positive cervical cancer is associated with impaired CD4+ T-cell immunity against early antigens E2 and E6. *Cancer Res.* (2004) 64:5449–55. doi: 10.1158/0008-5472.CAN-04-0831

72. van Poelgeest MI, Nijhuis ER, Kwappenberg KM, Hamming IE, Wouter Drijfhout J. Distinct regulation and impact of type 1 T-cell immunity against HPV16 L1, E2 and E6 antigens during HPV16-induced cervical infection and neoplasia. *Int J Cancer*. (2006) 118:675–83. doi: 10.1002/ijc.21394
73. van Poelgeest MI, van Seters M, van Beurden M, Kwappenberg KM, Heijmans-Antonissen C, Drijfhout JW, et al. Detection of human papillomavirus (HPV) 16-specific CD4+ T-cell immunity in patients with persistent HPV16-induced vulvar intraepithelial neoplasia in relation to clinical impact of imiquimod treatment. *Clin Cancer Res*. (2005) 11:5273–80. doi: 10.1158/1078-0432.CCR-05-0616
74. Welters MJ, van der Logt P, van den Eeden SJ, Kwappenberg KM, Drijfhout JW, Fleuren GJ, et al. Detection of human papillomavirus type 18 E6 and E7-specific CD4+ T-helper 1 immunity in relation to health versus disease. *Int J Cancer*. (2006) 118:950–6. doi: 10.1002/ijc.21459
75. Coleman HN, Moscicki AB, Farhat SN, Gupta SK, Wang X, Nakagawa M. CD8 T-cell responses in incident and prevalent human papillomavirus types 16 and 18 infections. *ISRN Obstet Gynecol*. (2012) 2012:854237. doi: 10.5402/2012/854237
76. Piersma SJ, Jordanova ES, van Poelgeest MI, Kwappenberg KM, van der Hulst JM, Drijfhout JW, et al. High number of intraepithelial CD8+ tumor-infiltrating lymphocytes is associated with the absence of lymph node metastases in patients with large early-stage cervical cancer. *Cancer Res*. (2007) 67:354–61. doi: 10.1158/0008-5472.CAN-06-3388
77. Carter JJ, Koutsky LA, Wipf GC, Christensen ND, Lee SK, Kuypers J, et al. The natural history of human papillomavirus type 16 capsid antibodies among a cohort of university women. *J Infect Dis*. (1996) 174:927–36. doi: 10.1093/infdis/174.5.927
78. Tong Y, Ermel A, Tu W, Shew M, Brown DR. Association of HPV types 6, 11, 16, and 18 DNA detection and serological response in unvaccinated adolescent women. *J Med Virol*. (2013) 85:1786–93. doi: 10.1002/jmv.23664
79. Beachler DC, Viscidi R, Sugar EA, Minkoff H, Strickler HD, Cranston RD, et al. A longitudinal study of human papillomavirus 16 L1, e6, and e7 seropositivity and oral human papillomavirus 16 infection. *Sex Transm Dis*. (2015) 42:93–7. doi: 10.1097/OLQ.0000000000000236
80. Safaeian M, Porras C, Schiffman M, Rodriguez AC, Wacholder S, Gonzalez P, et al. Epidemiological study of anti-HPV16/18 seropositivity and subsequent risk of HPV16 and−18 infections. *J Natl Cancer Inst*. (2010) 102:1653–62. doi: 10.1093/jnci/djq384
81. Franceschi S, Baussano I. Naturally acquired immunity against human papillomavirus (HPV): why it matters in the HPV vaccine era. *J Infect Dis*. (2014) 210:507–9. doi: 10.1093/infdis/jiu143
82. Castellsagué X, Naud P, Chow SN, Wheeler CM, Germar MJ, Lehtinen M, et al. Risk of newly detected infections and cervical abnormalities in women seropositive for naturally acquired human papillomavirus type 16/18 antibodies: analysis of the control arm of PATRICIA. *J Infect Dis*. (2014) 210:517–34. doi: 10.1093/infdis/jiu139
83. Beachler DC, Jenkins G, Safaeian M, Kreimer AR, Wentzensen N. Natural acquired immunity against subsequent genital human papillomavirus infection: a systematic review and meta-analysis. *J Infect Dis*. (2016) 213:1444–54. doi: 10.1093/infdis/jiv753
84. Dobson SR, McNeil S, Dionne M, Dawar M, Ogilvie G, Krajden M, et al. Immunogenicity of 2 doses of HPV vaccine in younger adolescents vs 3 doses in young women: a randomized clinical trial. *JAMA*. (2013) 309:1793–802. doi: 10.1001/jama.2013.1625
85. Meites E, Kempe A, Markowitz LE. Use of a 2-dose schedule for human papillomavirus vaccination - updated recommendations of the advisory committee on immunization practices. *MMWR Morb Mortal Wkly Rep*. (2016) 65:1405–8. doi: 10.15585/mmwr.mm6549a5
86. Markowitz LE, Dunne EF, Saraiya M, Chesson HW, Curtis CR, Gee J, et al. Human papillomavirus vaccination: recommendations of the advisory committee on immunization practices (ACIP). *MMWR Recomm Rep*. (2014) 63:1–30.
87. Stanley M, Pinto LA, Trimble C. Human papillomavirus vaccines—immune responses. *Vaccine*. (2012) 30 (Suppl. 5):F83–7. doi: 10.1016/j.vaccine.2012.04.106
88. Suzich JA, Ghim SJ, Palmer-Hill FJ, White WI, Tamura JK, Bell JA, et al. Systemic immunization with papillomavirus L1 protein completely prevents the development of viral mucosal papillomas. *Proc Natl Acad Sci USA*. (1995) 92:11553–7. doi: 10.1073/pnas.92.25.11553
89. Roden RB, Hubbert NL, Kirnbauer R, Breitburd F, Lowy DR, Schiller JT. Papillomavirus L1 capsids agglutinate mouse erythrocytes through a proteinaceous receptor. *J Virol*. (1995) 69:5147–51. doi: 10.1128/JVI.69.8.5147-5151.1995
90. GlaxoSmithKline Vaccine HPV-007 Study Group, Romanowski B, de Borba PC, Naud PS, Roteli-Martins CM, De Carvalho NS, et al. Sustained efficacy and immunogenicity of the human papillomavirus (HPV)-16/18 AS04-adjuvanted vaccine: analysis of a randomised placebo-controlled trial up to 6.4 years. *Lancet*. (2009) 374:1975–85. doi: 10.1016/S0140-6736(09)61567-1
91. Schwarz TF, Galaj A, Spaczynski M, Wysocki J, Kaufmann AM, Poncelet S, et al. Ten-year immune persistence and safety of the HPV-16/18 AS04-adjuvanted vaccine in females vaccinated at 15-55 years of age. *Cancer Med*. (2017) 6:2723–31. doi: 10.1002/cam4.1155
92. Garland SM, Hernandez-Avila M, Wheeler CM, Perez G, Harper DM, Leodolter S, et al. Quadrivalent vaccine against human papillomavirus to prevent anogenital diseases. *N Engl J Med*. (2007) 356:1928–43. doi: 10.1056/NEJMoa061760
93. Pedersen C, Petaja T, Strauss G, Rumke HC, Poder A, Richardus JH, et al. Immunization of early adolescent females with human papillomavirus type 16 and 18 L1 virus-like particle vaccine containing AS04 adjuvant. *J Adolesc Health*. (2007) 40:564–71. doi: 10.1016/j.jadohealth.2007.02.015
94. Joura EA, Giuliano AR, Iversen OE, Bouchard C, Mao C, Mehlsen J, et al. A 9-valent HPV vaccine against infection and intraepithelial neoplasia in women. *N Engl J Med*. (2015) 372:711–23. doi: 10.1056/NEJMoa1405044
95. Arbyn M, Xu L. Efficacy and safety of prophylactic HPV vaccines. A Cochrane review of randomized trials. *Expert Rev Vaccines*. (2018) 17:1085–91. doi: 10.1080/14760584.2018.1548282
96. Hildesheim A, Wacholder S, Catteau G, Struyf F, Dubin G, Herrero R, et al. Efficacy of the HPV-16/18 vaccine: final according to protocol results from the blinded phase of the randomized Costa Rica HPV-16/18 vaccine trial. *Vaccine*. (2014) 32:5087–97. doi: 10.1016/j.vaccine.2014.06.038
97. Palefsky JM, Giuliano AR, Goldstone S, Moreira ED Jr, Aranda C, Jessen H, et al. HPV vaccine against anal HPV infection and anal intraepithelial neoplasia. *N Engl J Med*. (2011) 365:1576–85. doi: 10.1056/NEJMoa1010971
98. Giuliano AR, Palefsky JM, Goldstone S, Moreira ED Jr, Penny ME, Aranda C, et al. Efficacy of quadrivalent HPV vaccine against HPV Infection and disease in males. *N Engl J Med*. (2011) 364:401–11. doi: 10.1056/NEJMoa0909537
99. Lehtinen T, Söderlund-Strand A, Petäjä T, Eriksson T, Jokiranta S, Natunen K, et al. Human Papillomavirus (HPV) Prevalence in Male Adolescents 4 Years After HPV-16/18 Vaccination. *J Infect Dis*. (2017) 216:966–8. doi: 10.1093/infdis/jix415
100. Safaeian M, van Doorslaer K, Schiffman M, Chen Z, Rodriguez AC, Herrero R, et al. Lack of heterogeneity of HPV16 E7 sequence compared with HPV31 and HPV73 may be related to its unique carcinogenic properties. *Arch Virol*. (2010) 155:367–70. doi: 10.1007/s00705-009-0579-2
101. Marth C, Landoni F, Mahner S, McCormack M, Gonzalez-Martin A, Colombo N, et al. Cervical cancer: ESMO Clinical Practice Guidelines for diagnosis, treatment and follow-up. *Ann Oncol*. (2017) 28(Suppl. 4):iv72-iv83. doi: 10.1093/annonc/mdx220
102. Hoffman SR, Le T, Lockhart A, Sanusi A, Dal Santo L, Davis M, et al. Patterns of persistent HPV infection after treatment for cervical intraepithelial neoplasia (CIN): a systematic review. *Int J Cancer*. (2017) 141:8–23. doi: 10.1002/ijc.30623
103. Vermaelen K. Vaccine strategies to improve anti-cancer cellular immune responses. *Front Immunol*. (2019) 10:8. doi: 10.3389/fimmu.2019.00008
104. Chabeda A, Yanez RJR, Lamprecht R, Meyers AE, Rybicki EP, Hitzeroth II. Therapeutic vaccines for high-risk HPV-associated diseases. *Papillomavirus Res*. (2018) 5:46–58. doi: 10.1016/j.pvr.2017.12.006
105. Yang L, Mohr I, Fouts E, Lim DA, Nohaile M, Botchan M. The E1 protein of bovine papilloma virus 1 is an ATP-dependent DNA helicase. *Proc Natl Acad Sci USA*. (1993) 90:5086–90. doi: 10.1073/pnas.90.11.5086
106. Flickinger JC Jr, Rodeck U, Snook AE. Listeria monocytogenes as a vector for cancer immunotherapy: current understanding and progress. *Vaccines*. (2018) 6:E48. doi: 10.3390/vaccines6030048
107. Maciag PC, Radulovic S, Rothman J. The first clinical use of a live-attenuated Listeria monocytogenes vaccine: a Phase I safety study of Lm-LLO-E7 in

patients with advanced carcinoma of the cervix. *Vaccine*. (2009) 27:3975–83. doi: 10.1016/j.vaccine.2009.04.041
108. Ferraro B, Morrow MP, Hutnick NA, Shin TH, Lucke CE, Weiner DB. Clinical applications of DNA vaccines: current progress. *Clin Infect Dis*. (2011) 53:296–302. doi: 10.1093/cid/cir334
109. Kim TJ, Jin HT, Hur SY, Yang HG, Seo YB, Hong SR, et al. Clearance of persistent HPV infection and cervical lesion by therapeutic DNA vaccine in CIN3 patients. *Nat Commun*. (2014) 5:5317. doi: 10.1038/ncomms6317
110. Samuels S, Marijne Heeren A, Zijlmans HJMAA, Welters MJP, van den Berg JH, Philips D, et al. HPV16 E7 DNA tattooing: safety, immunogenicity, and clinical response in patients with HPV-positive vulvar intraepithelial neoplasia. *Cancer Immunol Immunother*. (2017) 66:1163–73. doi: 10.1007/s00262-017-2006-y
111. Trimble CL, Peng S, Kos F, Gravitt P, Viscidi R, Sugar E, et al. A phase I trial of a human papillomavirus DNA vaccine for HPV16+ cervical intraepithelial neoplasia 2/3. *Clin Cancer Res*. (2009) 15:361–7. doi: 10.1158/1078-0432.CCR-08-1725
112. Bagarazzi ML, Yan J, Morrow MP, Shen X, Parker RL, Lee JC, et al. Immunotherapy against HPV16/18 generates potent TH1 and cytotoxic cellular immune responses. *Sci Transl Med*. (2012) 4:155ra138. doi: 10.1126/scitranslmed.3004414
113. Trimble CL, Morrow MP, Kraynyak KA, Shen X, Dallas M, Yan J, et al. Safety, efficacy, and immunogenicity of VGX-3100, a therapeutic synthetic DNA vaccine targeting human papillomavirus 16 and 18 E6 and E7 proteins for cervical intraepithelial neoplasia 2/3: a randomised, double-blind, placebo-controlled phase 2b trial. *Lancet*. (2015) 386:2078–88. doi: 10.1016/S0140-6736(15)00239-1
114. Rosales R, López-Contreras M, Rosales C, Magallanes-Molina JR, Gonzalez-Vergara R, Arroyo-Cazarez JM, et al. Regression of human papillomavirus intraepithelial lesions is induced by MVA E2 therapeutic vaccine. *Hum Gene Ther*. (2014) 25:1035–49. doi: 10.1089/hum.2014.024
115. Çuburu N, Kim R, Guittard GC, Thompson CD, Day PM, Hamm DE, et al. A prime-pull-amplify vaccination strategy to maximize induction of circulating and genital-resident intraepithelial CD8+ memory T cells. *J Immunol*. (2019) 202:1250–64. doi: 10.4049/jimmunol.1800219
116. Arbyn M, Redman CWE, Verdoodt F, Kyrgiou M, Tzafetas M, Ghaem-Maghami S, et al. Incomplete excision of cervical precancer as a predictor of treatment failure: a systematic review and meta-analysis. *Lancet Oncol*. (2017) 18:1665–79. doi: 10.1016/S1470-2045(17)30700-3
117. Ghaem-Maghami S, Sagi S, Majeed G, Soutter WP. Incomplete excision of cervical intraepithelial neoplasia and risk of treatment failure: a meta-analysis. *Lancet Oncol*. (2007) 8:985–93. doi: 10.1016/S1470-2045(07)70283-8
118. Ghaem-Maghami S, De-Silva D, Tipples M, Lam S, Perryman K, Soutter W. Determinants of success in treating cervical intraepithelial neoplasia. *BJOG*. (2011) 118:679–84. doi: 10.1111/j.1471-0528.2010.02770.x
119. Arbyn M, Kyrgiou M, Simoens C, Raifu AO, Koliopoulos G, Martin-Hirsch P, et al. Perinatal mortality and other severe adverse pregnancy outcomes associated with treatment of cervical intraepithelial neoplasia: meta-analysis. *BMJ*. (2008) 18:a1284. doi: 10.1136/bmj.a1284
120. Kyrgiou M, Athanasiou A, Paraskevaidi M, Mitra A, Kalliala I, Martin-Hirsch P, et al. Adverse obstetric outcomes after local treatment for cervical preinvasive and early invasive disease according to cone depth: systematic review and meta-analysis. *BMJ*. (2016) 28:i3633. doi: 10.1097/01.ogx.0000508341.95858.c5
121. Bruno MT, Cassaro N, Garofalo S, Boemi S. HPV16 persistent infection and recurrent disease after LEEP. *Virol J*. (2019) 16:148. doi: 10.1186/s12985-019-1252-3
122. Strander B, Hällgren J, Sparén P. Effect of ageing on cervical or vaginal cancer in Swedish women previously treated for cervical intraepithelial neoplasia grade 3: population based cohort study of long term incidence and mortality. *BMJ*. (2014) 348:f7361. doi: 10.1136/bmj.f7361
123. Ebisch RMF, Rutten DWE, IntHout J, Melchers WJG, Massuger LFAG, Bulten J, et al. Long-lasting increased risk of human papillomavirus-related carcinomas and premalignancies after cervical intraepithelial neoplasia grade 3: a population-based cohort study. *J Clin Oncol*. (2017) 35:2542–50. doi: 10.1200/JCO.2016.71.4543
124. Swedish KA, Factor SH, Goldstone SE. Prevention of recurrent high-grade anal neoplasia with quadrivalent human papillomavirus vaccination of men who have sex with men: a nonconcurrent cohort study. *Clin Infect Dis*. (2012) 54:891–8. doi: 10.1093/cid/cir1036
125. Kang WD, Choi HS, Kim SM. Is vaccination with quadrivalent HPV vaccine after loop electrosurgical excision procedure effective in preventing recurrence in patients with high-grade cervical intraepithelial neoplasia (CIN2-3)? *Gynecol Oncol*. (2013) 130:264–8. doi: 10.1016/j.ygyno.2013.04.050
126. Ghelardi A, Parazzini F, Martella F, Pieralli A, Bay P, Tonetti A, et al. SPERANZA project: HPV vaccination after treatment for CIN2. *Gynecol Oncol*. (2018) 151:229–34. doi: 10.1016/j.ygyno.2018.08.033
127. Hildesheim A, Gonzalez P, Kreimer AR, Wacholder S, Schussler J, Rodriguez AC, et al. Impact of human papillomavirus (HPV) 16 and 18 vaccination on prevalent infections and rates of cervical lesions after excisional treatment. *Am J Obstet Gynecol*. (2016) 215:212.e1–5. doi: 10.1016/j.ajog.2016.02.021
128. Swedish KA, Goldstone SE. Prevention of anal condyloma with quadrivalent human papillomavirus vaccination of older men who have sex with men. *PLoS ONE*. (2014) 9:e93393. doi: 10.1371/journal.pone.0093393
129. Kreuter A, Waterboer T, Wieland U. Regression of cutaneous warts in a patient with WILD syndrome following recombinant quadrivalent human papillomavirus vaccination. *Arch Dermatol*. (2010) 146:1196–7. doi: 10.1001/archdermatol.2010.290
130. Moscato GM, Di Matteo G, Ciotti M, Di Bonito P, Andreoni M, Moschese V. Dual response to human papilloma virus vaccine in an immunodeficiency disorder: resolution of plantar warts and persistence of condylomas. *J Eur Acad Dermatol Venereol*. (2016) 30:1212–3. doi: 10.1111/jdv.13133
131. Lee HJ, Kim JK, Kim DH, Yoon MS. Condyloma accuminatum treated with recombinant quadrivalent human papillomavirus vaccine (types 6, 11, 16, 18). *J Am Acad Dermatol*. (2011) 64:e130–2. doi: 10.1016/j.jaad.2010.12.032
132. Petry KU, Bollaerts K, Bonanni P, Stanley M, Drury R, Joura E, et al. Estimation of the individual residual risk of cervical cancer after vaccination with the nonavalent HPV vaccine. *Hum Vaccin Immunother*. (2018) 14:1800–6. doi: 10.1080/21645515.2018.1450125
133. Poynten IM, Tabrizi SN, Jin F, Templeton DJ, Machalek DA, Cornall A, et al. Vaccine-preventable anal human papillomavirus in Australian gay and bisexual men. *Papillomavirus Res*. (2017) 3:80–4. doi: 10.1016/j.pvr.2017.02.003
134. Ong JJ, Walker S, Grulich A, Hoy J, Read TRH, Bradshaw C, et al. Incidence, clearance, and persistence of anal human papillomavirus in men who have sex with men living with human immunodeficiency virus: implications for human papillomavirus vaccination. *Sex Transm Dis*. (2019) 46:229–33. doi: 10.1097/OLQ.0000000000000958
135. Rodríguez-Carunchio L, Soveral I, Steenbergen RD, Torné A, Martinez S, Fusté P, et al. HPV-negative carcinoma of the uterine cervix: a distinct type of cervical cancer with poor prognosis. *BJOG*. (2015) 122:119–27. doi: 10.1111/1471-0528.13071
136. Tao X, Zheng B, Yin F, Zeng Z, Li Z, Griffith CC, et al. Polymerase chain reaction human papillomavirus (HPV) detection and HPV genotyping in Invasive cervical cancers with prior negative HC2 test results. Am *J Clin Pathol*. (2017) 147:477–83. doi: 10.1093/ajcp/aqx027
137. Petry KU, Liebrich C, Luyten A, Zander M, Iftner T. Surgical staging identified false HPV-negative cases in a large series of invasive cervical cancers. *Papillomavirus Res*. (2017) 4:85–9. doi: 10.1016/j.pvr.2017.10.003
138. Tjalma W. HPV negative cervical cancers and primary HPV screening. *Facts Views Vis Obgyn*. (2018) 10:107–13.
139. Pirog EC, Lloveras B, Molijn A, Tous S, Guimerà N, Alejo M, et al. HPV prevalence and genotypes in different histological subtypes of cervical adenocarcinoma, a worldwide analysis of 760 cases. *Mod Pathol*. (2014) 27:1559–67. doi: 10.1038/modpathol.2014.55
140. Pirog EC. Cervical adenocarcinoma: diagnosis of human papillomavirus-positive and human papillomavirus-negative tumors. *Arch*

Pathol Lab Med. (2017) 141:1653–67. doi: 10.5858/arpa.2016-0356-RA

141. Kusanagi Y, Kojima A, Mikami Y, Kiyokawa T, Sudo T, Yamaguchi S, et al. Absence of high-risk human papillomavirus (HPV) detection in endocervical adenocarcinoma with gastric morphology and phenotype. *Am J Pathol.* (2010) 177:2169–75. doi: 10.2353/ajpath.2010.100323

142. Park KJ, Kiyokawa T, Soslow RA, Lamb CA, Oliva E, Zivanovic O, et al. Unusual endocervical adenocarcinomas: an immunohistochemical analysis with molecular detection of human papillomavirus. *Am J Surg Pathol.* (2011) 35:633–46. doi: 10.1097/PAS.0b013e31821534b9

6

Susceptibility to *Plasmodium falciparum* Malaria: Influence of Combined Polymorphisms of IgG3 Gm Allotypes and Fc Gamma Receptors IIA, IIIA and IIIB

Abdou Khadre Dit Jadir Fall[1], Celia Dechavanne[1], Audrey Sabbagh[1], Evelyne Guitard[2], Jacqueline Milet[1], André Garcia[1], Jean-Michel Dugoujon[2], David Courtin[1†] and Florence Migot-Nabias[1†]*

[1] Université de Paris, Institut de Recherche pour le Développement (IRD), UMR 261 MERIT, Paris, France, [2] CNRS UMR 5288 Laboratoire d'Anthropologie Moléculaire et d'Imagerie de Synthèse (AMIS), Université Paul Sabatier Toulouse III, Toulouse, France

***Correspondence:**
Florence Migot-Nabias
florence.migot-nabias@ird.fr

[†]These authors have contributed equally to this work

The binding of immunoglobulin (Ig) to Fc gamma receptors (FcgR) at the immune cell surface is an important step to initiate immunological defense against malaria. However, polymorphisms in receptors and/or constant regions of the IgG heavy chains may modulate this binding. Here, we investigated whether polymorphisms located in FcgR and constant regions of the heavy chain of IgG are associated with susceptibility to *P. falciparum* malaria. For this purpose, a clinical and parasitological follow-up on malaria was conducted among 656 infants in southern Benin. G3m allotypes (from total IgG3) were determined by a serological method of hemagglutination inhibition. FcgRIIA 131R/H and FcgRIIIA 176F/V genotypes were determined using the TaqMan method and FcgRIIIB NA1/NA2 genotypes were assessed by polymerase chain reaction using allele-specific primers. Association analyses between the number of malaria infections during the follow-up and polymorphisms in IgG G3m allotypes and FcgR were studied independently by zero inflated binomial negative regression. The influence of combinations of G3m allotypes and FcgRIIA/FcgRIIIA/FcgRIIIB polymorphisms on the number of *P. falciparum* infections, and their potential interaction with environmental exposure to malaria was assessed by using the generalized multifactor dimensionality reduction (GMDR) method. Results showed that individual carriage of G3m24 single allotype and of G3m5,6,10,11,13,14,24 phenotype was independently associated with a high risk of malaria infection. A risk effect for G3m6 was observed only under high environmental exposure. FcgRIIIA 176VV single genotype and combined carriage of FcgRIIA 131RH/FcgRIIIA 176VV/FcgRIIIB NA1NA2, FcgRIIA 131HH/FcgRIIIA 176FF/FcgRIIIB NA1NA1, FcgRIIA 131HH/FcgRIIIA 176VV/FcgRIIIB NA2NA2 and FcgRIIA 131HH/FcgRIIIA 176VV/FcgRIIIB NA1NA2 genotypes were related to a high number of malaria infections. The risk was accentuated for FcgRIIIA 176VV when considering the influence of environmental exposure to malaria. Finally, the GMDR analysis including environmental exposure showed strengthened associations with a malaria risk when

FcgRIIA/FcgRIIIA/FcgRIIIB genotypes were combined to G3m5,6,11,24 and G3m5,6,10,11,13,15,24 phenotypes or G3m10 and G3m13 single allotypes. Our results highlight the relevance of studying IgG heavy chain and FcgR polymorphisms, independently as well as in combination, in relation to the individual susceptibility to *P. falciparum* infection. The intensity of individual exposure to mosquito bites was demonstrated to impact the relationships found.

Keywords: malaria, IgG polymorphism, Gm allotypes, Fc gamma receptor, Benin, generalized multifactor dimensionality reduction

INTRODUCTION

Malaria remains the most lethal parasitic disease in the world. According to the latest world malaria report in 2019, 228 million estimated cases of malaria occurred in 2018 while the estimated number of deaths remained a concern, 429 000 in 2017 and 405 000 in 2018 (1). Data for the 2015–2018 period highlight that no significant progress in reducing global malaria cases was made. Therefore, it seems urgent to identify new targets and new tools to fight the disease.

The pioneering work of Cohen et al. in 1960 demonstrated that IgG from malaria immune Gambian adults contributed to diminish the *P. falciparum* parasitemia when transferred to non-immune African infected children (2). Since then, there has been an increased interest in exploring the role of IgG in malaria immunity. Namely, the same experimentation was made with IgG from malaria immune African adults passively transferred to Thai patients, demonstrating that efficacy was independent of the type of infecting isolate (3). Further studies established that firstly, cytophilic IgG1 and IgG3 isotypes were mostly associated with *P. falciparum* malaria protection (4–6) including protection of the newborn partly conferred by transplacental transfer of malaria-specific IgG3 (7). Secondly, they showed that it was crucial to investigate the functionality, and not only the levels of IgG directed to asexual stages of *P. falciparum* when evaluating malaria protection parameters (8).

IgG can act on *P. falciparum* in two ways: directly by agglutinating the parasites and therefore preventing their reinvasion of red blood cells and indirectly by binding to Fc gamma receptors (FcgR) expressed at the surface of immune cells such as monocytes, macrophages, or neutrophils (9). This fixation triggers cell activation signals and immune response (opsonization, phagocytosis, reactive oxygen species-ROS, and nitric oxide-NO production). FcgR are important in providing a significant link between the humoral and cellular immunity by bridging the interaction between specific antibodies and effector cells. Nevertheless, genetic variability in constant regions of IgG heavy chains (10) and in FcgR (11) could modulate the susceptibility to malaria infections.

Indeed, most of the interactions between FcgR and IgG involve constant regions (CH1, CH2, and CH3) of the heavy IgG chains. Allelic variations found in the CH1, CH2, and CH3 IgG chains can lead to variations in the amino acid sequences of IgG subclasses and therefore in their efficiency to bind to their receptors. These amino acid changes are responsible for antigenic determinants named human immunoglobulin Gm (gamma markers) allotypes. There are four allotypes for IgG1 in the CH1 and CH3 constant domains called G1m [1, 2, 3, 17], one allotype for IgG2 in the CH2 constant domain called G2m23 and thirteen allotypes for IgG3 in the CH2 and CH3 constant domains called G3m [5, 6, 10, 11, 13, 14, 15, 16, 21, 24, 26, 27, 28] (12, 13). The most polymorphic G3m allotypes are distinguished by variations on nine amino acids (13, 14). Gm allotypes, which are inherited in fixed combinations called haplotypes, vary qualitatively and quantitatively according to human population groups (15).

Facer (16) was the first author to highlight the relationship between Gm allotypes and malaria. She showed, in a sample of Gambian children with past or acute *P. falciparum* malaria, a preferential expression of G3m10, G3m11, and G3m14 allotypes associated with a risk of anemia (16). According to Pandey et al. (17), G3m6 carrying haplotypes may explain the difference in susceptibility to malaria infection between the Fulani and Masaleit ethnic groups in Sudan. Indeed, a lower frequency of G3m6 in Fulani was associated with a lower parasitamia compared to Masaleit. Migot-Nabias et al. (10) demonstrated the existence of an inverse relationship between the carriage of the Gm5,6,13,14; 1,17 phenotype (G3m; G1m) and the presence of uncomplicated malaria in Benin, while for Giha et al. (18) the Gm5,6,13,14; 1,17 phenotype was associated with a higher incidence of malaria in Sudan. Finally, Pandey et al. (19) showed that the carriage of Gm5,13,14; 3; 23 phenotype (G3m; G1m; G2m) was associated with a high level of IgG1 to *P. vivax* *Pv*MSP1-19 and *Pv*AMA-1 antigens, response considered as protective against malaria.

The FcgRs are key components of the immune response, by operating on activation and modulation of the pro-inflammatory and cytotoxic pathways, by influencing the number of white blood cells as well as the transport of circulating antibodies (20, 21). In the family of FcgR receptors, FcgRIIA, FcgRIIIA, and FcgRIIIB appear to play an important role in malaria susceptibility.

FcgRIIA initiates endocytosis, phagocytosis, and the release of inflammatory mediators. There are two variants for FcgRIIA, 131R (Arginine) and 131H (Histidine) firstly described according to their IgG2 binding efficiency, which is more affine for the 131H variant (22). Binding affinity for IgG is more important for IgG3 and IgG1 than for IgG4 and IgG2 (23). Ouma et al. (24) showed that 131R homozygosity confers protection against high parasite densities in contrast to 131H homozygosity.

FcgRIIIA receptor plays an important role in phagocytosis and degranulation and presents two allotypes variants consisting in either F (Phenylalanine) or V (Valine) in position 176, the 176V variant offering a better affinity for IgG1 (25).

FcgRIIIB is a C-terminus linked glycosylphosphatidylinositol (GPI) receptor expressed at the surface of neutrophils and eosinophils. A strong affinity for IgG1 and IgG3 was described (11). The FcgRIIIB presents a polymorphism named NA1/NA2 that refers to neutrophil antigen (NA) 1 and 2 forms which differ in amino acids at positions 65 and 82 in two extra-glycosylation sites (11, 26, 27). The FcgRIIIB NA1 form is capable of better ingestion of IgG1 or IgG3 opsonized particles than the NA2 form (28). The FcgRIIA and FcgRIIIB receptors play an important role in phagocytosis and degranulation. Indeed, in order of decreasing affinity, we have for FcgRIIA, IgG3 > IgG1 > IgG2 = IgG4, for FcgRIIIA, IgG3 > IgG1 >> IgG4 > IgG2 while FcgRIIIB binds generally IgG1 and IgG3 and not IgG2 and IgG4 (23).

Various studies have investigated the relationships between polymorphisms in FcgRIIA, FcgRIIIA, and FcgRIIIB receptors and malaria immunity. Omi et al. (29) showed an association between the FcgRIIIB NA2 allele and an increased susceptibility to cerebral malaria in Thailand. Those results were strengthened by the study of Adu et al. (30) which described an association between FcgRIIIB NA2 allele and a higher risk of malaria infection. Moreover, the authors showed that the FcgRIIA 131R allele was associated with protection against malaria. The presence of the FcgRIIA 131RH heterozygous polymorphism was associated with malaria protection in some studies (31, 32) while for Maiga et al. (33), a marginal protective effect on parasitemia was observed in a Fulani group from Mali harboring the 131RR genotype. Munde et al. (11) demonstrated that the FcgRIIA 131R-FcgRIIIA 176F-FcgRIIIB NA2 haplotype was important in conditioning susceptibility to malaria anemia (or increased levels of circulating parasites) in West Kenya. Ouma et al. (34) reinforced the results obtained from independent analysis of FcgR (31, 32) by showing a negative association between the FcgRIIA 131H-FcgRIIIB NA1 haplotype and severe malaria anemia and a positive one when considering the FcgRIIA 131H-FcgRIIIB NA2 haplotype.

As presented above, the individual susceptibility to malaria has yet been related to polymorphisms located either in the constant domains of the IgG heavy chain or in several FcgR, considered independently. We can hypothesize that the anchoring of IgG on its cellular receptors can be favored according to the respective variants on both sides. For this purpose, the present study investigated the combination of polymorphisms at both IgG constant domains and FcgR with the aim to evaluate their joint impact on susceptibility to *P. falciparum* malaria. More precisely, the relationships between FcgRIIA 131R/H, FcgRIIIA 176 F/V, FcgRIIIB NA1/NA2, Gm allotypes, and malaria phenotypes were determined in a cohort of Beninese infants.

METHODS

Study Area and Design

The study was conducted in three health centers from the district of Tori Bossito located in southwest Benin, where 656 infants were included at birth (35) and 567 of them followed up from birth to 18 months of age (36). Health workers performed an active follow-up of these infants. It consisted of scheduled home visits every week to detect fever. In case of axillary temperature higher than 37.5°C, a questionnaire was fulfilled and both a *Plasmodium* rapid diagnostic test (RDT) and a thick blood smear examination (TBS) by optical microscopy were performed.

A symptomatic malaria infection was defined by the combined presence of an axillary temperature >37.5°C and a positive RDT and/or a positive TBS. In this case, an antimalarial treatment was administered according to the national guidelines that were applied at the time of the study. It consisted in an artemisinin-based combination therapy (artemether and lumefantrine). TBS were also performed every month to detect asymptomatic malaria infections. In addition, mothers were invited to bring their infants to the health center, at any time, in case of fever (suspected by the mother) or clinical signs, whether or not they were related to malaria, and the same protocol was applied.

Venous blood samples were collected quarterly for hematological and immunological measurements. Venous blood was centrifuged for plasma isolation, and genomic DNA extraction was performed from buffy coat using the QIAamp® DNA blood Mini Kit (QIAGEN) according to the manufacturer's instructions.

To assess the environmental risk of malaria exposure, environmental (information on house characteristics and its immediate surrounding) and geographical data (satellite images, soil type, watercourse nearby, vegetation index, rainfall) were recorded. Throughout the study, every 6 weeks, human landing catches were performed in several points of the villages to evaluate spatial and temporal variations of *Anopheles* density. Altogether, these data allowed modeling, for each child included in the follow-up, an individual risk of exposure to *Anopheles* bites by means of a space- and time-dependent variable (37).

IgG Gm Allotypes

The Gm allotype determination was performed for 501 infants (all singletons) for whom a sufficient quantity of plasma (200 µl) was available at 15 months of age. Indeed, plasma samples collected earlier in the follow-up (3, 6, 9, and 12 months) were not suitable for this determination due 1) to a possible presence of IgG from maternal origin bearing their own Gm allotypes and 2) to an insufficient quantity of infant neo-synthesized IgG.

In order to guarantee a highly reliable result, Gm allotype determinations for infants were confirmed by means of their consistency (inheritance) with those of both biological parents. Thereby, Gm determinations of 71 infants were discarded due to the lack of either the paternal (n = 62) or the maternal sample (n = 9).

From the 430 residual samples for whom trios of Gm determinations could be constituted, inconsistent determinations within the father-mother-child trio were observed for 23 cases (5.3%), leading to Gm data for 407 infants that were retained for further analysis.

G1m [1, 2, 3, 17] and G3m [5, 6, 10, 11, 13, 14, 15, 16, 21, 24, 28] allotypes were determined in plasma samples by a standard hemagglutination inhibition method (38). All infants carried the G1m1,17 allele. Considering G3m allotypes, no child presented G3m16 or G3m21, both on the CH2 domain, and absent in populations of sub-Saharan Africa (13). Similarly, due to the uncertain location of the Gm28 allotype on either IgG1 or IgG3 sub-classes among sub-Saharan Africans (13), this allotype was discarded from the analysis. Therefore, the differentiation of infants was based on the remaining G3m allotypes combined into four G3m alleles mostly encountered in Africa, that are G3m5,10,11,13,14, G3m5,6,11,24, G3m5,6,10,11,14, and G3m10,11,13,15 (13, 15). The homozygous or heterozygous carriage of these alleles led to the ten following possible G3m phenotypes: G3m5,10,11,13,14; G3m5,6,10,11,14; G3m5,6,10,11,13,14; G3m5,6,11,24; G3m5,6,10,11,13,14,24; G3m5,6,10,11,14,24; G3m10,11,13,15; G3m5,10,11,13,14,15; G3m5,6,10,11,13,14,15; and G3m5,6,10,11,13,15,24.

FcgRIIA, FcgRIIIA, and FcgRIIIB Genotyping

Genomic DNA was available for 369 out of the 407 infants for whom Gm data were retained. Among these 369 infants, 368 Gm data were available, while all were genotyped for FcgRIIA, 365 for FcgRIIIA and 353 for FcgRIIIB. However, multivariate models using the four complete FcgR polymorphisms and G3m phenotypes determinations were done on 350 infants.

FcgRIIA and FcgRIIIA Genotyping

Single nucleotide polymorphisms (SNP) corresponding to FcgRIIA rs1801274 and FcgRIIIA rs396991 were genotyped by the Applied Biosystems TaqMan SNP Genotyping Assay using predesigned primer/probe sets (C_9077561_20 and C_25815666_10). PCR was performed using the 7900HT Real-time PCR System (Applied Biosystems) according to the following conditions: one cycle at 92°C for 10 min, 40 cycles at 92°C for 15 s, and 60°C for 60 s. The results were then analyzed using the SDS software.

FcgRIIIB Genotyping

Two different PCR were performed for the detection of FcgRIIIB NA1 and NA2 alleles, using allele-specific oligonucleotides described previously by Hans and Mehta (39). Regarding NA1, the 5'-CAG TGG TTT CAC AAT GTG AA-3' (forward) and 5' CAT GGA CTT CTA GCT GCA CCG 3' (reverse) primers were used to amplify a DNA fragment of 142 pb. Genomic DNA (100 ng) was added to the reaction mixture containing 100 μM $MgCl_2$, 1X buffer solution, 16 μM dNTPs, 2.8 μM sense and antisense primers and 0.5 unit of Taq polymerase. PCR reaction conditions included 1 cycle at 95°C for 5min, followed by 30 cycles at 95°C for 30 s, 55°C for 30 s, and 72°C for 45 s. For NA2, the 5'-CTTC AAT GGT ACA GCG TGC TT-3' (forward) and 5'-CTG TAC TCT CCA CTG TCG TT-3' (reverse) primers were used to amplify a DNA sequence of 169 pb. Genomic DNA (100 ng) was added to the reaction mixture containing 45 μM $MgCl_2$, 1X buffer solution, 16 μM dNTPs, 1.39 μM sense and antisense primers, and 0.5 unit of Taq polymerase. PCR reaction conditions included one cycle at 95°C for 5min, followed by 30 cycles at 95°C for 30 s, 60°C for 30 s, and 72°C for 45 s. The products of 142 pb and 169 pb were revealed on a 2% agarose gel.

Statistical Analysis

The clinical phenotype of interest was the number of *P. falciparum* infections per individual during the follow-up. No discrimination was made between symptomatic and asymptomatic infections since the total of symptomatic infections was greater than that of asymptomatic infections (597 *versus* 200 out of 797 infections) and there were more infants presenting only symptomatic infections (n = 153) than infants presenting only asymptomatic infections (n = 14).

The Chi-square test was used to examine differences between proportions and the Mann-Whitney *U*-test was used for comparisons of demographic and clinical characteristics between groups. The genotypic frequencies of FcgRIIA 131R/H, FcgRIIIA 176F/V and FcgRIIIB NA1/NA2 were tested for Hardy-Weinberg equilibrium (HWE).

First, association analyses between the number of malaria infections during the 18-month follow-up and polymorphisms in FcgR and IgG G3m allotypes were studied by zero-inflated binomial negative regression with adjustment on covariates (age of mothers in years and of infants in months, number of antenatal visits, bednet use, birthweight, and environmental exposure). Environmental exposure was categorized into low *versus* high exposure, taking the median as the threshold value. Univariate analyzes on each of the covariates were made and only those with a P value < 0.20 in the univariate model were included in the final multivariate model.

The statistical analysis was carried out using the Stata software version 13.

Finally, to evaluate the influence of combinations of G3m allotypes, FcgRIIA, FcgRIIIA, and FcgRIIIB polymorphisms on the number of *P. falciparum* infections during the follow-up, and their potential interaction with mosquito exposure, we performed multivariate analyses by using the generalized multifactor dimensionality reduction (GMDR) method (40). This non-parametric and genetic model-free approach overcomes some of the limitations of the traditional statistical methods (i.e. sample size limitation) to detect and characterize gene-gene and gene-environment interactions. GMDR is very similar to the original MDR method. However, instead of using the counts of individuals, the GMDR method uses a residual-based score in order to classify the individuals, thus allowing adjustment for discrete and continuous covariates.

Since the GMDR software requires a complete dataset with no missing values for analysis, we removed individuals with missing genotype data for at least two polymorphisms and those with unknown number of antenatal visits (n = 21). The remaining missing data for FcgR polymorphisms were imputed using the R package MICE (Multivariate Imputation by Chained Equations) (41), a multivariate imputation approach that takes into consideration patterns in the data such as linkage disequilibrium.

We performed an exhaustive search of all possible genotype combinations of one to four polymorphisms among those studied (G3m allotypes, FcgRIIA 131R/H, FcgRIIIA 176F/V, and FcgRIIIB NA1/NA2), and model selection and evaluation was carried out using ten-fold cross-validation. Briefly, a GMDR model was developed using 9/10th of the data and a classification error was estimated from this training set. Then, cross-validation methods were used to estimate the prediction error of the selected GMDR model using 1/10th of the data as evaluation data. This procedure was repeated for each of the ten pieces of the data and the classification and prediction errors were averaged across all ten runs. Two parameters were used to evaluate the best models: (a) the testing balanced accuracy (TBA), which is a measure of the degree of accuracy to which the selected interaction correctly predicts the number of malaria infections in the testing sets (value averaged across all ten sets), with 1.00 indicating perfect prediction, and (b) the cross-validation consistency (CVC), which indicates how many times a set of loci is identified across the cross-validation subsets.

Besides TBA and CVC statistics, GMDR also provides a measure of the significance of the identified model, the signal test, a robust nonparametric test implemented in this extension to MDR (40). The model with the highest TBA, the maximum CVC score, and 0.05 or lower P value derived from the sign test was considered as the best model.

In the first round of analysis, the environmental variable quantifying mosquito exposure at individual level was included as a covariate in the GMDR models as well as the following variables: mother and child ages, bednet use, and number of antenatal visits. In the second round of analysis, this environmental variable was tested for its interaction with the gene polymorphisms to detect gene-environment interactions (only four covariates in the GMDR models).

A linear regression analysis was performed for the significant models found in the GMDR analysis to estimate the effect of the combinations on malaria infections.

Ethics

The University of Abomey-Calavi's institutional review board and the IRD's Consultative Ethics Committee approved the study protocol. All women in this study signed an informed consent before enrollment (which also included their infants) with the possibility to withdraw at any time.

RESULTS

Participants Characteristics

As presented in **Table 1**, the study was conducted in a sample of Beninese infants presenting malaria infections (n = 260, 70%) or not (n = 109, 30%). The number of infants who had symptomatic and asymptomatic infections during the follow-up was respectively 245 and 106. A majority of infants presenting malaria infections had less than four infections (n = 201, 77.3%), 51 infants (19.6%) had between five and eight infections and eight infants (3.1%) had more than eight infections during the follow-up.

Infants belonged mostly to the Tori ethnic group and no difference appeared between ethnic groups regarding malaria infection (P = 0.156). There were almost as many girls as boys and infants distributed equally in *P. falciparum* infected and non-infected groups (P = 0.842).

TABLE 1 | Characteristics of the 369 study participants.

Characteristics of mothers and infants	*P. falciparum* infections in infants		P-value
	No (n = 109)	Yes (n = 260)	
Mothers			
Mother age (mean ± SD in years)	30 (6.07)	26 (5.20)	**0.001**[a]
Number of antenatal visits (mean ± SD)	4.20 (2.22)	3.43 (1.58)	0.443[a]
Placental malaria (n, %)			0.189[b]
No	99 (27.0)	224 (61.2)	
Yes	9 (2.5)	34 (9.3)	
Maternal education (n, %)			0.781[b]
No education	94 (25.5)	221 (59.9)	
Partial primary	11 (3.0)	25 (6.8)	
Complete primary or more	4 (1.0)	14 (3.8)	
Primigravidae (n, %)			0.078[b]
No	98 (28.5)	215 (58.3)	
Yes	11 (3.0)	45 (12.2)	
Infants			
Birth weight (mean ± SD in g)	3049 (418)	2976 (392)	0.589[a]
Infant age (mean ± SD in months)	12 (3.54)	14 (3.06)	**<0.001**[a]
Sex (n, %):			
Male	55 (50.4)	129 (49.6)	0.882[b]
Female	54 (49.5)	131 (50.4)	
Ethnic group (n, %)[c]:			
Tori	77 (70.6)	195 (51.9)	0.156[b]
Fon	9 (8.2)	27 (10.4)	
Others	23 (21.1)	34 (13.1)	
Bednet use (mean of use ± SD)	0.77 (0.41)	0.71 (0.45)	**0.023**[a]
Mosquito exposure (mean of exposure ± SD)	0.42 (0.50)	0.53 (0.50)	**0.048**[a]
***P. falciparum* infections in infants (n, %)**			
1 to 4 infections	–	201 (77.3)	
5 to 8 infections		51(19.6)	
9 to 16 infections		8 (3.1)	

[a] *Statistical significance determined using Mann-Whitney U-test.*
[b] *Statistical significance determined by χ^2 analysis.*
[c] *4 missing values.*
In bold: significant P value at the 0.05 threshold.

Interestingly, infants from the non-infected group were younger (P < 0.001), had more bednet use (P = 0.023), and were less exposed to mosquitoes (P = 0.048) and their mothers were older (P = 0.001) than infants from the *P. falciparum* infected group.

G3m Allotypes and Malaria Infection

Distribution of G3m Phenotypes in the Study Group

Nine G3m phenotypes were observed in the study population, among which six presented a frequency above 5% and were G3m5,10,11,13,14 (n = 110, 29.9%), G3m5,6,10,11,13,14,24 (n = 106, 28.8%), G3m5,6,10,11,13,14 (n = 49, 13.3%), G3m5,10,11,13,14,15 (n = 41, 11.1%), G3m5,6,11,24 (n = 26, 7.1%), and G3m5,6,10,11,13,15,24 (n = 19, 5.2%) (**Figure 1**). The three remaining combinations were G3m5,6,10,11,13,14,15 (n = 8, 2.2%), G3m5,6,10,11,14 (n = 8, 2.2%), and G3m5,6,10,11,14,24 (n = 1, 0.3%).

G3m Allotypes and Malaria Infections

Carriage of G3m allotypes both in single form and in combinations was analyzed through a zero-inflated binomial regression model in order to explain the number of malaria infections per infant during the follow-up. We introduced a term of interaction between the genetic and the environmental variables in the model in order to explore the potential effect of G3m allotypes varying according to the intensity of individual exposure to mosquito bites.

Association Between G3m Allotypes and Malaria Infections

The six most prevalent G3m phenotypes (frequency above 5%) were analyzed.

Only G3m5,6,10,11,13,14,24 was associated with a greater risk of malaria infections (n = 106, IRR = 1.295, 95% CI = 1.093;1.535, P = 0.003, **Table 2**).

The analysis of the carriage of single G3m6, G3m10, G3m13, G3m14, G3m15 and G3m24 allotypes showed that G3m24 is associated with an increased risk of malaria infections (n = 152, IRR = 1.195, 95% CI = 1.016;1.406, P = 0.031, **Table 2**).

To explore the potential role of environmental exposure on this effect, we introduced an interaction term in the analyses.

Interaction Between G3m Allotypes—Environmental Exposure and Malaria Infections

Table 3 confirmed that under conditions of high level of environmental exposure to mosquito bites, G3m5,6,10,11,13,14,24 is associated with an increased risk of malaria infection (n = 56, IRR = 1.648, 95% CI = 1.312;2.070, P < 0.001) as well as the carriage of G3m6 (n = 116, IRR = 1.350, 95% CI = 1.059;1.720, P = 0.015) and of G3m24 (n = 78, IRR = 1.479, 95% CI = 1.183;1.850, P = 0.001).

FcgRIIA 131R/H, FcgRIIIA 176 F/V, and FcgRIIIB NA1/NA2 Polymorphisms

Distribution of FcgR Polymorphisms in the Study Group

The observed distribution of FcgRIIA 131R/H and FcgRIIIA 176F/V genotypes in the whole study group showed consistency with HWE (both P > 0.10). The FcgRIIIB NA1/NA2 genotype distribution revealed significant deviation from HWE

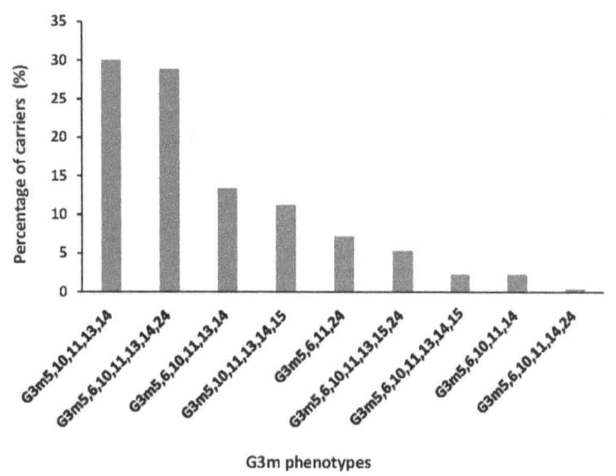

FIGURE 1 | Distribution of G3m phenotypes in the study group.

TABLE 2 | Association between G3m allotypes and malaria infections.

G3m allotypes	n	IRR	CI 95%	P value
G3m phenotypes with frequency at least 5%				
G3m5,10,11,13,14	110	0.952	0.793; 1.149	0.626
G3m5,6,10,11,13,14,24	**106**	**1.295**	**1.093; 1.535**	**0.003**
G3m5,6,10,11,13,14	49	0.821	0.646; 1.043	0.100
G3m5,10,11,13,14,15	41	0.252	0.653; 1.171	0.370
G3m5,6,11,24	26	0.938	0.674; 1.302	0.708
G3m5,6,10,11,13,15,24	19	0.853	0.577; 1.259	0.424
G3m single allotypes				
G3m6	217	1.089	0.918; 1.292	0.323
G3m10	342	1.065	0.765; 1.482	0.708
G3m13	333	1.016	0.777; 1.330	0.903
G3m14	323	1.109	0.858; 1.433	0.426
G3m15	68	0.855	0.684; 1.069	0.171
G3m24	**152**	**1.195**	**1.016; 1.406**	**0.031**

This table presents the zero inflated negative binomial model obtained through the control variables mother age (in years), child age (in months), bednet use, environmental exposure, and number of antenatal visits. The reference groups were the absence of the respective models for each G3m phenotype or single allotype. G3m5 and G3m11 were not analyzed individually because the whole population group carries them.
In bold: significant P value at the 0.05 threshold.

expectations which was also observed by Munde et al. (11) (P < 0.001, **Table 4**).

FcgR Polymorphisms and Malaria Infections

Association between FcgRIIA 131R/H, FcgRIIIA 176F/V, and FcgRIIIB NA1/NA2 polymorphisms and the number of malaria infections was determined using zero-inflated binomial regression models (with and without the interaction between the genetic and environmental variables).

Association Between FcgR Polymorphisms and Malaria Infections

We determined if individual FcgR polymorphisms were associated with malaria infections (**Table 5**). None of the FcgRIIA 131RH, 131RR, nor 131HH genotypes was associated with the number of malaria infections. However, infants carrying FcgRIIIA 176VV compared to FcgRIIIA 176FF had a higher risk of infection (n = 35, IRR = 1.344, 95% CI = 0.303;3.308, P = 0.035) while the FcgRIIIB NA1NA2 was associated with a lower number of infections compared to NA2NA2 (n = 131, IRR = 0.812, 95% CI = 0.670;0.985, P = 0.035).

Finally, we analyzed the influence of FcgRIIA/RIIIA/RIIIB genotype combinations on the occurrence of malaria infections. The distribution of these combinations is shown in **Figure 2**, where 25 out of the 27 possible combinations are present in the study group, the three most prevalent of them being 131RH/176FV/NA2NA2 (10.6%), 131RH/176FV/NA1NA1 (9.1%), and 131RH/176FF/NA1NA1 (8.9%). No individual presented the 131RR/176VV/NA1NA1 and 131RR/176VV/NA2NA2 genotype combinations. Compared to the reference 131RR/176FF/NA2NA2, a higher risk of malaria infection was found for carriers of the following genotype combinations: 131RH/176VV/NA1NA2 (n = 4, IRR = 2.035, 95% CI = 1.126;3.677, P = 0.019), 131HH/176VV/NA1NA2 (n = 9, IRR = 1.842, 95% CI =

TABLE 3 | Interaction between G3m allotypes—environmental exposure and malaria infections.

G3m allotypes*exposure to malaria	n	IRR	95% CI	P value
G3m phenotypes with frequency at least 5%				
Ref. No G3m5,10,11,13,14*low exposure				
G3m5,10,11,13,14*low exposure	61	0.893	0.677; 1.179	0.427
G3m5,10,11,13,14*high exposure	49	1.209	0.927; 1.577	0.160
Ref. No G3m5,6,10,11,13,14,24*low exposure				
G3m5,6,10,11,13,14,24*low exposure	50	1.056	0.803; 1.389	0.693
G3m5,6,10,11,13,14,24*high exposure	**56**	**1.648**	**1.312; 2.070**	**<0.0001**
Ref. No G3m5,6,10,11,13,14*low exposure				
G3m5,6,10,11,13,14*low exposure	19	1.097	0.750; 1.605	0.632
G3m5,6,10,11,13,14*high exposure	30	0.932	0.685; 1.269	0.659
Ref. No G3m5,10,11,13,14,15*low exposure				
G3m5,10,11,13,14,15*low exposure	21	1.042	0.658; 1.651	0.859
G3m5,10,11,13,14,15*high exposure	20	1.018	0.695; 1.491	0.925
Ref. No G3m5,6,11,24*low exposure				
G3m5,6,11,24*low exposure	12	1.095	0.656; 1.828	0.728
G3m5,6,11,24*high exposure	14	1.059	0.682; 1.644	0.797
Ref. No G3m5,6,10,11,13,15,24*low exposure				
G3m5,6,10,11,13,15,24*low exposure	11	0.784	0.420; 1.466	0.448
G3m5,6,10,11,13,15,24*high exposure	8	1.119	0.674; 1.859	0.663
G3m single allotypes				
Ref. No G3m6*low exposure				
G3m6*low exposure	101	1.087	0.837; 1.411	0.529
G3m6*high exposure	**116**	**1.350**	**1.059; 1.720**	**0.015**
Ref. No G3m10*low exposure				
G3m10*low exposure	171	0.895	0.537; 1.491	0.671
G3m10*high exposure	171	1.137	0.685; 1.886	0.618
Ref. No G3m13*low exposure				
G3m13*low exposure	167	0.807	0.540; 1.206	0.297
G3m13*high exposure	166	1.048	0.706; 1.555	0.814
Ref. No G3m14*low exposure				
G3m14*low exposure	160	1.056	0.703; 1.585	0.792
G3m14*high exposure	163	1.336	0.895; 1.993	0.156
Ref. No G3m15*low exposure				
G3m15*low exposure	37	0.897	0.623; 1.241	0.465
G3m15*high exposure	31	1.053	0.775; 1.432	0.737
Ref. No G3m24*low exposure				
G3m24*low exposure	74	1.020	0.789; 1.317	0.878
G3m24*high exposure	**78**	**1.479**	**1.183; 1.850**	**0.001**

This table presents the zero inflated negative binomial model obtained through the control variables mother age (in years), child age (in months), number of antenatal visits, and the use of bednet. The interaction between G3m allotypes and the environmental exposure was studied. The reference groups were indicated in each case.
In bold: significant P value at the 0.05 threshold.

1.016;3.339, P = 0.044), 131HH/176VV/NA2NA2 (n = 5, IRR = 1.933, 95% CI =1.087;3.437, P = 0.025) and 131HH/176FF/NA1NA1 (n = 7, IRR = 2.110, 95% CI = 1.039;4.283, P = 0.039) (**Table 6**). To explore the potential role of environmental exposure on this effect, we introduced an interaction term in the analyses.

Interaction Between FcgR Polymorphisms—Environmental Exposure and Malaria Infections

Results confirmed the higher risk of infection associated with FcgRIIIA 176VV compared to 176FF when exposed to high levels of mosquito bites (n = 17, IRR = 1.722, 95% CI = 1.213;2.445, P = 0.002). A similar pattern, barely significant, was observed for infants carrying FcgRIIIB NA2NA2 compared to FcgRIIIB NA1NA1 (n = 51, IRR = 1.372, 95% CI = 0.998;1.885, P = 0.051) (**Table 7**).

The analysis of the interaction between FcgRIIA/RIIIA/RIIIB combined genotypes and environmental exposure showed that infants carrying 131RH/176FV/NA1NA2 compared to 131RR/176FF/NA2NA2 have a trend towards a lower number of infections when exposed to low environmental risk levels (n = 13, IRR = 0.445, 95% CI = 0.194;1.017, P = 0.055). However, compared to the same reference, the carriage of 131HH/176FF/NA1NA1 was associated with a trend towards a higher risk of infection when exposed to low levels of exposure (n = 2, IRR = 2.622, 95% CI = 0.978;7.029, P = 0.055) (**Table 8**).

Detection of Gene-Gene and Gene-Environment Interactions by Generalized Multifactor Dimensionality Reduction (GMDR)

GMDR was used to screen the potential interactions among G3m and FcgR polymorphisms and to evaluate the impact of gene-exposure interaction on the risk of malaria infection.

Among all possible one- to four-locus models evaluated by the GMDR method, none reached the cut-off significance level of 0.05 when mosquito exposure was included as a covariate in the GMDR models, along with mother and child age, bednet use, and number of antenatal visits (data not shown). In contrast, when the exposure variable was combined with G3m and FcgR polymorphisms to detect potential gene-environment interactions, several models displayed significant results (**Table 9**).

The five-factor interaction model combining G3m, FcgRIIA, FcgRIIIA, FcgRIIIB polymorphisms, and mosquito exposure was the best model identified, with the maximum prediction accuracy of 62.70%, the maximum CV consistency of 10/10, and a sign test P-value of 0.001.

These results only hold for four G3m in single form and in combinations: G3m5,6,11,24, G3m5,6,10,11,13,15,24, G3m10, and G3m13. Models with lower prediction accuracies, though still significant, were obtained for G3m5,10,11,13,14,15 and G3m14 (TBA of 0.5602 and 0.6043, respectively; CVC = 10/10 and P = 0.011 for both). These results suggest significant gene-gene interactions between G3m and FcgR polymorphisms that are only revealed in an environment of high exposure to mosquito bites. The four-factor model including the three FcgR polymorphisms and mosquito exposure was the second best prediction model with a prediction accuracy of 60.82%, a maximum CV consistency of 10/10, and a sign test P-value of 0.001. The two-factor model involving the FcgRIIA 131R/H polymorphism and mosquito exposure (TBA of 0.604) reached an almost identical prediction accuracy.

We also conducted a linear regression analysis for the significant models associating G3m, FcgR and environmental exposure found in the GMDR analysis (**Table 9**, P in bold) in order to estimate the effect of such associations. GMDR analysis is

TABLE 4 | Distribution of FcgR genotypes in the study group.

Variations	FcgRIIA 131 R/H rs1801274			FcgRIIIA 176 F/V rs396991			FcgRIIIB NA1/NA2		
Genotypes	**HH**	**RH**	**RR**	**FF**	**FV**	**VV**	**NA1NA1**	**NA1NA2**	**NA2NA2**
Number of infants (%)	80 (21.7%)	194 (52.6%)	95 (25.7%)	165 (45.2%)	165 (45.2%)	35 (9.6%)	106 (30.0%)	131 (37.1%)	116 (32.9%)
Minor allele frequency (minor allele)		0.48 (H)			0.32 (V)			0.48 (NA1)	
HWE test [a] χ^2 (P-value, df = 2)		χ^2 = 1.04 (P > 0.10)			χ^2 = 0.46 (P > 0.10)			χ^2 = 23.35 (P < 0.001)	

[a]*Hardy-Weinberg equilibrium test.*

TABLE 5 | Association between each FcgRIIA, FcgRIIIA, and FcgRIIIB genotype and malaria infections.

FcgR polymorphisms	n	IRR	95% CI	P value
FcgRIIA 131 R/H model				
131RR (reference)	95			
131RH	194	1.168	0.955; 1.429	0.129
131HH	80	8.435	0.929; 1.523	0.929
FcgRIIIA 176 F/V model				
176FF (reference)	165			
176FV	165	0.948	0.200; 1.069	0.071
176VV	**35**	**1.344**	**0.303; 3.308**	**0.035**
FcgRIIIB NA1/NA2 model				
NA2NA2 (reference)	116			
NA1NA2	**131**	**0.812**	**0.670; 0.985**	**0.035**
NA1NA1	106	0.903	0.735; 1.109	0.332

This table presents the zero inflated negative binomial individual models obtained through the control variables mother age (in years), child age (in months), number of antenatal visits, environmental exposure, and bednet use. The references are indicated for FcgRIIA R/H, FcgRIIIA F/V, and FcgRIIIB NA1/NA2.
In bold: significant P value at the 0.05 threshold.

TABLE 6 | Association between FcgRIIA/FcgRIIIA/FcgRIIIB combined genotypes and malaria infections.

FcgR polymorphisms combination models	n	IRR	95% CI	P value
131RR/176FF/NA2NA2 (reference)	21			
131RR/176FF/NA1NA2	30	1.091	0.684; 1.739	0.713
131RR/176FF/NA1NA1	9	1.456	0.842; 2.520	0.179
131RR/176FV/NA2NA2	12	1.426	0.819; 2.481	0.209
131RR/176FV/NA1NA2	10	0.495	0.214; 1.148	0.102
131RR/176FV/NA1NA1	4	0.980	0.397; 2.415	0.965
131RR/176VV/NA1NA2	1	1.053	0.306; 3.616	0.934
131RH/176FF/NA2NA2	22	1.459	0.934; 2.279	0.096
131RH/176FF/NA1NA2	26	1.036	0.655; 1.639	0.878
131RH/176FF/NA1NA1	31	1.331	0.854; 2.075	0.206
131RH/176FV/NA2NA2	37	1.365	0.879; 2.119	0.165
131RH/176FV/NA1NA2	23	1.014	0.624; 1.649	0.953
131RH/176FV/NA1NA1	32	1.186	0.748; 1.881	0.467
131RH/176VV/NA2NA2	6	0.866	0.295; 2.539	0.795
131RH/176VV/NA1NA2	**4**	**2.035**	**1.126; 3.677**	**0.019**
131RH/176VV/NA1NA1	5	0.684	0.203; 2.307	0.541
131HH/176FF/NA2NA2	5	1.919	0.922; 3.995	0.081
131HH/176FF/NA1NA2	6	0.628	0.214; 1.839	0.397
131HH/176FF/NA1NA1	**7**	**2.110**	**1.039; 4.283**	**0.039**
131HH/176FV/NA2NA2	7	1.064	0.453; 2.496	0.886
131HH/176FV/NA1NA2	20	1.180	0.727; 1.917	0.501
131HH/176FV/NA1NA1	14	0.780	0.436; 1.395	0.403
131HH/176VV/NA2NA2	**5**	**1.933**	**1.087; 3.437**	**0.025**
131HH/176VV/NA1NA2	**9**	**1.842**	**1.016; 3.339**	**0.044**
131HH/176VV/NA1NA1	4	1.838	0.877; 3.851	0.106

This table presents the zero inflated negative binomial model obtained through the control variables age (mother and child), antenatal visits, mosquito exposure, and mosquito net possession for the FcgRIIA/FcgRIIIA/FcgRIIIB genotype models. The reference was the absence of HH/FF/NA2NA2.
In bold: significant P value at the 0.05 threshold.

based on linear regression. Therefore, using linear regression models was perfectly suited to quantify the effect detected by GMDR analysis. Consistent with the GMDR analysis, the linear regression models showed a higher risk of malaria infection in carriers of 131RR/176FF/NA2NA2/G3m5,6,11,24 and 131HH/176VV/NA1NA2/G3m5,6,10,11,13,15,24 combinations, when exposed to a high-risk environment (regression coefficient = 4.804, P = 0.032 and regression coefficient = 5.444, P = 0.015, respectively) (**Supplementary Table 1**). Linear models confirmed, also, a higher risk of malaria infection in carriers of G3m10 and G3m13 combined to 131HH/176FF/NA1NA1 in a low-risk environment with a regression coefficient of 6.160 (P = 0.039) and 6.248 (P = 0.044), respectively (**Supplementary Table 2**). The genotype combination 131HH/176FF/NA1NA1 indeed showed a trend towards a higher risk of infection in a low-risk environment (**Table 8**).

DISCUSSION

We studied the combined impact of FcgRIIA, FcgRIIIA, and FcgRIIIB polymorphisms and IgG G3m allotypes on malaria susceptibility in early life in Benin. First, we studied separately the influence of IgG G3m allotypes and of FcgRs polymorphisms on the number of *P. falciparum* infections during an 18 months clinical and parasitological follow-up of newborns. Second, the influence of combined IgG G3m allotypes and FcgRs polymorphisms was assessed. We identified an increased risk of *P. falciparum* infection in infants carrying particular FcgRIIA 131R/H – FcgRIIIA 176F/V – FcgRIIIB NA1/NA2 genotypes combined to G3m5,6,11,24 or G3m5,6,10,11,13,15,24 phenotypes or to G3m10 or G3m13 single allotypes. These

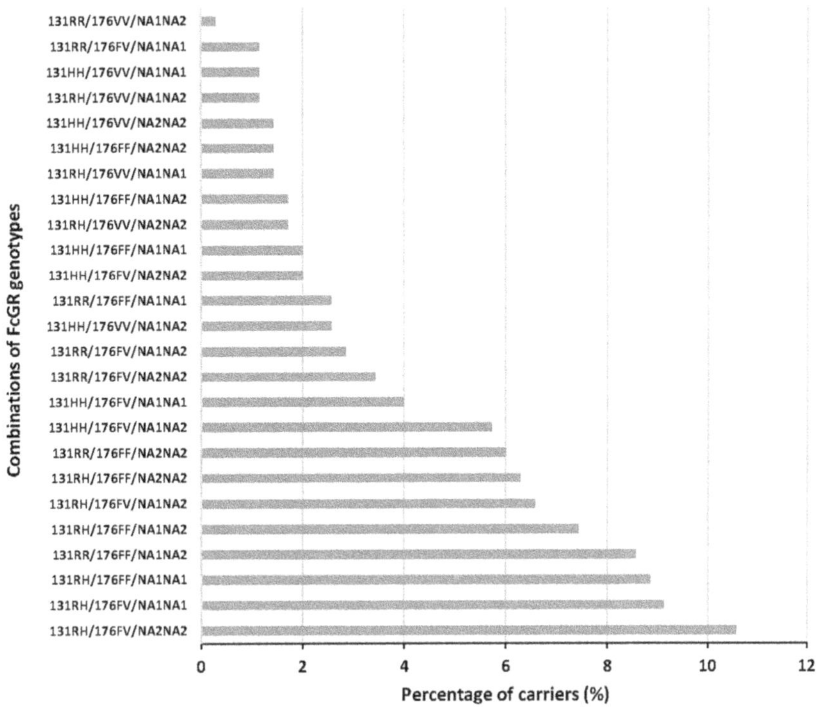

FIGURE 2 | Distribution of FcgRIIA/FcgRIIIA/FcgRIIIB phenotypes in the study group.

observations were reinforced by the application of two complementary statistical approaches (GMDR method and linear regression analysis), allowing to take into account the individual risk of exposure to malaria. **Figure 3** presents a summary of the main results.

No diversity was observed among infants for the G1m allotypes, since all infants were G1m1 and G1m17 positive; therefore, the analysis focused on the G3m diversity present on IgG3. Our results showed an increased risk of malaria infections associated with the carriage of the G3m5,6,10,11,13,14,24 phenotype. It should be pointed out that the presence of G3m24 in this combination could play an important role as it was also associated with a higher risk to be infected by *P. falciparum* when considered as a single allotype. The risk effect of some allotypes was accentuated when infants were highly exposed to mosquito bites. For example, the effect of G3m6 appeared only when the interaction with the exposure variable was considered. These results suggest that the G3m6 effect is accentuated in conditions of high mosquito exposure and the risk associated with G3m5,6,10,11,13,14,24 could be linked to the presence of both G3m6 and G3m24.

The interactions observed between G3m allotypes and mosquito exposure could be related to the quantity of anti-malarial IgG3 that increased following repeated infections with *P. falciparum*. IgG3 antibodies were shown to be protective against malaria and they can act directly by limiting host cell invasion or indirectly *via* their Fc-mediated effector functions (8, 42). Therefore, an increased level of IgG3 harboring specific G3m allotypes, in case of high mosquito exposure, could facilitate the identification of the risk effect linked to these characteristics. Of note, IgG allotypes were found to correlate with serum IgG levels (19, 43) but also with the switching between IgG isotypes suggesting that IgG allotypes may affect the humoral antibody response. Moreover, it was recently demonstrated that allotypic variants within the IgG3 subclass substantially affect FcgRIIIA binding and Antibody-Dependent Cellular Cytotoxicity (44). To our knowledge, no work has previously shown associations between Gm phenotypes comprising G3m24 or G3m24 alone with a higher risk of malaria infections, while G3m24 is prevalent among sub-Saharan African populations (45, 46). In contrast, Gm phenotypes including G3m6 have been already associated with malaria susceptibility (10, 17, 18). Indeed, the G3m5,6,13,14 phenotype was associated with a higher incidence of uncomplicated malaria (18). It is interesting to note that G3m6 allotype is rare among Fulani, who are less susceptible to malaria than other sympatric ethnic groups (17). However, we also demonstrated the existence of an inverse relationship between the carriage of the G3m5,6,13,14 phenotype and the presence of uncomplicated malaria (10) in the Fon ethnic group. Given that both polymorphisms in the IgG3 heavy chain gene and FcgR can influence the IgG binding on immunoglobulin Fc-receptors and impact immunity to malaria through ADCC, ADCI, or phagocytosis of malaria parasites, the interpretation of results coming from separate investigations of these distinct polymorphisms remains challenging.

TABLE 7 | Interaction between FcgRIIA, FcgRIIIA, and FcgRIIIB genotypes—environmental exposure and malaria infections.

FcgR genotypes*exposure to malaria	n	IRR	95% CI	P value
FcgRIIA model				
FcgRIIA 131RR*low exposure (reference)	46			
FcgRIIA 131RR*high exposure	49	0.824	0.587; 1.155	0.263
FcgRIIA 131RH*low exposure	104	0.885	0.668; 1.173	0.399
FcgRIIA 131RH*high exposure	90	1.266	0.970; 1.652	0.081
FcgRIIA 131HH*low exposure	34	0.972	0.656; 1.440	0.890
FcgRIIA 131HH*high exposure	46	1.213	0.892; 1.650	0.218
FcgRIIIA model				
FcgRIIIA 176FF*low exposure (reference)	76			
FcgRIIIA 176FF*high exposure	89	1.072	0.847; 1.357	0.559
FcgRIIIA 176FV*low exposure	78	0.833	0.640; 1.083	0.174
FcgRIIIA 176FV*high exposure	87	1.124	0.884; 1.430	0.337
FcgRIIIA 176VV*low exposure	18	1.022	0.646; 1.616	0.924
FcgRIIIA 176VV*high exposure	**17**	**1.722**	**1.213; 2.445**	**0.002**
FcgRIIIB model				
FcgRIIIB NA2NA2*low exposure (reference)	65			
FcgRIIIB NA2NA2*high exposure	51	1.227	0.932; 1.617	0.144
FcgRIIIB NA1NA2*low exposure	66	0.814	0.610; 1.085	0.161
FcgRIIIB NA1NA2*high exposure	65	0.997	0.764; 1.299	0.983
FcgRIIIB NA1NA1*low exposure	48	0.894	0.649; 1.233	0.497
FcgRIIIB NA1NA1*high exposure	58	1.115	0.847; 1.468	0.436
FcgRIIIB NA1NA1*low exposure (reference)	48			
FcgRIIIB NA2NA2*high exposure	51	1.372	0.998; 1.885	0.051

This table presents the zero inflated negative binomial model obtained through the control variables mother age (in years), child age (in months), number of antenatal visits mosquito, and bednet use. The interaction between FcgR polymorphisms and environmental exposure was studied. The reference was the absence of estimations in FcgRIIA R/H, FcgRIIIA F/V, and FcgRIIIB NA1/NA2.

In bold: significant P value at the 0.05 threshold; underlined: trend of significance at the P value threshold of 0.05.

FcgRs provide a crucial link between the humoral and cellular immune responses. Polymorphisms which alter the affinity of FcgRs in binding IgG subclasses have been described. In human, FcgRII and FcgRIII are known to bind IgG subclasses. Regarding FcgRIIA 131R/H polymorphisms, our results revealed no significant association with malaria infections whether or not the mosquito exposure factor was taken into account. On the other side, a malaria risk associated with the FcgRIIIA 176VV genotype was observed, which was strengthened in conditions of high exposure to mosquitoes. These results differed from those of Omi et al. (47) who found no relation between FcgRIIIA 176F/V polymorphism and the severity of malaria in Thai people (47) and of Munde et al. (11) who showed no relation between FcgRIIIA 176F/V and severe malarial anemia (SMA) (11). The differences in the size of the population groups, the ethnic origin and genetic diversity of the populations and the clinical definition of malaria used, may preclude a rigorous comparison between studies. In other cases, the FcgRIIIA 176V allele was identified as a genetic risk factor for the development of atopic diseases (48) or for generalized aggressive periodontitis (39). It has been shown that the 176V variant improved the FcgRIIIA affinity for IgG1 and IgG2 (49). Regarding our results, this same variant could be associated with a lower affinity to IgG3, thus reducing the effectiveness of the antimalarial response. Finally, our results showed an association between the FcgRIIIB NA1NA2 genotype and protection against malaria when compared to the carriage of NA2NA2, while in conditions of high mosquito exposure, the NA2NA2 genotype was associated with a higher risk compared to NA1NA1. The polymorphic expression of FcgRIIIB NA1/NA2 influences the phagocytic capacity of neutrophils and Salmon et al. (50) already showed a decreased phagocytosis in relation to NA2NA2 compared to NA1NA1 (50). In line with these results, other studies showed a risk for malaria (30) or cerebral malaria (29) associated with the carriage of the FcgRIIIB NA2 variant.

TABLE 8 | Interaction between FcgRIIA/RIIIA/RIIIB combined genotypes—environmental exposure and malaria infections.

FcgR genotypes combinations*exposure to malaria	n	IRR	95% CI	P value
131RR/176FF/NA2NA2*low exposure (reference)	9			
131RR/176FF/NA2NA2*high exposure	12	0.737	0.356; 1.524	0.411
131RR/176FF/NA1NA2*low exposure	10	0.947	0.498; 1.801	0.869
131RR/176FF/NA1NA2*high exposure	16	0.729	0.354; 1.503	0.393
131RR/176FF/NA1NA1*low exposure	5	1.078	0.508; 2.284	0.844
131RR/176FF/NA1NA1*high exposure	4	1.293	0.573; 2.917	0.535
131RR/176FV/NA2NA2*low exposure	7	1.052	0.513; 2.158	0.889
131RR/176FV/NA2NA2*high exposure	5	1.230	0.486; 3.113	0.662
131RR/176FV/NA1NA2*low exposure	3	0.219	0.028; 1.692	0.146
131RR/176FV/NA1NA2*high exposure	7	0.488	0.185; 1.286	0.147
131RR/176FV/NA1NA1*low exposure	3	0.880	0.284; 2.726	0.825
131RR/176FV/NA1NA1*high exposure	1	0.621	0.138; 2.793	0.535
131RR/176VV/NA1NA2*low exposure	1	0.796	0.224; 2.821	0.724
131RH/176FF/NA2NA2*low exposure	14	1.018	0.536; 1.933	0.955
131RH/176FF/NA2NA2*high exposure	8	1.385	0.728; 2.634	0.320
131RH/176FF/NA1NA2*low exposure	11	0.801	0.403; 1.595	0.529
131RH/176FF/NA1NA2*high exposure	15	0.883	0.464; 1.680	0.706
131RH/176FF/NA1NA1*low exposure	10	0.998	0.478; 2.084	0.997
131RH/176FF/NA1NA1*high exposure	21	1.176	0.638; 2.169	0.602
131RH/176FV/NA2NA2*low exposure	23	0.952	0.504; 1.799	0.881
131RH/176FV/NA2NA2*high exposure	14	1.287	0.685; 2.418	0.431
131RH/176FV/NA1NA2*low exposure	13	0.445	0.194; 1.017	0.055
131RH/176FV/NA1NA2*high exposure	10	1.147	0.598; 2.201	0.679
131RH/176FV/NA1NA1*low exposure	17	0.752	0.381; 1.484	0.412
131RH/176FV/NA1NA1*high exposure	15	1.207	0.629; 2.318	0.571
131RH/176VV/NA2NA2*low exposure	5	0.642	0.206; 2.001	0.445
131RH/176VV/NA1NA2*low exposure	3	1.778	0.720; 4.386	0.211
131RH/176VV/NA1NA2*high exposure	3	1.675	0.761; 3.688	0.200
131RH/176VV/NA1NA1*low exposure	2	0.381	0.049; 2.933	0.355
131RH/176VV/NA1NA1*high exposure	3	0.733	0.164; 3.280	0.685
131HH/176FF/NA2NA2*low exposure	2	1.013	0.286; 3.591	0.983
131HH/176FF/NA2NA2*high exposure	3	1.855	0.746; 4.609	0.183
131HH/176FF/NA1NA2*low exposure	3	0.481	0.134; 1.719	0.260
131HH/176FF/NA1NA2*high exposure	3	0.454	0.058; 3.496	0.449
131HH/176FF/NA1NA1*low exposure	2	2.622	0.978; 7.029	0.055
131HH/176FF/NA1NA1*high exposure	5	1.332	0.498; 3.559	0.567
131HH/176FV/NA2NA2*high exposure	7	0.943	0.375; 2.371	0.901
131HH/176FV/NA1NA2*low exposure	10	1.033	0.504; 2.118	0.927
131HH/176FV/NA1NA2*high exposure	10	0.955	0.486; 1.876	0.895
131HH/176FV/NA1NA1*low exposure	6	0.362	0.103; 1.275	0.114
131HH/176FV/NA1NA1*high exposure	8	0.791	0.381; 1.641	0.530
131HH/176VV/NA2NA2*low exposure	2	1.520	0.535; 4.319	0.431
131HH/176VV/NA2NA2*high exposure	3	1.724	0.835; 3.559	0.140
131HH/176VV/NA1NA2*low exposure	4	0.366	0.047; 2.828	0.336
131HH/176VV/NA1NA2*high exposure	5	1.888	0.922; 3.867	0.082
131HH/176VV/NA1NA1*low exposure	2	1.328	0.430; 4.099	0.622
131HH/176VV/NA1NA1*high exposure	2	1.752	0.673; 4.562	0.251

This table presents the zero inflated negative binomial model, with the interaction between FcgR and environmental exposure obtained through the control variables mother age (in years), child age (in months), number of antenatal visits, and use of bednet.

Underlined: trend of significance at the P value threshold of 0.05.

TABLE 9 | Association between FcgR polymorphisms, G3m phenotypes, and malaria infections: Results of the GMDR analysis when considering environmental exposure as an interaction variable.

No. of variables considered	Best model	Testing balanced accuracy(TBA)	Sign test P-value	Cross-validation consistency (CVC)
1	environmental exposure	0.6161	**0.0107**	10/10
2	FcgRIIA, environmental exposure	0.6038	**0.0010**	9/10
3	FcgRIIA, FcgRIIIA, environmental exposure	0.4871	0.6230	5/10
4	FcgRIIA, FcgRIIIA, FcgRIIIB, environmental exposure	0.6082	**0.0010**	10/10
5	G3m†, FcgRIIA, FcgRIIIA, FcgRIIIB, environmental exposure	0.6270	**0.0010**	10/10

All models are adjusted for mother age (in years), child age (in months), bednet use, and number of antenatal visits.

†These results were obtained only for the four following G3m allotypes and allotype combinations: G3m5,6,11,24, G3m5,6,10,11,13,15,24, G3m10, and G3m13 (each considered as presence/absence). The five-factor models were also significant for G3m5,10,11,13,14,15 (TBA = 0.5602; CVC = 10/10) and G3m14 (TBA = 0.6043; CVC = 10/10) although at a lesser degree (sign test P = 0.0107 in both cases).

In bold: significant P value at the 0.05 threshold.

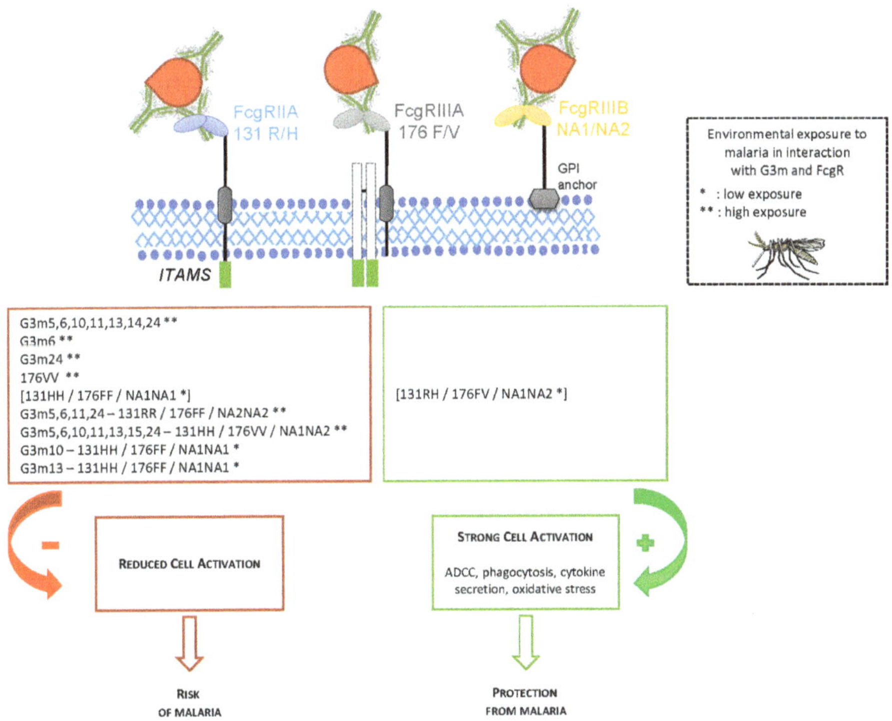

FIGURE 3 | Summary of the main findings of the study.

FcgR receptors act synergistically by crosslinking. The additive effects of the host FcgRIIA/FcgRIIIA/FcgRIIIB genotypes might impact the immune response to *P. falciparum* and therefore affect the outcome of the disease. This synergy function results in phagocytosis of immunoglobulin-opsonized immune complexes and in the stimulation of neutrophils degranulation, which leads to the production of reactive oxygen species (ROS). The absence in our study of relationship with malaria infection involving FcgRIIA/FcgRIIIA genotype combinations compared to FcgRIIA/FcgRIIIA/FcgRIIIB ones may reflect a particular synergy between FcgRIIA and FcgRIIIB receptors (**Table 9**). Indeed, it has been shown that FcgRIIA and FcgRIIIB can interact functionally to trigger neutrophils by means of an IgG mediated response (51–53). Moreover, FcgRIIA is considered essential for the induction of effector functions, and the abundance of FcgRIIIB can guarantee an effective interaction with IgG complexes (54). As already suggested, the HWE deviation observed for FcgRIIIB could be due to unidentified mutations likely resulting from disease-related evolutionary selection pressure exerted by *P. falciparum* and potentially by other infectious diseases occurring in the population (11).

It has been shown that FcgRIIA 131H contributes to an efficient binding to IgG2 and IgG3 as opposed to 131R (23) and also that IgG2 and IgG3 contribute to individual resistance to malaria (8). The 131H variant was found more prevalent in the Fulani people of Daraweesh, a village in eastern Sudan, who are less affected by clinical malaria (55). The same variant was associated with protection from malaria infection in Indian individuals at least 5 years old (56) and with protection against high parasitemia both in African and Asian people (31). However it was associated with a higher risk in a cohort of Gambian children less than 5 years (57). In comparison, the 131R variant has been shown to play a major role in ADRB (58, 59) and is associated with a low phagocytic activity and poor immune complex clearance (60). In genotype analysis, the higher risk associated with 131RH/176VV/NA1NA2, 131HH/176VV/NA2NA2, 131HH/176VV/NA1NA2 and 131HH/176FF/NA1NA1 carriage compared to 131RR/176FF/NA2NA2 may be explained by the presence of FcgRIIIA 176VV in the three first genotype combinations. Moreover, the joint presence of FcgRIIA 131H variant in all combinations is in line with results from some of the studies reported above, according to which this variant is less protective than the 131R one (57).

Since G3m and FcgR polymorphisms act individually on malaria infections, it is plausible that their combined polymorphisms act in synergy against malaria infections. This aspect has never been studied before and the MDR method was used to precisely explore it. The G3m5,6,11,24 - 131RR/176FF/NA2NA2 and G3m5,6,10,11,13,15,24 - 131HH/176VV/NA1NA2 combinations were the most significant G3m/FcgR ones associated with malaria (at risk according to the linear regressions) when taking into account the interaction with the environmental variable of exposure to mosquito bites, according to the GMDR analysis. This is particularly interesting in view of the preceding results, indicative of a cumulative risk linked to the double carriage of G3m6 and G3m24 joined to either FcgRIIIA 176VV or FcgRIIIB NA2NA2. Moreover, linear regression of these interactions showed high regression coefficients (4.804 and 5.444). Thus, these interactions are at risk under conditions of high exposure to mosquito bites because of the cumulative presence of G3m6 and G3m24 in one hand and of the FcgRIIIA 176VV and FcgRIIIB NA2NA2 genotypes in another hand. The malaria risk under conditions of low exposure involving G3m10 - FcgRIIA 131HH/FcgRIIIA 176FF/FcgRIIIB NA1NA1 and G3m13 - FcgRIIA 131HH/FcgRIIIA 176FF/FcgRIIIB NA1NA1 is interesting to note since at the individual level, G3m10 and G3m13 did not show any significant association. Thus, this result could reflect the fact that the effect found is only due to the influence of the FcgR association. Moreover, the linear regression showed that the FcgR associations concerned were defined at risk in the previous results.

The efficacy of IgG3 response can be explained by FcgR affinity but also by the nature of targeted antigens. High concentrations of AMA1, MSP1, MSP2-FC27, MSP3, GLURP-R2-specific IgG3 were found in infants able to control asymptomatic infections (61). Of course, other key antigens expressed during the different steps of the *P. falciparum* cycle life probably participate to the control of the parasite growth. Functional assays will clarify the mechanisms and antigens involved in malaria protection. These answers can probably also vary depending immune system cells. For example, FcgRIIIB is present on neutrophils and not monocytes, natural killers react more with FcgRIIIA compared to FcgRIIA, while monocytes and macrophages present both FcgRIIA and FcgRIIIA.

This study showed the importance of polymorphisms in both FcgR and IgG in the modulation of the risk of malaria infections in Beninese infants. It would then be interesting to look at the CNV (Copy Number Variations) of these polymorphisms and their influence on risk or protection against malaria. CNV are polymorphisms represented by DNA segments that differ among individuals due to suppression, insertion, inversion, duplication, or complex recombination (62). Recent studies have highlighted the relationship between CNV and disease: FcgRIIIB low CNV was associated with systemic lupus erythematosus risk (63) while for Chen et al. (64) a low FcgRIIIA CNV was positively associated with lupus and rheumatoid arthritis and a low FcgRIIIB CNV, with a risk of lupus but not rheumatoid arthritis (64). It would be interesting, thus, to explore the role of CNV in FcgR receptors in individual variation of malaria susceptibility.

In summary, the current study demonstrates that some combined G3m-FcgR polymorphisms are associated with a malaria risk and that this risk is even more pronounced in case of high mosquito exposure. The results highlight the relevance of studying combined IgG heavy chain/FcgR polymorphisms in relation to *P. falciparum* malaria as one or the other, or both, may influence the individual susceptibility to infection. Understanding the functional diversity within IgG subclasses may shed light on associations found with infectious diseases or auto-immune diseases and potentially initiate new strategies to improve therapeutic antibodies.

ETHICS STATEMENT

The studies involving human participants were reviewed and approved by the Abomey-Calavi's institutional review board and the IRD's Consultative Ethics Committee. Written informed consent to participate in this study was provided by the participants' legal guardian/next of kin.

AUTHOR CONTRIBUTIONS

CD, DC, and FM-N conceived and designed the project. AF, EG, DC, and FM-N performed the laboratory experiments. JM and J-MD brought technical support or result validation. AF, CD, AS, AG, DC, and FM-N performed statistical analysis. AF, CD, DC, and FM-N wrote the paper. All authors contributed to the article and approved the submitted version.

ACKNOWLEDGMENTS

The authors are grateful to all women and infants of Tori Bossito who agreed to participate in this project, to field supervisors and community health workers of contributing villages, to midwives, nurses, and health auxiliaries of the three health centers, as well as to laboratory technicians of Tori Bossito for their collaboration. The authors would like to thank the Faculté des Sciences de la Santé (FSS), the Institut des Sciences Biomédicales Appliquées de Cotonou (ISBA), the Programme National de Lutte contre le Paludisme (PNLP) for their institutional support.

REFERENCES

1. World Health Organization. (2019). Available at: https://www.who.int/malaria/publications/world-malaria-report-2018/report/fr/ (Accessed December 2019).
2. Cohen S, Carrington S, McGregor IA. Gamma-globulin and acquired immunity to human malaria. *Nature* (1961) 192:733–7. doi: 10.1038/192733a0
3. Sabchareon A, Burnouf T, Ouattara D, Attanath P, Bouharoun-Tayoun H, Chantavanich P, et al. Parasitologic and clinical human response to immunoglobulin administration in falciparum malaria. *Am J Trop Med Hyg* (1991) 45:297–308. doi: 10.4269/ajtmh.1991.45.297
4. Aribot G, Rogier C, Sarthou JL, Trape JF, Balde AT, Druilhe P, et al. Pattern of immunoglobulin isotype response to Plasmodium falciparum blood-stage antigens in individuals living in a holoendemic area of Senegal (Dielmo, west Africa). *Am J Trop Med Hyg* (1996) 54:449–57. doi: 10.4269/ajtmh.1996.54.449
5. Beck HP, Felger I, Genton B, Alexander N, Al-Yaman F, Anders RF, et al. Humoral and cell-mediated immunity to the Plasmodium falciparum ring-infected erythrocyte surface antigen in an adult population exposed to highly endemic malaria. *Infect Immun* (1995) 63:596–600. doi: 10.1128/IAI.63.2.596-600.1995
6. Ferreira MU, Kimura EAS, Katzin AM, Santos-Neto LL, Ferrari JO, Villalobos JM, et al. The IgG-subclass distribution of naturally acquired antibodies to Plasmodium falciparum, in relation to malaria exposure and severity. *Ann Trop Med Parasitol* (1998) 92:245–56. doi: 10.1080/00034989859807
7. Dechavanne C, Dechavanne S, Sadissou I, Lokossou AG, Alvarado F, Dambrun M, et al. Associations between an IgG3 polymorphism in the binding domain for FcRn, transplacental transfer of malaria-specific IgG3, and protection against Plasmodium falciparum malaria during infancy: a birth cohort study in Benin. *PloS Med* (2017) 14:e1002403. doi: 10.1371/journal.pmed.1002403
8. Courtin D, Oesterholt M, Huismans H, Kusi K, Milet J, Badaut C, et al. The quantity and quality of African children's IgG responses to merozoite surface antigens reflect protection against Plasmodium falciparum malaria. *PloS One* (2009) 4:e7590. doi: 10.1371/journal.pone.0007590
9. Beeson JG, Drew DR, Boyle MJ, Feng G, Fowkes FJ, Richards JS. Merozoite surface proteins in red blood cell invasion, immunity and vaccines against malaria. *FEMS Microbiol Rev* (2016) 40:343–72. doi: 10.1093/femsre/fuw001
10. Migot-Nabias F, Noukpo JM, Guitard E, Doritchamou J, Garcia A, Dugoujon JM. Imbalanced distribution of GM immunoglobulin allotypes according to the clinical presentation of Plasmodium falciparum malaria in Beninese children. *J Infect Dis* (2008) 198:1892–5. doi: 10.1086/593210
11. Munde EO, Okeyo WA, Raballah E, Anyona SB, Were T, Ong'echa JM, et al. Association between Fcg receptor IIA, IIIA and IIIB genetic polymorphisms and susceptibility to severe malaria anemia in children in western Kenya. *BMC Infect Dis* (2017) 17:289. doi: 10.1186/s12879-017-2390-0
12. De Lange GG. Polymorphisms of human immunoglobulins: Gm, Am, Em and Km allotypes. *Exp Clin Immunogenet* (1989) 6:7–17.
13. Lefranc MP, Lefranc G. Human Gm, Km, and Am allotypes and their molecular characterization: a remarkable demonstration of polymorphism. *Methods Mol Biol* (2012) 882:635–80. doi: 10.1007/978-1-61779-842-9_34
14. Lefranc M-P, Giudicelli V, Duroux P, Jabado-Michaloud J, Folch G, Aouinti S. IMGT®, the international ImMunoGeneTics information system® 25 years on. *Nucleic Acids Res* (2015) 43(Database issue):D413–22. doi: 10.1093/nar/gku1056
15. Dugoujon JM, Hazout S, Loirat F, Mourrieras B, Crouau-Roy B, Sanchez-Mazas A. GM haplotype diversity of 82 populations over the world suggests a centrifugal model of human migrations. *Am J Phys Anthropol* (2004) 125:175–92. doi: 10.1002/ajpa.10405
16. Facer CA. Direct antiglobulin reactions in Gambian children with P. falciparum malaria. III. Expression of IgG subclass determinants and genetic markers and association with anaemia. *Clin Exp Immunol* (1980) 41:81–90.
17. Pandey JP, Nasr A, Rocca KM, Troye-Blomberg M, Elghazali G. Significant differences in GM allotype frequencies between two sympatric tribes with markedly differential susceptibility to malaria. *Parasite Immunol* (2007) 29:267–9. doi: 10.1111/j.1365-3024.2007.00938.x
18. Giha HA, Nasr A, Iriemenam NC, Arnot D, Troye-Blomberg M, Theander TG, et al. Antigen-specific influence of GM/KM allotypes on IgG isotypes and association of GM allotypes with susceptibility to Plasmodium falciparum malaria. *Malar J* (2009) 8:306. doi: 10.1186/1475-2875-8-306
19. Pandey JP, Morais GC, Fontes JFC, Braga EM. Immunoglobulin GM 3 23 5,13,14 phenotype is strongly associated with IgG1 antibody responses to Plasmodium vivax vaccine candidate antigens PvMSP1-19 and PvAMA-1. *Malar J* (2010) 9:229. doi: 10.1186/1475-2875-9-229
20. Ravetch J. In vivo veritas: the surprising roles of Fc receptors in immunity. *Nat Immunol* (2010) 11:183–5. doi: 10.1038/ni0310-183
21. Hogarth PM, Pietersz GA. Fc receptor-targeted therapies for the treatment of inflammation, cancer and beyond. *Nat Rev Drug Discovery* (2012) 11:311–31. doi: 10.1038/nrd2909
22. Parren PW, Warmerdam PA, Boeije LC, Arts J, Westerdaal NA, Vlug A, et al. On the interaction of IgG subclasses with the low affinity Fc gamma RIIa (CD32) on human monocytes, neutrophils, and platelets. Analysis of a functional polymorphism to human IgG2. *J Clin Invest* (1992) 90:1537–46. doi: 10.1172/JCI116022
23. Vidarsson G, Dekkers G, Rispens T. IgG subclasses and allotypes : from structure to effector functions. *Front Immunol* (2014) 5:520:520. doi: 10.3389/fimmu.2014.00520
24. Ouma C, Keller CC, Opondo DA, Were T, Otieno RO, Otieno MF, et al. Association of FCgamma receptor IIA (CD32) polymorphism with malarial anemia and high-density parasitemia in infants and young children. *Am J Trop Med Hyg* (2006) 74:573–7. doi: 10.4269/ajtmh.2006.74.573
25. Yoo EM, Morrison S. "Antibody Engineering", in Encyclopedia of Industrial Biotechnology, Bioprocess, Bioseparation, and Cell Technology, ed. John Wiley & Sons. (2010) 1:332–43. doi: 10.1002/9780470054581.eib044
26. Huizinga TW, Kleijer M, Tetteroo PA, Roos D, von dem Borne AE. Biallelic neutrophil Na-antigen system is associated with a polymorphism on the phospho-inositol-linked Fc gamma receptor III (CD16). *Blood* (1990) 75:213–7. doi: 10.1182/blood.V75.1.213.bloodjournal751213
27. Bux J, Kissel K, Hofmann C, Santoso S. The use of allele-specific recombinant Fc gamma receptor IIIb antigens for the detection of granulocyte antibodies. *Blood* (1999) 93:357–62. doi: 10.1182/blood.V93.1.357.401k39_357_362
28. Huizinga TW, Kerst M, Nuyens JH, Vlug A, von dem Borne AE, Roos D, et al. Binding characteristics of dimeric IgG subclass complexes to human neutrophils. *J Immunol* (1989) 142:2359–64.
29. Omi K, Ohashi J, Patarapotikul J, Hananantachai H, Naka I, Looareesuwan S, et al. Fcgamma receptor IIA and IIIB polymorphisms are associated with susceptibility to cerebral malaria. *Parasitol Int* (2002) 51:361–6. doi: 10.1016/s1383-5769(02)00040-5
30. Adu B, Dodoo D, Adukpo S, Hedley PL, Arthur FK, Gerds TA, et al. Fc g receptor IIIB (FcgRIIIB) polymorphisms are associated with clinical malaria in Ghanaian children. *PloS One* (2012) 7:e46197. doi: 10.1371/journal.pone.0046197
31. Zhao J, Ma L, Chen S, Xie Y, Xie L, Deng Y, et al. Association between Fc-gamma receptor IIa (CD32) gene polymorphism and malaria susceptibility: a meta-analysis based on 6928 subjects. *Infect Genet Evol* (2014) 23:169–75. doi: 10.1016/j.meegid.2014.02.011
32. Grant AV, Roussilhon C, Paul R, Sakuntabhai A. The genetic control of immunity to Plasmodium infection. *BMC Immunol* (2015) 16:14. doi: 10.1186/s12865-015-0078-z
33. Maiga B, Dolo A, Toure O, Dara V, Tapily A, Campino S, et al. Fc gamma receptor IIa-H131R polymorphism and malaria susceptibility in sympatric ethnic groups, Fulani and Dogon of Mali. *Scand J Immunol* (2014) 79:43–50. doi: 10.1111/sji.12122
34. Ouma C, Davenport GC, Garcia S, Kempaiah P, Chaudhary A, Were T, et al. Functional haplotypes of Fc gamma (Fcg) receptor (FcgRIIA and FcgRIIIB) predict risk to repeated episodes of severe malarial anemia and mortality in Kenyan children. *Hum Genet* (2012) 131:289–99. doi: 10.1007/s00439-011-1076-8
35. Le Port A, Cottrell G, Martin-Prevel Y, Migot-Nabias F, Cot M, Garcia A. First malaria infections in a cohort of infants in Benin : biological, environmental and genetic determinants. Description Study Site Population Methods Prelim Results *BMJ Open* (2012) 2:e000342. doi: 10.1136/bmjopen-2011-000342
36. Dechavanne C, Sadissou I, Bouraima A, Ahouangninou C, Amoussa R, Milet J, et al. Acquisition of natural humoral immunity to P. falciparum in early life in Benin: impact of clinical, environmental and host factors. *Sci Rep* (2016) 6:33961. doi: 10.1038/srep33961

37. Cottrell G, Kouwaye B, Pierrat C, Le Port A, Bourama A, Fonton N, et al. Modeling the influence of local environmental factors on malaria transmission in Benin and its implications for cohort study. *PloS One* (2012) 7:e28812. doi: 10.1371/journal.pone.0028812
38. Field LL, Dugoujon JM. Immunoglobulin allotyping GM, KM of GAW5 families. *Genet Epidemiol* (1989) 6:31–3. doi: 10.1002/gepi.1370060108
39. Hans VM, Mehta DS. Genetic polymorphism of Fcγ-receptors IIa, IIIa and IIIb in South Indian patients with generalized aggressive periodontitis. *J Oral Sci* (2011) 53:467–74. doi: 10.2334/josnusd.53.467
40. Lou XY, Chen GB, Yan L, Ma JZ, Zhu J, Elston R, et al. A generalized combinatorial approach for detecting gene-by-gene and gene-by-environment interactions with application to nicotine dependence. *Am J Hum Genet* (2007) 80:1125–37. doi: 10.1086/518312
41. Van Buuren S, Groothuis-Oudshoorn K. mice: Multivariate Imputation by Chained Equations in R. *J Stat Software* (2011) 45:1–67. doi: 10.18637/jss.v045.i03
42. Roussilhon C, Oeuvray C, Müller-Graf C, Tall A, Rogier C, Trape JF, et al. Long-term clinical protection from falciparum malaria is strongly associated with IgG3 antibodies to merozoite surface protein 3. *PloS Med* (2007) 13:e320. doi: 10.1371/journal.pmed.0040320
43. Pandey JP, French MA. GM phenotypes influence the concentrations of the four subclasses of immunoglobulin G in normal human serum. *Hum Immunol* (1996) 51:99–102. doi: 10.1016/s0198-8859(96)00205-4
44. De Taeye SW, Bentlage AEH, Mebius MM, Meesters JI, Lissenberg-Thunnissen S, Falck D, et al. FcγR Binding and ADCC Activity of Human IgG Allotypes. *Front Immunol* (2020) 11:740. doi: 10.3389/fimmu.2020.00740
45. Damelang T, Rogerson SJ, Kent SJ, Chung AW. Role of IgG3 in infectious diseases. *Trends Immunol* (2019) 40:197–211. doi: 10.1016/j.it.2019.01.005
46. Dard P, Lefranc MP, Osipova L, Sanchez-Mazas A. DNA sequence variability of IGHG3 alleles associated to the main G3m haplotypes in human populations. *Eur J Hum Genet* (2001) 9:765–72. doi: 10.1038/sj.ejhg.5200700
47. Omi K, Ohashi J, Patarapotikul J, Hananantachai H, Naka I, Looareesuwan S, et al. Absence of association between the Fc gamma receptor IIIA-176F/V polymorphism and the severity of malaria in Thai. *Jpn J Infect Dis* (2002) 55:167–9.
48. Zeyrek D, Tanac R, Altinoz S, Berdeli A, Gulen F, Koksoy H, et al. FcγRIIIa-V/F 158 polymorphism in Turkish children with asthma bronchiale and allergic rhinitis. *Pediatr Allergy Immunol* (2008) 19:20–4. doi: 10.1111/j.1399-3038.2007.00553.x
49. Bruhns P, Iannascoli B, England P, Mancardi DA, Fernandez N, Jorieux S, et al. Specificity and affinity of human Fcgamma receptors and their polymorphic variants for human IgG subclasses. *Blood* (2009) 113:3716–25. doi: 10.1182/blood-2008-09-179754
50. Salmon JE, Edberg JC, Kimberly RP. Fc gamma receptor III on human neutrophils. *Allelic Variants Have Function Distinct Capacities J Clin Invest* (1990) 85:1287–95. doi: 10.1172/JCI114566
51. Salmon JE, Millard SS, Brogle NL, Kimberly RP. Fc gamma receptor IIIb enhances Fc gamma receptor IIa function in an oxidant-dependent and allele-sensitive manner. *J Clin Invest* (1995) 95:2877–85. doi: 10.1172/JCI117994
52. Vossebeld PJ, Homburg CH, Roos D, Verhoeven AJ. The anti-Fc gamma RIII mAb 3G8 induces neutrophil activation via a cooperative action of Fc gamma RIIIb and Fc gamma RIIa. *Int J Biochem Cell Biol* (1997) 29:465–73. doi: 10.1016/s1357-2725(96)00160-4
53. Edberg JC, Kimberly RP. Modulation of Fc gamma and complement receptor function by the glycosyl-phosphatidylinositol-anchored form of Fc gamma RIII. *J Immunol* (1994) 152:5826–35.
54. Van Sorge NM, Van der Pol WL, Van de Winkel JG. FcgammaR polymorphisms: implications for function, disease susceptibility and immunotherapy. *Tissue Antigens* (2003) 61:189–202. doi: 10.1034/j.1399-0039.2003.00037.x
55. Nasr A, Iriemenam NC, Troye-Blomberg M, Giha HA, Balogun HA, Osman OF, et al. Fc gamma receptor IIa (CD32) polymorphism and antibody responses to asexual blood-stage antigens of Plasmodium falciparum malaria in Sudanese patients. *Scand J Immunol* (2007) 66:87–96. doi: 10.1111/j.1365-3083.2007.01947.x
56. Sinha S, Mishra SK, Sharma S, Patibandla PK, Mallick PK, Sharma SK, et al. Polymorphisms of TNF-enhancer and gene for FcgammaRIIa correlate with the severity of falciparum malaria in the ethnically diverse Indian population. *Malar J* (2008) 7:13. doi: 10.1186/1475-2875-7-13
57. Cooke GS, Aucan C, Walley AJ, Segal S, Greenwood BM, Kwiatkowski DP, et al. Association of Fcgamma receptor IIa (CD32) polymorphism with severe malaria in West Africa. *Am J Trop Med Hyg* (2003) 69:565–8. doi: 10.4269/ajtmh.2003.69.565
58. Pleass RJ, Ogun SA, McGuinness DH, Van de Winkel JG, Holder AA, Woof JM. Novel antimalarial antibodies highlight the importance of the antibody Fc region in mediating protection. *Blood* (2003) 102:4424–30. doi: 10.1182/blood-2003-02-0583
59. Shi J, McIntosh RS, Adame-Gallegos J, Dehal PK, Van Egmond M, Van de Winkel J, et al. The generation and evaluation of recombinant human IgA specific for Plasmodium falciparum merozoite surface protein 1-19 (PfMSP1 19). *BMC Biotechnol* (2011) 11:77. doi: 10.1186/1472-6750-11-77
60. Warmerdam PA, van de Winkel JG, Gosselin EJ, Capel PJ. Molecular basis for a polymorphism of human Fc gamma receptor II (CD32). *J Exp Med* (1990) 172:19–25. doi: 10.1084/jem.172.1.19
61. Adamou R, Dechavanne C, Sadissou I, d'Almeida T, Bouraima A, Sonon P, et al. Plasmodium falciparum merozoite surface antigen-specific cytophilic IgG and control of malaria infection in a Beninese birth cohort. *Malar J* (2019) 18:194–204. doi: 10.1186/s12936-019-2831-x
62. Redon R, Ishikawa S, Fitch KR, Feuk L, Scherer SW, Hurles ME, et al. Global variation in copy number in the human genome. *Nature* (2006) 444:444–54. doi: 10.1038/nature05329
63. Molokhia M, Fanciulli M, Petretto E, Patrick AL, McKeigue P, Roberts AL, et al. FCGR3B copy number variation is associated with systemic lupus erythematosus risk in Afro-Caribbeans. *Rheumatol (Oxford)* (2011) 50:1206–10. doi: 10.1093/rheumatology/keq456
64. Chen JY, Wang CM, Chang SW, Cheng CH, Jan Wu YJ, Lin JC, et al. Association of FCGR3A and FCGR3B copy number variations with systemic lupus erythematosus and rheumatoid arthritis in Taiwanese patients. *Arthritis Rheumatol* (2014) 66:3113–21. doi: 10.1002/art.38813

7

Short-Lived Immunity After 17DD Yellow Fever Single Dose Indicates that Booster Vaccination may be Required to Guarantee Protective Immunity in Children

Ana Carolina Campi-Azevedo[1*†], *Laise Rodrigues Reis*[1†], *Vanessa Peruhype-Magalhães*[1], *Jordana Grazziela Coelho-dos-Reis*[1], *Lis Ribeiro Antonelli*[1], *Cristina Toscano Fonseca*[1], *Christiane Costa-Pereira*[1], *Elaine Maria Souza-Fagundes*[2], *Ismael Artur da Costa-Rocha*[1], *Juliana Vaz de Melo Mambrini*[1], *Jandira Aparecida Campos Lemos*[3], *José Geraldo Leite Ribeiro*[4], *Iramaya Rodrigues Caldas*[1], *Luiz Antônio Bastos Camacho*[5], *Maria de Lourdes de Sousa Maia*[6], *Tatiana Guimarães de Noronha*[6], *Sheila Maria Barbosa de Lima*[6], *Marisol Simões*[6], *Marcos da Silva Freire*[6], *Reinaldo de Menezes Martins*[6], *Akira Homma*[6], *Pedro Luiz Tauil*[7], *Pedro Fernando Costa Vasconcelos*[8], *Alessandro Pecego Martins Romano*[9], *Carla Magda Domingues*[10], *Andréa Teixeira-Carvalho*[1] and *Olindo Assis Martins-Filho*[1*]

[1] Instituto René Rachou, Fundação Oswaldo Cruz – FIOCRUZ-Minas, Belo Horizonte, Brazil, [2] Departamento de Fisiologia e Biofísica, Universidade Federal de Minas Gerais, Belo Horizonte, Brazil, [3] Secretaria Municipal de Saúde de Belo Horizonte, Belo Horizonte, Brazil, [4] Secretaria do Estado de Saúde de Minas Gerais, Belo Horizonte, Brazil, [5] Escola Nacional de Saúde Pública – FIOCRUZ, Rio de Janeiro, Brazil, [6] Instituto de Tecnologia em Imunobiológicos Bio-Manguinhos – FIOCRUZ, Rio de Janeiro, Brazil, [7] Faculdade de Medicina, Universidade de Brasília, Brasilia, Brazil, [8] Instituto Evandro Chagas, Ananindeua, Brazil, [9] Departamento de Imunização e Doenças Transmissíveis (DEIDT) – Secretaria de Vigilância em Saúde, Ministério da Saúde, Brasilia, Brazil, [10] Programa Nacional de Imunizações – Secretaria de Vigilância em Saúde, Ministério da Saúde, Brasilia, Brazil

***Correspondence:**
Ana Carolina Campi-Azevedo
campiazevedo@gmail.com
Olindo Assis Martins-Filho
oamfilho@gmail.com

† These authors have contributed equally to this work

The Yellow Fever (YF) vaccination is recommended for people living in endemic areas and represents the most effective strategy to reduce the risk of infection. Previous studies have warned that booster regimens should be considered to guarantee the long-term persistence of 17DD-YF-specific memory components in adults living in areas with YF-virus circulation. Considering the lower seroconversion rates observed in children (9–12 months of age) as compared to adults, this study was designed in order to access the duration of immunity in single-dose vaccinated children in a 10-years cross-sectional time-span. The levels of neutralizing antibodies (PRNT) and the phenotypic/functional memory status of T and B-cells were measured at a baseline, 30–45 days, 1, 2, 4, 7, and 10 years following primary vaccination. The results revealed that a single dose induced 85% of seropositivity at 30–45 days and a progressive time-dependent decrease was observed as early as 2 years and declines toward critical values (below 60%) at time-spans of ≥4-years. Moreover, short-lived YF-specific cellular immunity, mediated by memory T and B-cells was also observed after 4-years. Predicted probability and resultant memory analysis emphasize that correlates of protection (PRNT; effector memory $CD8^{+}$ T-cells; non-classical memory B-cells) wane to critical values within ≥4-years after primary vaccination. Together, these results clearly demonstrate the decline of 17DD-YF-specific memory response along time in children primarily vaccinated at 9–12 months of age and support the need of booster regimen to guarantee the long-term persistence of memory components for children living in areas with high risk of YF transmission.

Keywords: yellow fever, 17DD vaccine, children, neutralizing antibodies, cellular memory

INTRODUCTION

The Yellow fever (YF) is an acute viral hemorrhagic disease caused by a single-stranded RNA Flavivirus that is endemic in Africa, South America and Central America (1, 2). YF is considered to be a re-emerging public health problem due to increasing number of outbreaks reported in the recent years worldwide (3).

The live attenuated YF vaccine has been an effective and safe control measure available to prevent YF since the 1930s (4). The YF vaccination is recommended for travelers and residents of endemic areas as the most effective strategy to reduce the risk of infection (5). The maintenance of high levels of immunity to YF is necessary to prevent the spread of the disease and large scale access to YF vaccines is critical to establish and maintain high levels of immunity amongst adult and children (3).

According to the World Health Organization, a single dose of YF vaccine is sufficient to provide lifelong protection in the general population (5, 6). However, previous studies have warned that the levels of neutralizing antibodies and the cellular immune responses elicited by YF vaccination decline considerably after primary vaccination (7–14).

Considering that the seroconversion rates observed in children following primary vaccination at 9-12 month of age are already lower than those observed in adults (15), it is expected that the duration of immunity in children would be even shorter as compared to adults. The present study was designed to assess the duration of humoral and cellular immunity following a single dose of 17DD-YF vaccine in children in a 10-year cross-sectional time-span. The quantification of neutralizing antibodies titers (PRNT) and the assessment of phenotypic/functional status of cellular memory were measured at baseline, 30–45 days, 1, 2, 4, 7, and 10 years following primary vaccination. These parameters have been considered relevant proxies of protection and can allow the monitoring of YF-specific immunological memory induced by the 17DD-YF vaccine (16–18).

This study aims to cover the gap in information about the duration of neutralizing antibodies and 17DD-specific T and B-cell memory overtime following the primary vaccination regimen in children. The data presented here bring original insights to support the importance of 17DD-YF booster vaccination in children to restore the YF-specific immune response elicited by primary vaccination.

METHODS

Study Oversight

This study was sponsored by the Programa Nacional de Imunizações-PNI, Ministry of Health, Brazil. The protocol was approved by the research ethics committee at the Escola Nacional de Saúde Pública (CAAE 0014.0.031.000-10, February 20th 2010) as well as at Instituto René Rachou (CAAE 0023.0.245.000-10, February 11th 2011 and CAAE 25315213.6.0000.5091, May 23rd 2015) and registered at the Clinicaltrials.gov (NCT 02990182, January 9th 2015). Written informed consent was obtained from the parents of the participants in this study.

Study Participants and Design

The study population consisted of 673 healthy children, from both genders, with ages ranging from 9 months to 12 years. Participants resided in two municipalities: Contagem and Ribeirão das Neves at Minas Gerais State, Brazil, and these two municipalities had no reports of YF cases for several decades prior the study onset. Moreover, the surveillance for epizootic events had not detected the circulation of YF virus amongst non-human primates in the State of Minas Gerais at the time of the study development. All participants have received, at 9–12 months of age, a single dose of the 17DD-YF substrain vaccine, produced by Instituto de Tecnologia em Imunobiológicos Bio-Manguinhos (FIOCRUZ, Brazil), from the seed lot 993FB013Z. The study was designed and supervised by the authors and structured into "two non-concurrent arms": (i) the first arm was a paired longitudinal analysis to identify early correlates of protection and included two groups, referred as "NV(day 0)"—non-vaccinated children at baseline, $n = 47$ and "PV(day 30–45)"—vaccinees at 30–45 days after primary vaccination, $n = 47$; (ii) the second arm was a cross-sectional analysis comprising of five groups, categorized according to the time after 17DD-YF primary vaccination: "PV(year 1)"—vaccinees at 1 year (8–18 months) after primary vaccination, $n = 141$; "PV(year 2)"—vaccinees at 2 years (19–30 months) after primary vaccination, $n = 114$; "PV(year 4)"—vaccinees at 4 years (31–69 months) after primary vaccination, $n = 128$; "PV(year 7)"—vaccinees at 7 years (75–99 months) after primary vaccination, $n = 116$ and "PV(year 10)"—vaccinees at 10 years (101–142 months) after primary vaccination, $n = 127$.

Heparinized blood samples (7 mL) were collected at health units at Contagem and Ribeirão das Neves (MG, Brazil) and transported to Grupo Integrado de Pesquisas em Biomarcadores at Instituto René Rachou-FIOCRUZ-Minas in Belo Horizonte (MG, Brazil). Blood samples were centrifuged to obtain the plasma that was aliquoted into cryovials and stored at −80°C for further analysis of neutralizing antibodies against yellow fever virus by plaque-reduction neutralization test (PRNT). Mononuclear cells were also isolated to quantify the levels of 17DD-YF specific cellular memory response by *in vitro* phenotypic and functional analyses. In addition to blood collection, a questionnaire was applied to obtain demographic data. The vaccination status and the date of YF immunization was verified in the vaccination card. Current health status, the use of prescribed medicine, pathological conditions, and any travel history after 17DD-YF vaccination was registered. Eligibility criteria included children of both genders with primary 17DD-YF vaccination at 9–12 months of age, with post-vaccination time ranging from 30–45 days to 10 years. Exclusion criteria encompassed the presence of autoimmune diseases, hemoglobinopathies and transient/permanent immunomodulatory condition. Children with previous history of blood transfusion and therapy based on hyperimmune serum up to 90 days before peripheral blood collection were not recruited to this study. All tests were carried out in a blind fashion without knowing whether the samples were from the first or second arm.

Testing Procedures

YF-Specific Neutralizing Antibodies

Heparin plasma samples were obtained from each volunteer and submitted to Ecteola-cellulose pre-treatment to remove heparin, as previously described by Campi-Azevedo et al. (19), for subsequent use in the PRNT assay. Ecteola-cellulose treated samples were assayed by the micro-PRNT$_{50}$ test according to Simões et al. (20). For the present study, the performances (sensitivity, specificity, and global accuracy) of micro-PRNT$_{50}$ and micro-PRNT$_{90}$ were defined for children samples and the cut-off 1:10 in reciprocal of serum dilution and the micro-PRNT$_{50}$ were selected as the most accurate condition. The micro-PRNT$_{50}$ was performed at the Laboratório de Tecnologia Virológica, Bio-Manguinhos (LATEV, FIOCRUZ-RJ, Brazil). The results were expressed as reverse of sample dilution, considering seropositivity as PRNT titers higher than 1:10 sample dilution.

YF-Specific Phenotypic and Functional Memory

The analysis of 17DD-YF specific cellular memory response was carried out as previously described by Campi-Azevedo et al. (8). Briefly, *in vitro* 17DD-YF-specific peripheral blood lymphoproliferative assay were conducted in two separate batches, referred as: non-stimulated Control Culture and 17DD-YF Culture. After the long-term incubation (144 h), cultured cells were harvested and stained with Live/Dead Dye (Life Technologies, Carlsbad, CA, USA) and a mix of monoclonal antibodies (mAbs) to identify memory T-cell subpopulations (anti-CD4/RPA-T4/FITC; anti-CD8/SK1/PerCP-Cy5.5; anti-CD27/M-T271/PE, and anti-CD45RO/UCHL1/PE-Cy7) and memory B-cell subsets (anti-IgD/IA6-2/FITC, anti-CD27/M-T271/PE, and anti-CD19/HIB19/PerCP). In a parallel, an aliquot of cultured cells were incubated with Live/Dead Dye, labeled with anti-CD8/SK1/PerCP and after pre-fix/permeabilization procedure re-incubated with a cocktail of anti-cytokine mAbs (anti-TNF-α/MAb11/PE-Cy7; anti-IFN-γ/B27/Alexa-Fluor488, and anti-IL-5/JES1-39D10/PE). All monoclonal antibodies were purchased from BD Biosciences (San Jose, CA, USA). Stained cells were washed, fixed and the data was acquired (100,000 lymphocytes/test) on a BD LSRFortessa Flow Cytometer (BD Biosciences, San Diego, CA, USA). FlowJo software (version 9.3.2, TreeStar, San Diego, CA, USA) was used to establish distinct gating strategies to quantify the memory T and B-cells subpopulations as previously described (8), including: "T-cell memory subsets:" Naïve T-cells/(NCD4;NCD8)/CD27$^+$CD45RO$^-$; early Effector Memory T-cells/(eEfCD4;eEfCD8)/CD27$^-$CD45RO$^-$; Central Memory T-cells/(CMCD4;CMCD8)/CD27$^+$CD45RO$^+$ and Effector Memory T-cells/(EMCD4;EMCD8)/CD27$^-$CD45RO$^+$ and "B-cell memory subsets:" Naïve B-cells/(NCD19)/CD27$^-$IgD$^+$; Non-classical Memory B-cells/(nCMCD19)/CD27$^+$IgD$^+$ and Classical Memory B-cells/(CMCD19)/CD27$^+$IgD$^-$. The percentage of cytokine$^+$ CD8$^+$ T-cells was also quantified. The results were reported as 17DD-YF-stimulated Culture/non-stimulated Control Culture Index, calculated as the ratio of results observed in the 17DD-YF-stimulated Cultures divided by the respective non-stimulated Control Culture.

Data Analysis

The GraphPad Prism software, Version 5.0 (San Diego, CA, USA) was employed to perform all statistical analyses. Kolmogorov-Smirnov, D'Agostino and Pearson omnibus and Shapiro-Wilk normality tests were used to check data distribution. Multiple strategies were employed for data analysis. Kruskal-Wallis test followed by Dunn's post-test were employed for intergroup comparative analysis. The Chi-square test was used to compare seropositivity rates, biomarker signatures, descriptive analysis of selected biomarkers and analysis of resultant memory. Spearman's correlation test was carried out to determine the PRNT wane along time continuum. In all cases, significant differences were considered at $p < 0.05$.

Biomarker signature analysis was carried out using the 75th percentile (3rd quartile) values for each biomarker (17DD-YF-stimulated Culture/non-stimulated Control Culture Index) as the cut-off edge to identify subjects with high biomarker levels. Those biomarkers with more than 25% of subjects above the cut-off were considered for comparative analysis amongst groups. Venn diagram analysis (http://bioinformatics.psb.ugent.be/webtools/Venn/) was employed to identify biomarkers observed selectively in PV (days 30–45), referred as correlates of protection. Overlay of ascendant biomarker signatures were employed for comparative analysis of time-depended changes in immunological profile after primary vaccination.

Logistic and multinomial regression models were constructed to evaluate the association between time after vaccination and changes in the biomarker levels. Following this, the fitted regression model was employed to calculate the predicted probabilities for each biomarker (isolated or combined) along time continuum. The Receiver Operating-Characteristic curves (ROC) were was constructed to estimate the capacity of time as a predictor of changes in biomarkers levels to monitor the 17DD-YF memory after primary vaccination in children. The Area Under the ROC Curve (AUC) was used for comparative analysis of predictive capacity amongst biomarkers (isolated or combined).

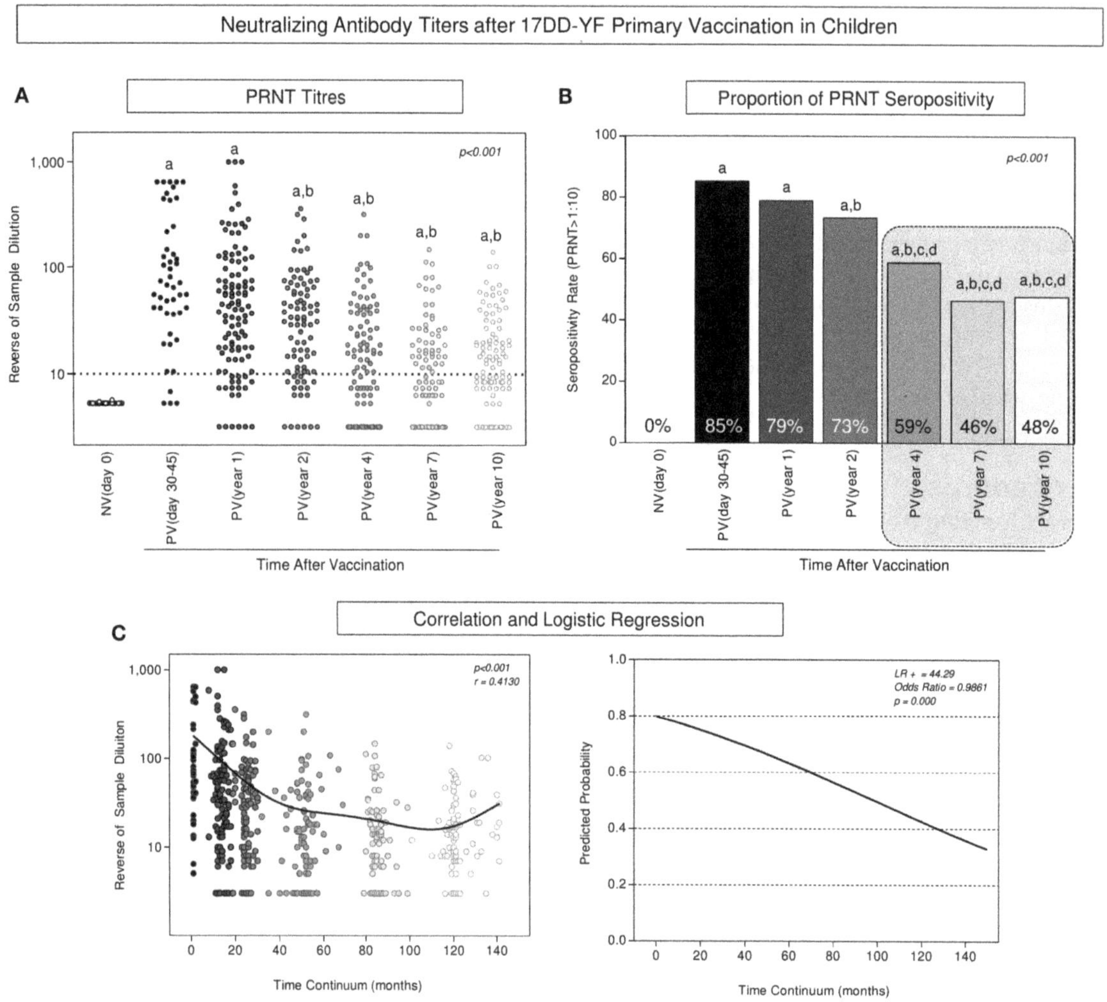

FIGURE 1 | Neutralizing antibody titers after 17DD-YF primary vaccination in children. PRNT titers were measured in Ecteola-treated plasma samples (19) from non-vaccinated children at baseline NV(day 0)/(○, $n = 47$) and at different times after primary vaccination: PV(day 30–45)/(●, $n = 47$), PV(year 1)/(●, $n = 141$), PV(year 2)/(●, $n = 114$), PV(year 4)/(●, $n = 128$), PV(year 7)/(●, $n = 116$), and PV(year 10)/(○, $n = 127$), as described previously by Simões et al. (20). **(A)** The PRNT levels were expressed in reverse of serum dilution. **(B)** Proportion of PRNT seropositivity (PRNT>1:10) were calculated for each group and the results expressed as seropositivity rates at baseline NV(day 0) [□] and at different times after primary vaccination: PV(day 30–45) [■], PV(year 1) [■], PV(year 2) [■], PV(year 4) [■], PV(year 7) [□], and PV(year 10) [□], considering the serum dilution >1:10 as the cut-off (dashed line). **(C)** Correlation and logistic regression were employed to determine the wane of PRNT levels along time continuum and the results expressed as reverse of serum dilution and predicated probability, respectively. Statistical analysis was carried out as described in Methods. In all cases, significant differences at $p < 0.05$ were underscored by using letters "a," "b," "c," and "d" for comparisons with NV(day 0), PV(day 30–45), PV(year 1), and PV(year 2), respectively and the *p*-values provide in the figure. Spearman correlation indices as well as Likelihood and Odds ratio are provided in the figure. Gray rectangle highlights the critical decrease of PRNT seropositivity rates ≥4 years after primary vaccination.

RESULTS

Progressive Time-Dependent Decrease in Neutralizing Antibody Titers Is Observed After 17DD-YF Primary Vaccination in Children

The levels of neutralizing antibodies, the proportion of PRNT seropositivity along with the correlation between PRNT levels and the logistic regression analysis of PRNT levels along time continuum are presented in the **Figure 1**. Data analysis revealed that primary vaccination induced a significant increase in the PRNT levels (**Figure 1A**) reaching a seropositivity rate of 85% in PV(day 30–45) as compared to NV(day 0) (**Figure 1B**). A progressive decrease in the PRNT levels was observed along time as early as 2 years after primary vaccination as compared to PV(days 30–45) (**Figure 1A**). Critical seropositivity rates (below 60%) were observed amongst vaccinees, particularly ≥4 years after primary vaccination (**Figure 1B**, gray dashed rectangle). Correlation analysis further supports the waning phenomenon observed in the PRNT levels along time after primary vaccination in children (**Figure 1C**). Furthermore, the outstanding likelihood ratio ($LR^+ = 44.29$) and odds ratio (OR = 0.9861, 95% CI = 0.9819–0.9903) reinforce the abrupt and progressive decline month to month in PRNT levels along time continuum, which reached values of 0.8454, 0.6025, and 0.1865 at 12, 36, and 120 months, respectively (**Figure 1C**).

Primary 17DD-YF Vaccination in Children Elicits Short-Lived YF-Specific Cellular Memory Mediated by Effector CD4$^+$ and CD8$^+$ T-Cells and Non-classical B-Cells

The analysis of YF-specific phenotypic and functional biomarkers was evaluated upon *in vitro* 17DD-YF antigen recall and the results are presented in **Figure 2**. An increase of memory T-cells (eEfCD4, eEfCD8, EMCD4, and EMCD8) as well as nCMCD19 cells along with an up-regulation of TNF-α and IFN-γ produced by CD8$^+$ T-cells is observed in PV(day 30–45) as compared to NV(day 0) (**Figures 2A,B**). Moreover, a significant decrease in these biomarkers occurs along the time, particularly ≥4 years after primary vaccination when almost all these attributes decline as compared to PV(days 30–45) (**Figure 2**).

Biomarker Signatures Emphasize the Short-Term Persistence of Phenotypic Effector Memory and Functional Activity of CD8$^+$ T-Cells

In order to accomplish the characterizing of the duration of phenotypic and functional memory induced by the 17DD-YF primary vaccination in children, the biomarker signatures were built for comparative analyses along time. To accomplish this goal, initially overlaid biomarkers signatures of NV(day 0) vs. PV(days 30–45) were assembled to identify attributes selectively observed in PV(day 30–45), further referred as correlates of protection in children (**Figure 3A**). Venn diagram analysis indicated that besides three common attributes (eEfCD4, eEfCD8, and CMCD19), five biomarkers (EMCD4, EMCD8, nCMCD19, TNFCD8, and IFNCD8) were tagged to be employed as selective correlates of protection for follow-up analysis overtime after primary 17DD-YF vaccination (**Figure 3B**).

Once the correlates of protection for follow-up analysis were selected, overlaid biomarker signatures were constructed to verify changes along time upon 17DD-YF primary vaccination (**Figure 3C**). Data analysis pointed out that all five biomarkers were persistently observed in PV(day 30–45) and PV(year 1). Although some attributes were not observed in PV(year 2), the lack of EMCD8, considered one of the top biomarkers to monitor the immunological memory to 17DD-YF vaccine (9) was noticed in PV(year 4), PV(year 7), and PV(year 10) (**Figure 3C**).

Descriptive Analysis Confirms the Time-Dependent Decrease of Proxies of Protection Upon 17DD-YF Primary Vaccination in Children

The biomarkers tagged as correlates of protection (EMCD4, EMCD8, nCMCD19, TNFCD8, and IFNCD8) were employed together with the neutralizing antibody levels to carry out a descriptive analysis to monitor the YF-specific memory along time after 17DD-YF primary vaccination. For this purpose, the proportion of subjects displaying biomarkers levels above the 75th percentile cut-off and PRNT levels >1:10 were calculated and data reported for each group (**Figure 4A**). Data demonstrated that in NV(day 0) there is a predominance of subjects displaying 0–1 biomarkers above that cut-off. Conversely, in the PV(day 30–45) there is a significantly higher prevalence of subjects displaying 3 biomarkers above that cut-off. In PV(year 1) and PV(year 2) there was a balanced proportion of subjects displaying 1–2 biomarkers above that cut-off. Notably, in PV(year 4), PV(year 7), and PV(year 10) there was a higher prevalence confined in only one biomarker above that cut-off (**Figure 4A**). Complementary analysis further revealed that the median number of biomarkers above that cut-off found in PV(day 30–45), PV(year 1), and PV(year 2) was higher as compared to NV(day 0). Although in PV(year 4), the median value still differed from that observed in NV(day 0), it was lower as compared to PV(days 30–45). Additionally, a critical median number of biomarkers above that cut-off was observed in PV(year 7) and PV(year 10) as compared to PV(days 30–45) that did not differ from those found in NV(day 0) (**Figure 4B**). Based on these findings, the vaccinees were distributed into two major groups referred as PV(≤year 2) and PV(≥year 4). The results showed that both groups presented higher median number of biomarkers above the cut-off as compared to NV(day 0), although the PV(≥year 4) group exhibited lower values as compared to PV(≤year 2) (**Figure 4B**).

Predicted Probability Analysis Emphasizes That Neutralizing Antibody Levels (PRNT), EMCD8, and nCMCD19 Are the Top Biomarkers to Monitor the 17DD-YF Memory After Primary Vaccination in Children

Logistic and multinomial regression models were constructed and the fitted regression model employed to calculate the predicted probabilities for each biomarker previously tagged as correlates of protection (EMCD4, EMCD8, nCMCD19, TNFCD8, and IFNCD8) to monitor the 17DD-YF memory after primary vaccination along time continuum. The ROC curves were constructed for comparative analysis of predicted capacity amongst biomarkers (isolated or combined). Based on the global accuracy (Area Under the ROC Curve—AUC), the neutralizing antibody levels (PRNT), EMCD8, and nCMCD19 presented moderate performance when employed isolated as a single parameter to monitor the 17DD-YF memory after primary vaccination in children (AUC = 0.6777; 0.5601, and 0.5770, respectively) (**Figure 5A**). The combined analysis of neutralizing antibody levels (PRNT), and EMCD8 and nCMCD19 further improved the predictive capacity of using these biomarkers to monitor the 17DD-YF memory after primary vaccination in children (AUC = 0.9201) (**Figure 5B**).

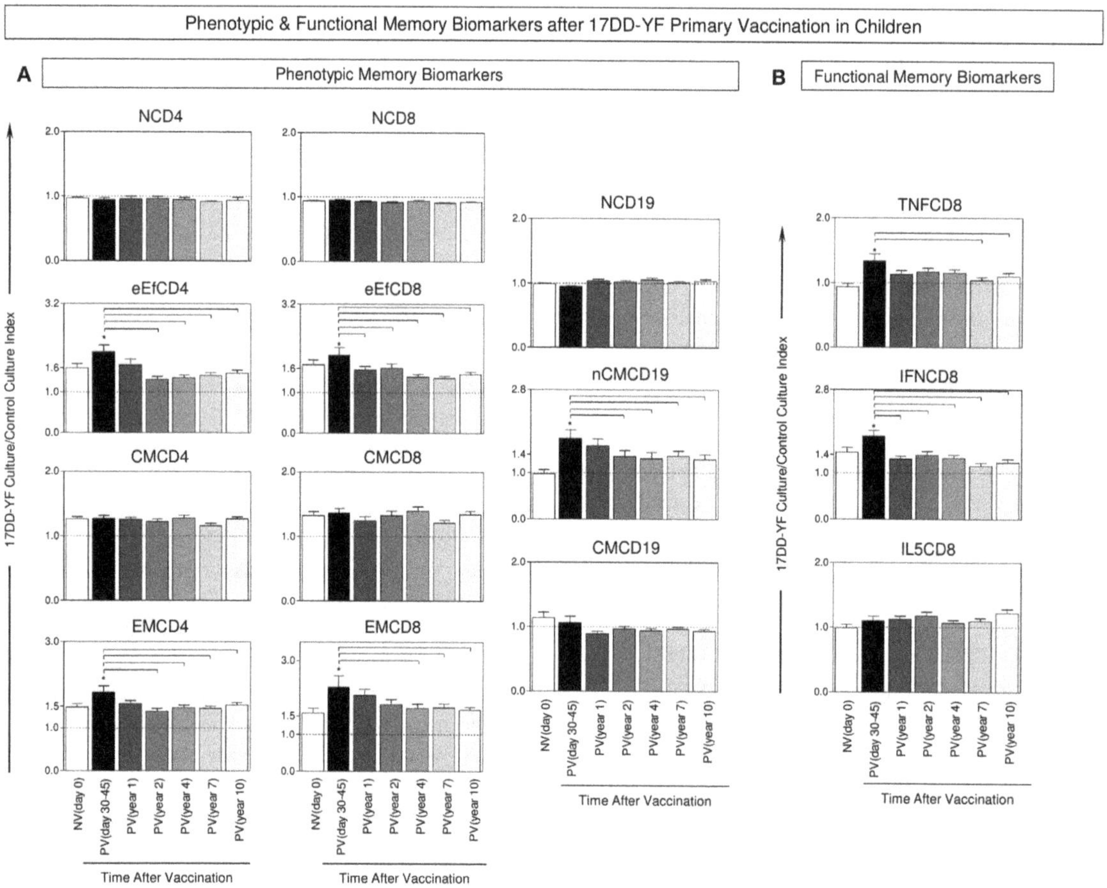

FIGURE 2 | Phenotypic and functional memory biomarkers after 17DD-YF primary vaccination in children. The analysis of 17DD-YF-specific memory was measured upon *in vitro* 17DD-YF antigen recall as described previously by Campi-Azevedo et al. (8) for non-vaccinated children at baseline NV(day 0)/(□, $n = 47$) and at different times after primary vaccination: PV(day 30–45)/(■, $n = 47$), PV(year 1)/(■, $n = 141$), PV(year 2)/(■, $n = 114$), PV(year 4)/(■, $n = 128$), PV(year 7)/(■, $n = 116$), and PV(year 10)/(□, $n = 127$). **(A)** Flow cytometric staining were used to quantify phenotypic features of T-cell memory subsets: Naïve T-cells/(NCD4;NCD8)/$CD27^{+}CD45RO^{-}$; early Effector Memory T-cells/(eEfCD4;eEfCD8)/$CD27^{-}CD45RO^{-}$ Central Memory T-cells/(CMCD4;CMCD8)/$CD27^{+}CD45RO^{+}$ Effector Memory T-cells/(EMCD4;EMCD8)/$CD27^{-}CD45RO^{+}$ and B-cell memory subsets: Naïve B-cells/(NCD19)/$CD27^{-}IgD^{+}$; Non-classical Memory B-cells/(nCMCD19)/$CD27^{+}IgD^{+}$ and Classical Memory B-cells/(CMCD19)/$CD27^{+}IgD^{-}$. **(B)** Flow cytometric staining were also performed to quantity functional $CD8^{+}$ T-cells producing TNF-α, IFN-γ and IL-5. The data were reported as median values ± inter-quartile range for 17DD-YF-stimulated Culture/non-stimulated Control Culture Index as described in Methods, highlighting the equivalence ratio by dashed line (Index = 1.0). Significant differences at $p < 0.05$ were underscored by using asterisk (*) to identify differences between NV(day 0) vs. PV(day 30–45) and intergroup differences identified by connecting lines.

The Resultant Memory (PRNT, EMCD8, or NCMCD19) Wanes Overtime Reaching Critical Values at 4 or More Years After 17DD-YF Primary Vaccination in Children

The results of neutralizing antibody levels (PRNT), EMCD8, and nCMCD19 profiles were combined at individual level to build a memory matrix and calculate the resultant YF-specific memory, comprising of humoral (PRNT) and cell-mediated (EMCD8 or nCMCD19) immunity. Then, each volunteer was classified as they present "None," "PRNT," "EMCD8 and/or nCMCD19," or "Both" attributes above the cut-off threshold, i.e., PRNT positivity at serum dilution >1:10, EMCD8 (17DD-YF-stimulated Culture/non-stimulated Control Culture >2.19) or nCMCD19 (17DD-YF Culture/Control Culture >1.66). The results demonstrated that 17DD-YF primary vaccination was able to guarantee persistent resultant memory in 79% of children included into PV(≤year 2). Conversely, a clear decline in the resultant memory down to 55% was observed into PV(≥year 4). Specifically, the resultant memory initially observed in 96% of children in PV(day 30–45) decrease to 77% in PV(year 1) and 73% in PV(year 2) followed by a marked shift down to 53, 55, and 58% in PV(year 4), PV(year 7) and PV(year 10), respectively (**Figure 6**).

DISCUSSION

The YF vaccination is currently recommended as a single dose for residents of disease risk areas and people traveling from or to those areas, who aged 9 months or older (5, 6,

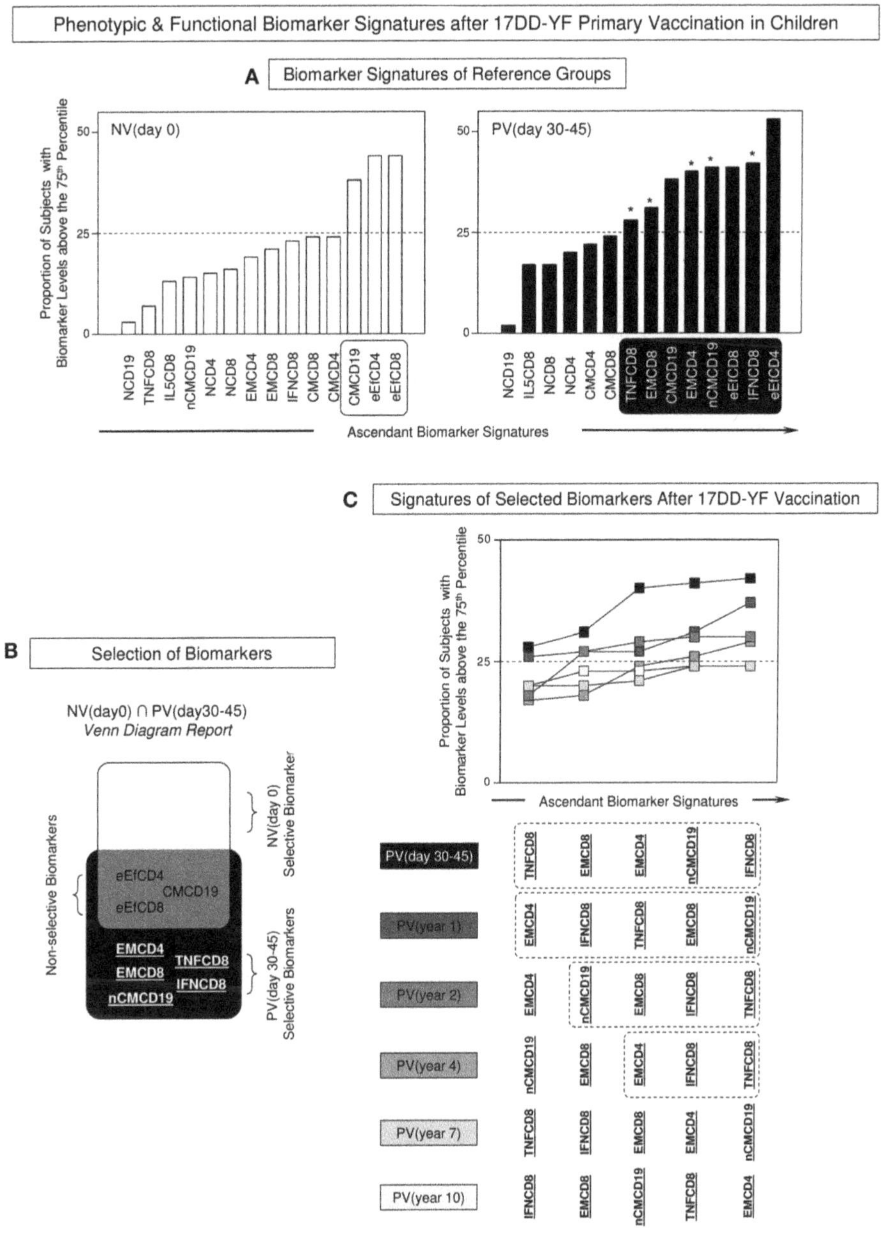

FIGURE 3 | Phenotypic and functional biomarker signatures after 17DD-YF primary vaccination in children. **(A)** Biomarker signatures of reference groups NV(day 0) [□] and PV(day 30–45) [■] were assembled to select biomarkers above the 75th percentile with proportions higher than the 25% in each group (white/black background rectangles). The selected biomarkers were underscored by asterisk (*) to identify differences between NV(day 0) vs. PV(day 30–45). **(B)** Venn diagram report was employed to identify the set of biomarkers selectively increased in [PV(day 30–45) vs. NV(day 0)]. The attributes EMCD4, EMCD8, nCMCD19, TNFCD8, and IFNCD8 were underscored as PV (day 30–45)-selective biomarkers. These attributes were tagged in bold underline format and employed for follow-up analysis overtime after 17DD-YF primary vaccination. Biomarkers with proportion higher than the 25% were underscored by asterisk (*) to identify differences between NV(day 0) vs. PV(day 30–45). **(C)** Overlaid signatures of selected biomarkers were assembled to identify changes in the 17DD-YF specific phenotypic and functional features at different times after primary vaccination: PV(day 30–45) [■], PV(year 1) [■], PV(year 2) [■], PV(year 4) [■], PV(year 7) [□], and PV(year 10) [□]. Dashed rectangles underscore the critical decline of selected biomarkers overtime after primary vaccination with absence of EMCD8 ≥ 4 years after primary vaccination.

21–23). According to the WHO, very few primary vaccine failures following YF vaccination have been reported. It has been proposed that, in addition to neutralizing antibodies, both innate and cell-mediated immunity also contribute to the initial immune response. Defining the parameters that modulate vaccine responses is relevant to increase vaccine effectiveness. It has been proposed that several factors may affect the YF vaccine response including: genetic background, gender,

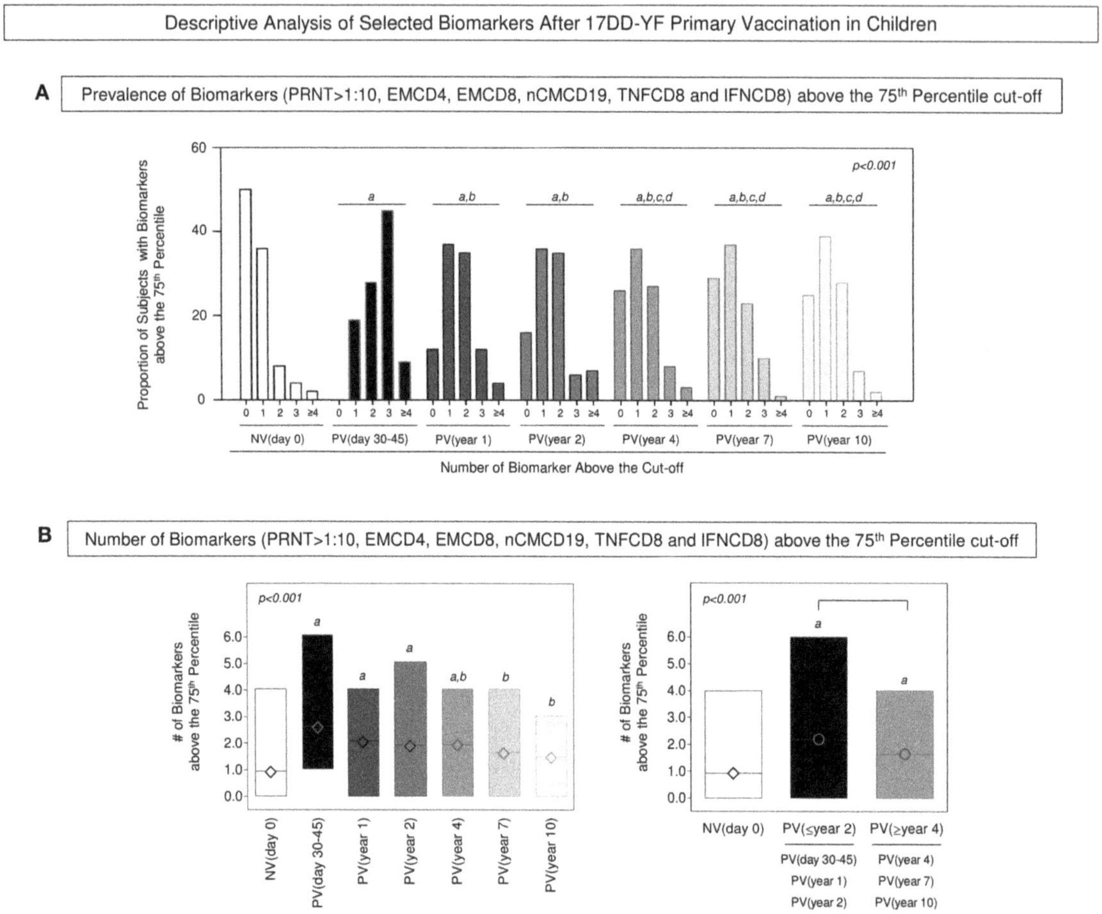

FIGURE 4 | Descriptive analysis of selected biomarkers after 17DD-YF primary vaccination in children. **(A)** Prevalence of Biomarkers (PRNT>1:10, EMCD4, EMCD8, nCMCD19, TNFCD8, and IFNCD8) above the 75th percentile cut-off. Data are presented as proportion of subjects with biomarkers above the cut-off at baseline NV(day 0) [□] and at different times after primary vaccination: PV(day 30–45) [■], PV(year 1) [■], PV(year 2) [■], PV(year 4) [■], PV(year 7) [□], and PV(year 10) [□]. **(B)** Number of Biomarkers (PRNT>1:10, EMCD4, EMCD8, nCMCD19, TNFCD8, and IFNCD8) above the 75th Quartile cut-off. Data are presented as mean (min to max) number of biomarkers above the cut-off at baseline NV(day 0) [◇] and at different times after primary vaccination: PV(day 30–45) [◆], PV(year 1) [◆], PV(year 2) [◇], PV(year 4) [◇], PV(year 7) [◇], and PV(year 10) [◇] as well as PV(≤year 2) [●], PV(≥year 4) [●]. Significant differences at $p < 0.05$ are underscored by using letters "a," "b," "c," and "d" for comparisons with NV(day 0), PV(day 30–45), PV(year 1), and PV(year 2), respectively. Intergroup differences are identified by connecting lines. The *p*-values are provided in the figure.

age, and environmental differences. Muyanja et al. (24) have proposed that host-specific immune response microenvironment may contribute to the effectiveness of the 17D-YF vaccine. These authors have suggested that an activated immune microenvironment prior to vaccination impedes the efficacy of the 17D-YF vaccine in an African cohort and suggest that booster regimens should be proposed to improve efficient immunity after YF vaccination. Other studies have suggested that the ability of YF-17D vaccine to infect dendritic cells and activate multiple Toll-like receptors seems to be essential for generating a potent immune response after vaccination (17, 25). A distinct hypothesis have been tested to explain the lower seropositivity rates after YF vaccination in children. An observational multicenter study, carried out by the Collaborative Group for Studies on Yellow Fever Vaccines has reported that the 17DD-YF vaccine reached distinct seroconversion rates in children according to the age at vaccination (26). Moreover, it has been demonstrated that simultaneous administration of other viral vaccines reduces significantly the response to YF vaccine in children (15). Conversely, no association between seroconversion rates and the maternal immunity status to YF has been observed (27). Our group have previously observed that children non-responsive to primary 17DD-YF vaccine presented a striking lack of innate immunity pro-inflammatory response, specially low levels of IL-12$^+$ and TNF-α$^+$ neutrophils and monocytes, along with an increased regulatory profile in the adaptive response, including higher levels of IL-4$^+$CD4$^+$ T cells as well as IL-10$^+$ and IL-5$^+$CD8$^+$ T cells (28). Interestingly, the revaccination of children with primary vaccination failure was able to restore the innate and adaptive immunity toward a balanced pro-inflammatory/regulatory profile.

Some studies that investigated the impact of booster doses on the status of YF-specific immune response in adults postulated that booster vaccination did not increase the titers of YF-specific

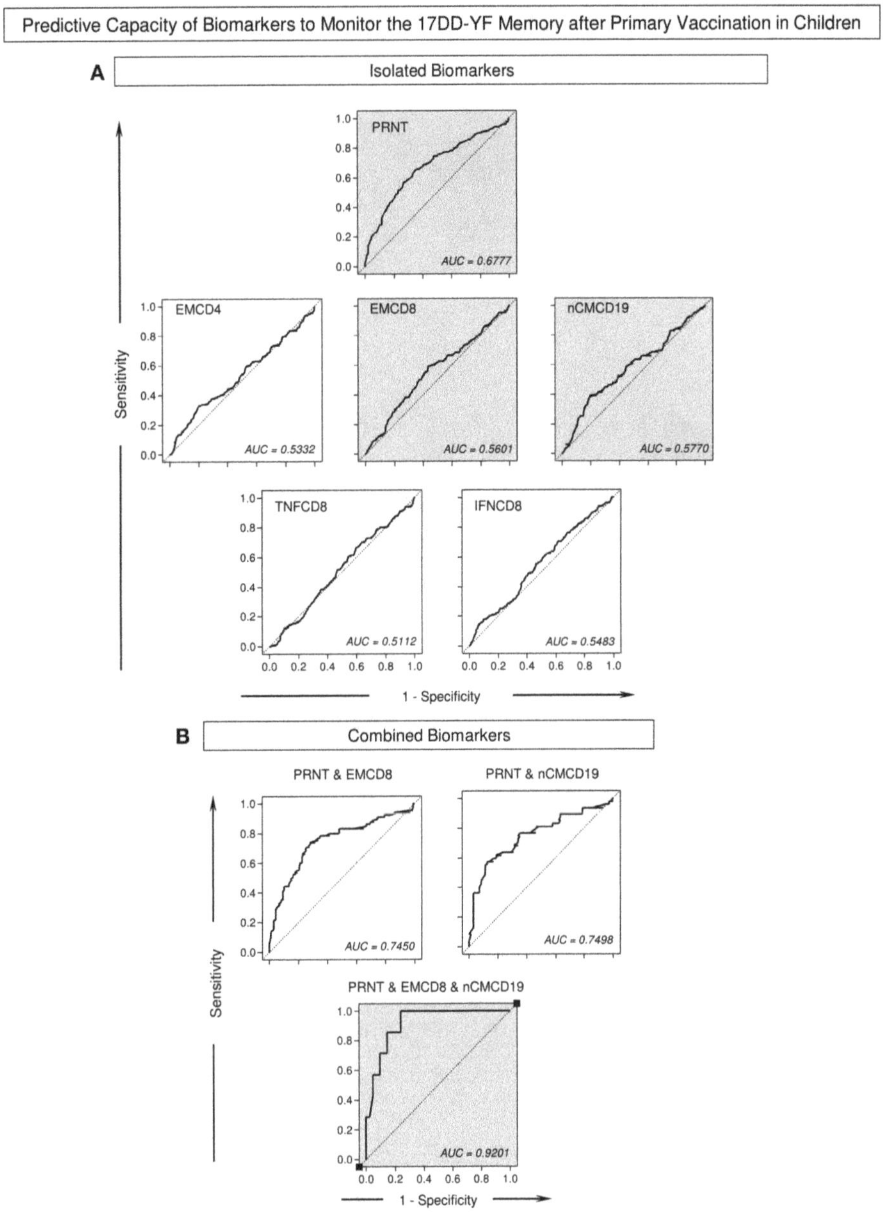

FIGURE 5 | Predictive capacity of biomarkers to monitor the 17DD-YF memory after primary vaccination in children. The Receiver Operating Characteristic (ROC) curves were used to estimate the capacity of time as a predictor of changes in biomarker levels to monitor the 17DD-YF memory after primary vaccination in children. Logistic and multinomial regression models were constructed to evaluate the association between time after vaccination and changes in the biomarker levels. Following, the fitted regression model was employed to calculate the predicted probabilities for each biomarker **(A)** isolated or **(B)** combined along time continuum. The Area Under the ROC Curves (AUC) were employed for comparative analysis of predictive capacity amongst biomarkers and the values provided in the figure. The gray background highlights the top three isolated biomarkers and the best combination of predictor biomarkers to monitor the 17DD-YF memory after primary vaccination in children.

antibodies nor induced or altered the phenotypes of $CD8^+$ T-cells and the immune responses observed following revaccination were reduced compared to primary responses (23, 29, 30). However, other studies have demonstrated that booster doses are relevant to guarantee the long-term persistence of 17DD-YF-specific memory components in travelers (31) and in residents of areas with YF-virus circulation (32, 33). Therefore, the single dose recommendations for YF vaccines have been considered controversial.

The decision to no longer recommend booster vaccination may especially have a direct impact on children, given that besides higher primary vaccination failures (15), there is no evidence for the long-term persistence of protective immunity in primary vaccinated children. Our group has already described the occurrence of time-dependent loss of YF-immunity in primary vaccinated adults (7–9). If this scenario also occurs in children it would contribute to worsening the setting in which a large proportion of individuals would become exposed to potential

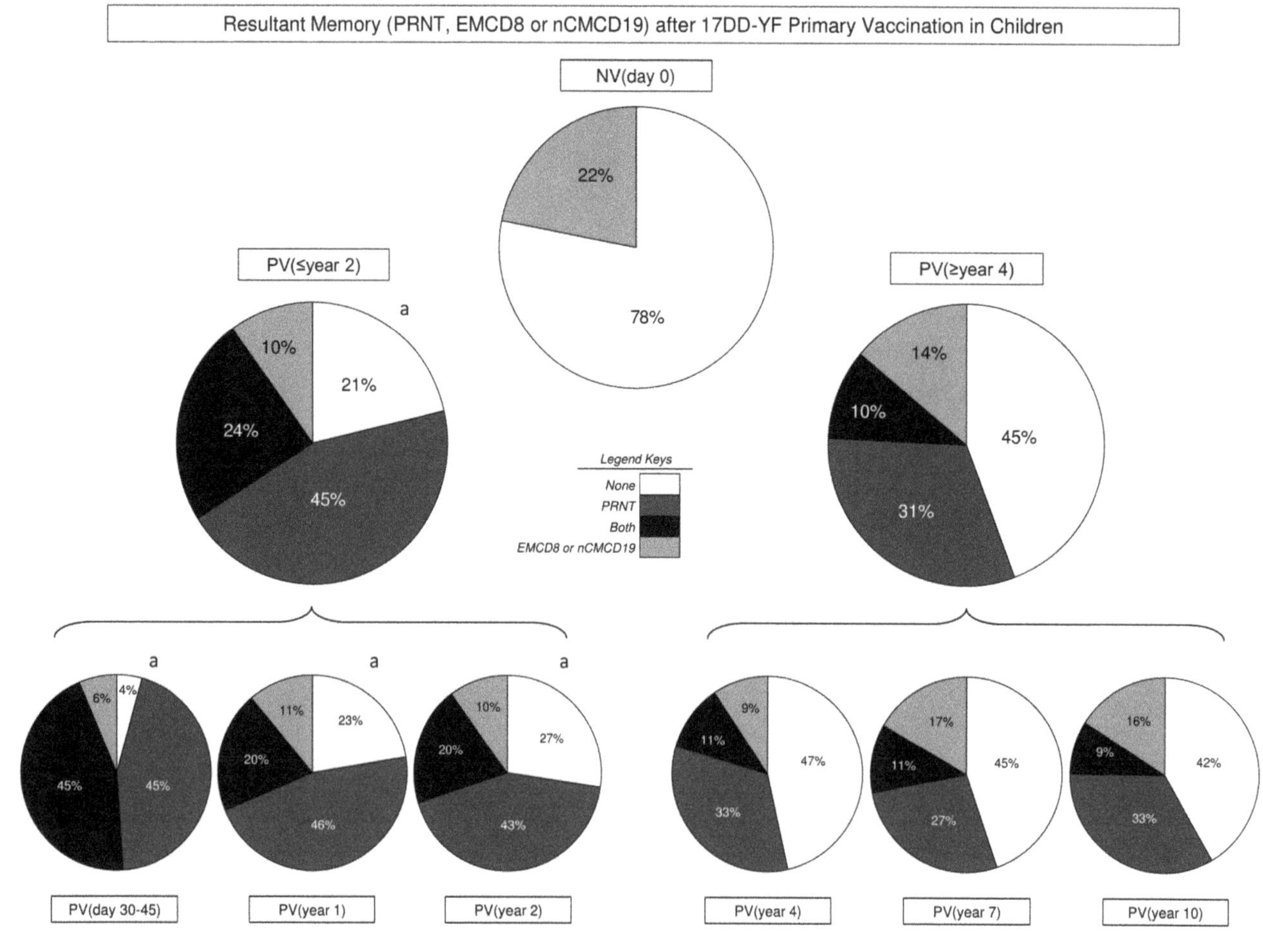

FIGURE 6 | Resultant memory (PRNT, EMCD8, or nCMCD19) after 17DD-YF Primary vaccination in children. The resultant memory status (PRNT, EMCD8, or nCMCD19) were assessed at individual level to define the overall proportion of subjects presenting None (◔), PRNT (◕), cellular memory "EMCD8 and/or nCMCD19" (◔) or both attributes "PRNT and cellular memory" (◕) at distinct time-points before/after primary 17DD-YF vaccination, including: NV(day 0), PV(≤year 2), PV(≥year 4) as well as PV(day 30–45), PV(year 1), PV(year 2), PV(year 4), PV(year 7), and PV(year 10). Significant differences ($p < 0.05$) of resultant memory status amongst study groups were assessed by Chi-square test and represented by letter "a" as compared to NV(day 0).

risk of YF infection, especially in endemic areas of high virus circulation. As indicated by the results of the present study, a substantial proportion of children could be susceptible to YF-virus infection, especially in endemic areas.

The studies that evaluated the timeline kinetics of correlates of protection after 17D-YF and 17DD-YF vaccination in adults have demonstrated that both humoral and cellular-mediated YF-specific immunity display a relevant decline overtime in single dose recipients of YF vaccines and that the booster doses efficiently improve the immunological status in re-vaccinated recipients (29–33). Recent studies from our group have shown that secondary or multiple vaccination regimens in adults are able to further improve the immunity parameters triggered by primary 17DD-YF vaccination and restore the resultant YF-specific memory in 100% of the volunteers. Moreover, it was observed that all vaccinees had at least one or both proxy of protection detectable at ≥10 years post-secondary vaccination (33).

Previous studies from our group have compared the cytokine-mediated immune response triggered by 17D-213/77-YF or 17DD-YF vaccines in children submitted to primary vaccination at 9–12 month of age with those non-responders to primary vaccination and also with those that received (28, 34). The results demonstrated that all children that received a booster dose 1 year after primary vaccination failure seroconverted and shifted the overall cytokine signatures toward a balanced pro-inflammatory/regulatory response of innate and adaptive immunity, overcoming the striking lack of innate immunity pro-inflammatory response observed in non-responder children (28, 34). These studies clearly indicated that booster regimens are relevant to guarantee the persistence of long-term immunity in areas with high risk of yellow fever transmission.

Data about the duration of YF-specific immunity in children following primary vaccination is still scarce and can provide supporting evidence to support the public health programs for

YF control worldwide. In this sense, the present investigation was designed to explore the duration of humoral and cellular immunity in primary vaccinated children in a 10-years cross-sectional timeline.

Our findings indicate that a substantial proportion of children lose their antiviral humoral immunity at 4 or more years after 17DD-YF primary vaccination. The PRNT has been considered the classical gold standard to measure post-vaccination immunity to YF for decades and generally regarded as the most appropriate parameter for monitoring protection by YF vaccine (6, 16). Reports from Niedrig et al. (16) regarding the timeline kinetics of YF-neutralizing antibody after 17D-YF vaccination in adults demonstrated that seropositivity rates (>1:10) significantly decrease from 94.0 to 74.5% from 1 to 10 years, respectively. In fact, upon closer inspection, the data clearly showed that antibody titers declined more rapidly during the first 1–4 years after 17D-YF vaccination and that seropositivity rates (>1:10) reached 69% when vaccinees are grouped together from 5 to 35 years post vaccination (13, 16). This rapid decline in neutralizing antibodies early after YF vaccination was also in a study by Hepburn et al. (29), which demonstrated that antibody levels decayed within 3–4 years in approximately half of the adult vaccines, even after booster vaccination.

Short-lived persistence of cell-mediated immunity has also been observed in memory T and B-cells (EMCD4; EMCD8; TNFCD8; IFNCD8; nCMCD19) after 4-years after a 17DD-YF single dose. Complementary predicted probability analysis together with resultant memory assessment highlighted that besides neutralizing antibody levels (PRNT), the levels of EMCD8 and nCMCD19 also decline to critical values at ≥4-years after primary vaccination. Several studies strongly suggested that $CD8^{+}T$ cells are relevant for immune protection upon YF after primary or secondary vaccination (8, 9, 17, 35). The role of nCMCD19 cells has not been completely elucidated in YF-vaccinated recipients. It is known that the maintenance of long-lived plasma cells that secrete antigen-specific antibodies, as well as memory B-cells, is essential for protection against pathogens, and is the basis of successful vaccinations (36). The nCMCD19 cells ($IgD^{+}CD27^{+}CD19^{+}$) are known as unclass-switched cells with similar functions compared to classical switched memory B-cells ($IgD^{-}CD27^{+}CD19^{+}$) and are not in the process of transition from naive to memory B cells. These nCMCD19 cells are believed to play an important role in secondary immune response in early phases of infection (37).

The current study further indicates that booster vaccination regimen may be required to guarantee protective immunity in children. The rapid and expressive loss of humoral and cellular immunity in a subpopulation of primary vaccinated children suggests that the first booster dose of vaccine should be administered within 4–5 years after primary vaccination instead of 10 years after vaccination as proposed previously for adults (32, 33).

The study's limitations include the cross-sectional representation of the average immune status of several birth cohorts, which assumed they differ only in time after vaccination, although this seems a legitimate assumption given that the vaccine and immunization practices have remained unchanged in the time period of those cohorts. Another limitation could be the possibility of booster by natural infections, as those children lived in an area where YF vaccine is recommended. However, it is important to mention that the study participants lived in a metropolitan region where there had been no cases in humans and non human primates.

The inclusion of the YF vaccine into worldwide immunization program for children living in endemic areas represents an important measure to ensure the YF-immunization in infancy and guarantee the effective control of YF expansion. The knowledge about duration of correlates of protection following YF vaccination in children is relevant to support further decisions to be made regarding the need of revaccination and to define the precise time for booster regimens. The results presented here add scientific knowledge about the immune response induced by 17DD-YF vaccine and bring new insights and increase awareness for healthcare workers about the importance of YF vaccination/revaccination in childhood. Moreover, our results may support the revision of the recommendation for a single dose YF-vaccine and will certainly guarantee that a large contingent of children will be revaccinated, improving the prevention of YF. Altogether, these data would be helpful to define targets and indicators for protection and susceptibility, especially in endemic countries with high historical rates of YF virus circulation in continuous expansion.

ETHICS STATEMENT

This studies involving human participants were reviewed and approved by the research ethics committee at the Escola Nacional de Saúde Pública (CAAE 0014.0.031.000-10, February 20th 2010) as well as at Instituto René Rachou (CAAE 0023.0.245.000-10, February 11th 2011 and CAAE 25315213.6.0000.5091, May 23rd 2015) and registered at the Clinicaltrials.gov (NCT 02990182, January 9th 2015). Written informed consent to participate in this study was provided by the participants' legal guardian/next of kin.

AUTHOR CONTRIBUTIONS

AC-A, IC, LC, MM, MF, RM, AH, PT, PV, AR, CD, AT-C, and OM-F: designing research study. IC, LC, AR, CD, and OM-F: funding acquisition. AC-A, LR, VP-M, JC, LA, CF, CC-P, ES-F, TN, SL, and MS: conducting experiments. JL, JR, and LC: field study. AC-A, LA, SL, and MS: acquiring data. AC-A, LR, VP-M, JC, LA, CF, CC-P, IC-R, and JM: analyzing data. PT and PV: validation. AH, PT, and PV: advisory committee. AC-A, LR, JC, CC-P, IC-R, AT-C, and OM-F: writing the manuscript.

ACKNOWLEDGMENTS

The authors thank the Program for Technological Development in Tools for Health-RPT-FIOCRUZ for the use of the flow cytometry facility. This study was supported by Fundação de Amparo à Pesquisa do Estado de Minas Gerais (FAPEMIG), BioManguinhos/FIOCRUZ, PROEP/IRR/FIOCRUZ, Conselho Nacional de Desenvolvimento Científico e Tecnológico-CNPq, Programa Nacional de Imunizações (PNI), and Secretaria de Vigilância em Saúde (SVS)-Ministério da Saúde, Brazil. The authors acknowledge the Programa de Pós-Graduação em Ciências da Saúde do Instituto René Rachou-FIOCRUZ-Minas, supported by the Coordenação de Aperfeiçoamento de Pessoal de Nível Superior (CAPES), and Fundação Carlos Chagas Filho de Amparo à Pesquisa do Estado do Rio de Janeiro (FAPERJ). The authors are thankful to the nursing of Secretaria Estadual de Saúde de Minas Gerais: Velizete de Lima, Alessandra de Souza (in memoriam), Matildes Souza Neto, and Rosangela Azevedo. The authors are thankful to the Programa PRINT-FIOCRUZ-CAPES. LA, CF, ES-F, LC, PV, AT-C, and OM-F received fellowships from CNPq.

REFERENCES

1. *Areas with Risk of Yellow fever Virus Transmission in Africa and South America.* (2019). Available online at: https://www.cdc.gov/yellowfever/maps/index.html
2. World Health Organization. *Yellow Fever Fact Sheet.* (2019). Available online at: https://www.who.int/en/news-room/fact-sheets/detail/yellow-fever
3. The Lancet. Yellow fever: a major threat to public health. *Lancet.* (2018) 391:402. doi: 10.1016/S0140-6736(18)30152-1
4. World Health Organization. *Eliminate Yellow fever Epidemics (EYE): A Global Strategy 2017–2026.* (2017). Available online at: https://apps.who.int/iris/handle/10665/255703
5. World Health Organization. Vaccines and vaccination against yellow fever. WHO position paper – June 2013. *Wkly Epidemiol Record.* (2013) 88:269–83.
6. World Health Organization. Background paper on yellow fever vaccine. In: *Vaccine Position Papers.* Geneva, SAGE Working Group (2013).
7. Caldas IR, Camacho LA, Martins-Filho OA, Maia M de L, Freire M da S, Torres C de R, et al. Duration of post-vaccination immunity against yellow fever in adults. *Vaccine.* (2014) 32:4977–84. doi: 10.1016/j.vaccine.2014.07.021
8. Campi-Azevedo AC, Costa-Pereira C, Antonelli LR, Fonseca CT, Teixeira-Carvalho A, Villela-Rezende G, et al. Booster dose after 10 years is recommended following 17DD-YF primary vaccination. *Hum Vaccin Immunother.* (2016) 12:491–502. doi: 10.1080/21645515.2015.1082693
9. Costa-Pereira C, Campi-Azevedo AC, Coelho-dos-Reis JG, Peruhype-Magalhães V, Araújo MSS, Antonelli LRV, et al. Multi-parameter approach to evaluate the timing of memory status after primary 17DD-YF vaccination. *PLoS Neglec Trop Dis.* (2018) 12:e0006462. doi: 10.1371/journal.pntd.0006462
10. Vasconcelos PF. Single shot of 17D vaccine may not confer life-long protection against yellow fever. *Mem Inst Oswaldo Cruz.* (2018) 113:135–7. doi: 10.1590/0074-02760170347
11. Patel D, Simons H. Yellow fever vaccination: is one dose always enough? *Travel Med Infect Dis.* (2013) 11:266–73. doi: 10.1016/j.tmaid.2013.08.007
12. Grobusch MP, Goorhuis A, Wieten RW, Verberk JD, Jonker EF, van Genderen PJ, et al. Yellow fever revaccination guidelines change – a decision too feverish? *Clin Microbiol Infect.* (2013) 19:885–6. doi: 10.1111/1469-0691.12332
13. Amanna IJ, Slifka MK. Questions regarding the safety and duration of immunity following live yellow fever vaccination. *Expert Rev Vaccines.* (2016) 15:1519–33. doi: 10.1080/14760584.2016.1198259
14. Estofolete CF e Nogueira ML. Is a dose of 17D vaccine in the current context of Yellow Fever enough? *Braz J Microbiol.* (2018) 49:683–4. doi: 10.1016/j.bjm.2018.02.003
15. Nascimento Silva JR, Camacho LA, Siqueira MM, Freire Mde S, Castro YP, Maia Mde L, et al. Mutual interference on the immune response to yellow fever vaccine and a combined vaccine against measles, mumps and rubella. *Vaccine.* (2011) 29:6327–34. doi: 10.1016/j.vaccine.2011.05.019
16. Niedrig M, Lademann M, Emmerich P, Lafrenz M. Assessment of IgG antibodies against yellow fever virus after vaccination with 17D by different assays: neutralization test, haemagglutination inhibition test, immunofluorescence assay and ELISA. *Trop Med Int Health.* (1999) 4:867–71. doi: 10.1046/j.1365-3156.1999.00496.x
17. Querec TD, Akondy RS, Lee EK, Cao W, Nakaya HI, Teuwen D, et al. Systems biology approach predicts immunogenicity of the yellow fever vaccine in humans. *Nat Immunol.* (2019) 10:116–25. doi: 10.1038/ni.1688
18. Ahmed R, Akondy RS. Insights into human CD8(+) T-cell memory using the yellow fever and smallpox vaccines. *Immunol Cell Biol.* (2011) 89:340–5. doi: 10.1038/icb.2010.155
19. Campi-Azevedo AC, Peruhype-Magalhães V, Coelho-Dos-Reis JG, Costa-Pereira C, Yamamura AY, Lima SMB, et al. Heparin removal by ecteola-cellulose pre-treatment enables the use of plasma samples for accurate measurement of anti-Yellow fever virus neutralizing antibodies. *J Immunol Methods.* (2017) 448:9–20. doi: 10.1016/j.jim.2017.05.002
20. Simões M, Camacho LAB, Yamamura AMY, Miranda EH, Cajaraville ACRA, Freire MS. Evaluation of accuracy and reliability of the plaque reduction neutralization test (micro-PRNT) in detection of yellow fever virus antibodies. *Biologicals.* (2012) 40:399–404. doi: 10.1016/j.biologicals.2012.09.005
21. Poland JD, Calisher CH, Monath TP, Downs WG, Murphy K. Persistence of neutralizing antibody 30–35 years after immunization with 17D yellow fever vaccine. *Bull World Health Organ.* (1981) 59:895–900.
22. Gotuzzo E, Yactayo S, Córdova E. Review article: Efficacy and duration of immunity after yellow fever vaccination: systematic review on the need for a booster every 10 years. *Am J Trop Med Hyg.* (2013) 89:434–44. doi: 10.4269/ajtmh.13-0264
23. Wieten RW, Jonker EF, van Leeuwen EM, Remmerswaal EB, Ten Berge IJ, de Visser AW, et al. A single 17D yellow fever vaccination provides lifelong immunity; characterization of yellow-fever-specific neutralizing antibody and T-cell responses after vaccination. *PLoS One.* (2016) 11:e0149871. doi: 10.1371/journal.pone.0149871
24. Muyanja E, Ssemaganda A, Ngauv P, Cubas R, Perrin H, Srinivasan D, et al. Immune activation alters cellular and humoral responses to yellow fever 17D vaccine. *J Clin Invest.* (2014) 124:3147–58. doi: 10.1172/JCI75429
25. Gaucher D, Therrien R, Kettaf N, Angermann BR, Boucher G, Filali-Mouhim A, et al. Yellow fever vaccine induces integrated multilineage and polyfunctional immune responses. *J Exp Med.* (2008) 205:3119–31. doi: 10.1084/jem.20082292
26. Collaborative Group for Studies with Yellow Fever Vaccine. Randomized, double-blind, multicenter study of the immunogenicity and reactogenicity of 17DD and WHO 17D-213/77 yellow fever vaccines in children: implications for the Brazilian National Immunization Program. *Vaccine.* (2007) 25:3118–23. doi: 10.1016/j.vaccine.2007.01.053
27. Collaborative Group for Studies of Yellow Fever Vaccine. A randomized double-blind clinical trial of two yellow fever vaccines prepared with substrains 17DD and 17D-213/77 in children nine-23 months old. *Mem Inst Oswaldo Cruz.* (2015) 110:771–80. doi: 10.1590/0074-02760150176
28. Luiza-Silva M, Campi-Azevedo AC, Batista MA, Martins MA, Avelar RS, da Silveira Lemos D, et al. Cytokine signatures of innate and adaptive immunity in 17DD yellow fever vaccinated children and its association with the level of neutralizing antibody. *J Infect Dis.* (2011) 204:873–83. doi: 10.1093/infdis/jir439

29. Hepburn MJ, Kortepeter MG, Pittman PR, Boudreau EF, Mangiafico JA, Buck PA, et al. Neutralizing antibody response to booster vaccination with the 17d yellow fever vaccine. *Vaccine.* (2006) 24:2843–9. doi: 10.1016/j.vaccine.2005.12.055
30. Kongsgaard M, Bassi MR, Rasmussen M, Skjødt K, Thybo S, Gabriel M, et al. Adaptive immune responses to booster vaccination against yellow fever virus are much reduced compared to those after primary vaccination. *Sci Rep.* (2017) 7:662. doi: 10.1038/s41598-017-00798-1
31. Lindsey NP, Horiuchi KA, Fulton C, Panella AJ, Kosoy OI, Velez JO, et al. Persistence of yellow fever virus-specific neutralizing antibodies after vaccination among US travellers. *J Travel Med.* (2018) 25:1–6. doi: 10.1093/jtm/tay108
32. Collaborative group for studies on yellow fever vaccines. Duration of immunity in recipients of two doses of 17DD yellow fever vaccine. *Vaccine.* (2019) 37:5129–35. doi: 10.1016/j.vaccine.2019.05.048
33. Campi-Azevedo AC, Peruhype-Magalhães V, Coelho-dos-Reis JG, Antonelli LRV, Costa-Pereira C, Speziali E, et al. 17DD-Yellow Fever re-vaccination regimens are required for long-term persistence of neutralizing antibodies and memory $CD8^+$ T-cells in populations of endemic areas with high risk of yellow fever transmission. *Emerg Infec Dis.* (2019) 25:1511–21. doi: 10.3201/eid2508.181432
34. Campi-Azevedo AC, de Araújo-Porto LP, Luiza-Silva M, Batista MA, Martins MA, Sathler-Avelar R, et al. 17DD and 17D-213/77 yellow fever substrains trigger a balanced cytokine profile in primary vaccinated children. *PLoS ONE.* (2012) 7:e49828. doi: 10.1371/journal.pone.0049828
35. Reinhardt B, Jaspert R, Niedrig M, Kostner C, L'age-Stehr J. Development of viremia and humoral and cellular parameters of immune activation after vaccination with yellow fever virus strain 17D: a model of human flavivirus infection. *J Med Virol.* (1998) 56:159–67. doi: 10.1002/(SICI)1096-9071(199810)56:2<159::AID-JMV10>3.0.CO;2-B
36. Sarkander J, Hojyo S, Tokoyoda K. Vaccination to gain humoral immune memory. *Clin Transl Immunol.* (2016) 5:e120. doi: 10.1038/cti.2016.81
37. Shi Y, Agematsu K, Ochs HD, Sugane K. Functional analysis of human memory B-cell subpopulations: IgD^+CD27^+ B cells are crucial in secondary immune response by producing high affinity IgM. *Clin Immunol.* (2003) 108:128–37. doi: 10.1016/S1521-6616(03)00092-5

8

Single-Nucleotide Variants in the AIM2 – Absent in Melanoma 2 Gene (rs1103577) Associated with Protection for Tuberculosis

Mariana Brasil de Andrade Figueira[1,2*], *Dhêmerson Souza de Lima*[3], *Antonio Luiz Boechat*[1,2], *Milton Gomes do Nascimento Filho*[1], *Irineide Assumpção Antunes*[4], *Joycenéa da Silva Matsuda*[4], *Thaís Rodrigues de Albuquerque Ribeiro*[1], *Luana Sousa Felix*[1], *Ariane Senna Fonseca Gonçalves*[1], *Allyson Guimarães da Costa*[2,5], *Rajendranath Ramasawmy*[2,6,7], *Alessandra Pontillo*[3], *Mauricio Morishi Ogusku*[8] *and Aya Sadahiro*[1,2*]

[1] Laboratório de Imunologia Molecular, Departamento de Parasitologia, Universidade Federal do Amazonas (UFAM), Manaus, Brazil, [2] Programa de Pós-Graduação em Imunologia Básica e Aplicada, Universidade Federal do Amazonas, Manaus, Brazil, [3] Laboratório de Imunogenética, Departamento de Imunologia, Instituto de Ciências Biomédicas (ICB), Universidade de São Paulo (USP), São Paulo, Brazil, [4] Policlínica Cardoso Fontes – Secretaria de Estado da Saúde do Amazonas-SUSAM, Manaus, Brazil, [5] Diretoria de Ensino e Pesquisa, Fundação Hospitalar de Hematologia e Hemoterapia do Amazonas (HEMOAM), Manaus, Brazil, [6] Instituto de Pesquisa Clínica Carlos Borborema, Fundação de Medicina Tropical Dr. Heitor Vieira Dourado, Manaus, Brazil, [7] Faculdade de Medicina Nilton Lins, Universidade Nilton Lins, Manaus, Brazil, [8] Laboratório de Micobacteriologia, Instituto Nacional de Pesquisas da Amazônia (INPA), Manaus, Brazil

***Correspondence:**
Mariana Brasil de Andrade Figueira
mariana_brasil@hotmail.com
Aya Sadahiro
asadahiro@ufam.edu.br

Tuberculosis (TB) remains a serious public health burden worldwide. TB is an infectious disease caused by the *Mycobacterium tuberculosis* Complex. Innate immune response is critical for controlling mycobacterial infection. NOD-like receptor pyrin domain containing 3/ absent in melanoma 2 (NLRP3/AIM2) inflammasomes are suggested to play an important role in TB. NLRP3/AIM2 mediate the release of pro-inflammatory cytokines IL-1β and IL-18 to control *M. tuberculosis* infection. Variants of genes involved in inflammasomes may contribute to elucidation of host immune responses to TB infection. The present study evaluated single-nucleotide variants (SNVs) in inflammasome genes *AIM2* (rs1103577), *CARD8* (rs2009373), and *CTSB* (rs1692816) in 401 patients with pulmonary TB (PTB), 133 patients with extrapulmonary TB (EPTB), and 366 healthy control (HC) subjects with no history of TB residing in the Amazonas state. Quantitative Real Time PCR was performed for allelic discrimination. The SNV of *AIM2* (rs1103577) is associated with protection for PTB (*p*adj: 0.033, ORadj: 0.69, 95% CI: 0.49-0.97). *CTSB* (rs1692816) is associated with reduced risk for EPTB when compared with PTB (*p*adj: 0.034, ORadj: 0.50, 95% CI: 0.27-0.94). Serum IL-1β concentrations were higher in patients with PTB than those in HCs (p = 0,0003). The SNV rs1103577 of *AIM2* appeared to influence IL-1β release. In a dominant model, individuals with the CC genotype (mean 3.78 ± SD 0.81) appeared to have a higher level of

IL-1β compared to carriers of the T allele (mean 3.45 ± SD 0.84) among the patients with PTB (p = 0,0040). We found that SNVs of *AIM2* and *CTSB* were associated with TB, and the mechanisms involved in this process require further study.

Keywords: tuberculosis, inflammasome, SNV, *AIM2*, *CARD8*, *CTSB*

INTRODUCTION

Tuberculosis (TB) is an infectious disease caused by mycobacteria belonging to the *Mycobacterium tuberculosis* complex (MTBC) (1). The MTBC typically affects the lungs (pulmonary TB (PTB) but can also affect other tissues and organs (extrapulmonary TB (EPTB)) (2). Approximately 25% of the world's population is infected with *M. tuberculosis*, but only approximately 5% to 10% of *M. tuberculosis*-infected individuals subsequently develop TB (3). The complexity of TB is influenced by several factors, such as the immune status and genetic factors of host (4–8).

The innate immune response is the first line of host defense against mycobacteria infection (9, 10). Innate immune system senses pathogens via pattern-recognition receptors (PRRs) to recognize conserved microbial components known as pathogen-associated molecular patterns (PAMPs). PRR also function as innate sensors of host-derived danger signals, the danger-associated molecular patterns (DAMPs) and may assemble in inflammasomes (11). Inflammasomes are intracellular multimeric protein complexes that play key roles in the innate immune response (12, 13). Inflammasomes are essential for controlling bacterial growth through the activation of caspase-1 to process pro-inflammatory IL-1β and IL-18 into active cytokines (14, 15). Caspase-1 also induces a type of inflammatory cell death called pyroptosis (16).

Inflammasomes belonging to the NOD-like receptor (NLR) family are composed of at least three components, a sensor protein (NLRP1, NLRP3, NLRP6, NLRP12, NLRC4; PYHIN family (PYD-like and HIN domain-containing proteins) as AIM2 and TRIM family (Tripartite motif proteins) containing PYRIN), an inflammatory caspase (caspase-1, Caspase-11) and an adapter molecule such as the apoptosis-associated speck-like containing a CARD domain (ASC) (17). NLRP3-inflammasomes is the most studied compared to others (18). NLRP3 and AIM2 inflammasomes play important role in host defense against *M. tuberculosis* (9, 15, 19–22).

The *NLRP3* gene is located on human chromosome 1. Basically, member of NLR family of PRR consists of three domains: a leucine-rich repeat (LRR)-region that interacts with antigens, a central nucleotide-binding NACHT domain and an effector domain PYD or CARD (23). *AIM2* gene is located on human chromosome 1. AIM2 is composed of two domains: a N-terminal pyrin domain (PYD) and a C-terminal hematopoietic interferon-inducible nuclear protein with a 200-amino acid repeat (HIN200) domain. AIM2 is a cytosolic double-stranded DNA receptor (24, 25).

Principles of inflammasome activation in TB involve two signals. The first signal induces the expression of NLRP3 and/or AIM2 inflammasome, pro-IL-1β and pro-IL-IL-18 genes caused by Toll-like receptor (TLR) stimulation. The second signal results to oligomerization domain and formation of inflammasome complex consequent of activating stimuli. After that, the effector domain recruits ASC protein to assemble the inflammasome complex (PRR, ASC protein and procaspase-1). ASC protein recruits procaspase-1 through caspase recruitment domain (CARD) consequently it is cleaved into active caspase-1 (14).

Activating stimuli described for NLRP3 are mitochondrial factors (mitochondrial reactive oxygen species, mitochondrial DNA, cardiolipin), mycobacterial components, cathepsins after lysosomal rupture as Cathepsin B encoded by *CTSB* gene located on human chromosome 8, potassium efflux and extracellular ATP via the P2X7 purinergic receptor (26, 27) and AIM2 is cytosolic dsDNA (25, 28). CTSB is cysteine exo/endopeptidase enzymes pH dependent belonging members of the papain family seems to involvement roles in NLRP3-inflammasome activation as well as degradation or processing of lysosomal proteins (29–31). CARD8 adaptor protein is encoded by *CARD8* gene present on chromosome 19. CARD8 acts as a negative regulator during NLRP3 inflammasome activation for adequate functioning and balanced response (32, 33).

In animal models of TB, NLRP3 (34, 35) and AIM2 (19, 36) inflammasomes have been found to recognize cytosolic DNA. Recently, the importance of inflammasomes in TB (37) as well as the crucial role of IL1β in infection control independent of inflammasome activation have been highlighted (38). TB is complex and multifactorial and identification of genetic variants can improve our understanding of the pathogenesis of TB (39).

Several studies have shown a genetic predisposition to development of TB (40–44). Genetic variant in inflammasomes can change their physiological function and contribute to the susceptibility, severity, and outcomes of TB (45). Single-nucleotide variant (SNV) of *NLRP3* (rs10754558) and SNV of *P2X7* (rs2230911) are associated with TB. SNV of *NLRP3* (rs10754558) is associated with protection against PTB (41). The SNV of *P2X7* (rs2230911) is associated with susceptibility to PTB. SNVs of *CARD8* (rs2043211) and *NLRP3* (rs35829419) are associated with EPTB in Ethiopian population (46).

The important role of inflammasomes in immunity to TB prompted us to evaluate the associations of SNVs in genes encoding the AIM2 inflammasome, CARD8, and CTSB in patients with TB from Amazonas state of Brazil.

MATERIAL AND METHODS

Ethics Statement

This study was approved by Human Research Ethics Committee of Federal University of Amazonas (N°. CAAE: 57978916.3.0000.5020;

August 17, 2016). All patients and controls participating in this study provided written informed consent for collection of blood and sputum samples for analysis.

Study Population

This is a case–control study and is consisted of 401 patients with PTB, 133 patients with EPTB, and 366 healthy controls (HCs). The study population was recruited from Policlínica Cardoso Fontes, a sanitary pneumology center (Manaus, AM, Brazil). The patients with PTB were positive for *M. tuberculosis*, which was determined through a molecular rapid test (TRM, GeneXpert MTB/RIF) (47) or through sputum smears and PKO culture method (47, 48). The diagnosis of EPTB was based on recommendations of Brazilian National Guidelines for the Control of Tuberculosis (49). The patients with EPTB were either sputum MTB-positive or culture-positive and were molecularly characterized for MTBC. The clinical manifestations of EPTB were pleural cutaneous, ganglionic, intestinal, perianal, ocular, bone, and miliary.

HCs participating in study had no history of TB and were contacts of patients with TB. The HCs were devoid of TB symptoms and negative for *M. tuberculosis* in sputum and/or in culture tests. Exclusion criteria comprised current pregnancy, recipients of organ transplants, and presence of other comorbidities, such as cancer, diabetes, HIV positive, hepatitis, and autoimmune diseases.

DNA Isolation and SNV Genotyping

Genomic DNA was extracted from whole human blood (1 mL) using tetramethylammonium bromide salts protocol (50). SNVs were selected according to the minor allele frequency (MAF) of > to 10% in the global population from NCBI database, but also for background information on inflammasome complex in tuberculosis. Three SNVs in inflammasome genes *AIM2* T>C (rs1103577) situated on chromosome 1q15, *CARD8* T>C (rs2009373) on 19q48, and *CTSB* A> C (rs1692816) on 8q11 were selected and genotyped using TaqMan probes for allelic discrimination assay by Real-Time PCR System (Applied Biosystems). The technology is based on hydrolysis fluorescent probes. The fluorescent probes are allele-specific oligonucleotides sequences of target SNV labeled with either VIC or FAM fluorescence to discriminate the alleles. Thermal cycling conditions for PCR were a pre-read stage at 60°C for 30 sec and subsequently a hold stage at 95°C for 10 min followed by 50 cycles of denaturation at 95°C for 15 sec and annealing\ extension at 60°C for 01 sec and finally followed by a post-read stage at 60°C for 30 sec. The reaction mix contained 5 µL TaqMan Genotyping Master Mix 1X; 0,5 µL TaqMan® probes 20X of target SNV, 4,5 µL Milli-Q water and 2 µL DNA (50ng\uL). For each PCR plate, a negative control and three known positive controls of target SNV (rare homozygote, wild-type homozygote and heterozygote) were included to increase the reliability of assay. Of note, the SNV rs35130877 of the *AIM2* gene was previously studied in the same population (41). This was carried out using QuantStudio™ 3 (ThermoFisher Scientific) and Design & Analysis Software v.1.4.2. The probes used in experiment are shown in **Supplementary Table 1**.

Cytokine Measurements

Human IL-1β levels were measured in plasma sample from patients with PTB prior to start of drug therapy and HCs using a commercially available enzyme-linked immunosorbent assay (ELISA) kit (BioLegend ELISA MAX™ Deluxe Sets) following the manufacturer's instructions. 50 µL of plasma samples were added to each well of high binding plate and readings were performed on a BioRad spectrophotometer plate as recommended by kit, using the 450 nm filter. Samples and standards were analyzed in duplicate. The minimal detectable concentration of IL-1β for this kit was 0.5 pg/mL.

Statistical Analysis

For each SNVs analysis, alleles analysis was performed using on the link https://ihg.helmholtz-muenchen.de/ihg/snps.html and the associations between the allelic/genotype frequencies among patients with PTB, EPTB, and HCs were examined using the package "SNPassoc" version 1.9-2 (https://cran.r-project.org/web/packages/SNPassoc/index.html) for R software version 3.4.3 (www.r-project.org). The best genetic model was performed via Akaike information criterion (AIC). The Hardy-Weinberg equilibrium was evaluated for all SNVs. The results were shown as the odds ratio (OR) and 95% confidence intervals (95% CI) from multivariate logistic regression analyses. To control the potential confounding factors, adjusted OR (OR_{adj}) values for age and sex were provided. The multivariate logistic regressions were performed using STATA 15 (StataCorp Texas, USA) after adjusting for age and sex. To compare multiple means of cytokine levels, one-way analysis of variance was applied with the Tukey's post-hoc test adjusted for multiple comparisons. A *p*-value less than 0.05 was considered as statistically significant.

RESULTS

Characteristics of the Study Population

A total of 900 unrelated individuals born in the North of Brazil participated in this study. Of 900 individuals, 534 and 366 were patients with TB and HCs, respectively. Among those with TB, 401 had PTB and 133 had EPTB. The mean ages of patients with PTB, EPTB, and the HCs were 38.1 ± 13.7, 34.6 ± 14.1, and 32.9 ± 12.5, respectively. Of patients with PTB, EPTB, and HCs, 243 (60.6%), 75 (56.4%), and 180 (49.2%) were male, respectively. Patients with EPTB exhibited mostly pleural (55.6%), followed by cutaneous (17.3%) and ganglionic (16.5%). Intestinal, perianal, ocular, bone, and miliary TB accounted for 10.5%.

Analysis of the SNVs in Inflammasome Genes

All SNVs studied *AIM2* rs1103577, *CARD8* rs2009373 and *CTSB* rs1692816 were in the Hardy-Weinberg equilibrium (HWE) in both HCs and patients with TB. The frequencies of alleles and genotypes as well as the different comparisons are shown in **Tables 1–4**. Genotypes and the best inheritance modeling for *AIM2*, *CARD8* and *CTSB* genes are reported in **Supplementary Table 2**.

The distribution of SNV of *AIM2* (rs1103577) genotypes is slightly different between patients with PTB compared with HC (p_{adj}: 0.083). The frequency of genotype CC was slightly higher among patients with PTB (32%) than among HCs (27%). The SNV of *AIM2* (rs1103577) was associated with a reduced risk of developing PTB (p_{adj}: 0.027, OR_{adj}: 0.69, 95% CI: 0.50-0.96) in a dominant model (CC versus CT + TT) when compared with HCs (**Table 1**). Carriers of T allele had 31% less chances of developing PTB compared to individuals homozygous for C allele, suggesting homozygosity for C allele may be a risk factor for PTB.

The SNV of *CARD8* (rs2009373) showed a decrease risk in development of EPTB when compared to PTB in a recessive model (p_{adj}: 0.026, OR_{adj}: 0.48, 95% CI: 0.25-0.96) (**Table 2**). Bearers of C allele had 52% less chance of developing PTB. The frequency of genotype TT was predominant among the patients with PTB (22%) than in the EPTB group (12%). Individuals homozygous for T allele had twice chance of developing PTB than EPTB when compared with individuals homozygous for C allele (TT vs. CC p = 0.05, OR=2.1, 95% CI: 0.99-4.4) (The results of the different alleles were extracted on the link https://ihg.helmholtz-muenchen.de/ihg/snps.html). Of note, the frequencies of genotype were 31%, 49% and 20% for CC, CT and TT respectively, among HCs group (**Supplementary Table 2**). Comparisons between patients with EPTB and HCs revealed that carriers of C allele (CC +CT vs. TT) had 85% risk of developing EPTB (p=0.07, OR = 1.85, 95% CI: 0.94-3.7). No association was revealed when patients with PTB were compared with HCs.

Regarding the SNV of *CTSB* (rs1692816), an overdominant model indicated that heterozygous individuals have a lower risk of developing EPTB compared to patients with PTB (p: 0.022, OR: 0.50, 95% CI: 0.27-0.92) (**Supplementary Table 2**) and when adjusted for sex and age (p: 0.026, OR: 0.50, 95% CI: 0.27-0.94) (**Tables 3** and **4**). The frequencies were 23%, 50% and 27% for

TABLE 1 | Genetic models of association SNV rs1103577 of *AIM2* gene adjusted for sex and age in patients with pulmonary tuberculosis (PTB) and healthy control.

AIM2 Genetic Model	PTB n, %	Controls n, %	p value $_{adj}$	OR $_{adj}$ (95% CI)	AIC
Codominant			0.083	1.00	988.4
CC	124 (0.32)	95 (0.27)		–	
CT	180 (0.47)	180 (0.51)		0.68 (0.48-0.96)	
TT	81 (0.21)	76 (0.22)		0.72 (0.47-1.11)	
Dominant			**0.027**		986.5
CC	124 (0.32)	95 (0.27)		–	
CT-TT	261 (0.68)	256 (0.73)		0.69 (0.50- 0.96)	
Recessive			0.672		991.2
CT-CC	304 (0.79)	275 (0.78)		–	
TT	81 (0.21)	76 (0.22)		0.92 (0.64-1.33)	
Overdominant			0.096		988.6
CC-TT	205 (0.53)	171 (0.49)		–	
CT	180 (0.47)	180 (0.51)		0.78 (0.58-1.05)	
Log-Additive	385 (0.52)	351 (0.48)	0.096	0.84 (0.68-1.03)	988.6
0,1,2					

PTB (pulmonary tuberculosis); adjusted for sex and age (p value $_{adj}$, OR_{adj}); 95% confidence interval (CI); AIC, Akaike information criterion value.
The results statistically significant are highlight in bold characters.

TABLE 2 | Genetic models of association SNV rs2009373 of *CARD8* gene adjusted for sex and age in patients with extrapulmonary tuberculosis (EPTB) and pulmonary tuberculosis (PTB).

CARD8 Genetic Model	EPTB n, %	PTB n, %	p value $_{adj}$	OR $_{adj}$ (95% CI)	AIC
Codominant			0.083	˜1.00	462.3
CC	31 (0.34)	111 (0.30)		–	
CT	50 (0.54)	183 (0.49)		0.98 (0.59-1.64)	
TT	11 (0.12)	82 (0.22)		0.48 (0.23-1.01)	
Dominant			0.444		464.6
CC	31 (0.34)	111 (0.30)		–	
CT-TT	61 (0.66)	265 (0.71)		0.82 (0.50-1.35)	
Recessive			**0.026**		460.3
CT-CC	81 (0.88)	294 (0.78)		–	
TT	11 (0.12)	82 (0.22)		0.48 (0.25-0.96)	
Overdominant			0.322		464.2
CC-TT	42 (0.46)	193 (0.51)		–	
CT	50 (0.54)	183 (0.49)		1.26 (0.80-2.00)	
Log-Additive			0.084		462.2
0,1,2	92 (0.20)	376 (0.80)		0.75 (0.53-1.04)	

PTB (pulmonary tuberculosis); EPTB (extrapulmonary tuberculosis); adjusted for sex and age (p value $_{adj}$, OR_{adj}); 95% confidence interval (CI); AIC, Akaike information criterion value.
The results statistically significant are highlight in bold characters.

TABLE 3 | Genetic models of association SNV rs1692816 of *CTSB* gene adjusted for sex and age in patients with extrapulmonary tuberculosis (EPTB) and healthy control subjects.

CTSB Genetic Model	EPTB n, %	Controls n, %	p value $_{adj}$	OR $_{adj}$ (95% CI)	AIC
Codominant			0.120	1.00	310.8
AA	19 (0.37)	93 (0.27)		–	
AC	17 (0.33)	169 (0.48)		0.49 (0.24-1.00)	
CC	15 (0.29)	89 (0.25)		0.83 (0.39-1.73)	
Dominant			0.120		310.6
AA	19 (0.37)	93 (0.26)		–	
AC-CC	32 (0.63)	258 (0.74)		0.61 (0.33-1.13)	
Recessive			0.545		312.7
AA-AC	36 (0.70)	262 (0.75)		-	
CC	15 (0.30)	89 (0.25)		1.22 (0.64-2.34)	
Overdominant			**0.046**		309.1
AA-CC	34 (0.67)	182 (0.52)		–	
AC	17 (0.33)	169 (0.48)		0.54 (0.29-1.00)	
Log-Additive			0.543		312.7
0,1,2	51 (0.13)	351 (0.87)		0.88 (0.59-1.32)	

EPTB (extrapulmonary tuberculosis); adjusted for sex and age (p value $_{adj}$, OR_{adj}); 95% confidence interval (CI); AIC, Akaike information criterion value. The results statistically significant are highlight in bold characters.

TABLE 4 | Genetic models of association SNV rs1692816 of CTSB gene adjusted for sex and age in patients with extrapulmonary tuberculosis (EPTB) and pulmonary tuberculosis (PTB).

CTSB Genetic Model	EPTB n, %	PTB n, %	p value $_{adj}$	OR $_{adj}$ (95% CI)	AIC
Codominant			0.084	1.00	314.9
AA	19 (0.37)	103 (0.27)		–	
AC	17 (0.33)	193 (0.50)		0.50 (0.25-1.01)	
CC	15 (0.29)	89 (0.23)		0.98 (0.47-2.07)	
Dominant			0.177		316.1
AA	19 (0.37)	103 (0.27)		–	
AC-CC	32 (0.63)	282 (0.73)		0.65 (0.35-1.20)	
Recessive			0.269		316.7
AA-AC	36 (0.71)	296 (0.77)		–	
CC	15 (0.29)	89 (0.23)		1.46 (0.76-2.80)	
Overdominant			**0.026**		312.9
AA-CC	34 (0.67)	192 (0.50)		–	
AC	17 (0.33)	193 (0.50)		0.50 (0.27-0.94)	
Log-Additive			0.841		317.8
0,1,2	51 (0.12)	385 (0.88)		0.96 (0.64-1.45)	

PTB (pulmonary tuberculosis); EPTB (extrapulmonary tuberculosis); adjusted for sex and age (p value $_{adj}$, OR_{adj}); 95% confidence interval (CI); AIC, Akaike information criterion value. The results statistically significant are highlight in bold characters.

the CC, AC and AA genotypes, respectively among patients with PTB and similar pattern was observed among HCs (CC 25%, AC 48% and AA 27%). In contrast, the frequencies among patients with EPTB were 29%, 33%, and 37% for CC, AC and AA genotypes, respectively. Similarly, comparison between patients and HCs disclosed that heterozygous individuals have lower risk of developing EPTB (p: 0.045, p_{adj}: 0.046, OR: 0.54, 95% CI: 0.29-1.0).

Logistic regression analysis, including sex and age variables with SNVs, confirmed the association of *AIM2* rs1103577 (p:0.033, OR: 0.69, 95% CI: 0.49-0.97) and *CTSB* rs1692816 with a lower risk for EPTB (p: 0.034, OR: 0.50, 95% CI: 0.27-0.94) (**Table 5**).

Cytokine IL-1β in a Dominant Model of *AIM2*, *CARD8*, and *CTSB* Genotypes

IL-1β is an important inflammatory cytokine with major role in host immune response against *M.tuberculosis* infection. Next, we evaluated *in vivo* the plasma IL-1β concentrations in PTB and HCs. Plasma IL-1β was higher in patients with PTB compared to those in HC group (p = 0.0003) (**Supplementary Figure 1**). We analyzed the distribution of plasma IL1-β according to genotypes of *AIM2*, *CARD8*, and *CTSB* in a dominant model. *AIM2* rs1103577 appeared to have an effect on plasma cytokine IL-1β when CC carriers were compared to allele T carriers (CC vs. CT+TT) in patients with PTB (p = 0.0040). CARD8 rs2009373 and CTSB rs1692816 did not show any influence on levels of plasma IL-β (**Figure 1A**). A QQ plot was used to validate the distribution of IL-1β in genotypes (**Figure 1B**).

DISCUSSION

Genetics and environmental factors are crucial for host immune response against *M. tuberculosis*. The complex network of mechanisms from early infection to development of TB remains

TABLE 5 | Multivariate logistic regression analysis for variables sex and age, including three inflammasomes genes in the studied groups.

Variable	Tuberculosis vs Control		Pulmonary tuberculosis vs Control		Extrapulmonary tuberculosis vs Control		Pulmonary vs Extrapulmonary tuberculosis	
	p value	OR (95% CI)	*p* value	OR (95% CI)	*p* value	OR (95% CI)	*p* value	OR (95% CI)
AIM2 rs1103577	0.053	0.73 (0.53-1.00)	**0.033**	0.69 (0.49-0.97)	0.241	0.68 (0.35-1.29)	0.976	1.00 (0.53-1.90)
CARD8 rs2009373	0.825	0.95 (0.70-1.31)	0.652	0.92 (0.66-1.28)	0.539	1.21 (0.64-2.28)	0.279	1.41 (0.75-2.67)
CTSB rs1692816	0.229	0.83 (0.63-1.11)	0.597	1.08 (0.80-1.46)	0.066	0.55 (0.29-1.03)	**0.034**	0.50 (0.27-0.94)

odds ratio (OR) and 95% confidence interval (CI).
The results statistically significant are highlight in bold characters.

poorly understood. Since the identification of function of various inflammasomes, several studies of genetic variants of genes involved in assembling the multiprotein complex of inflammasomes have attempted to determine the reason of susceptibility of some individuals to develop diseases while others remain asymptomatic. In the early stage of infection, innate immune response is essential to ensure the success of control and elimination of bacilli. Subsequently, upon inflammasomes activation, proinflammatory cytokines are released to keep in check the invading pathogen (45). In this context, we have focus on one SNV in the *AIM2* inflammasome in tuberculosis together with two other SNVs, one in *CARD8* and one in *CTSB*, that are related to NLRP3 pathway.

Studies regarding human genetic variants of *AIM2* are rare in infectious diseases (41, 42, 45). Recently, we investigated another SNV of *AIM2* (rs35130877) in 288 patients with PTB and 288 HCs. None of participants had this SNV (41). In this study, we found that SNV of *AIM2* (rs1103577) was associated with protection against TB. Interestingly, immunological studies involving mice have demonstrated a protective role of AIM2 against *M. tuberculosis* infection (19, 51). Inhibition of inflammasomes decreased the survival of *M. tuberculosis* in mice (37) and suggested that a high level of IL-1β favored the survival of bacteria. Carriers homozygous for C allele have higher IL-1 concentrations compared to T allele carriers, and T allele is associated with protection in our study. Furthermore, modern lineages of MTBC have high multiplication rates, which correlates to high levels of IL-1β (52). However, some individuals are resistant to *M. tuberculosis* infection despite continuous exposure (53, 54), suggesting sterile clearance potentially due to a reflex of genetic background and immunity of individual.

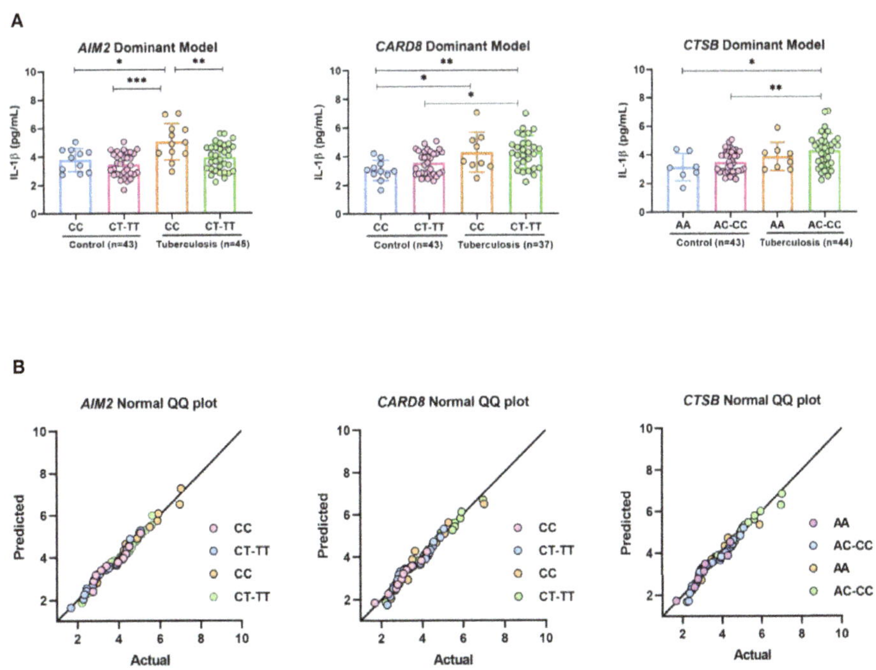

FIGURE 1 | IL-1β profile respective on genotypes of *AIM2*, *CARD8* and *CTSB* from pulmonary tuberculosis patients and control. **(A)** Serum concentrations of IL-1β distributed in *AIM2*, *CARD8* and *CTSB* dominant model genotypes. **(B)** Graphic Normal QQ plot for three SNV studied. Groups were further compared with each other using ANOVA test with Tukey's multiple comparisons test, *$p < 0,05$; **$p < 0,001$; ***$p < 0,0001$.

IL-1β is a proinflammatory cytokine and has been suggested to play key role in host protection against *M. tuberculosis* infection (55, 56). The protein ESAT of *M. tuberculosis* is cited as a potent activator of NLRP3\ASC inflammasome to liberate mature IL-1β (9). Patients with PTB also exhibit increased levels of IL-1βcompared to HCs. Patients with PTB also demonstrate higher levels of IL-1β (37, 38, 57), reinforcing an important role in the early innate immune response to control *M. tuberculosis* infection. We found that the serum concentrations of cytokine IL-1β were correlated according to genotypes CC versus CT-TT (*AIM2*) among patients with PTB in a dominant model. The T allele (TT +CT) correlated with low level of IL1 while homozygosity for the C allele with high level of IL-1β. The T allele is associated with protection to development of TB while individuals homozygous for C allele with susceptibility. Interestingly, excessive levels of IL-1β has been associated with severe TB and lung damage (57, 58).

NLRP3 and AIM2-inflammasome are suggested to play important role in host-defense against mycobacteria (19, 59). Recently, Souza de Lima et al. (22) have shown that NLRP3/IL-1ß/IL-18 pathway is strongly activated in a cathepsin-dependent form by virulent strain H37Rv and non-virulent BCG strains of *M. tuberculosis* in human macrophages, in vitro. Interestingly, the response was modulated according to macrophage donor genotype of SNV NLRP3 rs10754558 that correlated to level of IL-1β release (22). Of note, IL-1β is one among key proinflammatory cytokines essential for recruitment of immune cells to the site of *M. tuberculosis* infection (55). Several studies have demonstrated the role of AIM2-inflamasome in mycobacterial infection. Mice macrophages infected with pathogenic strain of *M. bovis* led to activation of AIM2-inflammasome and mature IL-1β release (60). Similarly, another study also demonstrated that THP-1 macrophages exposed to rBCG (Recombinant BCG ΔureC::hly) vaccine results in AIM2-inflammasome activation with increased production of IL-1β and IL-18 and autophagy, corroborating the role of AIM2-inflammasome in innate immune response (61).

AIM2-deficient mice infected with *Mycobacterium bovis* Bacillus Calmette-Guérin (BCG) showed a higher infection burden and developed severe disease due to simultaneous induction of reactive IFN-β and IFN-γ responses compared to wild-type mice (51). The AIM2 inflammasome appears to play a protective role through the induction of IL-1β and negative regulation of type I IFN induction. High production of type I IFNs reduces the IFN-γ response in TB infection (51). Interestingly, we showed that individuals homozygous for C allele had higher level of IL-1β compared to carriers of T allele and T allele is associated with protection to the development of TB. Higher level of IL-1β in the early stage might be important in keeping in check the pathogen but at a later stage might cause tissue damage.

The SNVs of *AIM2* (rs1103577), *CARD8* (rs2009373) and *CTSB* (rs1692816) are located in intronic region of respective gene. Although the functional role of these variants has not been elucidated, non-coding regions can affect gene expression resulting in different responses to presence of pathogens and can serve such as genetic markers (62). In future studies, it will be interesting to quantify the AIM2 messenger RNA (mRNA) from macrophages of different genotypes of *AIM2* (rs1103577) upon mycobacterial infection. Intronic regions have been highlighted for increasing the expression of mRNA in very diverse organisms (mammals, plants). Thus being an important regulator in the expression of proteins (63–66).

In this study, stratification of patients into PTB and EPTB suggested that *CARD8* rs2009373 and *CTSB* rs1692816 were associated with a lower risk of developing PTB. However, multivariate logistic regression analysis showed that only *CTSB* rs1692816 was associated with a reduced risk for EPTB. Indeed, we observed that heterozygosity for the variant provides lower risk for development of EPTB. CTSB is a member of cathepsin family localized in lysosomes and cytosol. CTSB promotes the degradation of protein in lysosomes and controls autophagy (67). Furthermore, the inhibition of CTSB blocks *M. tuberculosis*-induced NLRP3 inflammasome assembly, thereby leading to a decrease in IL-1βrelease, suggesting that the release of lysosomal CTSB and possibly other cathepsins are crucial for activation of NLRP3 to control *M. tuberculosis* infection (22, 30). Although, the function of this *CTSB* rs1692816 is not known, we can speculate that heterozygous individuals have an advantage in modulating the NLRP3 inflammasome in the release of IL-1β that is sufficient to keep in check the bacteria in comparison to homozygotes. Indeed, heterozygosity for some genes variant have been shown to provide an advantage to some infectious diseases. Heterozygosity for hemoglobin S is an advantage in Africa against *Plasmodium falciparum* malaria. Heterozygosity for the MAL/TIRAP variant in the TLRs pathway have been suggested to provide protection against invasive pneumococcal disease, malaria, tuberculosis and chagas disease (68, 69).

The SNV of *CARD8* (rs2009373) was not associated with TB in this study. However, other variants of *CARD8* (rs6509365 and rs2043211) have been associated with susceptibility to TB (41, 46, 70). CARD8 negatively regulates NLRP3 activation, and *CARD8* rs2043211 appears to have a loss of function. Interestingly, *NLRP3* (rs35829419)/*CARD8* (rs2043211) interaction is associated with levels of IL-1β (71).

Another important aspect is the variation in allele frequencies among populations. We found that some alleles were present in high or low frequencies or were entirely absent in specific populations, thereby indicating different evolutionary histories that are assumed are under selective pressure from prevalent diseases.

The distribution of MAF for rs1103577 of *AIM2* (T allele) in HCs (T = 0.47) is comparable to that of a European population (T = 0.40) and different from that of an African population (C = 0.09). The Amazonian population is an admixture of approximately 60% American, 50% European, and 10% African ancestry (72). The MAF of *CARD8* rs2009373 (T allele) in our group (T = 0.45) was similar to frequencies of South Asian (T = 0.46), European (T = 0.47), American (T = 0.41), and African (0.50) populations, but different from those of West Asian populations (C = 0.23). For rs1692816 of *CTSB*, both alleles A and C are frequent in different populations. The frequency of *CTSB* rs1692816 C allele was 0.49 in our population, compared to

African (0.56), American (0.59), and European (0.66) populations. However, the frequency of the rs1692816 C allele was similar to that of East (0.50) and South (0.53) Asian populations. The frequencies of the different alleles were extracted from http:// www.ensembl.org/. These frequencies indicate the importance of careful selection of cases and controls from same homogeneous population to avoid spurious associations.

The present study had some limitations. First, the sample size of the cases was small, especially for patients with EPTB. Second, we could not assay IL-1β in patients with EPTB due to a lack of biological samples. Additionally, the *NLRP3* data deviated from the HWE in both cases with TB and HCs; thus, they were excluded.

This result corroborates previous studies carried out by several researchers, both in an experimental model and in human cells infected by mycobacteria, which suggest the critical role of AIM2 in tuberculosis. We suggested *AIM2* rs1103577 was found to be associated with a lower risk of developing PTB and genotypes CC for AIM2 rs1103577 patients with PTB demonstrate higher levels of IL-1β. The *CARD8* and *CTSB* genes were also found to be important targets for TB, and other genetic variants should be investigated. Further studies are needed to confirm the association in other populations. Finally, it is indisputable that tuberculosis is a complex disease with a strong genetic link.

ETHICS STATEMENT

The studies involving human participants were reviewed and approved by The Human Research Ethics Committee of the Federal University of Amazonas (N°. CAAE: 57978916.3.0000.5020, August 17th, 2016). The patients/participants provided their written informed consent to participate in this study.

AUTHOR CONTRIBUTIONS

MBAF: realized the experiments, analyzed the data and wrote the paper. DL: analyzed the data and intellectual contribution. AB: analyzed the data and intellectual contribution. MGNF: Sample processing and intellectual contribution. IA: Contributed with samples and patient selection and intellectual contribution. JM: Contributed with samples and patient selection and intellectual contribution and intellectual contribution. TR: Sample processing and intellectual contribution. LF: Sample processing and intellectual contribution. AG: Sample processing and intellectual contribution. AC: intellectual contribution. RR: wrote the paper and intellectual contribution. AP: analyzed the data and intellectual contribution. MO: Sample processing, understanding of genotyping assays and intellectual contribution. AS: Analyzed the data, wrote the paper and intellectual contribution. All authors contributed to the article and approved the submitted version.

ACKNOWLEDGMENTS

We thank all subjects involved in the study, incluing pacients and to the staff of Policlínica Cardoso Fontes, Manaus, Amazonas, Brazil; Programa de Apoio à Pós-Graduação-Coordenação de Aperfeiçoamento de Pessoal de Nível Superior (PROAP/CAPES) and Fundação de Amparo à Pesquisa do Estado do Amazonas (FAPEAM).

REFERENCES

1. Galagan JE. Genomic insights into tuberculosis. *Nat Rev Genet* (2014) 15:5. doi: 10.1038/nrg3664
2. Pai M, Behr M, Dowdy D, Dheda K, Divangahi M, Boehme CC, et al. Tuberculosis. *Nat Rev Dis Primers* (2016) 2:16076. doi: 10.1038/nrdp.2016.76
3. World Health Organization. *Global Tuberculosis Report 2019* (2019). Geneva: World Health Organization. Available at: https://apps.who.int/iris/bitstream/handle/10665/329368/9789241565714-eng.pdf?ua (Accessed January 02, 2020).
4. Paramel GV, Sirsjö A, Fransén K. Role of genetic alterations in the NLRP3 and CARD8 genes in health and disease. *Mediators Inflamm* (2015) 2015:10. doi: 10.1155/2015/846782
5. Cadena AM, Fortune SM, Flynn JL. Heterogeneity in tuberculosis. *Nat Rev Immunol* (2017) 17:11. doi: 10.1038/nri.2017.69
6. Torrelles JB, Schlesinger LS. Integrating Lung Physiology, Immunology, and Tuberculosis. *Trends Microbiol* (2017) 25:8. doi: 10.1016/j.tim.2017.03.007
7. Cardona P-J. Pathogenesis of tuberculosis and other mycobacteriosis. *Enferm Infecc Microbiol Clin* (2018) 36:1. doi: 10.1016/j.eimce.2017.10.009
8. Batista LAF, Silva KJS, Silva LMC, Moura YF, Zucchi FCR. Tuberculosis: A granulomatous disease mediated by epigenetic factors. *Tuberculosis* (2020) 123:101943. doi: 10.1016/j.tube.2020.101943
9. Mishra BB, Moura-alves P, Sonawane A, Hacohen N, Griffiths G, Moita LF, et al. Mycobacterium tuberculosis protein ESAT-6 is a potent activator of the NLRP3/ASC inflammasome. *Cell Microbiol* (2010) 12:8. doi: 10.1111/j.1462-5822.2010.01450.x
10. Abdallah AM, Bestebroer J, Savage NDL, Punder K, Zon VM, Wilson L, et al. Mycobacterial secretion systems ESX-1 and ESX-5 play distinct roles in host cell death and inflammasome activation. *J Immunol* (2011) 187:9. doi: 10.4049/jimmunol.1101457
11. Franchi L, Muñoz-Planillo R, Núñez G. Sensing and reacting to microbes through the inflammasomes. *Nat Immunol* (2012) 13:4. doi: 10.1038/ni.2231
12. Martinon F, Burns K, Tschopp J. The Inflammasome: A molecular platform triggering activation of inflammatory caspases and processing of proIL-β. *Mol Cell* (2002) 10:2. doi: 10.1016/S1097-2765(02)00599-3
13. Strowig T, Henao-Mejia J, Elinav E, Flavell R. Inflammasomes in health and disease. *Nature* (2012) 481:7381. doi: 10.1038/nature10759
14. Guo H, Callaway JB, Ting JP-Y. Inflammasomes: mechanism of action, role in disease, and therapeutics. *Nat Med* (2015) 21:7. doi: 10.1038/nm.3893
15. Wawrocki S, Druszczynska M. Inflammasomes in Mycobacterium tuberculosis - Driven Immunity. *Can J Infect Dis Med Microbiol* (2017) 2017:2309478. doi: 10.1155/2017/2309478
16. Xue Y, Tuipulotu DE, Tan WH, Kay C, Man SM. Emerging Activators and Regulators of Inflammasomes and Pyroptosis. *Trends Immunol* (2019) 40:11. doi: 10.1016/j.it.2019.09.005
17. Yu C-H, Moecking J, Geyer M, Masters SL. Mechanisms of NLRP1-Mediated Autoinflammatory Disease in Humans and Mice. *J Mol Biol* (2018) 430:2. doi: 10.1016/j.jmb.2017.07.012
18. Yang Y, Wang H, Kouadir M, Song H, Shi F. Recent advances in the mechanisms of NLRP3 inflammasome activation and its inhibitors. *Cell Death Dis* (2019) 10:128. doi: 10.1038/s41419-019-1413-8
19. Saiga H, Kitada S, Shimada Y, Kamiyama N, Okuyama M, Makino M, et al. Critical role of AIM2 in Mycobacterium tuberculosis infection. *Int Immunol* (2012) 24:10. doi: 10.1093/intimm/dxs062
20. Wassermann R, Gulen MF, Sala C, Perin SG, Lou Y, Rybniker J, et al. Mycobacterium tuberculosis differentially activates cGAS-and inflammasome-dependent intracellular immune responses through ESX-1. *Cell Host Microbe* (2015) 17:6. doi: 10.1016/j.chom.2015.05.003
21. Xu F, Qi H, Li J, Sun L, Gong J, Chen Y, et al. Mycobacterium tuberculosis infection up-regulates MFN2 expression to promote NLRP3 inflammasome formation. *J Biol Chem* (2020) 295:51. doi: 10.1074/jbc.RA120.014077

22. Souza de Lima DS, Bomfim CC, Leal VN, Reis EC, Soares JLS, Fernandes FP, et al. Combining Host Genetics and Functional Analysis to Depict Inflammasome Contribution in Tuberculosis Susceptibility and Outcome in Endemic Areas. *Front Immunol* (2020) 11:550624. doi: 10.3389/fimmu.2020.550624
23. Awad F, Assrawi E, Louvrier C, Jumeau C, Georgin-Lavialle S, Grateau G, et al. Inflammasome biology, molecular pathology and therapeutic implications. *Pharmacol Ther* (2018) 187:133–49. doi: 10.1016/j.pharmthera.2018.02.011
24. Kesavardhana S, Kanneganti T-D. Mechanisms governing inflammasome activation, assembly and pyroptosis induction. *Int Immunol* (2017) 29:5. doi: 10.1093/intimm/dxx018
25. Wang B, Yin Q. AIM2 inflammasome activation and regulation: A structural perspective. *J Struct Biol* (2017) 200:3. doi: 10.1016/j.jsb.2017.08.001
26. Vanaja SK, Rathinam VA, Fitzgerald KA. Mechanisms of inflammasome activation: recent advances and novel insights. *Trends Cell Biol* (2015) 25:5. doi: 10.1016/j.tcb.2014.12.009
27. Jo EK, Kim J, Shin DM, Sasakawa C. Molecular mechanisms regulating NLRP3 inflammasome activation. *Cell Mol Immunol* (2016) 13:148159. doi: 10.1038/cmi.2015.95
28. Jin T, Perry A, Jiang J, Smith P, Curry JA, Unterholzner L, et al. Structures of the HIN domain: DNA complexes reveal ligand binding and activation mechanisms of the AIM2 inflammasome and IFI16 receptor. *Immunity* (2012) 36:4. doi: 10.1016/j.immuni.2012.02.014
29. Mort JS, Buttle DJ. Cathepsin B. *Int J Biochem Cell Biol* (1997) 29:5. doi: 10.1016/S1357-2725(96)00152-5
30. Amaral EP, Riteau N, Moayeri M, Maier N, Mayer-Barber KD, Pereira RM, et al. Lysosomal Cathepsin Release Is Required for NLRP3-Inflammasome Activation by Mycobacterium tuberculosis in Infected Macrophages. *Front Immunol* (2018) 9:1427. doi: 10.3389/fimmu.2018.01427
31. Campden RI, Zhang Y. The role of lysosomal cysteine cathepsins in NLRP3 inflammasome activation. *Arch Biochem Biophys* (2019) 670:32–42. doi: 10.1016/j.abb.2019.02.015
32. Razmara M, Srinivasula SM, Wang L, Poyet JL, Geddes BJ, DiStefano PS, et al. CARD-8 protein, a new CARD family member that regulates caspase-1 activation and apoptosis. *J Biol Chem* (2002) 277(16):13952–8. doi: 10.1074/jbc.M107811200
33. Ito S, Hara Y, Kubota T. CARD8 is a negative regulator for NLRP3 inflammasome, but mutant NLRP3 in cryopyrin-associated periodic syndromes escapes the restriction. *Arthritis Res Ther* (2014) 16:1. doi: 10.1186/ar4483
34. Abdalla H, Srinivasan L, Shah S, Mayer-Barber KD, Sher A, Sutterwala FS, et al. Mycobacterium tuberculosis infection of dendritic cells leads to partially caspase-1/11-independent IL-1β and IL-18 secretion but not to pyroptosis. *PloS One* (2012) 7:7. doi: 10.1371/journal.pone.0040722
35. Dorhoi A, Nouailles G, Jörg S, Hagens K, Heinemann E, Pradl L, et al. Activation of the NLRP3 inflammasome by Mycobacterium tuberculosis is uncoupled from susceptibility to active tuberculosis. *Eur J Immunol* (2012) 42:2. doi: 10.1002/eji.201141548
36. Shah S, Bohsali A, Ahlbrand SE, Srinivasan L, Rathinam VK, Vogel SN, et al. Cutting edge: Mycobacterium tuberculosis but not nonvirulent mycobacteria inhibits IFN-β and AIM2 inflammasome-dependent IL-1β production via its ESX-1 secretion system. *J Immunol* (2013) 191:7. doi: 10.4049/jimmunol.1301331
37. Subbarao S, Sanchez-garrido J, Kri N, Shenoy AR, Robert BD. Genetic and pharmacological inhibition of inflammasomes reduces the survival of Mycobacterium tuberculosis strains in macrophages. *Sci Rep* (2020) 10:3709. doi: 10.1038/s41598-020-60560-y
38. Mayer-Barber KD, Barber DL, Shenderov K, White SD, Wilson MS, Cheever A, et al. Cutting Edge: Caspase-1 Independent IL-1 Production Is Critical for Host Resistance to Mycobacterium tuberculosis and Does Not Require TLR Signaling In Vivo. *J Immunol* (2010) 184:7. doi: 10.4049/jimmunol.0904189
39. Briken V, Ahlbrand SE, Shah S. Mycobacterium tuberculosis and the host cell inflammasome: a complex relationship. *Front Cell Infect Microbiol* (2013) 3:62. doi: 10.3389/fcimb.2013.00062
40. Eklund D, Welin A, Andersson H, Verma D, Söderkvist P, Stendahl O, et al. Human gene variants linked to enhanced NLRP3 activity limit intramacrophage growth of mycobacterium tuberculosis. *J Infect Dis* (2014) 209:5. doi: 10.1093/infdis/jit572
41. Souza de Lima D, Ogusku MM, Sadahiro A, Pontillo A. Inflammasome genetics contributes to the development and control of active pulmonary tuberculosis. *Infect Genet Evol* (2016) 41:240–4. doi: 10.1016/j.meegid.2016.04.015
42. Liu C-W, Lin C-J, Hu H-C, Liu H-J, Chiu Y-C, Lee S-W, et al. The association of inflammasome and TLR2 gene polymorphisms with susceptibility to tuberculosis in the Han Taiwanese population. *Sci Rep* (2020) 10:10184. doi: 10.1038/s41598-020-67299-6
43. Souza de Lima D, Leal VNC, Ogusku MM, Sadahiro A, Pontillo A, Alencar BC. Polymorphisms in SIGLEC1 contribute to susceptibility to pulmonary active tuberculosis possibly through the modulation of IL-1ß. *Infect Genet Evol* (2017) 55:313–7. doi: 10.1016/j.meegid.2017.09.031
44. Barletta-Naveca RH, Naveca FG, de Almeida VA, Porto JIR, da Silva GAV, Ogusku MM, et al. Toll-like receptor-1 single-nucleotide polymorphism 1805T/G is associated with predisposition to multibacillary tuberculosis. *Front Immunol* (2018) 9:1455. doi: 10.3389/fimmu.2018.01455
45. Fernandes FP, Leal VNC, Souza de Lima D, Reis EC, Pontillo A. Inflammasome genetics and complex diseases: a comprehensive review. *Eur J Hum Genet* (2020) 28:13071321. doi: 10.1038/s41431-020-0631-y
46. Abate E, Blomgran R, Verma D, Lerm M, Fredrikson M. Polymorphisms in CARD8 and NLRP3 are associated with extrapulmonary TB and poor clinical outcome in active TB in Ethiopia. *Sci Rep* (2019) 9:3126. doi: 10.1038/s41598-019-40121-8
47. Brasil. Ministério da Saúde. *Secretaria de Vigilância em Saúde. Departamento de Vigilância das Doenças Transmissíveis. Rede de Teste Rápido para Tuberculose no Brasil: primeiro ano da implantação/Ministério da Saúde, Secretaria de Vigilância em Saúde, Departamento de Vigilância das Doenças Transmissíveis* (2015). Brasília: Ministério da Saúde. Available at: http://www.saude.gov.br/images/pdf/2016/janeiro/15/rtr-tb-15jan16-isbn-web.pdf (Accessed March 02, 2020).
48. Salem JI, Carvalho CM, Ogusku MM, Maia R. PKO – Alternative method for isolating mycobacteria from sputum. *Acta Amazonica* (2007) 37:3. doi: 10.1590/S0044-59672007000300013
49. Brasil. Ministério da Saúde *Secretaria de Vigilância em Saúde. Departamento de Vigilância das Doenças Transmissíveis. Manual de recomendações para o controle da tuberculose no Brasil / Ministério da Saúde, Secretaria de Vigilância em Saúde, Departamento de Vigilância das Doenças Transmissíveis* (2019). Brasília: Ministério da Saúde. Available at: http://bvsms.saude.gov.br/bvs/publicacoes/manual_recomendacoes_controle_tuberculose_brasil_2_ed.pdf (Accessed March 02, 2020).
50. Gustincich S, Manfioletti G, Del Sal G, Schneider C, Carninci P. A fast method for high-quality genomic DNA extraction from whole blood. *Biotechniques* (1991) 11:3.
51. Yan S, Shen H, Lian Q, Jin W, Zhang R, Lin X, et al. Deficiency of the AIM2-ASC Signal Uncovers the STING-Driven Overreactive Response of Type I IFN and Reciprocal Depression of Protective IFN-γ Immunity in Mycobacterial. *J Immunol* (2018) 200:3. doi: 10.4049/jimmunol.1701177
52. Romagnoli A, Petruccioli E, Palucci I, Camassa S, Carata E, Petrone L, et al. Clinical isolates of the modern Mycobacterium tuberculosis lineage 4 evade host defense in human macrophages through eluding IL-1β-induced autophagy. *Cell Death Dis* (2018) 9:624. doi: 10.1038/s41419-018-0640-8
53. Möller M, Kinnear CJ, Orlova M, Kroon EE, Helden PDV, Schurr E, et al. Genetic Resistance to Mycobacterium tuberculosis Infection and Disease. *Front Immunol* (2018) 9:2219. doi: 10.3389/fimmu.2018.02219
54. Simmons JD, Stein CM, Seshadri C, Campo M, Alter G, Fortune S, et al. Immunological mechanisms of human resistance to persistent Mycobacterium tuberculosis infection. *Nat Rev Immunol* (2018) 18:9. doi: 10.1038/s41577-018-0025-3
55. Yamada H, Mizumo S, Horai R, Yoichiro I, Sugawara I, et al. Protective Role of Interleukin-1 in Mycobacterial Infection in IL-1 α/β Double-Knockout Mice. *Lab Invest* (2000) 80(5):759–67. doi: 10.1038/labinvest.3780079
56. Fremond CM, Togbe D, Doz E, Rose S, Vasseur V, Maillet I, et al. IL-1 receptor-mediated signal is an essential component of MyD88-dependent innate response to Mycobacterium tuberculosis infection. *J Immunol* (2007) 179:2. doi: 10.4049/jimmunol.179.2.1178
57. Mishra BB, Rathinam VAK, Martens GW, Martinot AJ, Kornfeld H, Fitzgerald KA, et al. Nitric oxide controls the immunopathology of

tuberculosis by inhibiting NLRP3 inflammasome-dependent processing of IL-1beta. *Nat Immunol* (2013) 14:1. doi: 10.1038/ni.2474

58. Zhang G, Zhou B, Li S, Yue J, Yang H, Wen Y, et al. Allele-specific induction of IL-1β expression by C/EBPβ and PU. 1 contributes to increased tuberculosis susceptibility. *PloS Pathog* (2014) 10:10. doi: 10.1371/journal.ppat.1004426
59. Rathinam VAK, Jiang Z, Waggoner SN, Sharma S, Cole LE, Waggoner L, et al. The AIM2 inflammasome is essential for host-defense against cytosolic bacteria and DNA viruses. *Nat Immunol* (2010) 11:5. doi: 10.1038/ni.1864
60. Yang Y, Zhou X, Kouadir M, Shi F, Ding T, Liu C, et al. The AIM2 inflammasome is involved in macrophage activation during infection with virulent Mycobacterium bovis strain. *J Infect Dis* (2013) 208:11. doi: 10.1093/infdis/jit347
61. Saiga H, Nieuwenhuizen N, Gengenbacher M, Koehler AB, Schuerer S, Moura-Alves P, et al. The Recombinant BCG Δ ureC:: hly vaccine targets the AIM2 inflammasome to induce autophagy and inflammation. *J Infect Dis* (2015) 211:11. doi: 10.1093/infdis/jiu675
62. Zou H, Wu LX, Tan L, Shang FF, Zhou HH, et al. Significance of Single-Nucleotide Variants in Long Intergenic Non-protein Coding RNAs. *Front Cell Dev Biol* (2020) 8:347. doi: 10.3389/fcell.2020.00347
63. Chorev M, Carmel L. The function of introns. *Front Genet* (2012) 3:55. doi: 10.3389/fgene.2012.00055
64. Gallegos JE, Rose AB. The enduring mystery of intron-mediated enhancement. *Plant Sci* (2015) 237:8–15. doi: 10.1016/j.plantsci.2015.04.017
65. Shaul O. How introns enhance gene expression. *Int J Biochem Cell Biol* (2017) 91:145–55. doi: 10.1016/j.biocel.2017.06.016
66. Rigau M, Juan D, Valencia A, Rico D. Intronic CNVs and gene expression variation in human populations. *PloS Genet* (2019) 15:1. doi: 10.1371/journal.pgen.1007902
67. Man SM, Kanneganti TD. Regulation of lysosomal dynamics and autophagy by CTSB/cathepsin B. *Autophagy* (2016) 12:12. doi: 10.1080/15548627.2016.1239679
68. Khor CC, Chapman SJ, Vannberg FO, Dunne A, Murphy C, Ling EY, et al. A Mal functional variant is associated with protection against invasive pneumococcal disease, bacteremia, malaria and tuberculosis. *Nat Genet* (2007) 39:4. doi: 10.1038/ng1976
69. Ramasawmy R, Cunha-Neto E, Fae KC, Borba SCP, Teixeira PC, Ferreira SCP, et al. Heterozygosity for the S180L variant of MAL/TIRAP, a gene expressing an adaptor protein in the Toll-like receptor pathway, is associated with lower risk of developing chronic Chagas cardiomyopathy. *J Infect Dis* (2009) 199:12. doi: 10.1086/599212
70. Pontillo A, Carvalho MS, Kamada AJ, Moura R, Schindler HC, Duarte AJS, et al. Susceptibility to Mycobacterium tuberculosis infection in HIV-positive patients is associated with CARD8 genetic variant. *J Acquir Immune Defic Syndr* (2013) 63:2. doi: 10.1097/QAI.0b013e31828f93bb
71. Roberts RL, Van Rij AM, Phillips LV, McCormick SPA, Merriman TR, Jones GT, et al. Interaction of the inflammasome genes CARD8 and NLRP3 in abdominal aortic aneurysms. *Atherosclerosis* (2011) 218:1. doi: 10.1016/j.atherosclerosis.2011.04.043
72. Araujo FJ, Silva LDO, Mesquita TG, Pinheiro SK, Vital WDS, Chrusciak-Talhari A, et al. Polymorphisms in the TOLLIP Gene Influence Susceptibility to Cutaneous Leishmaniasis Caused by Leishmania guyanensis in the Amazonas State of Brazil. *Plos* (2015) 9:6. doi: 10.1371/journal.pntd.0003875

9

Humoral Immunity vs. *Salmonella*

Akiko Takaya[1], Tomoko Yamamoto[2] and Koji Tokoyoda[3]*

[1] Laboratory of Microbiology and Molecular Genetics, Graduate School of Pharmaceutical Sciences, Chiba University, Chiba, Japan, [2] Department of Infectious Diseases, Medical Mycology Research Center, Chiba University, Chiba, Japan, [3] Deutsches Rheuma-Forschungszentrum Berlin (DRFZ), A Leibniz Institute, Berlin, Germany

***Correspondence:** Koji Tokoyoda tokoyoda@drfz.de*

In primary infection with *Salmonella*, it has been reported—without consideration of *Salmonella*'s functions—that humoral immunity plays no role in the clearance of bacteria. In fact, *Salmonella* targets and suppresses several aspects of humoral immunity, including B cell lymphopoiesis, B cell activation, and IgG production. In particular, the suppression of IgG-secreting plasma cell maintenance allows the persistence of *Salmonella* in tissues. Therefore, the critical role(s) of humoral immunity in the response to *Salmonella* infection, especially at the late phase, should be re-investigated. The suppression of IgG plasma cell memory strongly hinders vaccine development against non-typhoidal *Salmonella* (NTS) because *Salmonella* can also reduce humoral immune memory against other bacteria and viruses, obtained from previous vaccination or infection. We propose a new vaccine against *Salmonella* that would not impair humoral immunity, and which could also be used as a treatment for antibody-dependent autoimmune diseases to deplete pathogenic long-lived plasma cells, by utilizing the *Salmonella*'s own suppression mechanism of humoral immunity.

Keywords: humoral immunity, antibody, plasma cells, IgG, *Salmonella*

INTRODUCTION

The immune system, i.e., innate and adaptive immunity, can overcome many types of bacterial infections. The frontline against infection with bacteria such as *Salmonella* is innate immunity. *Salmonella* infection leads to enteric fever or diarrhea, often resulting in death of humans and animals. The pathogenesis of infection should be separately considered as two dynamics of the immune system vs. *Salmonella*: firstly, bacterial growth within 1 week after infection and, secondly, if protected from death, bacterial clearance after 1 week after infection. Early bacterial growth in mice is controlled by the Nramp gene, expressed in macrophages (1), and is suppressed by a T-cell-independent host response which requires granuloma formation and production of nitric oxide and cytokines such as tumor necrosis factor α (TNFα), interleukin 12 (IL-12) and interferon γ (IFNγ) (2–6). For clearance of the bacteria, innate immunity, namely the complement system and phagocytosis by macrophages, neutrophils and dendritic cells, are the most critical responses against the bacterial pathogens, while IFNγ and antibodies resulting from adaptive immunity also dramatically enhance the innate immune response. It has been thought that adaptive immunity itself dominantly works for secondary infection except for IFNγ from T cells. However, it remains enigmatic how adaptive immunity contributes to the clearance of *Salmonella* in the primary infection. We herein discuss the roles of humoral immunity against *Salmonella* for the clearance of the bacteria.

DEVELOPING A VACCINE AGAINST *SALMONELLA*

Salmonella enterica is a Gram-negative intracellular bacterium with over 2,500 different serovars identified until now. *Salmonella* Typhi (*S.* Typhi) and *S.* Paratyphi cause typhoid fever, a systemic febrile illness only affecting humans. The other numerous NTS serovars such as *S.* Typhimurium and *S.* Enteritidis infect many different hosts and results in diarrheal disease. NTS also causes severe, extra-intestinal, invasive bacteremia, referred to as invasive NTS (iNTS) disease (7). Immunocompromised individuals, including those infected with human immunodeficiency virus (HIV) or malaria, and infants are particularly at risk of acquiring iNTS disease (8–12). iNTS disease is estimated to cause 3.4 million cases of illness and 681,316 deaths annually, with 63.7% of all cases occurring in children under the age of five (8). Thus, infection with NTS is still a serious health concern. Moreover, the emergence of multidrug-resistant strains of *Salmonella* calls into question the future use of antibiotics to treat infection and further emphasizes the need for the development of the safer and more effective vaccines. While a vaccine against NTS is not currently available, it has been reported that naturally acquired antibodies against NTS reduce the risk of iNTS disease (13, 14). In contrast, infection with *S.* Typhi can be prevented by vaccination with attenuated strains, e.g., Ty21a. However, effective vaccines preventing iNTS disease are likely to differ from those protecting against *S.* Typhi infections. Furthermore, it is known that *Salmonella* generates chronic carriers; a chronic carrier state has been identified in 2.2% of patients with reported NTS, lasting from 30 days to 8.3 years (15). Although *Salmonella* invades myeloid cells and escapes phagocytosis, it is unclear why humoral immunity does not contribute to the clearance of *Salmonella* which continuously transfers among short-lived myeloid cells. Overall, the lack of a vaccine and the presence of chronic carriers suggests that NTS suppresses long-lasting humoral immunity, i.e., humoral memory.

THE IMMUNE SYSTEM VS. *SALMONELLA*

Infection of susceptible Nramp^{-} mice with *S.* Typhimurium provides a murine model for typhoid fever which bears many similarities to human *S.* Typhi infection. This *S.* Typhi model is ultimately fatal due to the inability of such mice to restrict bacterial growth *in vivo*. Administration of attenuated strains of *S.* Typhimurium as a model of vaccination resulted in the generation of immune memory against *Salmonella* and protection against death from challenge with a virulent strain of the bacteria (16, 17). The murine model infected with virulent *S.* Typhimurium showed similar pathogenesis on the early growth of bacteria. However, it seems unclear whether the model with attenuated *S.* Typhimurium really mimics the clearance of *Salmonella*, i.e., whether *S.* Typhi and *S.* Typhimurium are excluded from their hosts in a similar way. Many studies have discussed typhoidal disease using NTS strains based on the assumption that *S.* Typhi and *S.* Typhimurium utilize the same invasion system in the hosts. However, it is impossible to compare the mechanism on the clearance of *Salmonella in vivo*, because *S.* Typhi is not infectious in mice. If *S.* Typhi and *S.* Typhimurium are excluded by distinct bacterial clearances, the difference may affect the ability to generate vaccines against *S.* Typhi and *S.* Typhimurium.

Innate cells can have several roles to play during the early stage of an infection, including controlling bacterial replication and producing cytokines and chemokines that activate and recruit inflammatory cells to the site of infection. Macrophages, neutrophils and dendritic cells increase in number early after *Salmonella* infection and produce cytokines that are important for host survival, such as TNFα. All three phagocytic cell types also harbor bacteria during infection. IFNγ from natural killer cells at the very early infection phase and from T cells at the late infection phase can activate macrophages and promote phagocytosis (18). In addition to innate cells, the clearance of bacteria from the tissues also requires functional CD4 T cells (19), resulting in long-lasting specific immunity to re-challenge infection (20). Susceptible mice can resolve a primary infection with attenuated *Salmonella* strains which requires a functioning immune system that can develop a T-bet-dependent Th1 cell response and IFNγ production to activate infected macrophages (19, 21). Similarly, mice lacking IL-12, IFNγ, reactive oxygen species, or inducible nitric oxide, all have deficiencies in primary clearance of *Salmonella* (22, 23). In contrast, mice lacking B cells resolve primary infection with attenuated bacterial strains with similar kinetics to wildtype mice (24, 25), indicating that B-cell responses do not participate in the primary clearance of the bacteria. CD8 T cells are generally not thought to contribute to the primary clearance of attenuated *Salmonella*, based on studies using β2-microglobulin-deficient mice that lack class I-restricted CD8 T cells (19, 26). However, recent experiments in mice lacking classical MHC class Ia genes, perforin, or granzyme, show that CD8 T cells make a modest contribution to *Salmonella* clearance during the later stages of the primary response (27). Overall, these data suggest a primary role for CD4 Th1 cells, a modest role for CD8 T cells and no role for B cells in primary immunity to *Salmonella*. However, the roles of adaptive immunity were considered from the viewpoint of how the lymphocytes respond to the infection, without any consideration of how *Salmonella* may purposefully subvert the immune response for its own advantage.

HUMORAL IMMUNITY VS. *SALMONELLA*

Immunization and infection with *Salmonella* greatly affects hematopoiesis in a TNFα- and CXCL12-dependent manner (28, 29). *Salmonella* is known to activate myelopoiesis and suppress B lymphopoiesis (30). Interestingly, the disruption of B lymphopoiesis has been also reported on *Plasmodium* infection in mice (31), suggesting the similar mechanism to *Salmonella*. This dramatic change in cellular commitment/differentiation is very reasonable, because in the early phase of infection, the immune system requires as many innate cells as possible to fight against the infection. Expanded myeloid cells are able to kill a lot of *Salmonella*, but some become the host cells for *Salmonella* without phagocytosis. Furthermore, the provision of B cells to the periphery is impaired due to death of B cell precursors in the bone marrow (BM), resulting in an indirect advantage to *Salmonella* for their long-term persistence.

In general, antibodies can protect against bacteria mainly by facilitating the uptake of the pathogen by phagocytic cells, which then destroy the ingested bacteria. Antibodies do this in two ways: one is to coat the pathogen to be recognized by Fc receptors on phagocytic cells, which is called opsonization. Alternatively, antibodies binding to the surface of a pathogen can activate the proteins of the complement system. Complement activation results in opsonization of the pathogen by binding complement receptors on phagocytes. Other complement components recruit phagocytic cells to the site of infection, and the terminal components of complement can lyse certain microorganisms directly by forming pores in their membranes. Most intracellular pathogens spread by moving from cell to cell through the extracellular fluids. The extracellular spaces are protected by humoral immunity. Antibodies produced by plasma cells cause the destruction of extracellular microorganisms and therefore prevent the spread of intracellular infections. Phagocytes, *Salmonella*'s hosts, are short-lived and survive for 0.75 days (neutrophils, lifespan) (32), 18–20 h (phagocytic monocytes, half-life) (33), 1.5–2.9 days (dendritic cells, half-life) (34), and <7 days (peripheral macrophages, lifespan) (35). Therefore, in order to survive, *Salmonella* has to transfer into new host cells every 1–7 days passing through extracellular fluids containing antibodies. It is unknown how and why *Salmonella* can escape from antibodies in extracellular spaces when transferring into new host cells. In secondary immune responses, anti-*Salmonella* IgG are critical for the enhancement of phagocytosis. However, anti-*Salmonella* IgG in the late phase of the primary immune response does not contribute to the clearance of the bacteria (23). This raises the following questions: what is the difference of anti-*Salmonella* antibodies in the primary and secondary immune responses? Is the affinity and/or amount of antibodies important? What other functions of *Salmonella* have to be also considered in the subversion of the immune response?

The activation of B cells and their differentiation into long-lived plasma cells is triggered by antigen and usually requires CD4 T cell help, presenting antigen on MHC class II. Bayer-Santos and his colleagues showed that a *Salmonella* protein, SteD depletes surface MHC class II and inhibits T cell activation (36). SteD localized in the Golgi network and vesicles containing the E3 ubiquitin ligase MARCH8 and MHC class II causing MARCH8-dependent ubiquitination and depletion of surface MHC class II and B7-2. A subset of effector CD4 T cells, known as T follicular helper cells, also control isotype switching and have a role in initiating somatic hypermutation of antibody variable V-region genes for affinity maturation mainly in germinal centers (GCs) of the spleen. Cunningham et al. indicated that GC formation is delayed when infected with *Salmonella* (37). However, GC-lacking CD40L (CD154)-deficient mice can normally induce the clearance of *Salmonella* in tissues. The formation of GCs and the affinity of antibodies do not affect the clearance of the bacteria. Di Niro et al. showed that *Salmonella* induces random activation, generating only a small fraction (0.5–2%) of *Salmonella*-specific plasma cells, and somatic hypermutation occurred efficiently at extrafollicular sites (38). Although it should be investigated how the abnormal induction consequently affects the immune responses, it is very intriguing why *Salmonella* does not allow immune cells to utilize the standard immune activation/maturation pathways. Following GC formation, B cells can differentiate into either short-lived plasma cells, memory B cells, or long-lived plasma cells. Memory B cells persist and are important for secondary immune responses against the same pathogen. Short-lived plasma cells temporally provide IgG, but do not survive for long periods of time. In contrast, long-lived plasma cells, or their precursors, migrate into the BM and persist in CXCL12-expressing stromal cells (39, 40). In general, IgG is the most critical antibody isotype for the clearance of bacteria and greatly contributes to the clearance of bacteria at least in the late phase of infection. In contrast, in the clearance of *Salmonella*, no role of B cells which has a potential to differentiate into IgG-secreting plasma cells has been reported. The distinction led to a possibility of *Salmonella*-specific suppression of humoral immunity, in particular IgG production as described below.

SALMONELLA ATTACKS THE MAIN SOURCE OF IGG

McSorley and Jenkins showed (i) that *Salmonella* can similarly survive in the tissues of naive wild-type and B cell-deficient mice until day 35 after infection, suggesting that antibodies and B cells are not necessary for the clearance of *Salmonella*, and (ii) that injection of heat-killed *Salmonella* induces a provision of anti-*Salmonella* IgG from day 20, although data of anti-*Salmonella* IgG titers in mice infected with live *Salmonella* are lacking (24). However, if *Salmonella* actively suppresses B cell functions, the necessity of B cells for fighting the infection therefore fails to be evaluated by these studies. Very recently, we have shown that *Salmonella* inhibits the persistence of IgG-secreting plasma cells in the BM of mice, which are the main source of serum IgG, by secreting a *Salmonella* protein known as SiiE (41) (**Figure 1**). Mice infected with a SiiE-deficient strain markedly enhanced the provision of anti-*Salmonella* IgG and promoted the clearance of *Salmonella*, even in the primary infection. Given these results, the roles of antibodies and B/plasma cells therefore have to be re-evaluated.

SiiE is known as an adhesin, binding to carbohydrates in a lectin-like manner, thereby promoting attachment of *Salmonella* to polarized epithelial cells and enabling colonization (42, 43). SiiE is secreted by *Salmonella* and remains surface-associated during bacterial invasion (44). SiiE mediates the first direct contact to the host cell through binding to glycostructures containing N-acetyl-glucosamine and/or α2, 3-linked sialic acid (45). Recently, Li et al. suggested that MUC1, the transmembrane mucin that is highly expressed at mucosal surfaces including the stomach and the intestinal tract, is a receptor for SiiE that enables apical invasion into enterocytes (46).

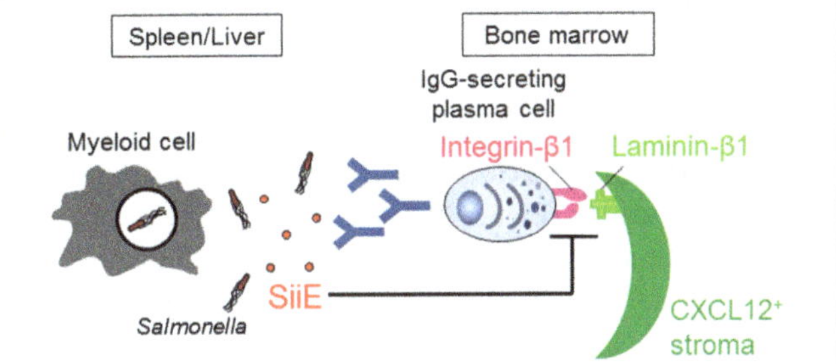

FIGURE 1 | *Salmonella* SiiE suppresses the retention of IgG-secreting plasma cells in BM survival niches by competing with laminin β1. SiiE secreted by *Salmonella* competes with laminin β1 to interact with integrin β1. The competition induces the detachment and then deletion of IgG-secreting plasma cells from laminin $\beta1^{+}CXCL12^{+}$ survival niches of the BM.

SiiE is a large protein with a molecular weight of 595 kDa. It has 53 highly similar repeats of bacterial immunoglobulin (BIg) domains that determine the length and only short protein moieties of distinct structure at the very N- and C-terminal parts (43). The amino acid sequence from 129 to 168 in the short N-terminal moiety has high homology to murine laminin β1. The 236 amino acid residues in the short N-terminal moiety consist of eight heptad repeats with a coiled-coil structure that are flanked by regions with a predominantly β-sheet structure (43). The integrity of the coiled-coil structure is required for the proper retention of SiiE and thereby affects invasion of polarized cells, while the β-sheet domains appear to be essential for the control of release of SiiE. The central part of the coiled-coil structure, including amino acids 129–168, plays an especially essential role in the retention of SiiE (43). The homologous region in the C-terminal region of laminin β1 also has a coiled-coil structure, which is involved in the assembly of a laminin molecule (47). The C-terminal region also modulates the integrin binding affinities of laminins (48). We showed that SiiE can bind to integrin β1, a laminin receptor, on BM IgG-secreting plasma cells and competes with their adhesion to laminin (41). Only the SiiE-derived peptide which has high homology to murine laminin β1 was able to reduce the number of BM IgG-secreting plasma cells. Moreover, the attenuated SiiE-deficient *Salmonella* enhanced both the production of high titers of protective IgG against *Salmonella* and the memory response, suggesting that it may be a novel and efficient vaccine against *Salmonella*. Histological analyses of the BM revealed that IgG- but not IgM-secreting plasma cells bind to laminin β1. Thus, laminin $\beta1^{+}CXCL12^{+}$ stromal cells are an integral part of the survival niche for IgG-secreting plasma cells in the BM, a lesson learnt from *Salmonella*.

ROLES OF HUMORAL IMMUNITY AGAINST *SALMONELLA* AND NEW GENERATION OF VACCINES

Salmonella SiiE reduces the number of BM IgG-secreting plasma cells (41). This reduction may have led to the underestimation of the roles of B cells, especially antibodies, in the late phase of the primary infection with *Salmonella*. If IgG production is not suppressed by *Salmonella* SiiE, humoral immunity, in particular IgG, is required for the clearance of *Salmonella* in the late phase of the primary infection (41). Infection with SiiE-deficient strain into B cell-deficient and wildtype mice should be examined in order to determine the precise role of humoral immunity in the late phase of primary infection with *Salmonella*. Since vaccines against NTS are not yet available, SiiE-deficient *Salmonella* may be the first efficient vaccine against NTS. It still remains unclear why vaccines against *S.* Typhi, but not NTS are available. Intriguingly, the *siiE* gene in *S.* Typhi has been reported as two distinct ORFs, suggesting that it is a pseudogene (49). The presence of a functional SiiE gene may be a reason for the differences in availability of vaccines against the two strains of *Salmonella*. Furthermore, SiiE impairs the persistence of all IgG-secreting plasma cells in an antigen-specific independent manner. This non-specific depletion of IgG-secreting plasma cells may result in the loss of long-lived plasma cells secreting IgG against many kinds of bacteria and viruses generated by previous vaccination or infection. Therefore, generating vaccines against NTS may be essential to avoid such a loss of vital of humoral memory. Other pathogens may also have an ability to suppress humoral immunity. Recent studies indicated that respiratory syncytial virus (RSV) infection fails to induce in IgA^{+} memory B cells (50) and that measles causes elimination of 11–73% of the antibody repertoire and depletion of previously expanded B memory clones after infection (51, 52). However, cellular and molecular mechanisms on their suppression are still unknown and should be investigated, then comparing with the case of *Salmonella*.

TREATMENT OF ANTIBODY-MEDIATED DISEASES USING A *SALMONELLA*-DERIVED PEPTIDE

The SiiE peptide homologous to laminin β1 significantly reduced the number of anti-DNA IgG-secreting plasma cells in the BM in the NZB/W murine model of lupus nephritis (41). This property could therefore be further exploited for the treatment of autoimmune diseases. Autoimmune diseases with a substantial contribution of pathogenic IgG autoantibodies, like systemic lupus erythematosus, can be refractory to conventional treatment e.g., immunosuppressive drugs and anti-CD20 antibodies, because BM plasma cells secreting these autoantibodies are protected in their BM niches (53–55). Multiple myeloma is caused by redundant titers of antibodies generated from plasma cell myeloma in the BM. It has already been reported that myeloma cell lines preferentially contact laminin *in vitro* (56, 57), suggesting that targeting of adhesion molecules including laminin should be considered as novel therapy (58). The depletion of BM plasma cell myeloma by SiiE may directly ameliorate disease. SiiE peptide and the related products may contribute to a recovery for these antibody-mediated diseases without relapse.

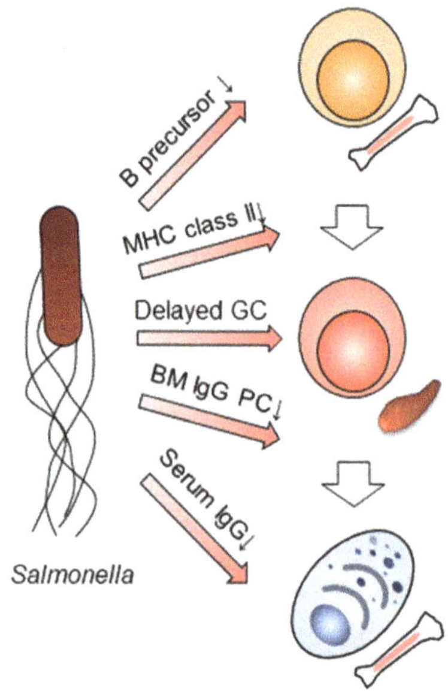

FIGURE 2 | Multilayer suppression of humoral immunity by *Salmonella* infection. *Salmonella* impairs humoral immunity at multiple stages; B cell lymphopoiesis, the expression of MHC class II in myeloid cells, germinal center (GC) formation, the persistence of BM IgG-secreting plasma cells (PC) and IgG titers in serum.

CONCLUSIONS AND PERSPECTIVES

Humoral immunity in the late phase of primary infection with *Salmonella* had been thought not to participate in the clearance of the bacteria. However, when taking into consideration *Salmonella*'s functions, it is clear that several aspects of humoral immunity, in particular the suppression of IgG production, does indeed contribute to the clearance of bacteria in the late phase of the primary infection (**Figure 2**). Using SiiE-deficient *Salmonella*, the collaboration between humoral immunity and other immune systems should be also re-evaluated. The function of other immune cells may be overestimated or underestimated due to the suppression of humoral immunity. Furthermore, the previous candidates of vaccines against NTS should be re-investigated by adding a mutation of SiiE. The combined mutations of *Salmonella* factors which interfere with immune systems may result in the development of the best vaccines against NTS. As infection with NTS may delete all IgG plasma cell memory gained by vaccination obtained from infancy, we therefore also alert to this danger and propose an obligatory use of vaccination against NTS in infancy.

AUTHOR CONTRIBUTIONS

AT and KT wrote the paper. TY supervised the work.

ACKNOWLEDGMENTS

We thank Mairi A. McGrath for your editing and scientific comments.

REFERENCES

1. Vidal SM, Malo D, Vogan K, Skamene E, Gros, P. Natural resistance to infection with intracellular parasites: isolation of a candidate for Bcg. *Cell.* (1993) 73:469–85. doi: 10.1016/0092-8674(93)90135-D
2. Umezawa K, Akaike T, Fujii S, Suga M, Setoguchi K, Ozawa A, et al. Induction of nitric oxide synthesis and xanthine oxidase and their roles in the antimicrobial mechanism against *Salmonella typhimurium* infection in mice. *Infect Immun.* (1997) 65:2932–40.
3. Kagaya K, Watanabe K, Fukazawa, Y. Capacity of recombinant gamma interferon to activate macrophages for *Salmonella*-killing activity. *Infect Immun.* (1989) 57:609–15.
4. Tite JP, Dougan G, Chatfield, SN. The involvement of tumor necrosis factor in immunity to *Salmonella* infection. *J Immunol.* (1991) 147:3161–4.
5. Kincy-Cain T, Clements JD, Bost KL. Endogenous and exogenous interleukin-12 augment the protective immune response in mice orally challenged with *Salmonella dublin. Infect Immun.* (1996) 64:1437–40.
6. Muotiala A, Makela PH. The role of IFN-γ in murine *Salmonella typhimurium* infection. *Microb Pathog.* (1990) 8:135–41. doi: 10.1016/0882-4010(90)90077-4
7. Feasey NA, Dougan G, Kingsley RA, Heyderman RS, Gordon MA. Invasive non-typhoidal salmonella disease: an emerging and neglected tropical disease in Africa. *Lancet.* (2012) 379:2489–99. doi: 10.1016/S0140-6736(11)61752-2
8. Ao TT, Feasey NA, Gordon MA, Keddy KH, Angulo FJ, Crump JA. Global burden of invasive nontyphoidal *Salmonella* disease, 2010. *Emerg Infect Dis.* (2015) 21:941–9. doi: 10.3201/eid2106.140999
9. Majowicz SE, Musto J, Scallan E, Angulo FJ, Kirk M, O'Brien SJ, et al. The global burden of nontyphoidal *Salmonella* gastroenteritis. *Clin Infect Dis.* (2010) 50:882–9. doi: 10.1086/650733
10. Crump JA, Heyderman RS. A perspective on invasive *Salmonella* disease in Africa. *Clin Infect Dis.* (2015) 61:S235–40. doi: 10.1093/cid/civ709
11. Uche IV, MacLennan CA, Saul A. A systematic review of the incidence, risk factors and case fatality rates of invasive nontyphoidal *Salmonella* (iNTS) disease in Africa (1966 to 2014). *PLoS Negl Trop Dis.* (2017) 11:e0005118. doi: 10.1371/journal.pntd.0005118
12. Park SE, Pak GD, Aaby P, Adu-Sarkodie Y, Ali M, Aseffa A, et al. The relationship between invasive nontyphoidal *Salmonella* disease, other bacterial bloodstream infections, and malaria in Sub-Saharan Africa. *Clin Infect Dis.* (2016) 62(Suppl. 1):S23–31. doi: 10.1093/cid/civ893
13. Gordon MA. Invasive nontyphoidal *Salmonella* disease: epidemiology, pathogenesis and diagnosis. *Curr Opin Infect Dis.* (2011) 24:484–9. doi: 10.1097/QCO.0b013e32834a9980
14. MacLennan CA, Gondwe EN, Msefula CL, Kingsley RA, Thomson NR, White SA, et al. The neglected role of antibody in protection against bacteremia caused by nontyphoidal strains of *Salmonella* in African children. *J Clin Invest.* (2008) 118:1553–62. doi: 10.1172/JCI33998
15. Marzel A, Desai PT, Goren A, Schorr YI, Nissan I, Porwollik S, et al. Persistent infections by nontyphoidal *Salmonella* in humans: epidemiology and genetics. *Clin Infect Dis.* (2016) 62:879–86. doi: 10.1093/cid/civ1221
16. Hoiseth SK, Stocker BA. Aromatic-dependent *Salmonella typhimurium* are non-virulent and effective as live vaccines. *Nature.* (1981) 291:238–9. doi: 10.1038/291238a0
17. Tennant SM, Levine MM. Live attenuated vaccines for invasive *Salmonella* infections. *Vaccine.* (2015) 33(Suppl. 3):C36–41. doi: 10.1016/j.vaccine.2015.04.029
18. Ingram JP, Brodsky IE, Balachandran, S. Interferon-γ in *Salmonella* pathogenesis: new tricks for an old dog. *Cytokine.* (2017) 98:27–32. doi: 10.1016/j.cyto.2016.10.009
19. Hess J, Ladel C, Miko D, Kaufmann SH. *Salmonella typhimurium* aroA^{-} infection in gene-targeted immunodeficient mice: major role of CD4^{+} TCR-αβcells and IFN-γin bacterial clearance independent of intracellular location. *J Immunol.* (1996) 156:3321–6.

20. Mastroeni P, Harrison JA, Hormaeche CE. Natural resistance and acquired immunity to *Salmonella*. *Fundam Clin Immunol.* (1994) 2:83–95.
21. Ravindran R, Foley J, Stoklasek T, Glimcher LH, McSorley SJ. Expression of T-bet by CD4 T cells is essential for resistance to *Salmonella* infection. *J Immunol.* (2005) 175:4603–10. doi: 10.4049/jimmunol.175.7.4603
22. Mastroeni P, Vazquez-Torres A, Fang FC, Xu Y, Khan S, Hormaeche CE, et al. Antimicrobial actions of the NADPH phagocyte oxidase and inducible nitric oxide synthase in experimental salmonellosis. II. Effects on microbial proliferation and host survival *in vivo*. *J Exp Med.* (2000) 192:237–48. doi: 10.1084/jem.192.2.237
23. Lehmann J, Bellmann S, Werner C, Schroder R, Schutze N, Alber G. IL-12p40-dependent agonistic effects on the development of protective innate and adaptive immunity against *Salmonella enteritidis*. *J Immunol.* (2001) 167:5304–15. doi: 10.4049/jimmunol.167.9.5304
24. McSorley SJ, Jenkins MK. Antibody is required for protection against virulent but not attenuated *Salmonella enterica* serovar Typhimurium. *Infect Immun.* (2000) 68:3344–8. doi: 10.1128/IAI.68.6.3344-3348.2000
25. Mastroeni P, Simmons C, Fowler R, Hormaeche CE, Dougan, G. *Igh-6*$^{-/-}$ (B-cell-deficient) mice fail to mount solid acquired resistance to oral challenge with virulent *Salmonella enterica* serovar Typhimurium and show impaired Th1 T-cell responses to *Salmonella* antigens. *Infect Immun.* (2000) 68:46–53. doi: 10.1128/IAI.68.1.46-53.2000
26. Lo WF, Ong H, Metcalf ES, Soloski MJ. T cell responses to Gram-negative intracellular bacterial pathogens: a role for CD8$^+$ T cells in immunity to *Salmonella* infection and the involvement of MHC class Ib molecules. *J Immunol.* (1999) 162:5398–406.
27. Lee SJ, Dunmire S, McSorley SJ. MHC class-I-restricted CD8 T cells play a protective role during primary *Salmonella* infection. *Immunol Lett.* (2012) 148:138–43. doi: 10.1016/j.imlet.2012.10.009
28. Ueda Y, Yang K, Foster SJ, Kondo M, Kelsoe G. Inflammation controls B lymphopoiesis by regulating chemokine CXCL12 expression. *J Exp Med.* (2004) 199:47–58. doi: 10.1084/jem.20031104
29. Ulich TR, del Castillo J, Ni RX, Bikhazi N. Hematologic interactions of endotoxin, tumor necrosis factor alpha (TNF alpha), interleukin 1, and adrenal hormones and the hematologic effects of TNF alpha in Corynebacterium parvum-primed rats. *J Leukoc Biol.* (1989) 45:546–57. doi: 10.1002/jlb.45.6.546
30. Slocombe T, Brown S, Miles K, Gray M, Barr TA, Gray D. Plasma cell homeostasis: the effects of chronic antigen stimulation and inflammation. *J Immunol.* (2013) 191:3128–38. doi: 10.4049/jimmunol.1301163
31. Bockstal V, Geurts N, Magez S. Acute disruption of bone marrow B lymphopoiesis and apoptosis of transitional and marginal zone B cells in the spleen following a blood-stage *Plasmodium chabaudi* infection in mice. *J Parasitol Res.* (2011) 2011:534697. doi: 10.1155/2011/534697
32. Pillay J, den Braber I, Vrisekoop N, Kwast LM, de Boer RJ, Borghans JA, et al. *In vivo* labeling with 2H2O reveals a human neutrophil lifespan of 5.4 days. *Blood.* (2010) 116:625–7. doi: 10.1182/blood-2010-01-259028
33. Italiani P, Boraschi D. From monocytes to M1/M2 macrophages: phenotypical vs. functional differentiation. *Front Immunol.* (2014) 5:514. doi: 10.3389/fimmu.2014.00514
34. Kamath AT, Henri S, Battye F, Tough DF, Shortman K. Developmental kinetics and lifespan of dendritic cells in mouse lymphoid organs. *Blood.* (2002) 100:1734–41. doi: 10.1182/blood.V100.5.1734.h81702001734_1734_1741
35. van Furth R. Origin and turnover of monocytes and macrophages. *Curr Top Pathol.* (1989) 79:125–50. doi: 10.1007/978-3-642-73855-5_6
36. Bayer-Santos E, Durkin CH, Rigano LA, Kupz A, Alix E, Cerny O, et al. The *Salmonella* effector SteD mediates MARCH8-dependent ubiquitination of MHC II molecules and inhibits T cell activation. *Cell Host Microbe.* (2016) 20:584–95. doi: 10.1016/j.chom.2016.10.007
37. Cunningham AF, Gaspal F, Serre K, Mohr E, Henderson IR, Scott-Tucker A, et al. *Salmonella* induces a switched antibody response without germinal centers that impedes the extracellular spread of infection. *J Immunol.* (2007) 178:6200–7. doi: 10.4049/jimmunol.178.10.6200
38. Di Niro R, Lee SJ, Vander Heiden JA, Elsner RA, Trivedi N, Bannock JM, et al. *Salmonella* infection drives promiscuous B cell activation followed by extrafollicular affinity maturation. *Immunity.* (2015) 43:120–31. doi: 10.1016/j.immuni.2015.06.013
39. Moser K, Tokoyoda K, Radbruch A, MacLennan I, Manz RA. Stromal niches, plasma cell differentiation and survival. *Curr Opin Immunol.* (2006) 18:265–70. doi: 10.1016/j.coi.2006.03.004
40. Tokoyoda K, Egawa T, Sugiyama T, Choi BI, Nagasawa, T. Cellular niches controlling B lymphocyte behavior within bone marrow during development. *Immunity.* (2004) 20:707–18. doi: 10.1016/j.immuni.2004.05.001
41. Manne C, Takaya A, Yamasaki Y, Mursell M, Hojyo S, Wu TY, et al. *Salmonella* SiiE prevents an efficient humoral immune memory by interfering with IgG$^+$ plasma cell persistence in the bone marrow. *Proc Natl Acad Sci USA.* (2019) 116:7425–30. doi: 10.1073/pnas.1818242116
42. Gerlach RG, Claudio N, Rohde M, Jackel D, Wagner C, Hensel M. Cooperation of *Salmonella* pathogenicity islands 1 and 4 is required to breach epithelial barriers. *Cell Microbiol.* (2008) 10:2364–76. doi: 10.1111/j.1462-5822.2008.01218.x
43. Wagner C, Polke M, Gerlach RG, Linke D, Stierhof YD, Schwarz H, et al. Functional dissection of SiiE, a giant non-fimbrial adhesin of *Salmonella enterica*. *Cell Microbiol.* (2011) 13:1286–301. doi: 10.1111/j.1462-5822.2011.01621.x
44. Morgan E, Bowen AJ, Carnell SC, Wallis TS, Stevens MP. SiiE is secreted by the *Salmonella enterica* Serovar Typhimurium Pathogenicity Island 4-encoded secretion system and contributes to intestinal colonization in cattle. *Infect Immun.* (2007) 75:1524–33. doi: 10.1128/IAI.01438-06
45. Wagner C, Barlag B, Gerlach RG, Deiwick J, Hensel M. The *Salmonella enterica* giant adhesin SiiE binds to polarized epithelial cells in a lectin-like manner. *Cell Microbiol.* (2014) 16:962–75. doi: 10.1111/cmi.12253
46. Li X, Bleumink-Pluym NMC, Luijkx Y, Wubbolts RW, van Putten JPM, Strijbis K. MUC1 is a receptor for the *Salmonella* SiiE adhesin that enables apical invasion into enterocytes. *PLoS Pathog.* (2019) 15:e1007566. doi: 10.1371/journal.ppat.1007566
47. Hohenester E. Structural biology of laminins. *Essays Biochem.* (2019) 63:285–95. doi: 10.1042/EBC20180075
48. Taniguchi Y, Ido H, Sanzen N, Hayashi M, Sato-Nishiuchi R, Futaki S, et al. The C-terminal region of laminin βchains modulates the integrin binding affinities of laminins. *J Biol Chem.* (2009) 284:7820–31. doi: 10.1074/jbc.M809332200
49. Main-Hester KL, Colpitts KM, Thomas GA, Fang FC, Libby SJ. Coordinate regulation of *Salmonella* pathogenicity island 1 (SPI1) and SPI4 in Salmonella enterica serovar Typhimurium. *Infect Immun.* (2008) 76:1024–35. doi: 10.1128/IAI.01224-07
50. Habibi MS, Jozwik A, Makris S, Dunning J, Paras A, DeVincenzo JP, et al. Impaired antibody-mediated protection and defective IgA B-cell memory in experimental infection of adults with respiratory syncytial virus. *Am J Respir Crit Care Med.* (2015) 191:1040–9. doi: 10.1164/rccm.201412-2256OC
51. Mina MJ, Kula T, Leng Y, Li M, de Vries RD, Knip M, et al. Measles virus infection diminishes preexisting antibodies that offer protection from other pathogens. *Science.* (2019) 366:599–606. doi: 10.1126/science.aay6485
52. Petrova VN, Sawatsky B, Han AX, Laksono BM, Walz L, Parker E, et al. Incomplete genetic reconstitution of B cell pools contributes to prolonged immunosuppression after measles. *Sci Immunol.* (2019) 4:aay6125. doi: 10.1126/sciimmunol.aay6125
53. Cheng Q, Mumtaz IM, Khodadadi L, Radbruch A, Hoyer BF, Hiepe F. Autoantibodies from long-lived 'memory' plasma cells of NZB/W mice drive immune complex nephritis. *Ann Rheum Dis.* (2013) 72:2011–7. doi: 10.1136/annrheumdis-2013-203455
54. Hoyer BF, Moser K, Hauser AE, Peddinghaus A, Voigt C, Eilat D, et al. Short-lived plasmablasts and long-lived plasma cells contribute to chronic humoral autoimmunity in NZB/W mice. *J Exp Med.* (2004) 199:1577–84. doi: 10.1084/jem.20040168
55. Hiepe F, Dorner T, Hauser AE, Hoyer BF, Mei H, Radbruch A. Long-lived autoreactive plasma cells drive persistent autoimmune inflammation. *Nat Rev Rheumatol.* (2011) 7:170–8. doi: 10.1038/nrrheum.2011.1
56. Kibler C, Schermutzki F, Waller HD, Timpl R, Muller CA, Klein G. Adhesive interactions of human multiple myeloma cell lines with different extracellular matrix molecules. *Cell Adhes Commun.* (1998) 5:307–23. doi: 10.3109/15419069809040300
57. Vande Broek I, Vanderkerken K, De Greef C, Asosingh K, Straetmans N, Van Camp B, et al. Laminin-1-induced migration of multiple myeloma cells involves the high-affinity 67 kD laminin receptor. *Br J Cancer.* (2001) 85:1387–95. doi: 10.1054/bjoc.2001.2078

10

Polymorphism in the Promoter Region of the *IL18* Gene and the Association with Severity on Paracoccidioidomycosis

Paula Keiko Sato [1,2*†], *Felipe Delatorre Busser* [1,2†], *Flávia Mendes da Cunha Carvalho* [1,3‡], *Alexandra Gomes dos Santos* [1,3], *Aya Sadahiro* [4], *Constancia Lima Diogo* [1,2], *Adriana Satie Gonçalves Kono* [5], *Maria Luiza Moretti* [6], *Olinda do Carmo Luiz* [7] and *Maria Aparecida Shikanai-Yasuda* [1,2,3*]

[1] *Laboratory of Medical Investigation in Immunology (LIM48), Faculdade de Medicina, Hospital das Clínicas, University of São Paulo, São Paulo, Brazil,* [2] *Institute of Tropical Medicine, Faculdade de Medicina, University of São Paulo, São Paulo, Brazil,* [3] *Department of Infectious and Parasitic Diseases, Faculdade de Medicina, University of São Paulo, São Paulo, Brazil,* [4] *Department of Parasitology, Instituto de Ciências Biológicas, Federal University of Amazonas, Manaus, Brazil,* [5] *Infectious Diseases Division, Hospital das Clínicas, University of São Paulo, São Paulo, Brazil,* [6] *Faculdade de Ciências Médicas, Hospital das Clínicas, State University of Campinas, Campinas, Brazil,* [7] *Department of Preventive Medicine, Faculdade de Medicina, University of São Paulo, São Paulo, Brazil*

Correspondence:
Paula Keiko Sato
paula.s@hc.fm.usp.br
Maria Aparecida Shikanai-Yasuda
masyasuda@yahoo.com.br

† *These authors have contributed equally to this work*

‡Present address:
Flávia Mendes da Cunha Carvalho, Structural Biology Unit, Laboratory of Medical Investigation in Immunopathology of Schistosomiasis and Other Parasitoses (LIM06), Faculdade de Medicina, Hospital das Clínicas, University of São Paulo, São Paulo, Brazil

Paracoccidioidomycosis (PCM) is an important endemic, systemic disease in Latin America caused by *Paracoccidioides* spp. This mycosis has been associated with high morbidity and sequels, and its clinical manifestations depend on the virulence of the infecting strain, the degree and type of immune response, infected tissues, and intrinsic characteristics of the host. The T helper(Th)1 and Th17/Th22 cells are related to resistance and control of infection, and a Th2/Th9 response is associated with disease susceptibility. In this study, we focused on interleukin(IL)-12p35 (*IL12A*), IL-18 (*IL18*), and IFN-γ receptor 1 (*IFNGR1*) genetic polymorphisms because their respective roles have been described in human PCM. Real-time PCR was employed to analyze *IL12A* -504 G/T (rs2243115), *IL18* -607 C/A (rs1946518), and *IFNGR1* -611 A/G (rs1327474) single nucleotide polymorphisms (SNP). One hundred forty-nine patients with the acute form (AF), multifocal chronic (MC), or unifocal chronic (UC) forms of PCM and 110 non-PCM individuals as a control group were included. In the unconditional logistic regression analysis adjusted by ethnicity and sex, we observed a high risk of the *IL18* -607 *A*-allele for both AF [$p = 0.015$; OR = 3.10 (95% CI: 1.24–7.77)] and MC groups [$p = 0.023$; OR = 2.61 (95% CI: 1.14–5.96)] when compared with UC. The *IL18* -607 *A*-allele associated risk for the AF and MC groups as well as the protective role of the *C*-allele in UC are possibly linked to higher levels of IL-18 at different periods of the course of the disease. Therefore, a novel role of *IL18* -607 C/A SNP is shown in the present study, highlighting its importance in the outcome of PCM.

Keywords: paracoccidioidomycosis, *Paracoccidioides* spp., single nucleotide polymophism, IL18, IL12A, IFNGR1, clinical forms of paracoccidioidomycosis

INTRODUCTION

Paracoccidioidomycosis (PCM) is one of the main endemic, systemic mycoses in Latin America, and it is caused by the thermally dimorphic fungi of the *Paracoccidioides brasiliensis* (*P. brasiliensis*) complex (*Paracoccidioides* spp.) and *Paracoccidioides lutzii*. PCM is associated with high morbidity and sequels; however, because it is not a compulsorily notified disease in Brazil, the actual data are based on reports of epidemiological surveys, case series, hospitalization, and mortality data (1). It is endemic in the southeast, central west, and south regions of Brazil and estimated at 0.71–2.70/100,000 inhabitants/year (2). Epidemic areas have been reported in the western Brazilian areas with a mean incidence of 9.4/100,000 and peaks of 37–39/100,000 inhabitants (3).

The inhalation of conidia of *Paracoccidioides* spp. can result in infection without symptoms, acute or chronic disease, or in sequelae. The clinical manifestations depend on the virulence of the infecting strain, the degree and type of immune response, infected tissues, and intrinsic characteristics of the host (4).

Some components of the innate immunity, such as neutrophils, dendritic cells, toll-like receptors, dectin-1, myeloid differentiation primary response 88 (MyD88), and NOD-like receptor P3 (NLRP3) inflammasome, have been evaluated in both experimental and human PCM (5–10). However, it is the adaptive response to *P. brasiliensis* that has been extensively studied with a well-established murine model and characterization of clinical forms of PCM by T helper (Th) responses and antibodies (11).

The acute form of PCM shows a mixed Th2/Th9 response: increased levels of IL-4, IL-5, IL-9, IL-10, TGF-β, and IL-27; low production of IFN-γ and TNF-α; and high levels of specific IgG4 and IgE antibodies. On the other hand, the chronic form presents a Th17/Th22 profile with high production of IL-17 and IL-22 and also secreting Th1-type cytokines, such as IFN-γ, TNF-α, and IL-2 as well as variable levels of IL-10 and IL-4 and increased levels of specific IgG1 antibodies (12, 13). Therefore, the Th2/Th9 responses can be associated with susceptibility to PCM, and the presence of Th1 and Th17/Th22 cells can contribute to more mild clinical manifestations with the axis IFN-γ/IL-12 directly associated with protection and control of the infection (11–16).

The high-affinity binding of IL-12 to its receptor results in the differentiation of naïve CD4 T cells into Th1 lymphocytes, which are the major producers of IFN-γ, alongside NK cells. In the presence of IL-12, IL-18 also stimulates the production of IFN-γ, inducing a Th1-mediated immune response; in the absence of IL-12, IL-18 can stimulate a Th2 response (17, 18).

Higher levels of IL-18 and sTNF-RII are described in the acute form of PCM when compared with the chronic form and controls, and IL-12 is also higher in patients than in controls (19). The same group reports higher levels of IL-18 during treatment and lower levels after antifungal treatment (20). As the disease is more severe in the acute form with high IL-18 levels, the authors suggest that this cytokine could be a useful marker of PCM severity.

Previous studies on murine PCM have shown that IL-12 and IL-18 secretions are associated with innate immunity factors. MyD88-deficient mice show a more severe disease after 8 weeks of infection with low levels of IL-12, and a protective role in murine pulmonary PCM was shown in the NLRP3 inflammasome, associated with IL-1β and IL-18 secretion and expansion of Th1 and Th17 cells and suppressive control of T-reg cells (7, 21).

The mechanisms controlling these effects are unclear, but reports on genetic background in both human and experimental disease have been shedding light on this matter. For instance, an autosomal dominant gene has been associated with resistance in murine PCM (22), and in human disease, reports show the influence of the human leukocyte antigen (HLA) in both susceptibility and outcomes. The HLA class I, HLA-B13, was found in a higher proportion in PCM patients compared to controls as well as a higher frequency of HLA-A9 in patients with the progressive pulmonary form (23). In parallel, increased risk of PCM development was associated with the presence of HLA-B40, which was found more in patients than in controls (24, 25). In 2011, the class II-HLA-DRB1*11 allele was reported in a higher frequency in patients with the more benign clinical presentation of this disease, the unifocal chronic (UC) form (26). Moreover, PCM patients were shown to have a higher proportion of the non-expressed C4B allele, C4B*Q0, of deficient C4 isotypes, suggesting to the authors a possible influence of different C4 isotype and allotype frequencies in the course of infection (27).

In addition, an enzyme phenotype (GLO-1 phenotype of glyoxalase I) was associated with PCM infection represented by a positive intradermic reaction, and a possible relationship with HLA antigens deserves further discussion because there is a close linkage between the GLO phenotype and HLA (28).

Our group and others have been studying single nucleotide polymorphisms (SNPs) and different mutations on cytokines and receptor genes. For instance, the inherited mutation Leu77Phe on the IL-12 receptor β1 subunit (IL-12Rβ1) gene (*IL12RB1*) associated with its loss of function and complete deficiency, resulting in a severe, acute form of PCM (29). Moreover, in Brazilian patients with PCM, reports of polymorphisms on IL-4 and IL-12Rβ1 genes have shown the relevance of *IL4* -590 C/T and *IL12RB1* 641 A/G SNPs in association with infection or clinical forms, contributing to a better understanding of the immunopathogenesis of this disease (30, 31).

Polymorphisms on the IFN-γ gene have also been described in infectious diseases, such as toxoplasmosis, tegumentar leishmaniasis, and PCM, and no association between alleles or genotypes and these diseases was observed (31–35). Furthermore, it is also necessary to consider that the expression of the IFN-γ receptor could be interfering in the axis IL-12/IFN-γ because its deficiency was already described in the more disseminated forms of histoplasmosis, coccidioidomycosis, mycobacteriosis, and disseminated BCG infection (36–39). This deficient expression could be associated with a mutation in the IFN-γ receptor 1 gene, such as the *IFNGR1* -611 A/G SNP, which has been associated with strong promoter activity and with decreased risk of pulmonary tuberculosis (40, 41).

IL-12p70, the bioactive form of IL-12, is a heterodimer of two subunits: p35 (encoded by the *IL12A* gene) and p40 (encoded by the *IL12B* gene). No association was found between *IL12B* +1188

A/C SNP and PCM (31). SNPs in the *IL12A* gene, on the other hand, have not yet been explored in this mycosis.

Studies show an association of *IL18* -607 C/A SNP (rs1946518) with protection or risk in several infections (42–45). However, as with the *IL12A* -504 G/T (rs2243115) and the *IFNGR1* -611 A/G (rs1327474) SNPs, there are still no studies associating this genetic polymorphism with systemic fungal infections.

Considering the interaction between IL-18, IL-12, and IFN-γ and the genetic aspects possibly involved in susceptibility to PCM and the lack of studies on this disease, the present study aimed to analyze the *IL18* -607 C/A (rs1946518), *IL12A* -504 G/T (rs2243115), and *IFNGR1* -611 A/G (rs1327474) SNPs, for the first time to our knowledge, in a cohort of Brazilian patients with PCM, also presenting a brief review of studies on these SNPs in infectious diseases.

MATERIALS AND METHODS

Subjects

A total of 149 patients with PCM from the General Infirmary and Systemic Mycosis Outpatient Clinic from the Infectious Diseases Division (Hospital das Clínicas, Faculdade de Medicina, University of São Paulo—HCFMUSP, São Paulo, SP, Brazil) were included in the study (**Table 2**). Thirty-nine patients had the acute form of PCM (AF) and 110 had the chronic form (CF); 93 had the multifocal chronic form (MC) and 17 had the UC form. This classification was performed according to Franco et al. (46). UC includes only patients with mild, restricted disease to the skin, mucosae, or lymph nodes without lung or cerebral involvement. The control group (CO) included 110 non-PCM subjects. The study protocol was approved by the ethics committee of HCFMUSP (CAPPesq 10273; Plataforma Brasil 123334/2013), and all subjects gave written informed consent in accordance with the Declaration of Helsinki.

The inclusion criteria were (a) patients with PCM: identification of *Paracoccidioides* spp. by mycological and/or histopathological examination and/or presence of anti-*P. brasiliensis* serum antibodies (titers ≥32 on counterimmunoelectrophoresis test) at the moment of enrollment or proven in the past; and (b) CO: individuals considered healthy without a previous history of the disease, not sensitized in lymphoproliferation assays against the 43-kDa glycoprotein of *P. brasiliensis*, and absence of serum anti-*P. brasiliensis* antibodies (by immunodiffusion test). Subjects with comorbidities, such as neoplasia and other acute or chronic systemic infectious diseases, were excluded.

DNA Extraction

Genomic DNA was obtained from peripheral blood leukocytes by the salt precipitation method (DTAB/CTAB; dodecyl trimethyl ammonium bromide/cetyltrimethyl ammonium bromide, both from Sigma-Aldrich, Merck, St. Louis, MO, USA) as previously described (47). The concentration and purity of the extracted DNA were evaluated by a UV spectrophotometer (Nanodrop LITE, Thermo Fisher Scientific, Carlsbad, CA, USA).

Detection of SNPs

The SNPs in the IL-12p35 (*IL12A* -504 G/T, rs2243115), IL-18 (*IL18* -607 C/A, rs1946518), and IFN-γ receptor 1 (*IFNGR1* -611 A/G, rs1327474) genes were investigated by real-time PCR using specific oligonucleotides and probes labeled with VIC (wild allele) or FAM (mutated allele) fluorochromes and TaqMan™ Genotyping Master Mix (all from Molecular Probes, Thermo Fisher Scientific, Carlsbad CA, USA). The assays and results were performed and analyzed with the StepOne Plus Real Time PCR System and software (Applied Biosystems, Thermo Fisher Scientific, Foster City, CA, USA).

Statistical Analysis

The deviations from the Hardy–Weinberg equilibrium and the distribution of genotypic and allelic frequencies of the SNPs on *IL12A*, *IL18*, and *IFNGR1* genes in the studied population were evaluated by Pearson's χ^2 test. To estimate the risk of patients with AF, MC, and UC PCM associated with genotypes and alleles, odds ratios (ORs) and 95% confidence intervals (95% CIs) were calculated as approximations of relative risk using unconditional logistic regression analysis. For ordered variables, tests for linear trend were done by categorizing the exposure variables and entering the scores as continuous. To verify the strength of association between the final events, we performed univariate and multivariate logistic analyses adjusted by ethnicity and sex with the STATA 14.0 software (StataCorp, College Station, TX, USA), and p-values $\leq$0.05 were considered statistically significant.

RESULTS

Considering the plausible role of genetic background in human PCM, we summarize all previously reported SNPs or mutations on immune-related genes and their main results on Brazilian patients in **Table 1**. Eight SNPs or mutations on DC-SIGN, HLA, IL-4, IL-10, IL-12Rβ1, and Vitamin D receptor genes were found to have an association with risk, outcome, or clinical forms of PCM. As the SNPs of this study had not yet been evaluated on PCM patients, we also compiled previous reports on the *IL18* (-607 C/A, rs1946518 and -137 G/C, rs187238), *IL12A* (-504 G/T, rs2243115), and *IFNGR1* (-611 A/G, rs13277474) SNPs and their association with diverse infectious diseases (**Supplementary Tables 1–3**, respectively).

This study evaluated the *IL18* -607 C/A, *IL12A* -504 G/T, and *IFNGR1* -611 A/G SNPs in 149 patients with the AF and CF of PCM and 110 control individuals (CO). The CF group is subclassified as MC and UC forms. There were no statistically significant differences between cases and controls in the distribution of ethnic groups or sex (data not shown). Regarding the different groups of patients (AF, MC, and UC), no differences in ethnic distribution were found (p = 0.476). However, in the univariate analysis of sex distribution, there was a significant difference between these groups with a male majority on a ratio of 17.6 in the MC group (**Table 2**).

Genotypic frequencies for the three evaluated SNPs were in Hardy–Weinberg equilibrium (data not shown). The distribution of genotypic and allelic frequencies of *IL12A* -504 G/T, *IL18* -607 C/A, and *IFNGR1* -611 A/G SNPs among patients and controls

TABLE 1 | Polymorphisms on immune-related genes in Brazilian patients with PCM.

Structure (gene)	Mutation (rs)	Main results	References
CTLA-4 (*CTLA4*)	−318 C/T and +49 A/G[a]	• No differences between patients and controls	(48)
DC-SIGN (*DCSIGN*)	rs4804803	• Genotype *DCSIGN-GG* on patients with oral PCM ($p = 0.032$)	(49)
FCγ-RIIa (*FCGR2A*)	rs1801274	• No differences between patients and controls	(49)
HLA (*HLA*)	HLA-DRB1 and HLA-DQB1 alleles[a]	• *HLA-DRB1*11* allele associated with UC form of PCM ($p = 0.039$)	(26)
IFN-γ (*IFNG*)	+874 T/A[a]	• No differences between patients and controls	(35)
	+874 T/A (rs2430561)	• No differences between patients and controls	(31)
		• No differences between clinical forms of PCM	
IL-4 (*IL4*)	−590 T/C[a]	• Patients with *C*-allele produce more IL-4 than those with *T*-allele ($p < 0.05$)	(35)
		• No differences between patients and controls	(30)
	Intron-3 microsatellite *RP1/RP2*[a]	• Genotypes *RP2/RP2* on patients and *RP1/RP1* on controls (with low IL-4 expression): $p = 0.0042$	(30)
IL-10 (*IL10*)	−1082 G/A[a]	• Genotypes *IL10-GG* on patients and *IL10-AA* on controls ($p = 0.0218$)	(34)
IL-12p40 (*IL12B*)	+1188 A/C (rs3212227)	• No differences between patients and controls	(31)
		• No differences between clinical forms of PCM	
IL-12Rβ1 (*IL12RB1*)	230 T/C Leu77Phe[a]	• Inherited IL-12Rβ1 deficiency leading to acute form of PCM	(29)
	641 A/G (rs11575834)	• No differences between patients and controls	(31)
		• Male patients: Genotype *IL12RB1-AA* on MC form and *IL12RB1-AG* on UC form ($p = 0.048$)	
JAK1	rs11208534	• No differences between patients and controls	(49)
TNF-α (*TNFA*)	−308 G/A[a]	• No differences between patients and controls	(34)
	rs1800629	• No differences between patients and controls	(49)
Vitamin D Receptor (*VDR*)	rs7975232	• Genotype *VDR-CC* ($p < 0.001$) and *C*-allele ($p = 0.027$) on patients	(49)

[a]*rs not informed or not applicable.*

TABLE 2 | Distribution (*n*), sex (M = Male; F = Female) and ethnicity (W = White; B = Black) ratio, and *p*-values among the groups of patients with acute, multifocal chronic and unifocal chronic forms of PCM.

Clinical forms of PCM	*n*	Sex ratio (M/F)	*p*	Ethnicity ratio (W/B)	*p*
Acute	39	1.8 (25/14)	0.000	1.2 (12/10)	0.476
Multifocal chronic	93	17.6 (88/5)		2.1 (57/27)	
Unifocal chronic	17	2.4 (12/5)		2.5 (10/4)	

and among AF and CF groups is shown in **Table 3**. We found no statistical significances in the univariate analysis of genotypic frequencies in the codominant, dominant, and recessive models nor in the distribution and frequencies of alleles.

In **Table 4**, we show the distribution of genotypic and allelic frequencies of *IL12A* -504 G/T, *IL18* -607 C/A, and *IFNGR1* -611 A/G SNPs among the groups of patients with the different clinical forms of PCM, analyzed by unconditional logistic regression with adjustments for ethnicity and sex. The comparison between AF, MC, and UC genotypic distribution did not result in a statistical difference.

Regarding the allelic distribution and frequencies of *IL18* -607 C/A SNP, unconditional logistic regression with adjustments for ethnicity and sex shows significant differences between AF and UC [$p = 0.015$; OR = 3.1 (95% CI: 1.24–7.77)] with a higher frequency of the *A*-allele in AF (53.8%) than in UC (26.5%) (**Tables 4**, **5**). The same is observed in the comparison between MC and UC [$p = 0.023$; OR = 2.61 (95% CI: 1.14–5.96)]. Concerning alleles of *IL12A* -504 G/T and *IFNGR1* -611 A/G SNPs, no statistical differences were found. Furthermore, **Table 5** shows the statistical data on sex and ethnicity as covariates of *IL18* -607 C/A SNP in the distribution of genotypes and alleles. There was a significant difference of sex distribution between AF and MC with a higher proportion of women in AF ($p = 0.000$); this is the opposite of the comparison between MC and UC, in which the proportion of female patients is significantly lower in the MC group ($p < 0.015$). This same effect occurred with the codominant, dominant, recessive, and allelic analyses, confirming and detailing the data of **Table 2**. There were no differences regarding sex distribution between AF and UC, and ethnicity had no statistically significant effect as a covariate in this analysis.

DISCUSSION

Genetic studies are relevant to understanding the mechanisms involved in the pathogenesis of diseases (50, 51). Some genetic polymorphisms are shown to directly interfere in cytokine expression, therefore directing the immune response of the host and possibly influencing the outcome of the disease.

TABLE 3 | Genotypic and allelic distributions and frequencies of *IL12A* -504 G/T, *IL18* -607 C/A, and *IFNGR1* -611 A/G SNPs, values of Odds Ratio (OR) and 95% Confidence Interval (95% CI) among the groups of Controls (*n* = 110) and Patients (*n* = 149), and among the groups of patients with Acute (*n* = 39) and Chronic (Multifocal + Unifocal) forms of PCM (*n* = 110).

SNP	Genotypes	Alleles	Groups—*n* (%)			Clinical forms of PCM—*n* (%)		
			Controls	Patients	OR (95% CI)	Acute	Chronic	OR (95% CI)
IL12A -564 G/T	GG		2 (1.8)	2 (1.3)	1.0	1 (2.6)	1 (0.8)	1.0
	GT		28 (25.5)	40 (26.9)	1.43 (0.19–10.76)	13 (33.4)	27 (24.6)	0.48 (0.03–8.32)
	TT		80 (72.7)	107 (71.8)	1.34 (0.18–9.7)	25 (64.0)	82 (74.6)	0.3 (0.02–5.05)
		G	32 (14.5)	44 (14.8)	1.0	15 (19.2)	29 (13.2)	1.0
		T	188 (85.5)	254 (85.2)	0.98 (0.6–1.61)	63 (80.8)	191 (86.8)	0.63 (0.32–1.26)
IL18 -607 C/A	CC		29 (26.4)	44 (29.5)	1.0	10 (25.7)	34 (30.9)	1.0
	CA		60 (54.5)	68 (45.6)	0.75 (0.42–1.34)	16 (41.0)	52 (47.3)	1.05 (0.43–2.58)
	AA		21 (19.1)	37 (24.8)	1.16 (0.57–2.37)	13 (33.3)	24 (21.8)	1.84 (0.7–4.89)
		C	118 (53.6)	156 (52.3)	1.0	36 (46.2)	120 (54.5)	1.0
		A	102 (46.4)	142 (47.7)	1.05 (0.74–1.49)	42 (53.8)	100 (45.5)	1.4 (0.83–2.35)
IFNGR1 -611 A/G	AA		14 (12.8)	21 (14.1)	1.0	4 (10.3)	17 (15.5)	1.0
	AG		47 (43.1)	66 (44.3)	0.93 (0.43–2.03)	19 (48.7)	47 (42.7)	0.58 (0.17–1.96)
	GG		48 (44.0)	62 (41.6)	0.86 (0.4–1.87)	16 (41.0)	46 (41.8)	0.67 (0.2–2.3)
		A	75 (34.4)	108 (36.2)	1.0	27 (34.6)	81 (36.8)	1.0
		G	143 (65.6)	190 (63.8)	0.92 (0.64–1.33)	51 (65.4)	139 (63.2)	1.1 (0.64–1.89)

In the present study, we investigated the possible association between the *IL12A* -504 G/T, *IL18* -607 C/A, and *IFNGR1* -611 A/G SNPs in Brazilian patients with PCM and disease susceptibility. The distribution of genotypes and alleles of the *IL12A* -504 G/T SNP was similar in all evaluated comparisons on our study. Although this SNP was related to immune responses against rubella vaccination and HBV and protection in tuberculosis, we did not observe a clear association with PCM (52–54).

As for *IFNGR1* -611 A/G SNP, genotypic and allelic distributions were similar in all evaluated comparisons, confirmed by unconditional logistic regression analysis (adjusted for sex and race). The absence of association with risk or protection reported here is similar to the data reported in tuberculosis and liver fibrosis progression due to recurrent hepatitis C (55–58). An association between tuberculosis and the *IFNGR1* -611 A/G and -56 T/C haplotype was observed by Bullak-Kardum et al. (41). In fact, the promoter activity is supposed to be stronger in -611 A/G than -56 T/C, and the variant *A* is estimated to decrease the binding of GATA-1 and TFIID factors to this site (40, 58). Because previous associations with risk or protection have been described in other SNPs, further studies should include the *IFNGR1* -611 A/G SNP.

In our analysis of the *IL18* -607 C/A SNP, we found no differences on allelic and genotypic distributions between patients and controls or between AF and CF groups of patients. On the other hand, the adjustment for sex and ethnicity in the unconditional regression logistic analysis confirmed the presence of the *A*-allele as a risk factor for the AF and MC groups when compared to the UC group.

The association of the *A*-allele/*AA*-genotype and higher risk is shown in various infectious diseases, such as chronic hepatitis B in Thailand and in India, gingivitis in the Czech Republic, pulmonary tuberculosis in China, Chagas disease in Colombia (mainly driven by rs360719), and infection by the hepatitis C virus in Egypt (37, 43, 52–62). Similarly to our results, the mutant allele/genotype of *IL18* -607 C/A is also associated with more severe outcomes in other infectious diseases: higher virus shedding of the severe acute respiratory syndrome-associated (SARS) coronavirus in Taiwan, lipodystrophy syndrome on HIV-positive Brazilian individuals, immune restoration disease on HIV–tuberculosis coinfected Indian patients, bacterial infections after liver transplantation in China, and hepatitis C–related hepatocellular carcinoma in Egypt (63–67).

The effect of the *A*-allele/*AA*-genotype on PCM and other infectious diseases could be explained by changes in IL-18 levels introduced by this mutant allele in the -607 position. In effect, the IL-18 human gene is composed of six exons and five introns with three very well-known SNPs in the promoter region: -656 G/T (rs1946519), -607 C/A (rs1946518), and -137 G/C (rs187238). Two of these positions, -607 and -137, are thought to be nuclear factor binding sites for cAMP responsive element binding protein and H4TF-1 nuclear factor, respectively, and mutation on both sites can affect the IL-18 levels (50).

The -607 *C*-allele/*CC*-genotype carriage has been associated with higher levels of IL-18 in the serum and/or of mRNA expression (50, 66, 68–70). In our study, we found higher *C*-allele carriage on patients with the UC form of PCM (73.5%), whereas the AF and MC groups (with 46.2 and 51.1% of *C*-allele carriage, respectively) had already been reported to have higher serum IL-18 levels than those from the former group (19, 20).

We hypothesize that the higher *C*-allele carriage on patients with the UC form of PCM may induce higher IL-18 levels at the early stages of infection, determining increased

TABLE 4 | Genotypic and allelic distributions and frequencies of *IL12A* -504 G/T, *IL18* -607 C/A, and *IFNGR1* -611 A/G SNPs, values of Odds Ratio (OR) and 95% Confidence Interval (95% CI) adjusted for sex and race by unconditional logistic regression analysis among the groups of patients with Acute (AF, $n = 39$), Multifocal Chronic (MC, $n = 93$) and Unifocal Chronic (UC, $n = 17$) forms of PCM.

SNP	Model	Genotypes	Alleles	Clinical Forms of PCM—*n* (%)			AF vs. MC[a]	AF vs. UC[b]	MC vs. UC[c]
				AF	MC	UC	OR (95% CI)	OR (95% CI)	OR (95% CI)
IL12A -504 G/T	Codominant	GG		1 (2.6)	1 (1.1)	0 (0.0)	1		
		GT		13 (33.4)	21 (22.6)	6 (35.3)	0.62 (0.04–10.78)	–	–
		TT		25 (64.0)	71 (76.3)	11 (64.7)	0.35 (0.02–5.84)	–	–
	Dominant	GG		1 (2.6)	1 (1.1)	0 (0.0)	1		
		GT + TT		38 (97.4)	92 (98.9)	17 (100.0)	0.41 (0.03–6.78)	–	–
	Recessive	GG + GT		14 (36.0)	22 (23.7)	6 (35.3)	1	1	1
		TT		25 (64.0)	71 (76.3)	11 (64.7)	0.55 (0.25–1.24)	0.97 (0.3–3.2)	1.76 (0.58–1.76)
			G	15 (19.2)	23 (12.4)	6 (17.6)	1	1	1
			T	63 (80.8)	163 (87.6)	28 (82.4)	0.59 (0.29–1.21)	0.90 (0.32–2.56)	1.52 (0.47–4.06)
IL18 -607 C/A	Codominant	CC		10 (25.7)	26 (28.0)	8 (47.1)	1		
		CA		16 (41.0)	43 (46.2)	9 (52.9)	0.97 (0.38–2.45)	–	–
		AA		13 (33.3)	24 (25.3)	0 (0.0)	1.41 (0.52–3.80)	–	–
	Dominant	CC		10 (25.7)	26 (28.0)	8 (47.1)	1	1	1
		CA + AA		29 (74.3)	67 (72.0)	9 (52.9)	1.13 (0.48–2.63)	2.58 (0.78–8.5)	2.29 (0.80–6.58)
	Recessive	CC + CA		27 (66.7)	69 (74.2)	17 (100.0)	1		
		AA		13 (33.3)	24 (25.8)	0 (0.0)	1.38 (0.63–3.11)	–	–
			C	36 (46.2)	95 (51.1)	25 (73.5)	1	1	1
			A	42 (53.8)	91 (48.9)	9 (26.5)	1.19 (0.69–2.07)	3.10 (1.24–7.77)	2.61 (1.14–5.96)
IFNGR1 -611 A/G	Codominant	AA		16 (41.0)	39 (41 9)	7 (41.2)	1	1	1
		AG		19 (48.7)	37 (39.8)	10 (58.8)	2.82 (0.84–9.52)	0.84 (0.2–3.52)	0.64 (0.19–2.18)
		GG		4 (10.3)	17 (18.3)	0 (0.0)	0.39 (0.03–4.22)	–	–
	Dominant	AA		16 (41.0)	39 (41.9)	7 (41.2)	1	1	1
		AG + GG		23 (59.0)	54 (85.1)	10 (58.8)	1.95 (0.61–6.22)	0.97 (0.24–3.92)	0.98 (0.29–3.25)
	Recessive	AA + AG		35 (89.7)	76 (81.7)	17 (100.0)	1		
		GG		4 (10.3)	17 (18.3)	0 (0.0)	0.23 (0.02–2.20)	–	–
			A	51 (65.4)	115 (61.8)	24 (70.6)	1	1	1
			G	27 (34.6)	71 (38.2)	10 (29.4)	0.86 (0.49–1.49)	1.27 (0.53–3.04)	1.48 (0.67–3.38)

[a]*Reference for AF vs. MC = MC.*
[b]*Reference for AF vs. UC = UC.*
[c]*Reference for MC vs. UC = UC.*

TABLE 5 | Association studies between the groups of patients with Acute (AF), Multifocal Chronic (MC), and Unifocal Chronic (UC) forms of PCM including sex, ethnicity, and the *IL18* -607 C/A SNP as covariates and results of *p*-values, Odds Ratio (OR), and 95% Confidence Interval (95% CI).

Covariates of *IL18* -607 C/A SNP	Comparisons								
	AF vs. MC[c]			AF vs. UC[d]			MC vs. UC[e]		
	p-value	OR	95% CI	*p*-value	OR	95% CI	*p*-value	OR	95% CI
Sex[a]	0.000	12.63	3.64–43.81	0.484	1.74	0.37–8.18	0.020	0.16	0.35–0.76
Ethnicity[b]	0.433	1.54	0.52–4.55	0.350	2.12	0.44–10.31	0.517	1.56	0.40–6.00
CC vs. CA vs. AA	0.546	1.25	0.60–2.62	0.070	3.06	0.91–10.27	0.164	1.89	0.77–4.65
Sex[a]	0.000	12.58	3.64–43.50	0.393	1.89	0.44–8.16	0.015	0.151	0.03–0.70
Ethnicity[b]	0.420	1.56	0.53–4.64	0.399	1.85	0.59–9.16	0.600	1.42	0.38–5.36
CC vs. CA + AA	0.755	1.13	0.48–2.63	0.769	2.58	0.78–8.5	0.724	2.29	0.80–6.58
Sex[a]	0.000	12.39	3.58–42.98	0.609	1.52	0.31–7.50	0.018	0.15	0.03–0.72
Ethnicity[b]	0.402	1.59	0.53–4.75	0.699	1.63	0.47–8.00	0.364	1.88	0.48–7.36
CC + CA vs. AA	0.569	1.38	0.63–3.11		Omitted			Omitted	
Sex[a]	0.000	12.6	3.64–43.80	0.484	1.74	0.37–8.31	0.020	0.16	0.03–0.76
Ethnicity[b]	0.430	1.54	0.52–0.30	0.350	2.12	0.44–10.31	0.517	1.56	0.40–6.00
C vs. A	0.528	1.19	0.69–2.07	0.015	3.10	1.24–7.77	0.023	2.61	1.14–5.96

[a] *Reference for sex = male.*
[b] *Reference for ethnicity = white.*
[c] *Reference for AF vs. MC = MC.*
[d] *Reference for AF vs. UC = UC.*
[e] *Reference for MC vs. UC = UC.*

levels of IFN-γ and a more efficient cellular response that controls fungal dissemination and the consequential tissular inflammation. In parallel, previous work in our lab shows that phytohemagglutinin-stimulated cells from *IL18* -607 *C*-allele-unifocal patients apparently produce more IFN-γ than *C*-allele carriers from the acute or the chronic multifocal groups, although without statistically significant difference (unpublished data). However, because both infection and disease in humans are recognized in a later and undefined period after fungal entrance, those initial events can only be evaluated in experimental PCM and have been elegantly shown in deficient mice models. The intravenous infection of IL-18-deficient mice ($IL\text{-}18^{-/-}$) with *P. brasiliensis* yeast cells resulted in a higher fungal burden in the lungs compared with wild-type (WT) animals and absence of granuloma formation (71). Furthermore, *P. brasiliensis* intratracheally infected mice deficient for NLRP3 inflammasome components ($Nlrp3^{-/-}$, $Casp1/11^{-/-}$, $Asc^{-/-}$) as well as deficient for the ATP receptor ($P2x7r^{-/-}$) also had a higher fungal burden in their lungs and liver; predominance of $CD4^{+}IL\text{-}4^{+}$, $CD4^{+}TGF\text{-}\beta^{+}$, and T-reg cells; a lower number of pulmonary PMN cells; and less IL-18 and IL-1β compared with their WT controls (7).

In this context, it is possible that patients with the less severe UC form of PCM present a more balanced IL-18/IL-12/IFN-γ axis, resulting in more localized and milder clinical manifestations compared with the other groups, in which the higher IL-18 levels are accompanied by other immunomodulating cytokines. The more severe form of PCM, the acute form, has been characterized by IL-4 with IL-18 inducing a Th2 immune response (high levels of IL-4, IL-5, and IL-13), by IL-4 and TGF-β inducing a Th9 pattern (high levels of IL-9), and both Th2 and Th9 inhibiting the Th1 response. Patients with chronic PCM were previously shown to have a mixed immune response of Th1 (IL-12 and IL-18 leading to IFN-γ production), Th17 (induced by IL-18, IL-1 and IL-23), and Th22 (induced by IL-18, IL-1, IL-23, and IL-21), which result in heterogeneous clinical symptoms (12, 13, 20).

In our study, the UC group included only patients with mild and restricted disease to the skin, mucosae, or lymph nodes. The exclusion of patients with lung involvement was based on the possible misclassification of MC patients who are more prone to develop pulmonary lesions. Although these criteria resulted in fewer patients in the UC group, it also revealed specific immunogenetic characteristics, such as the association of a more favorable outcome with the *IL18* -607 *C*-allele in the present study and the *IL12RB1* 641 *AG*-genotype and the HLA-DRB1*11 allele carriage, previously reported by our group (26, 31).

Additionally, the association of the *IL18* -607 *A*-allele with the more severe forms of PCM described herein collaborates with previous reports on different genes emphasizing the influence of genetic background on the outcome of this mycosis. The *GG*-genotype of *IL10* -1082 G/A SNP, the *RP2/RP2*-genotype of the intron-3 microsatellite polymorphism of the *IL4* gene, the *AA*-genotype of *IL12RB1* 641 A/G SNP, the *GG*-genotype of the *DCSIGN* rs4804803 A/G SNP, and the *CC*-genotype of the *VDR* rs7975232 A/C SNP have all been previously associated with susceptibility or the more severe outcome in PCM (26, 29–31, 34, 35, 49). In parallel, HLA class I antigens and the GLO-1 phenotype of the glyoxalase enzyme have been associated with the progression of disease (pulmonary form) or infection (23–25, 27, 28).

We reinforce that our present data and all the genetic associations previously described may be considered in the same context of association of autosomal gene dominance with resistance in murine PCM, which is a model that reproduces several characteristics of the human disease (22).

The comparison between patients and controls in our study shows a greater number of male than female subjects, particularly in the MC group. As previously described, there has been a male predominance among cases of chronic PCM (72–74). This mycosis manifests more frequently in male farmers who are constantly working in direct contact with the soil where *Paracoccidioides* spp. probably occurs (1). In addition, infected women are less likely to manifest the chronic form because of the putative role of estrogen (17-β-estradiol) as a protective factor that impairs conidia transformation into yeast form during murine infection (75–77). Although this effect has been less commonly registered in human PCM, epidemiological data reported in Brazil show that the disease is rare in adult females (4.3%) and usually occurring in the menopausal period (91.3%) (78). Contrarily, it has been demonstrated that 17-β-estradiol can exert an anti-inflammatory role by decreasing TNF-α and IL-6 while increasing IL-4 levels, which further results in a Th2 response (79). In oral PCM lesions, a positive correlation between the amount of estradiol receptors and the fungal burden was observed only in female patients (80). These recent findings may explain the more even distribution of the acute form of PCM among sexes, and the higher frequency of females in UC and lower in MC could be evidence of protection for women in developing the more severe chronic form of the disease.

Possible limitations in our study are the inclusion of only one health center, mixed ethnic groups in the Brazilian population, and lack of detection of IL-18 levels and functional analyses. Although reflecting the distribution of PCM in endemic areas, our cohort with a low number of patients with the UC form is also a limitation for further inquiry.

In summary, our study did not show an association between PCM and the evaluated *IL12A* and *IFNGR1* SNPs or between the acute and chronic forms or between multifocal and unifocal chronic forms. For the *IL18* -607 C/A SNP, no association was shown with infection or among acute and chronic forms. However, we show an association between the *IL18* -607 *A*-allele and the more severe clinical forms of PCM, acute and multifocal chronic forms, when compared to the UC form, the less severe form of this disease, associated with the *IL18* -607 *C*-allele. To the best of our knowledge, this is the first study that evaluates the association between *IL12A*, *IFNGR1*, and *IL18* SNPs and PCM.

The present data suggest a novel role of *IL18* -607 C/A SNP as a contributor to a more favorable outcome of this disease, potentially leading to a more balanced and more efficient cellular response for the control of fungal dissemination at the early stages of infection in UC. Furthermore, our work highlights the need for new studies with other SNPs on the *IL18* gene and on other components of the immune response for a better understanding of the pathophysiology and the clinical expression of PCM.

ETHICS STATEMENT

The studies involving human participants were reviewed and approved by Research and Ethics Committee of Hospital das Clínicas, Faculdade de Medicina, University of São Paulo - HCFMUSP, São Paulo, SP, Brazil (CAPPesq 10273; Plataforma Brasil 123334/2013). The patients/participants provided their written informed consent to participate in this study.

AUTHOR CONTRIBUTIONS

PS and MS-Y conceived and designed the experiments. MM and AK contributed with samples and patient selection. PS, FB, FC, CD, and AS performed the experiments. PS, AG, and OL analyzed the data. PS, FB, AG, FC, and MS-Y wrote the paper and/or performed bibliographic revision. PS, MS-Y, MM, AK, FB, FC, CD, AS, AG, and OL approved the paper. All authors contributed to the article and approved the submitted version.

ACKNOWLEDGMENTS

We thank Nídia P. O. Silva and Eron L. dos Santos for their contribution on DNA extraction of some of the samples and Marcia A. Ferreira, Carlos Jose Quinteiro, and Rodolfo E. Fujimori for providing older articles.

REFERENCES

1. Martinez R. New trends in paracoccidioidomycosis epidemiology. *J Fungi.* (2017) 3:1. doi: 10.3390/jof3010001
2. Martinez R. Epidemiology of paracoccidioidomycosis. *Rev Inst Med Trop São Paulo.* (2015) 57:11–20. doi: 10.1590/S0036-46652015000700004
3. Vieira G de D, Alves T da C, Lima SM, Camargo LM, Sousa CM. Paracoccidioidomycosis in a western Brazilian Amazon State: clinical-epidemiologic profile and spatial distribution of the disease. *Rev Soc Bras Med Trop.* (2014) 47:63–8. doi: 10.1590/0037-8682-0225-2013
4. Benard G. An overview of the immunopathology of human paracoccidioidomycosis. *Mycopathologia.* (2008) 165:209–21. doi: 10.1007/s11046-007-9065-0
5. Calich VL, Costa TA, Felonato M, Arruda C, Bernardino S, Loures FV, et al. Innate immunity to *Paracoccidioides brasiliensis* infection. *Mycopathologia.* (2008) 165:223–36. doi: 10.1007/s11046-007-9048-1
6. Calich VL, Pina A, Felonato M, Bernardino S, Costa TA, Loures FV. Toll-like receptors and fungal infections: the role of TLR2, TLR4 and MyD88 in paracoccidioidomycosis. *FEMS Immunol Med Microbiol.* (2008) 53:1–7. doi: 10.1111/j.1574-695X.2008.00378.x
7. Feriotti C, de Araújo EF, Loures FV, da Costa TA, Galdino NAL, Zamboni DS, et al. NOD-like receptor P3 inflammasome controls protective Th1/Th17 immunity against pulmonary paracoccidioidomycosis. *Front Immunol.* (2017) 10:786. doi: 10.3389/fimmu.2017.00786
8. Jannuzzi GP, de Almeida JRF, Amarante-Mendes GP, Romera LMD, Kaihami GH, Vasconcelos JR, et al. TLR3 is a negative regulator of immune

responses against *Paracoccidioides brasiliensis*. *Front Cell Infect Microbiol.* (2019) 8:426. doi: 10.3389/fcimb.2018.00426

9. Rodrigues DR, Fernandes RK, Balderramas H de A, Penitenti M, Bachiega TF, Calvi SA, et al. Interferon-gamma production by human neutrophils upon stimulation by IL-12, IL-15 and IL-18 and challenge with *Paracoccidioides brasiliensis*. *Cytokine.* (2014) 69:102–9. doi: 10.1016/j.cyto.2014.05.009
10. de Castro LF, Longhi LNA, Paião MR, Justo-Júnior ADS, de Jesus MB, Blotta MHSL, et al. NLRP3 inflammasome is involved in the recognition of *Paracoccidioides brasiliensis* by human dendritic cells and in the induction of Th17 cells. *J Infect.* (2018) 77:137–44. doi: 10.1016/j.jinf.2018.03.004
11. Calich VL, Vaz CA, Burger E. Immunity to *Paracoccidioides brasiliensis* infection. *Res Immunol.* (1998) 149:407–500. doi: 10.1016/S0923-2494(98)80764-5
12. Oliveira SJ, Mamoni RL, Musatti CC, Papaiordanou PM, Blotta MH. Cytokines and lymphocyte proliferation in juvenile and adult forms of paracoccidioidomycosis: comparison with infected and non-infected controls. *Microbes Infect.* (2002) 4:139–44. doi: 10.1016/S1286-4579(01)01521-0
13. de Castro LF, Ferreira MC, Silva RM, Blotta MHSL, Longhi LN, Mamoni RL. Characterization of immune response in human paracoccidioidomycosis. *J Infect.* (2013) 67:470–85. doi: 10.1016/j.jinf.2013.07.019
14. Calich VLG, Mamoni RL, Loures FV. Regulatory T cells in paracoccidioidomycosis. *Virulence.* (2018) 1:1–12. doi: 10.1080/21505594.2018.1483674
15. Benard G, Romano CC, Cacere CR, Juvenale M, Mendes-Giannini MJ, Duarte AJ. Imbalance of IL-2, IFN-gamma and IL-10 secretion in the immunosuppression associated with human paracoccidioidomycosis. *Cytokine.* (2001) 13:248–52. doi: 10.1006/cyto.2000.0824
16. Romano CC, Mendes-Giannini MJS, Duarte AJS, Benard G. The role of interleukin-10 in the differential expression of interleukin-12p70 and its β2 receptor on patients with active or treated paracoccidioidomycosis and healthy infected subjects. *Clin Immunol.* (2005) 114:86–94. doi: 10.1016/j.clim.2004.09.005
17. Nakanishi K, Yoshimoto T, Tsutsui H, Okamura H. Interleukin-18 is a unique cytokine that stimulates both Th1 and Th2 responses depending on its cytokine milieu. *Cytokine Growth Factor Rev.* (2001) 12:53–72. doi: 10.1016/S1359-6101(00)00015-0
18. Samarani S, Allam O, Sagala P, Aldabah Z, Jenabian MA, Mehraj V, et al. Imbalanced production of IL-18 and its antagonist in human diseases, and its implications for HIV-1 infection. *Cytokine.* (2016) 82:38–51. doi: 10.1016/j.cyto.2016.01.006
19. Corvino CL, Mamoni RL, Fagundes GZ, Blotta MH. Serum interleukin-18 and soluble tumour necrosis factor receptor 2 are associated with disease severity in patients with paracoccidioidomycosis. *Clin Exp Immunol.* (2007) 147:483–90. doi: 10.1111/j.1365-2249.2006.03308.x
20. Alves ABRM, David MA, de Castro LF, da Silva RM, Longhi LNA, Blotta MHSL, et al. Differential production of interleukin-1 family cytokines (IL-1β, IL-18, IL-33 and IL-37) in patients with paracoccidioidomycosis: correlation with clinical form and antifungal therapy. *Med Mycol.* (2018) 56:332–43. doi: 10.1093/mmy/myx050
21. Loures FV, Pina A, Felonato M, Feriotti C, de Araújo EF, Calich VL. MyD88 signaling is required for efficient innate and adaptive immune responses to *Paracoccidioides brasiliensis* infection. *Infect Immun.* (2011) 79:2470–80. doi: 10.1128/IAI.00375-10
22. Calich VL, Burger E, Kashino SS, Fazioli RA, Singer-Vermes LM. Resistance to *Paracoccidioides brasiliensis* in mice is controlled by a single dominant autosomal gene. *Infect Immun.* (1987) 55:1919–23. doi: 10.1128/IAI.55.8.1919-1923.1987
23. de Restrepo FM, Restrepo M, Restrepo A. Blood groups and HLA antigens in paracoccidioidomycosis. *Sabouraudia.* (1983) 21:35–9. doi: 10.1080/00362178385380061
24. Lacerda GB, Arce-Gomez B, Telles Filho FQ. Increased frequency of HLA-B40 in patients with paracoccidioidomycosis. *J Med Vet Mycol.* (1988) 26:253–6. doi: 10.1080/02681218880000351
25. Goldani LZ, Monteiro CM, Donadi EA, Martinez R, Voltarelli JC. HLA antigens in Brazilian patients with paracoccidioidomycosis. *Mycopathologia.* (1991) 114:89–91. doi: 10.1007/BF00436427
26. Sadahiro A, Roque AC, Shikanai-Yasuda MA. Generic human leukocyte antigen class II (DRB1 and DQB1) alleles in patients with paracoccidioidomycosis. *Med Mycol.* (2007) 45:35–40. doi: 10.1080/13693780600999132
27. de Messias IJ, Reis A, Brenden M, Queiroz-Telles F, Mauff G. Association of major histocompatibility complex class III complement components C2, BF, and C4 with Brazilian paracoccidioidomycosis. *Complement Inflamm.* (1991) 8:288–93. doi: 10.1159/000463198
28. Balarin MA, Freire-Maia DV. The association between glyoxalase I and paracoccidioidomycosis infection. *Rev Soc Bras Med Trop.* (1993) 26:141–3. doi: 10.1590/S0037-86821993000300002
29. Moraes-Vasconcelos D, Grumach AS, Yamaguti A, Andrade MEB, Fieschi C, Beaucoudrey L, et al. *Paracoccidioides brasiliensis* disseminated disease in a patient with inherited deficiency in the beta1 subunit of the interleukin (IL)-12/IL-23 receptor. *Clin Infect Dis.* (2005) 41:e31–7. doi: 10.1086/432119
30. Mendonça MS, Peraçolli TS, Silva-Vergara ML, Ribeiro SC, Oliveira RF, Mendes RP, et al. High interleukin-4 expression and interleukin-4 gene polymorphisms are associated with susceptibility to human paracoccidioidomycosis. *Mem Inst Oswaldo Cruz.* (2015) 110:781–5. doi: 10.1590/0074-02760150197
31. Carvalho FM, Busser FD, Freitas VL, Furucho CR, Sadahiro A, Kono AS, et al. Polymorphisms on *IFNG*, *IL12B* and *IL12RB1* genes and paracoccidioidomycosis in the Brazilian population. *Infect Genet Evol.* (2016) 43:245–51. doi: 10.1016/j.meegid.2016.05.025
32. Neves E de S, Curi AL, Albuquerque MC, Palhano-Silva CS, Silva LB, Bueno WF, et al. Genetic polymorphism for IFN-γ +874 T/A in patients with acute toxoplasmosis. *Rev Soc Bras Med Trop.* (2012) 45:751–60. doi: 10.1590/S0037-86822012000600020
33. Matos GI, Covas CJF, Bittar RC Gomes-Silva A, Marques F, Maniero VC, et al. *IFNG* +874 T/A polymorphism is not associated with American tegumentary leishmaniasis susceptibility but can influence *Leishmania* induced IFN-γ production. *BMC Infec Dis.* (2007) 7:33. doi: 10.1186/1471-2334-7-33
34. Bozzi A, Pereira PP, Reis BS, Goulart MI, Pereira MC, Pedroso EP, et al. Interleukin-10 and tumor necrosis factor-alpha single nucleotide gene polymorphism frequency in paracoccidioidomycosis. *Hum Immunol.* (2006) 67:931–9. doi: 10.1016/j.humimm.2006.07.014
35. Bozzi A, Reis BS, Pereira PP, Pedroso EP, Goes AM. Interferon-gamma and interleukin-4 single nucleotide gene polymorphisms in Paracoccidioidomycosis. *Cytokine.* (2009) 48:212–7. doi: 10.1016/j.cyto.2009.07.011
36. Jouanguy E, Dupuis S, Pallier A, Döffinger R, Fondanèche MC, Fieschi C, et al. In a novel form of IFN-gamma receptor 1 deficiency, cell surface receptors fail to bind IFN-gamma. *J Clin Invest.* (2000) 105:1429–36. doi: 10.1172/JCI9166
37. Zerbe CS, Holland SM. Disseminated histoplasmosis in persons with interferon-γ receptor 1 deficiency. *Clin Infect Dis.* (2005) 41:e38–41. doi: 10.1086/432120
38. Vinh DC, Masannat F, Dzioba RB, Galgianai JN, Holland SM. Refractory disseminated coccidioidomycosis & mycobacteriosis in interferon-γ receptor deficiency. *Clin Infect Dis.* (2009) 49:e62–5. doi: 10.1086/605532
39. Marazzi MG, Chapgier A, Defilippi A, Pistioia V, Mangini S, Savioli C, et al. Disseminated *Mycobacterium scrofulaceum* infection in a child with interferon-γ receptor 1 deficiency. *Int J Infect Dis.* (2010) 14:167–70. doi: 10.1016/j.ijid.2009.03.025
40. Rosenzweig SD, Schäffer AA, Ding L, Sullivan R, Enyedi B, Yim JJ, et al. Interferon-gamma receptor 1 promoter polymorphisms: population distribution and functional implications. *Clin Immunol.* (2004) 112:113–9. doi: 10.1016/j.clim.2004.03.018
41. Bulat-Kardum L, Etokebe GE, Knezevic J, Balen S, Matakovic-Mileusnic N, Zaputovic L, et al. Interferon-gamma receptor-1 gene promoter polymorphisms (G-611A; T-56C) and susceptibility to tuberculosis. *Scand J Immunol.* (2006) 63:142–50. doi: 10.1111/j.1365-3083.2005.01694.x
42. Anyona SB, Kempaiah P, Raballah E, Ouma C, Were T, Davenport GC, et al. Functional promoter haplotypes of interleukin-18 condition susceptibility to severe malarial anemia and childhood mortality. *Infect Immun.* (2011) 79:4923–32. doi: 10.1128/IAI.05601-11
43. Han M, Yue J, Lian YY, Zhao YL, Wang HX, Liu LR. Relationship between single nucleotide polymorphism of interleukin-18 and susceptibility to pulmonary tuberculosis in the Chinese Han population. *Microbiol Immunol.* (2011) 55:388–93. doi: 10.1111/j.1348-0421.2011.00332.x

44. Hirankarn N, Manonom C, Tangkijvanich P, Poovorawan Y. Association of interleukin-18 gene polymorphism (-607A/A genotype) with susceptibility to chronic hepatitis B virus infection. *Tissue Antigens.* (2007) 70:160–3. doi: 10.1111/j.1399-0039.2007.00865.x
45. Haas SL, Weiss C, Bugert P, Gundt J, Witt H, Singer MV, et al. Interleukin 18 promoter variants (−137G>C and −607C>A) in patients with chronic hepatitis C: association with treatment response. *J Clin Immunol.* (2009) 29:620–8. doi: 10.1007/s10875-009-9302-z
46. Franco M, Montenegro MR, Marques RS, Dillon L. Host-parasite relationship in Paracoccidioidomycosis. *J Med Vet Mycol.* (1987) 25:5–9. doi: 10.1080/02681218780000021
47. Gustincich S, Manfioletti G, Del Sal GS, Schneider G, Carninci PA. A fast method for high quality genomic DNA extraction from whole human blood. *Biotechniques.* (1991) 11:298–302.
48. Lozano VF, Lins TC, Teixeira MM, Vieira RG, Blotta MHS, Goes AM, et al. Polymorphism analysis of the CTLA-4 gene in paracoccidioidomycosis patients. *Mem Inst Oswaldo Cruz.* (2011) 106:220–6. doi: 10.1590/S0074-02762011000200017
49. Alves Pereira Neto T, Costa Pereira AA, Costa Hanemann JA, Coelho LFL, Malaquias LCC. *DC-SIGN* and *VDR* polymorphisms are associated with chronic form of paracoccidioidomycosis with oral manifestations. *Mycoses.* (2019) 62:186–92. doi: 10.1111/myc.12866
50. Giedraitis V, He B, Huang WX, Hillert J. Cloning and mutation analysis of the human IL-18 promoter: a possible role of polymorphisms in expression regulation. *J Neuroimmunol.* (2001) 112:146–52. doi: 10.1016/S0165-5728(00)00407-0
51. Cao W, Luo LL, Chen WW, Liang L, Zhang RR, Zhao YL, et al. Polymorphism in the *EREG* gene confers susceptibility to tuberculosis. *BMC Med Genet.* (2019) 20:7. doi: 10.1186/s12881-018-0729-z
52. Dhiman N, Haralambieva IH, Vierkant RA, Pankratz VS, Ryan JE, Jacobson RM, et al. Predominant inflammatory cytokine secretion pattern in response to two doses of live rubella vaccine in healthy vaccinees. *Cytokine.* (2010) 50:24–9. doi: 10.1016/j.cyto.2009.12.002
53. Pan L, Zhang W, Liang Z, Wu X, Zhu X, Li J, et al. Association between polymorphisms of the cytokine and cytokine receptor genes and immune response to hepatitis B vaccination in a Chinese Han population. *J Med Virol.* (2012) 84:26–33. doi: 10.1002/jmv.22251
54. Wang J, Tang S, Shen H. Association of genetic polymorphisms in the *IL12-IFNG* pathway with susceptibility to and prognosis of pulmonary tuberculosis in a Chinese population. *Eur J Clin Microbiol Infect Dis.* (2010) 29:1291–5. doi: 10.1007/s10096-010-0985-0
55. Awomoyi AA, Nejentsev S, Richardson A, Hull J, Koch O, Podinovskaia M, et al. No association between interferon-gamma receptor-1 gene polymorphism and pulmonary tuberculosis in a Gambian population sample. *Thorax.* (2004) 59:291–4. doi: 10.1136/thx.2003.013029
56. Velez DR, Hulme WF, Myers JL, Weinberg JB, Levesque MC, Stryjewskiet ME, et al. *NOS2A*, *TLR4*, and *IFNGR1* interactions influence pulmonary tuberculosis susceptibility in African-Americans. *Hum Genet.* (2009) 126:643–53. doi: 10.1007/s00439-009-0713-y
57. Shin JG, Park BL, Kim LH, Namgoong S, Kim JO, Chang HS, et al. Association study of polymorphisms in interferon-γ receptor genes with the risk of pulmonary tuberculosis. *Mol Med Rep.* (2015) 12:1568–78. doi: 10.3892/mmr.2015.3544
58. Falleti E, Fabris C, Toniutto P, Fontanini E, Cussigh A, Caldato M, et al. Genetic polymorphisms of inflammatory cytokines and liver fibrosis progression due to recurrent hepatitis C. *Interferon Cytokine Res.* (2007) 27:239–46. doi: 10.1089/jir.2006.0062
59. Karra VK, Gumma PK, Chowdhury SJ, Ruttala R, Polipalli SK, Chakravarti A, et al. IL-18 polymorphisms in hepatitis B virus related liver disease. *Cytokine.* (2015) 73:277–82. doi: 10.1016/j.cyto.2015.02.015
60. Vokurka J, Klapusová L, Pantuckova P, Kukletova M, Kukla L, Holla LI. The association of MMP-9 and IL-18 gene promoter polymorphisms with gingivitis in adolescents. *Arch Oral Biol.* (2009) 54:172–8. doi: 10.1016/j.archoralbio.2008.09.002
61. Leon Rodriguez DA, Carmona FD, Echeverría LE, González CI, Martin J. *IL18* gene variants influence the susceptibility to Chagas disease. *PLoS Negl Trop Dis.* (2016) 10:e0004583. doi: 10.1371/journal.pntd.0004583
62. Estfanous SZK, Ali SA, Seif SM, Soror SHA, Abdelaziz DHA. Inflammasome genes' polymorphisms in Egyptian chronic hepatitis c patients: influence on vulnerability to infection and response to treatment. *Mediators Inflamm.* (2019) 2019:3273645. doi: 10.1155/2019/3273645
63. Chen WJ, Yang JY, Lin JH, Fann CSJ, Osyetrov V, King CC, et al. Nasopharyngeal shedding of severe acute respiratory syndrome-associated coronavirus is associated with genetic polymorphisms. *Clin Infect Dis.* (2006) 42:1561–9. doi: 10.1086/503843
64. Castelar L, Silva MM, Castelli EC, Deghaide NHS, Mendes-Junior CT, Machado AA, et al. Interleukin-18 and interferon-gamma polymorphisms in Brazilian human immunodeficiency virus-1-infected patients presenting with lipodystrophy syndrome. *Tissue Antigens.* (2010) 76:126–30. doi: 10.1111/j.1399-0039.2010.01471.x
65. Affandi JS, Kumar M, Agarwal U, Singh S, Price P. The search for a genetic factor associating with immune restoration disease in HIV patients co-infected with *Mycobacterium tuberculosis*. *Dis Markers.* (2013) 34:445–9. doi: 10.1155/2013/246017
66. Shi BJ, Yu XY, Li H, Xing TH, Fan JW, Wang PW, et al. Association between donor and recipient interleukin-18 gene polymorphisms and the risk of infection after liver transplantation. *Clin Invest Med.* (2017) 40:E176–87. doi: 10.25011/cim.v40i5.28623
67. Bakr NM, Awad A, A Moustafa E. Association of genetic variants in the interleukin-18 gene promoter with risk of hepatocellular carcinoma and metastasis in patients with hepatitis C virus infection. *IUBMB Life.* (2018) 70:165–74. doi: 10.1002/iub.1714
68. Sakai K, Kita M, Sawai N, Shiomi S, Sumida Y, Kanemasa K, et al. Levels of interleukin-18 are markedly increased in *Helicobacter pylori*-infected gastric mucosa among patients with specific *IL18* genotypes. *J Infect Dis.* (2008) 197:1752–61. doi: 10.1086/588196
69. Rezaeifar A, Eskandari-Nasab E, Moghadampour M, Kharazi-Nejad E, Hasani SSA, Asadi-Saghandi A, et al. The association of interleukin-18 promoter polymorphisms and serum levels with duodenal ulcer, and their correlations with bacterial CagA and VacA virulence factors. *Scand J Infect Dis.* (2013) 45:584–92. doi: 10.3109/00365548.2013.794301
70. Hasan FT, Naif HM. Association of gene polymorphisms and serum levels of IL-18 with the susceptibility to infection with hepatitis B virus. *J Infect Dis Med.* (2017) 2:3. doi: 10.4172/2576-1420.1000117
71. Ketelut-Carneiro N, Silva GK, Rocha FA, Milanezi CM, Cavalcanti-Neto FF, Zamboni DS, et al. IL-18 triggered by the Nlrp3 inflammasome induces host innate resistance in a pulmonary model of fungal infection. *J Immunol.* (2015) 194:4507–17. doi: 10.4049/jimmunol.1402321
72. Blotta MHSL, Mamoni RL, Oliveira SJ, Nouér SA, Papaiordanou PMO, Goveia A, et al. Endemic regions of paracoccidioidomycosis in Brazil: a clinical and epidemiologic study of 584 cases in the southeast region. *Am J Trop Med Hyg.* (1999) 61:390–4. doi: 10.4269/ajtmh.1999.61.390
73. Belissimo-Rodrigues F, Machado AA, Martinez R. Paracoccidioidomycosis epidemiological features of 1000-cases series from a hyperendemic area on the Southeast of Brazil. *Am J Trop Med Hyg.* (2011) 85:546–50. doi: 10.4269/ajtmh.2011.11-0084
74. Shikanai-Yasuda MA, Mendes RP, Colombo AL, Queiroz-Telles F, Kono ASG, Paniago AMM, et al. Brazilian guidelines for the clinical management of paracoccidioidomycosis. *Rev Soc Bras Med Trop.* (2017) 50:715–40. doi: 10.1590/0037-8682-0230-2017
75. Aristizabal BH, Clemons KV, Stevens DA, Restrepo A. Morphological transition of *Paracoccidioides brasiliensis* conidia to yeast cells: *in vivo* inhibition in females. *Infect Immun.* (1998) 66:5587–91. doi: 10.1128/IAI.66.11.5587-5591.1998
76. Pinzan CF, Ruas LP, Casabona-Fortunato AS, Carvalho FC, Roque-Barreira MC. Immunological basis for the gender differences in murine *Paracoccidioides brasiliensis* infection. *PLoS ONE.* (2010) 5:e10757. doi: 10.1371/journal.pone.0010757
77. Shankar J, Wu TD, Clemons VK, Monteiro JP, Mirels LF, Stevens DA. Influence of 17-beta-estradiol on gene expression of *Paracoccidioides* during mycelia-to-yeast transition. *PLoS ONE.* (2011) 6:e28402. doi: 10.1371/journal.pone.0028402
78. Severo LC, Roesch EW, Oliveira EA, Rocha MM, Londero AT. Paracoccidioidomycosis in women. *Rev Iberoam Micol.* (1998) 15:88–9.

11

Design and Development of a Novel Peptide for Treating Intestinal Inflammation

Lulu Zhang[1], Xubiao Wei[1], Rijun Zhang[1], Jim N. Petitte[2], Dayong Si[1], Zhongxuan Li[1], Junhao Cheng[1] and Mengsi Du[1]*

[1] *Laboratory of Feed Biotechnology, State Key Laboratory of Animal Nutrition, College of Animal Science and Technology, China Agricultural University, Beijing, China,* [2] *Prestage Department of Poultry Science, North Carolina State University, Raleigh, NC, United States*

***Correspondence:**
Rijun Zhang
rjzhang@cau.edu.cn

Intestinal inflammatory disorders, such as inflammatory bowel disease (IBD), are associated with increased pro-inflammatory cytokine secretion in the intestines. Furthermore, intestinal inflammation increases the risk of enteric cancer, which is a common malignancy globally. Native anti-inflammatory peptides are a class of anti-inflammatory agents that could be used in the treatment of several intestinal inflammation conditions. However, potential cytotoxicity, and poor anti-inflammatory activity have prevented their development as anti-inflammatory agents. Therefore, in this study, we designed and developed a novel hybrid peptide for the treatment of intestinal inflammation. Eight hybrid peptides were designed by combining the active centers of antimicrobial peptides, including LL-37 (13-36), YW12D, innate defense regulator 1, and cathelicidin 2 (1-13) with thymopentin or the active center of thymosin alpha 1 (Tα1) (17-24). The hybrid peptide, LL-37-Tα1 (LTA), had improved anti-inflammatory activity with minimal cytotoxicity. LTA was screened by molecule docking and *in vitro* experiments. Likewise, its anti-inflammatory effects and mechanisms were also evaluated using a lipopolysaccharide (LPS)-induced intestinal inflammation murine model. The results showed that LTA prevented LPS-induced impairment in the jejunum epithelium tissues and infiltration of leukocytes, which are both histological markers of inflammation. Additionally, LTA decreased the levels of tumor necrosis factor-alpha, interferon-gamma, interleukin-6, and interleukin-1β. LTA increased the expression of zonula occludens-1 and occludin, and reduced permeability and apoptosis in the jejunum of LPS-treated mice. Additionally, its anti-inflammatory effect is associated with neutralizing LPS, binding to the Toll-like receptor 4-myeloid differentiation factor 2 (TLR4/MD-2) complex, and modulating the nuclear factor-kappa B signal transduction pathway. The findings of this study suggest that LTA may be an effective therapeutic agent in the treatment of intestinal inflammation.

Keywords: anti-inflammatory activity, toll-like receptor, molecular dynamics simulation, lipopolysaccharide neutralization, intestinal barrier, NF-κB

INTRODUCTION

Intestinal inflammation is a defensive response against infections and damage caused by microbiological toxins or noxious substances (1). Clinical symptoms of intestinal inflammation include abdominal pain, diarrhea, rectal bleeding, weight loss, malnutrition, and fever (2). Furthermore, intestinal patients, such as those with inflammatory bowel disease (IBD), have an increased risk of developing colorectal and small intestinal cancers (3–5). The mechanisms of intestinal inflammation as well as its progression to intestinal cancer have been extensively studied, focusing on dysregulation within the immune response and breakdown of the mucosal barrier (6).

Intestinal inflammation is treated with corticosteroids, specifically glucocorticoids (7, 8). This treatment can successfully decrease the production of pro-inflammatory cytokines and chemokines, cell adhesion molecules, and other key mediators of inflammation (9); however, prolonged use of corticosteroids is related to side effects, including impaired wound healing, mild hirsutism, linear growth inhibition, myopathy, osteoporosis, osteonecrosis, peptic ulcers, pancreatitis, and candidiasis (10, 11). Therefore, there is a need to identify and develop new drugs that have both the desired efficiency and improved safety.

In recent years, antimicrobial peptides (AMPs) have been reported to have anti-inflammatory effects (12–14). AMPs can not only directly interact with lipopolysaccharide (LPS) to inhibit the release of inflammatory cytokines (15, 16), but can also inhibit the translocation of nuclear factor-kappa B (NF-κB) to dampen the inflammatory response (13). As a result, AMPs are especially appealing candidates for the treatment of inflammatory disorders. LL-37 and YW12D effectively neutralize LPS; consequently, they have considerable potential for the treatment of LPS-induced inflammation (15, 17, 18). Cathelicidin 2 (CATH-2), a highly cationic (11^+) chicken heterophil-derived peptide, inhibits IL-1β, and nitric oxide production in LPS-induced HD11 cells (19). Innate defense regulator (IDR)-1, one type of synthetic innate defense regulators, has protective activity against LPS-induced inflammation mediated by modulating NF-κB and mitogen-activated protein kinase (MAPK) signaling pathways (13, 20). Based on their previous anti-inflammatory activity observed, LL-37, IDR-1, CATH2, and YW12D were selected for further study.

Thymopentin (TP5) is a synthetic peptide consisting of five amino acid residues (21), and thymosin alpha 1 (Tα1) is a 28-amino acid peptide produced by thymic stromal cells (22, 23). Both TP5 and Tα1 exhibit similar immunoregulatory activity. They play an important role in regulating immunity, tolerance, and inflammation (24–26). TP5 and Tα1 exert their immune-modulating effect by interacting with Toll-like receptors (TLRs) and intracellular signaling pathways, such as NF-κB, MAPK, and myeloid differentiation primary response 88 (MyD88) pathways (27–29) Additionally, TP5 and Tα1 can counteract a pro-inflammatory cytokine storm and autoimmunity (24, 30, 31). Overall, TP5 and Tα1 exhibit immunoregulatory activity and low cytotoxicity (30, 32). Thus, they are commonly used in the clinic to treat various types of inflammatory diseases, such as cancer and infectious disease (21, 24, 33, 34).

The development of AMPs as potential anti-inflammatory drugs has faced several obstacles that are mainly attributed to their significant cytotoxicity toward eukaryotic cells, hampering their clinical development (19, 35, 36). In contrast, TP5 and Tα1 exhibit low cytotoxicity but relatively weak anti-inflammatory activity (30, 32). To improve the anti-inflammatory activity and reduce undesirable cytotoxic effects of native peptides, hybridization has been put forward. Hybridization is a simple and effective strategy for developing novel therapeutic peptides that combines the advantages of different native peptides (37). It has been reported that LL-37 (13-36) and CATH2 (1-13), which are the short peptides derived from native AMP, can effectively attenuate antigen- and pathogen-induced inflammation (19, 38, 39). Tα1 (17-24) also exhibited good immunoregulatory activity (40, 41). Thus, in the present study, we designed eight hybrid peptides by combining AMPs, including YW12D and IDR-1, or the active center of AMPs, including LL-37 (13-36) and CATH2 (1-13) with TP5 or the active center of Tα1 (17-24). The hybrid peptides were evaluated based on their anti-inflammatory activity and cytotoxicity. The best hybrid, based on these criteria, was screened by molecule docking and *in vitro* experiments. Likewise, its anti-inflammatory effect and mechanism were also evaluated using an LPS-induced murine model of intestinal inflammation.

MATERIALS AND METHODS

Hybrid Peptide Design

The hybrid peptides were constructed by combining the active center of LL-37, YW12D, IDR-1, and CATH2 with the TP5 or the active center of Tα1.The amino acid sequences of the parental and hybrid peptides are listed in the **Table 1**.

Sequence Analysis of Hybrid Peptides

The mean hydrophobicity was calculated online using ProParam (ExPASy Proteomics Server: http://www.expasy.org/tools/protparam.html). The 3D structures of hybrid peptides LL-37-TP5 (LTP), LL-37-Tα1 (LTA), YW12D-TP5 (YTP), YW12D-Tα1 (YTA), IDR-1-TP5 (ITP), IDR-1-Tα1 (ITA), CATH2-TP5 (CTP),

Abbreviations: AMPs, antimicrobial peptides; IDR, innate defense regulator; CATH2, cathelicidin 2; TP5, Thymopentin; Tα1, Thymosin alpha 1; LPS, lipopolysaccharide; LTA, LL-37-Tα1; TNF-α, tumor necrosis factor-alpha; IFN-γ, interferon-gamma; IL-6, interleukin-6; TLR4/MD-2, Toll-like receptor 4/myeloid differentiation factor 2; NF-κB, nuclear factor-kappa B; IBD, inflammatory bowel diseases; UJ, ulcerative jejunitis; TLRs, Toll-like receptors; MAPK, mitogen-activated protein kinase; MyD88, myeloid differentiation primary response 88; LTP, LL-37-TP5; YTP, YW12D-TP5; YTA, YW12D-Tα1; ITP, IDR-1-TP5; ITA, IDR-1-Tα1; CTP, CATH2-TP5; CTA, CATH2-Tα1; DMEM, Dulbecco's modified Eagle's medium; FBS, fetal bovine serum; CCK-8, Cell Counting Kit-8; SPF, specific pathogen free; PMB, Polymyxin B; H&E, hematoxylin-eosin; HRP, horse-radish peroxidase; DAB, 3, 3′diaminobenzidine; DAPI, 4,6-diamidino-2-phenylindole; TUNEL, deoxynucleotidyl transferase mediated dUTP nick end labeling; PPs, Peyer's patches; TEM, Transmission electron microscopy; TJ, tight junctions; TEER, transepithelial electrical resistance; PD, potential difference; Isc, short-circuit current; RT, total electrical resistance; MPO, myeloperoxidase; ZO-1, zonula occluden-1; CE TAL, Chromogenic End-point Tachypleus Amebocyte Lysate; MD, Molecular Dynamics; NPT, number, pressure, and temperature; NVT, number, volume, and temperature; MM-PBSA, Poisson-Boltzmann accessible surface area; IBD, inflammatory bowel diseases.

TABLE 1 | Key physicochemical parameters of parental and hybrid peptides.

Peptides	Sequence	H[a]
LL-37	LLGDFFRKSKEKIGKEFKRIVQRIKDFLRNLVPRTES	−0.559
YW12D	YVKLWRMIKFLR	0.167
IDR-1	KSRIVPAIPVSLL	1.046
CATH2	RWGRFLRKIRRFRPKVTITIQGSARF	−0.638
TP5	RKDVT	−1.608
Tα1	SDAAVDTSSEITTKDLKEKKEVVEEAEN	−1.029
LTP	IGKEFKRIVQRIKDFLRNLVPRTERKDVT	−0.8
LTA	IGKEFKRIVQRIKDFLRNLVPRTEKEKKEVVE	−0.894
YTP	YVKLWRMIKFLRRKDVT	−0.376
YTA	YVKLWRMIKFLRKEKKEVVE	−0.59
ITP	KSRIVPAIPVSLLRKDVT	0.289
ITA	KSRIVPAIPVSLLKEKKEVVE	−0.09
CTP	RWGRFLRKIRRFRRKDVT	−1.61
CTA	RWGRFLRKIRRFRKEKKEVVE	−1.635

[a] *The mean hydrophobicity (H) is the total hydrophobicity (sum of all residue hydrophobicity indices) divided by the number of residues.*

and CATH2-Tα1 (CTA) were built using I-TASSER (http://zhanglab.ccmb.med.umich.edu/I-TASSER/).

Hybrid Peptides Scan by Molecule Docking

The constructed 3D structures of the hybrid peptides were then subjected to molecular docking. The initial structure for myeloid differentiation factor 2 (MD-2) was extracted from the crystal structure of the TLR4/MD-2 complex (PDB code: 2Z64). The initial MD-2/hybrid peptide complex was generated by ZDOCK3.0.2. For each hybrid peptide, a total of 3600 decoy structures were predicted through the rigid-binding option in ZDOCK; among these, the decoy with the lowest energy was chosen for the following flexible docking study. For each molecule, 100 docking runs were performed by flexpepdock (http://flexpepdock.furmanlab.cs.huji.ac.il/). The most plausible docking confirmation with the lowest score, which is calculated by the total Rosetta energy, was selected for scanning of the hybrid peptide.

Peptides Synthesis

The hybrid peptides, LTP, LTA, CTP, and YTP, which were selected via molecule docking, and their parental peptides, LL-37, CATH2, YW12D, TP5, and Tα1, were synthesized and purified by KangLong Biochemistry (Jiangsu, China). The purity of all peptides was higher than 95%, as determined by high performance liquid chromatography (HPLC) and mass spectrometry. The peptides were dissolved in endotoxin-free water and stored at −80°C.

Cell Culture

Mouse macrophage cell line (RAW264.7) was purchased from the Shanghai Cell Bank, the Institute of Cell Biology, China Academy of Sciences (Shanghai, China). The cells were cultured in Dulbecco's modified Eagle's medium (DMEM; Hyclone) supplemented with 10% (v/v) fetal bovine serum (FBS; Bioscience) and 1% (v/v) penicillin/streptomycin (Hyclone) at 37°C in a moist atmosphere (5% CO_2, 95% air).

Cell Viability Assay

The viability of peptide-treated RAW264.7 cells was determined using the Cell Counting Kit-8 (CCK-8) Assay Kit (Dojindo) (42). RAW264.7 cells were pre-seeded on a 96-well plate at a density of 3 × 10^4 cells/mL in 100 μL DMEM medium overnight. The cells were either treated with various concentrations of peptides or without peptides at 37°C and 5% CO_2 for 24 h. Each well was incubated with 10 μL CCK-8 solution for 4 h in the darkness. Then, the absorbance at 450 nm was measured using a microplate reader. Cell viability was calculated as:

$$Cell\ viability\ (\%) = (OD450\ (sample)/OD450(control)) \times 100\%$$

where $OD_{450(sample)}$ is the absorbance at 450 nm of the cells with peptides treated and $OD_{450(control)}$ is the absorbance at 450 nm of the cells without peptides treated.

Animal Model

Seventy-two C57/BL6 male mice (6–8 weeks of age) were purchased from Charles River (Beijing, China). Mice were maintained in a specific pathogen free (SPF) environment at 22 ± 1°C with relative 55 ± 10% humidity, and the assays were performed in conformity with the laws and regulations for live animal treatment at China Agricultural University.

The mice were randomly distributed into six groups (n = 12 each): control, LPS (*E. coli*, O111:B4, Sigma-Aldrich, USA) treatment, LL-37 pretreatment followed by LPS treatment (LL-37 + LPS), Tα1 pretreatment followed by LPS treatment (Tα1 + LPS), LTA pretreatment followed by LPS treatment (LTA + LPS). Different peptides (10 mg/kg mouse weight) were injected intraperitoneally once daily for 7 days, whereas an equal volume of sterile saline was injected intraperitoneally to the control and LPS-treated groups. On day 7, mice in LPS, LL-37 + LPS, Tα1 + LPS, and LTA + LPS groups were intraperitoneally injected with LPS (10 mg/kg mouse weight) 1h after saline or the peptides treatment, and the control group was intraperitoneally injected with an equal volume of saline. The mice were then euthanized by cervical dislocation 6 h after intraperitoneal injection of LPS or saline, and samples of the intestines were collected for analysis. The body weights of the mice were recorded before and after the experiment.

Histopathology and Immunohistochemistry

Intestinal tissues samples from the jejunum were fixed in 4% paraformaldehyde immediately after the mice were euthanized. After embedding, the tissues were sectioned (5 μm) using an RM2235 microtome (Leica) and stained with hematoxylin-eosin (H&E). Images were acquired using a DM3000 microscope. LPS-induced intestinal injury was evaluated using Chiu's score (43) according to changes of the villus and glands of the jejunal mucosa. Villus height and crypt depth were measured using CaseViewer software.

For immunohistochemical analysis of $CD177^+$, nonspecific binding sites were blocked with PBS containing 1% w/v BSA for 1 h. Anti-$CD177^+$ antibodies (Santa, USA) were added at a dilution of 1:100 and incubated overnight at 4°C. Samples were washed five times in PBS and treated with horse-radish peroxidase (HRP)-conjugated rabbit anti-goat IgG (JIR, USA) at ratio of 1:100; samples were left to incubate at 4°C for 1 h. After washing with PBS, 3,3′-diaminobenzidine (DAB; DAKO, USA) was added, and the slides were counterstained with Harris hematoxylin. Finally, the samples were dehydrated in an alcohol gradient (70–100%), and cleared in xylene. All slides were mounted in neutral balsam.

The apoptotic cells in the jejunal sections were detected via a commercial the terminal deoxynucleotidyl transferase mediated dUTP nick end labeling (TUNEL) staining kit according to the manufacturer's instruction (Roche, Indianapolis, IN, USA). The sections were co-stained with the DAPI (Servicebio, Wuhan, China). The number of apoptotic cells was counted in four to six randomly selected fields at 200× magnification.

Transmission Electron Microscopy (TEM)

The tight junctions (TJs) between gut epithelial cells were observed by TEM. A jejunum specimen was excised with a scalpel and fixed in 2.5% glutaraldehyde for 4 h at 4°C. Afterwards, the specimens were treated with osmic acid and embedded in epon. Ultrathin sections were acquired using a diamond knife, and stained with uranyl acetate and lead citrate before visualization by TEM (Model H-7650, HITACHI, Japan).

Measurement of Transepithelial Electrical Resistance (TEER)

The TEER values of intestinal membranes were assessed by an *in vitro* diffusion chamber method using stripped mouse jejunal membranes. The underlying muscularis of the jejunal membranes were removed, and the jejunal segments were mounted in a diffusion chamber with an exposed surface area of 1.78 cm^2. Using chambers were equipped with two pairs of electrodes connected to the chambers by 3 M KCl/3.5% agar bridges. Each side of the chamber was bubbled with a mixture of 5% CO_2 and 95% O_2 to maintain the viability of the jejunal membranes. The temperature was maintained at 37°C during the experiment by a circulating water bath. The potential difference (PD) and the short-circuit current (Isc) were measured, and then, total electrical resistance (RT) was calculated by Ohm's law, that is RT = PD/Isc (44).

ELISA

RAW264.7 cells were treated with or without 10 μg/mL peptides for 1h before the addition of 100 ng/mL LPS and further incubation for 12 h at 37°C. Levels of tumor necrosis factor-alpha (TNF-α), interleukin-6 (IL-6), and IL-1β were detected in culture supernatant and jejunum, respectively. In addition, the level of interferon-gamma (IFN-γ) was detected in the jejunum. ELISA was performed using a commercial ELISA kit (eBioscience, San Diego, USA).

The activities of myeloperoxidase (MPO) in the jejunum were detected using ELISA kits (Boster Wuhan, China) according to the manufacturer's instructions.

Western Blotting

Whole protein of intestinal tissues was obtained with the whole protein extraction kit (KeyGEN Biotech, Nanjing, China) according to the manufacturer's instructions. The protein concentration was measured via the BCA kit (KeyGEN Biotech, Nanjing, China). Protein samples (40 μg protein/lane) were separated by 10% sodium dodecyl sulfate-polyacrylamide gel electrophoresis (SDS-PAGE) and transferred to polyvinylidene difluoride (PVDF) membranes (Bio-Rad). The membranes were blocked with 5% nonfat dried milk in 0.05% TBST and immunoblotted with primary specific antibodies against inhibitor of κB (IκB)-α, p-IκB-α, IκB kinase (IKK)-β, p-IKK-β, NF-κB (p65), p-NF-κB (p-p65), zonula occluden-1 (ZO-1), occludin, and β-actin (Santa Cruz, CA, USA). After washing with TBST, membranes were incubated with anti-mouse/rabbit HRP-conjugated secondary antibodies (HuaAn, Hangzhou China). The proteins were detected with SuperSignal West Femto maximum sensitivity substrate (Pierce Biotechnology) and

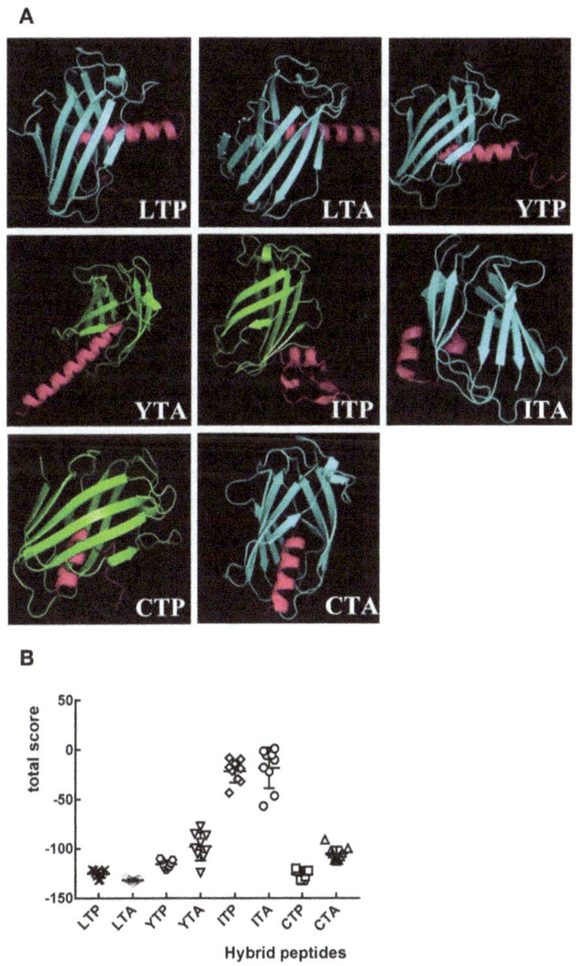

FIGURE 1 | The overall structure of hybrid peptide-MD-2 Complex. **(A)** Shows the views of the hybrid peptides (red) binding to MD-2 (blue or green). **(B)** An energy plot with 10 out of 100 decoy structures from an MD-2 docking study by Flexpepdock. Data are given as mean values ± standard.

visualized using a ChemiDoc MP Imaging System (Bio-Rad, Hercules, CA, USA).

Neutralization of LPS

The neutralization of LPS by the peptides was assessed using a quantitative Chromogenic End-point Tachypleus Amebocyte Lysate (CE TAL) assay via the QCL-1000 kit (Xiamen, China). A constant concentration of LPS (1.0 EU/mL final concentration; *E. coli*, O111:B4, Sigma-Aldrich, USA) was incubated with various concentrations of the peptides or polymyxin B (PMB) (0–64 μg/mL final concentration; Sigma-Aldrich, USA) at 37°C for 15 min in the wells of pyrogenic sterile microliters plates. The 100 μL aliquots concentrate of limulus amebocyte lysate reagent was added and incubated at 37°C for 6 min. On the addition of chromogenic substrate, yellow color appeared. The reactions were stopped by adding 25% HCl, and then the absorbances measured at 540 nm (45).

The level of LPS in the plasma were detected using QCL-1000 kit (Xiamen, China) according to the manufacturer's instructions.

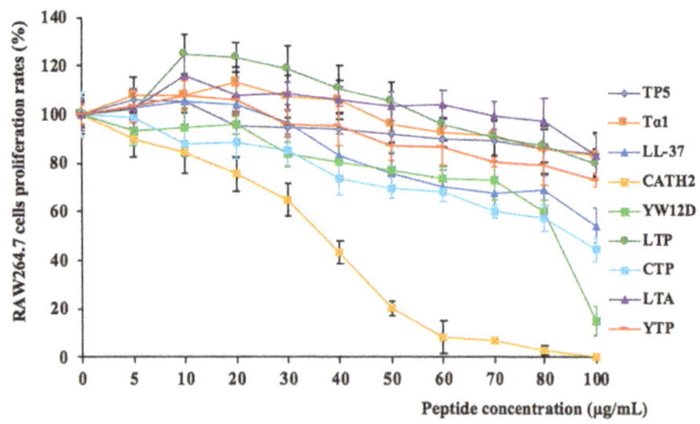

FIGURE 2 | Cell proliferation rates of RAW264.7 cells in the absence or presence of parental peptides and hybrid peptides. RAW264.7 cells were pre-seeded in DMEM medium overnight. The cells were treated with various concentrations of peptides or without peptides at 37°C and 5% CO_2 for 24 h. They were incubated with CCK-8 solution for 4 h, and then, they were measured at 450 nm. Data are given as mean values ± standard deviation from 8 biological replicates.

Molecular Dynamics Simulation

The crystallographic structure of the TLR4/MD-2 complex was taken from PDB bank (PDB code: 2Z64), and the initial structure for MD-2 was extracted from the crystal structure of the TLR4/MD-2 complex. The missing hydrogen atoms were added under pH 7.0 by Maestro (46). The docking pose was determined by RosettaDock (version 3.5), and the pose with the lowest score (total Rosetta energy for this model) was selected for further analysis.

The best binding pose of LTA with MD-2 was refined using a molecular dynamics (MD) simulation with AMBER14 (47, 48). The force fields used for the simulation were GAFF and FF14SB, and the system was solvated with TIP3P water molecules in a cubic box with a minimum distance of 10 Å between the protein

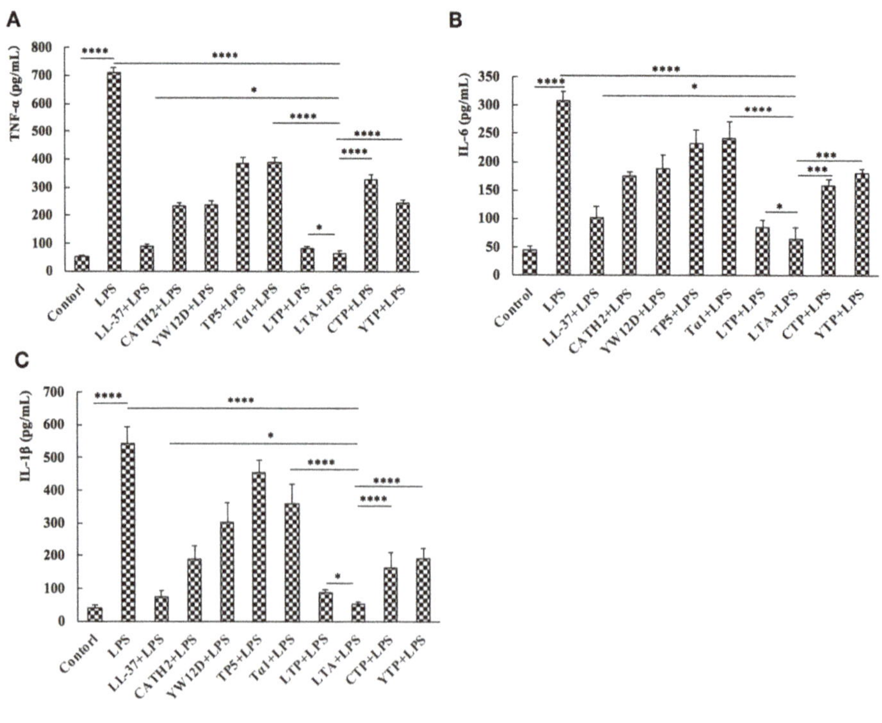

FIGURE 3 | Hybrid peptides suppress the LPS-induced cytokine secretion. 12 h after treatment with 100 ng/mL LPS in the presence or absence of peptides, protein levels of TNF-α **(A)**, IL-6 **(B)**, and IL-1β **(C)** in RAW264.7 cells were quantified by ELISA. Data are given as mean values ± standard deviation from 3 biological replicates. NS: $P > 0.05$, $^{*}P \leq 0.05$, $^{***}P \leq 0.001$, and $^{****}P \leq 0.0001$.

and the edge of the box. Na^+ and Cl^- atoms were added to mimic the physiological conditions and neutralize the system. The system was first minimized with 5000 steps by the conjugate gradient algorithm, following by heating gradually over 100 ps. Subsequently, the volume of the system was adjusted under a constant number, pressure, and temperature (NPT) ensemble. Afterwards, a 60 ns MD simulation was performed under constant number, volume, and temperature (NVT) ensemble.

Based on the 300 snapshots extracted from the last 40 ns of the equilibrated MD simulation, the long-range electrostatic interactions were calculated by the Particle-mesh Ewald (PME) method (49), and the binding energy was calculated by the molecular mechanics Poisson-Boltzmann accessible surface area (MM-PBSA) method (50).

Flow Cytometry

RAW264.7 cells were treated with PBS, anti-mouse mAbTLR4/MD-2 complex (MTS510 Ab) (eBioscience, San Diego, USA) or isotype control (IgG) (eBioscience, San Diego, USA) for 1 h at 4°C before staining with 10 µg/mL N-terminus fluorescein isothiocyanate (FITC)-labeled LTA. The cells were then harvested by trypsin and washed five times with PBS. The average FITC intensity of the cells was measured via flow cytometry.

Analysis of Confocal Laser-Scanning Microscopy

To verify TLR4/MD-2 as the pattern recognition receptor, RAW264.7 cells were treated with PBS, MTS510 Ab or isotype control (IgG) (eBioscience, San Diego, USA) for 1 h at 4°C. Afterwards, RAW264.7 cells were incubated with N-terminus FITC-LTA at 10 µg/mL for 1 h at 4°C in the dark. Then, the cells were washed with PBS, fixed with paraformaldehyde, and rinsed twice with PBS. The cell nuclei were stained with DAPI (diluted 1:500 in PBS) (Sigma, USA) for 5 min, and the cells were rinsed six times with PBS. The above cells were spread on a glass slide, fixed, and observed via a Leica TCA sp5 confocal microscope (Germany).

Statistics

All data are expressed as mean values ± standard deviation from at least 3 independent experiments. Statistical comparisons were carried out by Student's t test and ANOVA test with GraphPad Prism v6 software (La Jolla, California). Significance was claimed with P values ≤ 0.05. NS: $P > 0.05$, $^{*}P \leq 0.05$, $^{**}P \leq 0.01$, $^{***}P \leq 0.001$, and $^{****}P \leq 0.0001$.

RESULTS

Selection of Anti-inflammatory Peptides by Molecular Docking

As an initial screen of the anti-inflammatory peptides, the binding modes of the eight hybrid peptides to MD-2 were analyzed by molecular docking. As shown in **Figures 1A,B**, of the eight hybrid peptides, LTP, LTA, YTP, and CTP had more favorable docking scores to MD-2, and the total social of them was lower than −100.

Cytotoxicity on RAW264.7 Macrophage Cells

The cytotoxic activity of the peptides on RAW264.7 macrophage cells was evaluated by CCK-8 assay, and the results are shown in **Figure 2**. Among the initial selected hybrid peptides and their parental peptides, LTP, and LTA exhibited the lowest cytotoxic activity, and the cell viability of the lower doses LTP- and LTA-treated cells was greater than 100%. Meanwhile, all the selected hybrid peptides showed lower cytotoxicity than their parental peptides. The cell viability of the peptide-treated RAW264.7 cells was greater than 80%. These data indicated that at a concentration of 10 µg/mL, all of the peptides were minimally cytotoxic to RAW264.7 cells and suitable for the following experiments.

Inhibition of Cytokine Release From LPS-Stimulated RAW264.7 Cells

To evaluate the anti-inflammatory effect of the hybrid peptides, the mouse macrophage cell line, RAW264.7, was used as a model. ELISA results show that all parental peptides and hybrid peptides were potent inhibitors of pro-inflammatory cytokine release (**Figure 3**). LPS caused a significant elevation in TNF-α, IL-6, and IL-1β levels compared to untreated RAW264.7 cells. Compared to the other tested peptides, 10 µg/mL of LTA in the presence of LPS caused a remarkable decrease in the release of TNF-α (**Figure 3A**), IL-6 (**Figure 3B**), and IL-1β (**Figure 3C**). Collectively, these data suggest that LTA is suitable for further anti-inflammatory experiments.

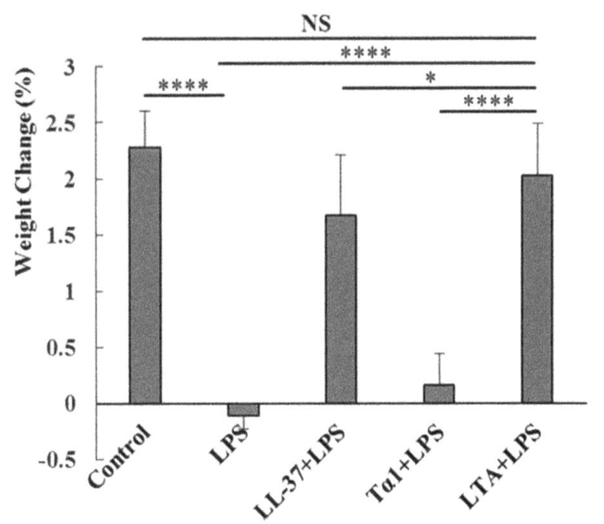

FIGURE 4 | Protective effects of LTA on body weight. Different peptides (10 mg/kg) were injected into the mice once daily for 6 days, whereas the control and LPS-treated groups were injected with an equal volume of sterile saline. On day 6, mice in the LPS and peptide-pretreated groups were injected with LPS (10 mg/kg) 1 h after the peptide or saline treatment. The control group was injected with an equal volume of saline. The body weights of the mice were recorded before and after the experiment. Data are given as mean values ± standard deviation from 12 biological replicates. NS: $P > 0.05$, $^{*}P \leq 0.05$, and $^{****}P \leq 0.0001$.

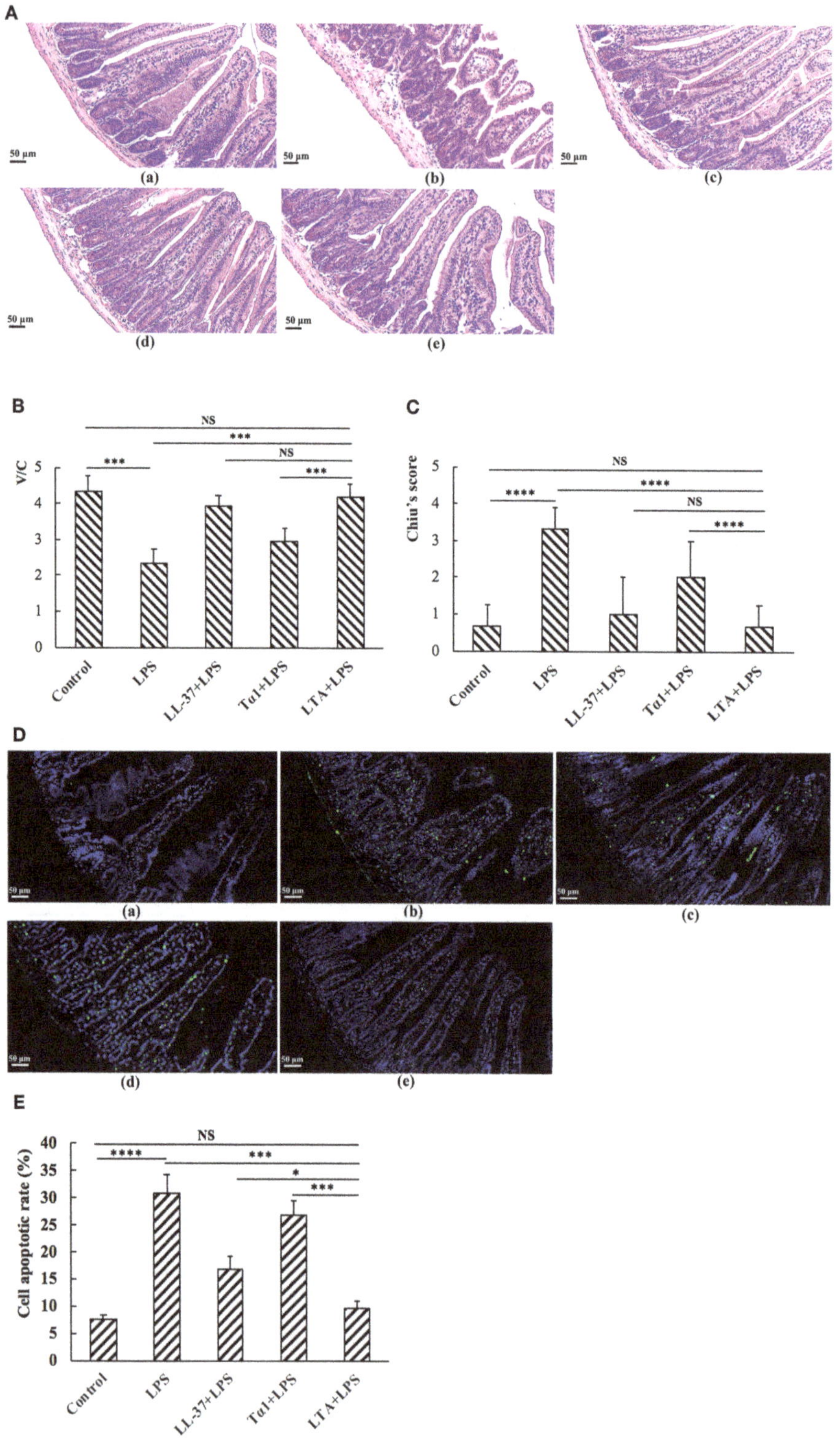

FIGURE 5 | The protective effects of LTA against LPS-induced clinical symptoms in mouse jejunum. Representative H&E-stained sections from (**A**,a) control, (**A**,b) LPS, (**A**,c) LL-37 + LPS, (**A**,d) Tα1 + LPS, (**A**,e) LTA + LPS. Original magnification 200 ×. **(B)** The effect of LTA on Chiu's scores. Chiu's score is comprised of changes of the villus and glands of the jejunal mucosa **(C)** The effect of LTA on the ratio of villus height to crypt depth (V/C) of the jejunum. **(D)** TUNEL staining of jejunal tissues. Original magnification 200 ×. (**D**,a) Control, (**D**,b) LPS, (**D**,c) LL-37 + LPS, (**D**,d) Tα1 + LPS, (**D**,e) LTA + LPS. **(E)** The number of apoptotic cells in 4–6 randomly selected fields was counted according to the number of positive green cells and the average calculated. Data are given as mean values ± standard deviation from 12 biological replicates. NS: $P > 0.05$, $^{*}P \leq 0.05$, $^{***}P \leq 0.001$, and $^{****}P \leq 0.0001$.

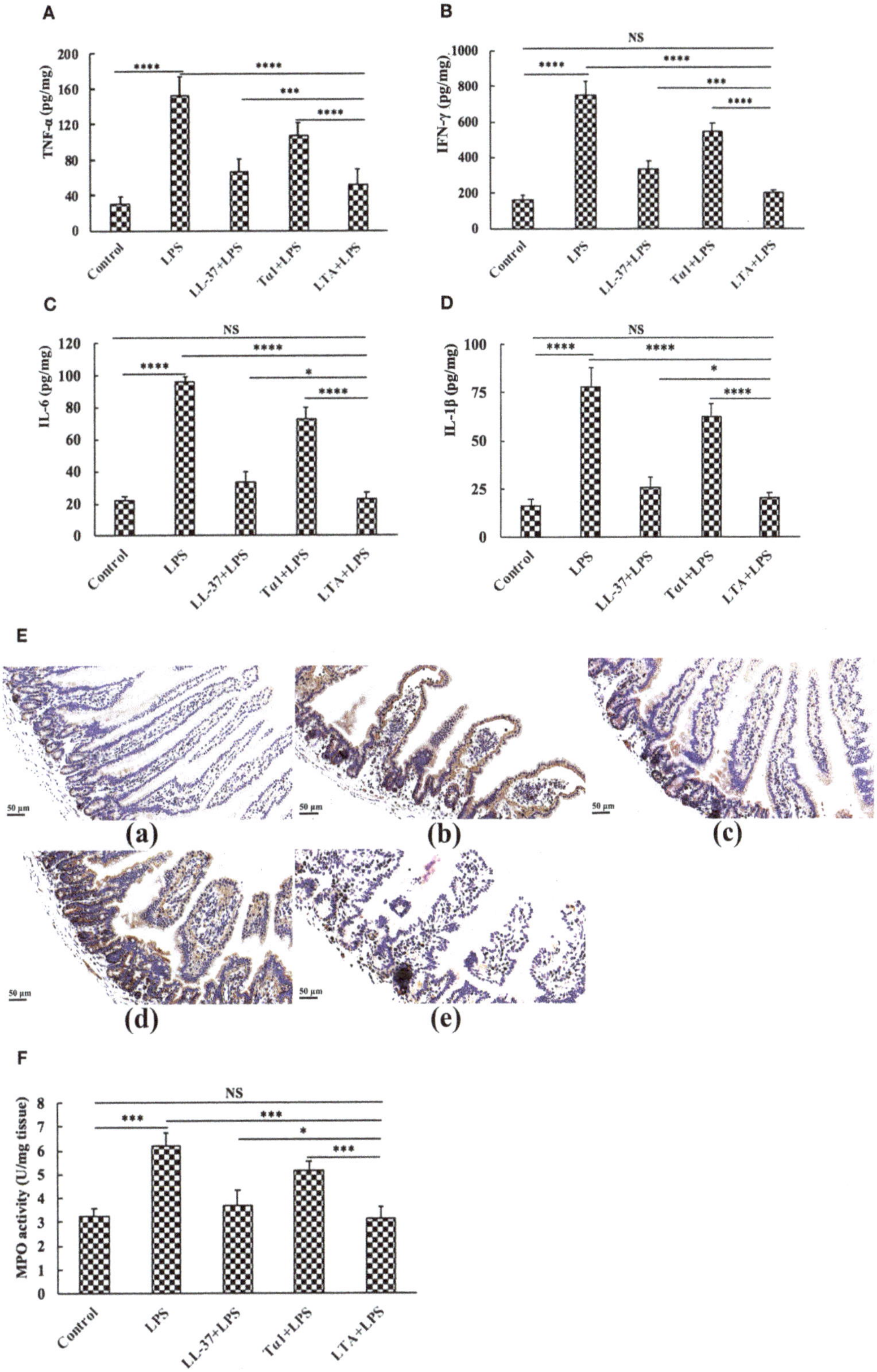

FIGURE 6 | The protective effects of LTA on the inflammatory response. ELISA for TNF-α **(A)**, IFN-γ **(B)**, IL-6 **(C)**, and IL-1β **(D)** in jejunal tissues. **(E)** Representative images of CD177+. Original magnification 400 ×. Formalin-fixed, paraffin-embedded 5-mm cross-sections were stained with a primary Ab to CD177+. (**E**,a) control, (**E**,b) LPS, (**E**,c) LL-37+LPS, (**E**,d) Tα1+LPS, (**E**,e) LTA+LPS. Enzymatic activities of MPO were measured **(F)**. Data are given as mean values ± standard deviation from 12 biological replicates. NS: $P > 0.05$, $^{*}P \leq 0.05$, $^{***}P \leq 0.001$, and $^{****}P \leq 0.0001$.

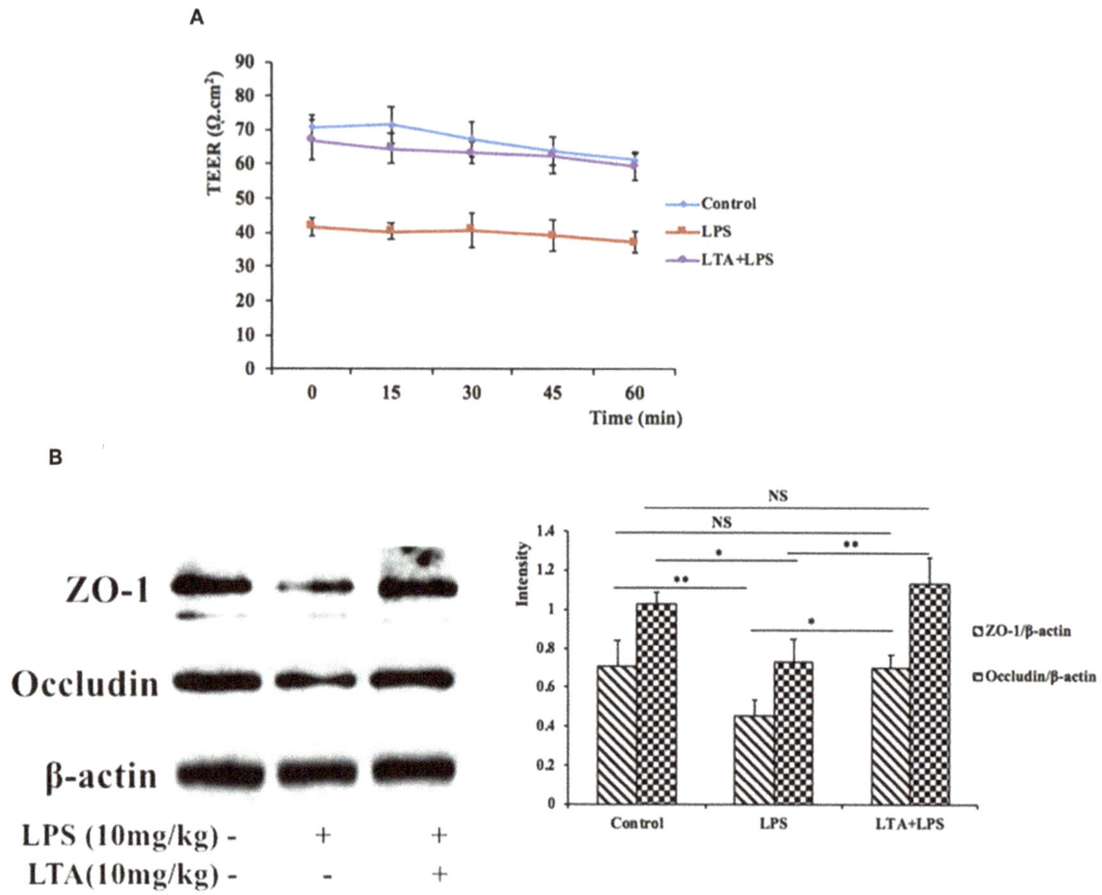

FIGURE 7 | The protective effects of LTA on the intestinal barrier. **(A)** TEER of mouse jejunal epithelium was measured *ex vivo* in Ussing chambers. **(B)** Expression of TJ proteins was determined by western-blot. Data are given as mean values ± standard deviation from at least 3 biological replicates. NS: $P > 0.05$, $^{*}P \leq 0.05$, and $^{**}P \leq 0.01$.

Effect of Hybrid Peptides on Body Weight

As expected, LPS treatment resulted in weight loss. Mice in the LPS-treated group showed significant weight loss compared to the control group. Mice in the LTA-pretreated group recovered their weight loss rapidly (**Figure 4**). Based on the weight-loss recovery, the hybrid peptide, LTA, appears to be more potent than the parental peptides (**Figure 4**).

The Protective Effects of LTA Against LPS-Induced Damage in Jejunum Tissue

Mice in the LPS group had significantly more macroscopic inflammation than those in the control and LTA-pretreated groups. Compared to the control, histological examination of the jejunum tissue in the LPS group showed considerable tissue injury (**Figure 5A**) and a decreased villus height to crypt depth (V/C) ratio (**Figure 5C**). Overall, the LPS-induced intestinal damage was significantly attenuated by LTA pretreatment; Chiu's score was restored from 3.33 ± 0.58 to 0.67 ± 0.58, and the V/C value was restored from 2.35 ± 0.389 to 4.19 ± 0.364 ($p \leq 0.05$) (**Figure 5B**). Based on the Chiu's score, the newly designed hybrid peptide appears to be more potent than the parental peptides (**Figure 5B**). In addition, the V/C value in the LTA-pretreated group was markedly increased compared to that in the Tα1-pretreated group. No statistical significance was found among the LTA-pretreated group compared to the LL-37-pretreated group (**Figure 5C**).

As shown by TUNEL staining, apoptosis of the LPS-treated group was significantly higher than that of the control group, as quantified by the apoptosis index (**Figures 5D,E**). Compared to the LPS-treated group, pretreatment with LTA in LPS-administered mice significantly reduced the apoptosis index (**Figures 5D,E**). In addition, the apoptosis index in the LTA-pretreated group was markedly decreased compared to the parental peptides.

To characterize the protective effect of LTA against inflammation in LPS-induced mice, the secretion of the inflammatory markers, TNF-α, IFN-γ, IL-6, and IL-1β were evaluated by ELISA. Administration of LPS caused a significant elevation of these pro-inflammatory cytokines in the jejunum compared to the control group (**Figures 6A–D**). **Figures 6A–D** shows that all peptides attenuated TNF-α, IFN-γ, IL-6, and IL-1β secretion. Meanwhile, mice in the LTA-pretreated group had

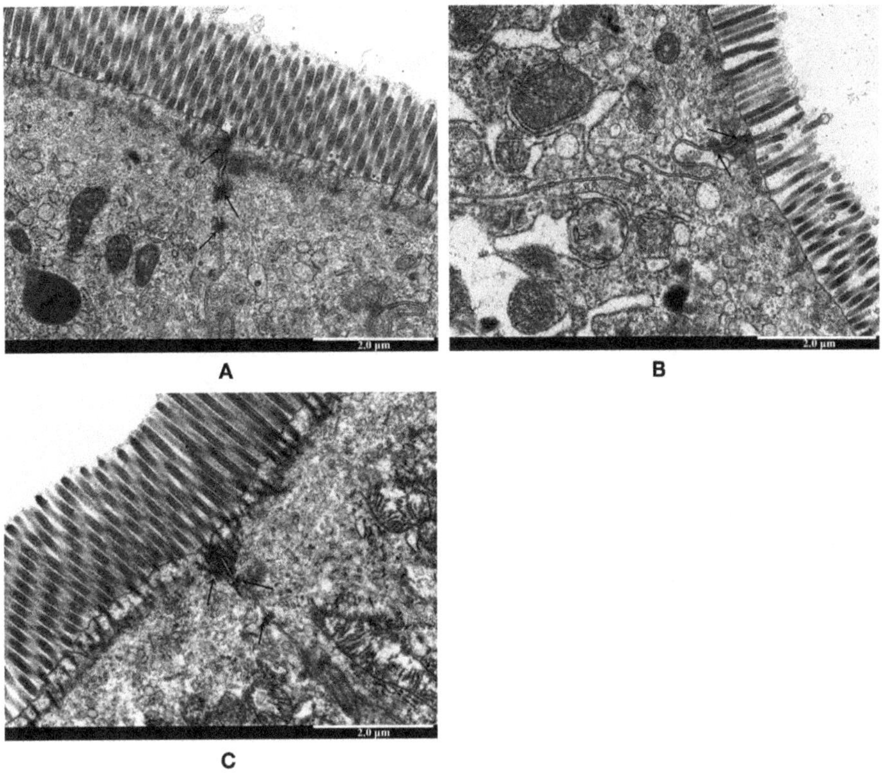

FIGURE 8 | The protective effects of LTA on intestinal TJs structure. TJs structure in the jejunal epithelium was confirmed by transmission electron microscope (TEM). Original magnification 20000 × **(A)** control, **(B)** LPS, **(C)** LTA+LPS. The wider intervals (black arrowheads) between the intestinal epithelial cells are indicated.

significantly lower TNF-α, IFN-γ, IL-6, and IL-1β concentrations than those in the Tα1- or LL-37-pretreated groups.

The infiltration of $CD177^+$ cells into jejunal tissue was detected via immunohistochemistry. In contrast to minimal infiltration of neutrophils into the jejunum of control mice, LPS triggered increased infiltration of $CD177^+$ neutrophils into the jejunal lesion area (**Figure 6E**). Pretreatment with the peptides reduced the infiltration of neutrophils compared to the group treated with LPS alone (**Figure 6E**). LTA, the most active peptide, reduced this effect to the basal level.

MPO (an indicator of jejunal infiltration by leukocytes) activity in the jejunum tissue from LPS treated mice was significantly increased compared to control mice. LTA pretreatment showed markedly decreased MPO activity compared to the LPS-treated group (**Figure 6F**). Moreover, MPO activity in the LTA-pretreated group was markedly decreased compared to Tα1 and LL-37 pretreatment (**Figure 6F**). Collectively, all of these results support the assertion that LTA is the most active peptide against LPS-induced impairment of mice, and it is suitable for further experiments.

LTA Prevented the LPS-Stimulated Disruption of Intestinal TJ Structure and Function

To assess the functional integrity of mouse intestinal epithelium under *ex vivo* conditions, TEER measurements were performed for 60 min. Compared to the control group, the TEER values in the LPS-treated group declined remarkably (**Figure 7A**), indicating an increase in permeability. However, pretreatment with LTA resulted in a significant protective effect; the TEER values in the LTA-pretreated group were similar to those in the control group (**Figure 7A**). These results suggest that LTA minimizes LPS-induced intestinal epithelial hyper permeability.

To investigate the protective effects of LTA on the LPS-stimulated disruption of TJs, TJ marker (ZO-1 and Occludin) levels were determined by western blotting. Compared to control group, the expression of ZO-1 and Occludin was down-regulated in mice treated with LPS alone (**Figure 7B**). However, the expression of these TJ markers in the LTA-pretreated group was significantly higher than that in the LPS-group (**Figure 7B**). These data suggest that LTA maintains the integrity of the junction complex. In addition, TEM, which was used to determine the TJs between gut epithelial cells, supported the protective effect of LTA against LPS-induced damage in jejunum tissues (**Figure 8**).

LTA Effects on the NF-κB Signaling Pathway in LPS-Induced Mice

Next, we investigated the NF-κB signaling pathway in LPS-induced mice pretreated with or without LTA to determine the mechanism by which LTA induces its anti-inflammatory

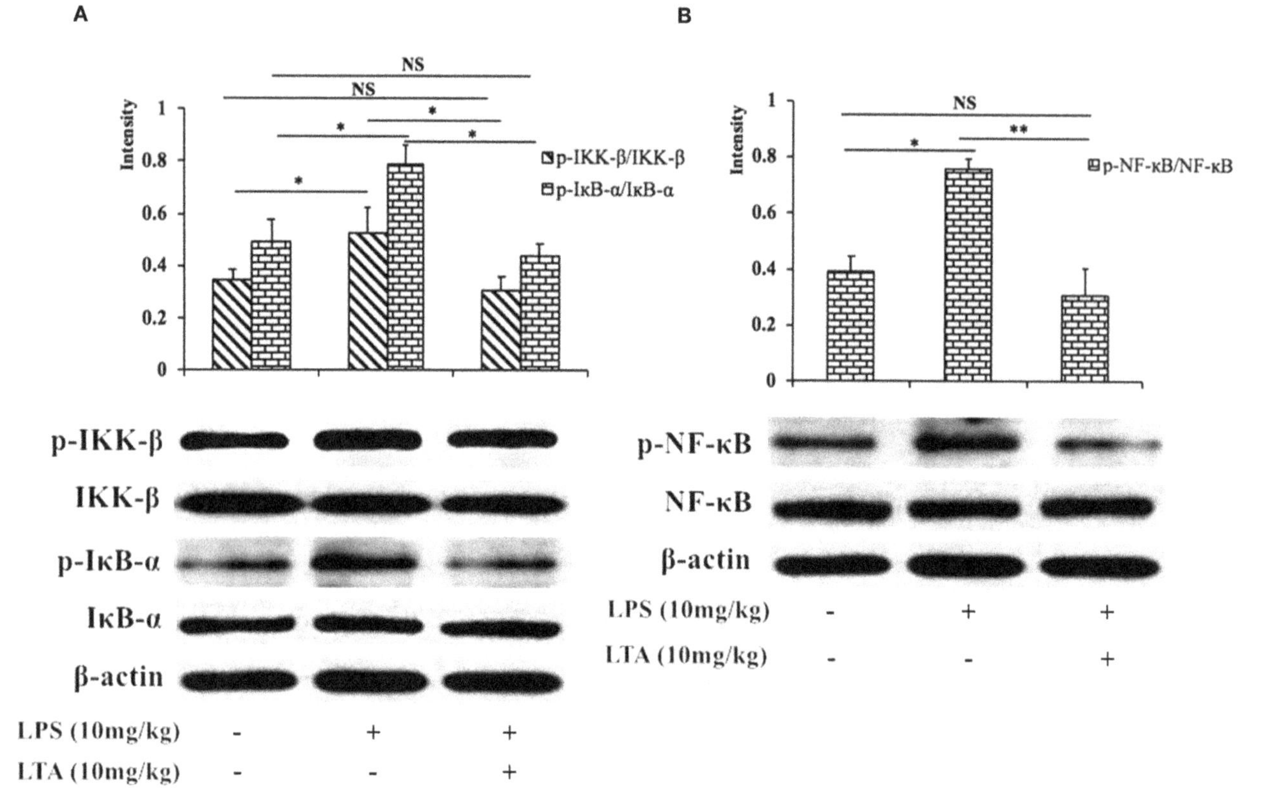

FIGURE 9 | Inhibitory effect of LTA on the NF-κB signaling pathways in mice. Phosphorylated and total protein levels of IKK-β and IκB-α **(A)**, NF-κB **(B)**, and β-actin from jejunal tissues were measured by western blot analyses. Data are given as mean values ± standard deviation from 3 biological replicates. NS: $P > 0.05$, $^{*}P \leq 0.05$, and $^{**}P \leq 0.01$.

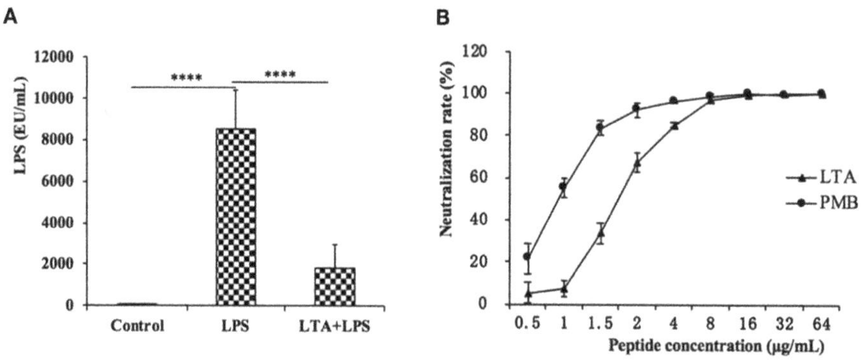

FIGURE 10 | LPS neutralization activity of LTA *in vitro* and *in vivo*. **(A)** The LPS concentration in the mice plasma. **(B)** *In vitro* LPS neutralization by LTA. Binding of LTA (shown as triangles) or PMB (shown as a circle) binding to LPS was determined using the chromogenic *in vitro* TAL assay. Data are given as mean values ± standard deviation from 3 biological replicates. NS: $P > 0.05$, $^{****}P \leq 0.0001$.

activity. The phosphorylation of IKK-β, IκB-α, and NF-κB increased significantly after stimulation with LPS, but the phosphorylation decreased in the group pretreated with LTA (**Figure 9**). These results suggest that one mechanism by which LTA modulates the immune system in mice is via the NF-κB pathway.

LPS Neutralization Activity of LTA *in vitro* and *in vivo*

The plasma LPS concentration in the mice was evaluated by the CE TAL test. In the LPS-treated group, the plasma LPS level sharply increased, but LTA significantly reduced the plasma LPS level (**Figure 10A**).

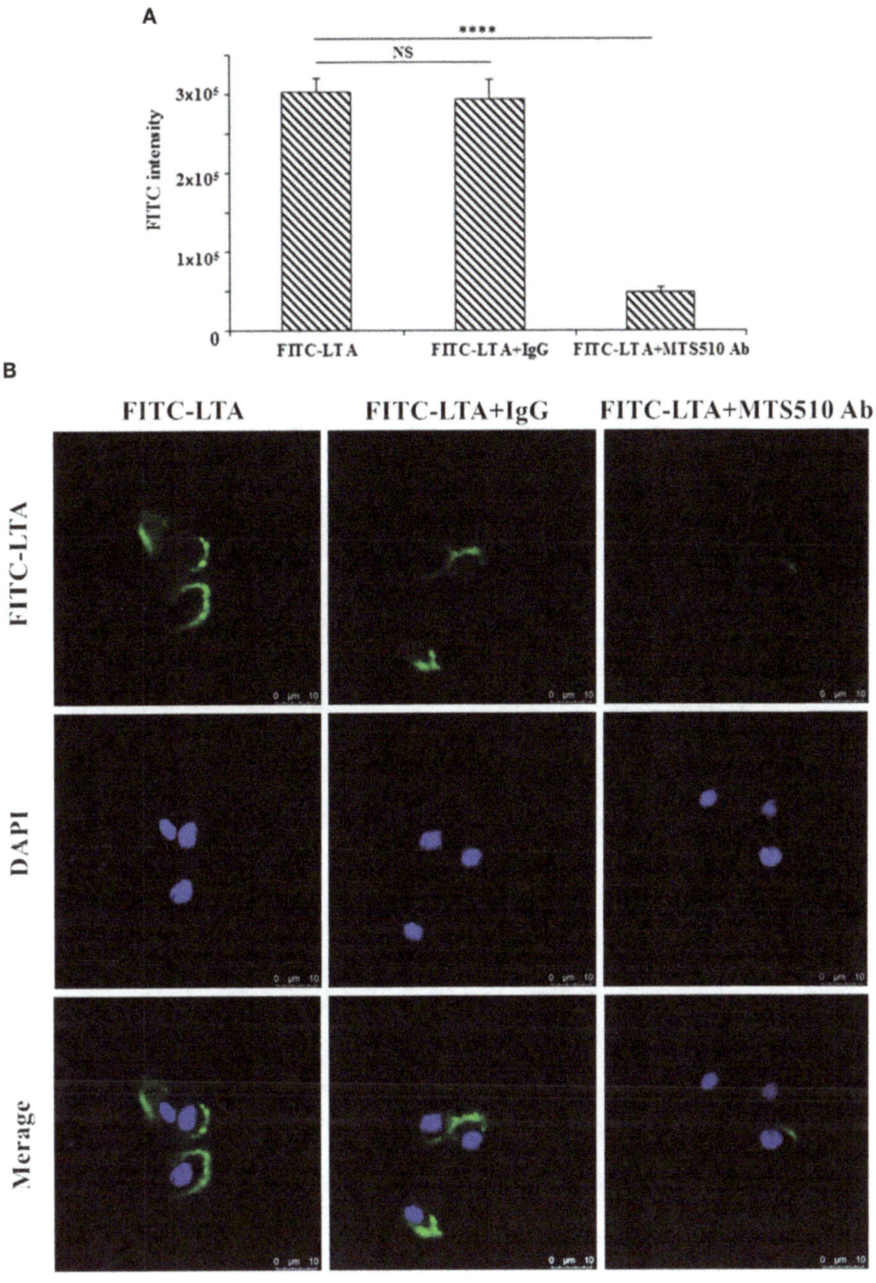

FIGURE 11 | TLR4/MD-2-dependent staining of RAW264.7 cells with FITC-LTA. **(A)** RAW264.7 cells were treated with PBS, anti-mouse mAbTLR4/MD-2 complex (MTS510 Ab) or isotype control (IgG) for 1 h at 4°C before staining with 10 μg/mL. The cells were then harvested by trypsin and washed five times with PBS. The above cells were analyzed by the flow cytometry. **(B)** Cells were treated with PBS, MTS510 Ab, or IgG before FITC-LTA staining for confocal laser scanning microscopy analysis. Bar, 10 μm. Data are given as mean values ± standard deviation from 3 biological replicates. NS: $P > 0.05$, $^{****}P \leq 0.0001$.

To test whether LTA neutralized LPS, an LPS neutralization activity was performed *in vitro*. As shown in **Figure 10B**, LTA inhibited the activation of tachypleus amebocyte lysate in a dose-dependent manner. The LPS neutralization activity LTA is similar to PMB, a cyclic hydrophobic peptide known to bind LPS (51), and LTA could completely neutralize LPS at 8 ug/mL or more.

The Specific Binding of LTA to TLR4/MD-2

To determine the recognition receptor, a binding assay of LTA to a receptor on the plasma membrane was performed via flow cytometry (**Figure 11A**) and confocal laser-scanning microscopy (**Figure 12B**). FITC-LTA caused a significant increase in the fluorescence intensity of RAW264.7 cells compared to the intensity of cells blocked with an

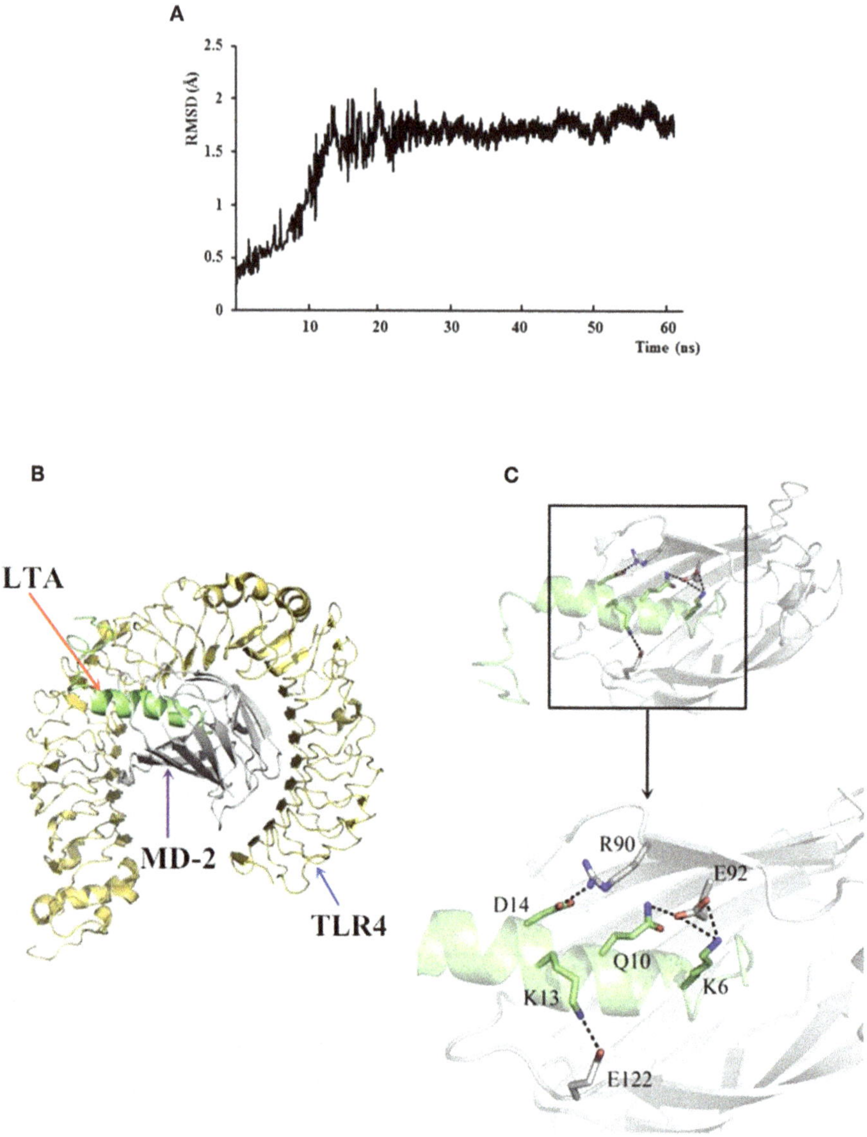

FIGURE 12 | The docking results of LTA to the TLR4/MD-2 complex. **(A)** Time evolution of RMSD during molecular dynamics simulation. **(B)** LTA is bound to the hydrophobic pocket of MD2. The yellow ribbons represented TLR4, gray ribbons represented MD2, and green ribbons represented LTA. **(C)** A close-up view of LTA binding to the MD-2. Residues involved in the interaction between LTA and MD-2 are displayed.

anti-mouse TLR4/MD-2 mAb. Meanwhile, this increased fluorescence intensity was not attenuated by IgG (**Figure 12A**). Similar results were also seen via confocal laser-scanning microscopy (**Figure 11B**).

To further predict binding of LTA to the TLR4/MD-2 complex, MD simulations were performed. Based on the root-mean square deviation (RMSD) values of TLR4/MD-2 (**Figure 12A**), the MD simulation was fully equilibrated during the full 60 ns. A total of 300 snapshots was taken from the last stable 40 ns of the MD simulation. The calculated binding free energy, which was well correlated with the determined binding affinities, is shown in **Table 2**. The binding energy of LTA to MD-2 calculated by MM-PBSA method was −996.2 kJ/mol. The interface of MD-2 that is bound to LPS was compared to that of LTA. There was a common hydrophobic pocket on MD-2 where both LPS (52) and LTA interacted with the protein (**Figures 12B,C**). The interaction between LTA and MD-2 was principally mediated by salt-bridges and hydrogen bonds between Asp14 (LTA) - Arg 90 (MD-2), Lys 6 and Gln 10 (LTA) - Glu 92 (MD-2), and Lys 13 (LTA) – Glu 122 (MD-2) (**Table 3**). This is consistent with the flow cytometry and confocal laser-scanning microscopy results that suggest that LTA blocks LPS binding to TLR4/MD2 complex, resulting in the LPS-antagonizing effects.

TABLE 2 | Key parameters of interactions between LTA and MD-2.

Interaction pair	Number of salt-bridges	Number of hydrogen bonds	Interaction surface (Å^2)	Binding free energy (kj/mol)
MD2...LTA	4	5	343	−996.2

TABLE 3 | Distances and salt-bridges between the binding residues of LTA and MD-2.

Interaction pair MD2...LTA	Distance (Å)	Salt-bridges
R_{90}-NH_2...D_{14}-OD_1	3.30	+
E_{122}-OE_2...K_{13}-NZ	3.00	+
E_{122}-OE_1...K_{13}-NZ	2.94	+
E_{92}-OE_1...Q_{10}-NE_2	3.00	-
E_{92}-OE_1...K_6-NZ	3.03	+
E_{92}-OE_2...K_6-NZ	3.19	+

The distance and salt-bridges of interaction pairs are extrapolated from the LTA/MD-2 molecular dynamics simulation. "+" means existence, and "−" means not determined.

DISCUSSION

LPS, a major component of the cell wall of Gram-negative bacteria, is released by antibiotic intake and can lead to intestinal inflammation. Intestinal inflammation is a chronic inflammatory disease associated with engagement of the immune response by increased pro-inflammatory cytokine secretion in the intestines (53, 54). Historically, intestinal inflammation is more common in western countries than Asia; the increasing incidence in Asia is likely due to the influence of a high-fat diet (55). Notably, intestinal inflammation increases the risk of enteric cancer, which is a commonly malignancy globally (56).

Native anti-inflammatory peptides are a class of anti-inflammatory agents that may be useful in the treatment of a range of inflammatory diseases (13, 18, 25). However, several concerns, such as potential cytotoxicity (35), poor anti-inflammatory activity based on peptide concentration, and weak physiological stability (57), have weakened their development as anti-inflammatory therapeutics. Hybridizing different anti-inflammatory peptides is one of the most successful approaches to obtain a novel anti-inflammatory peptide with increased activity but minimized cytotoxicity (58, 59). Based on previous findings, we designed several hybrid peptides comprising the active center of AMPs, including LL-37 (13-36), YW12D (1-12), IDR-1 (1-13), and CATH2 (1-13), with TP5 or the active center of Tα1 (17-24).

It has been well established that LPS mediates its immune response in macrophages via TLR4 (60). MD-2, an accessory protein of TLR4, is responsible for recognizing LPS; in turn, LPS interacts with the Toll/Interleukin-1 receptor (TIR) domain on TLR4 and induces the inflammatory effects (61, 62). Therefore, targeting MD-2 is an important therapeutic strategy for the attenuation of the inflammatory response (62–64). Initially, molecular docking was used to simply and effectively scan the binding mode of the anti-inflammatory peptides. LTP, LTA, YTP, and CTP were the hybrid peptides selected for further study, and the anti-inflammatory activities of these four hybrid peptides were assessed in RAW264.7 cells. The four hybrid peptides showed higher anti-inflammatory activity than their parental peptides. LTA, the most active peptide, was selected for a comprehensive analysis.

The hybrid peptides designed in our study were aimed to fight inflammatory disorders with reduced cytotoxicity. Because cytotoxicity is often thought to be a bottleneck for the therapeutic use of these peptides, it was important to evaluate toxicity. In this study, the proliferation assays showed that the hybrid peptides had lower cytotoxic than their parental peptides. Presumably, this decreased cytotoxic activity was due to the rational hydrophobicity of these hybrid peptides, which is similar to that described in other studies (59). The low cytotoxic activity at relatively high peptide concentrations combined with modified anti-inflammatory activity is an excellent combination from the parental peptides.

The present study showed that murine models of intestinal inflammation induced by LPS have characteristics similar to human IBD (14, 65), such as weight loss, neutrophil infiltration, histological features of multiple erosions, and inflammatory intestinal mucosal changes, including crypt abscess. However, LTA treatment significantly reverses weight loss and reduce histological damage such as ulceration of the epithelial and decreased villus height to crypt depth ratio, in the LPS-induced intestinal inflammation experimental model. The infiltration of activated neutrophils is one of the most representative histological features observed in intestinal inflammation, because neutrophils generate superoxide anions and other reactive species (66). The infiltration of activated was significantly increased in LPS-treated mice; however, mice pre-treated with LTA did not show the same effect. The activity of MPO is directly proportional to the neutrophil concentration in the inflamed tissue. Therefore, MPO activity is an index of neutrophil infiltration and inflammation (67). Consistent with this, jejunal MPO activity was markedly increased in LPS-treated mice, but pretreatment with LTA significantly reduced this effect. In addition, MPO activity in the LTA-pretreated group was markedly decreased compared to the Tα1 and LL-37 pretreated groups. Apoptosis is one of the ulcerogenic processes associated with intestinal inflammation (68). In this study, TUNEL staining showed that LPS markedly increased the number of apoptotic cells in the jejunal mucosa, while administration of LTA decreased the extent of apoptosis.

Excessive production of inflammatory cytokines, such as TNF-α, which can amplify the inflammatory cascade by triggering the accumulation and activation of leukocytes, is often seen in intestinal inflammation (69). In the present study, we found that pretreatment with LTA reduced the levels of TNF-α, IFN-γ, IL-6, and IL-1β in the jejunum. Moreover, the levels of TNF-α, IFN-γ, IL-6, and IL-1β in LTA-pretreated group were markedly decreased compared to the Tα1- and LL-37-pretreated groups.

Collectively, these results support the deduction that LTA is the most active peptide that prevents LPS-induced impairment

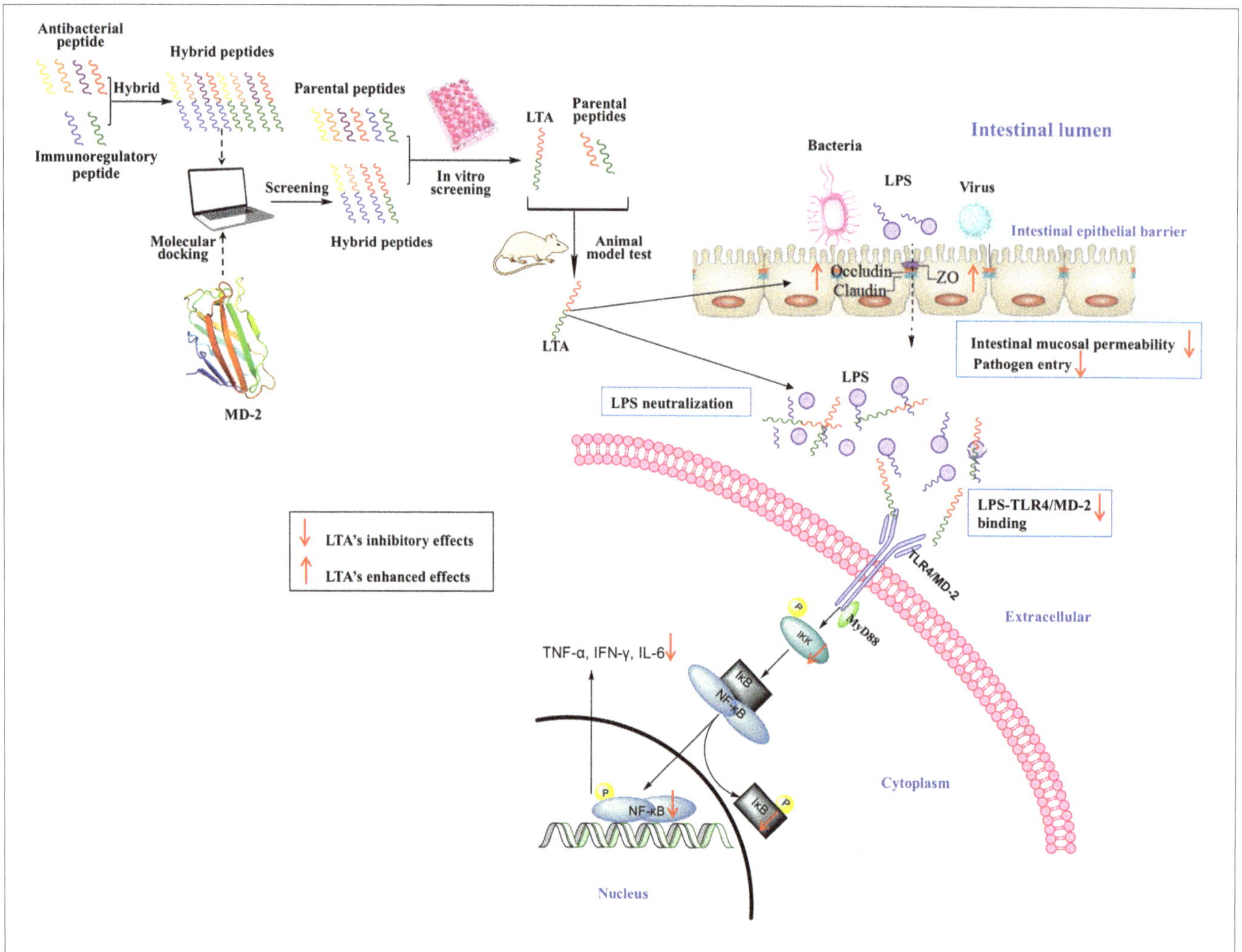

FIGURE 13 | Schematic illustration of design and development of the novel hybrid peptide, LTA for the treatment of intestinal inflammation.

in mice. To identify the mechanisms of the observed anti-inflammatory effects in LPS-treated mice, a comprehensive and detailed analysis was conducted.

LPS can upregulate ~100 different genes, including pro-inflammatory cytokines, signaling molecules, and transcriptional regulators; thus, it can induce several functional responses that contribute to immunity (70). LPS has high biological activity and plays an important role in the pathogenesis of intestinal inflammation (14). In this study, we found that LTA-pretreated mice had significantly reduced plasma LPS levels compared to the LPS-only treated. *In vitro* experiments showed that LTA can almost completely neutralize LPS at a concentration of 8 μg/mL. By neutralizing LPS, LTA could significantly attenuate the intestinal inflammatory effects by reducing the binding of LPS to the TLR4 receptor in the immune cells *in vivo*.

The intestinal mucosa forms a physical and metabolic barrier against toxins and pathogens from the lumen into the circulatory system (71). Deterioration of the intestinal epithelial barrier increases host susceptibility to luminal pathogens and antigens, leading to the chronic intestinal immune response (72). This deterioration is also a key contributing factor in the pathogenesis of intestinal inflammation (73). First, we evaluated the effect of LTA on gut epithelial barrier function via the TEER tests and the results showed that LTA alleviated LPS-induced permeability. The intestinal epithelial barrier is formed by an interplay between different types of barrier components, such as intercellular TJ proteins (74). TJs are responsible for limiting the paracellular movement of compounds across the intestinal mucosa (75). Regions of increased permeability in the TJs are major sites for both infections and the initiation of inflammation in the gut (76). Our data indicated that the expression of two major TJ proteins, Occludin and ZO-1, was regulated by LTA. In addition, TEM was used to determine the TJs between gut epithelial cells, and its results support the protective effect of LTA against LPS-induced damage in jejunum tissues. The effect of LTA on the epithelial barrier suggests that LTA could protect the host by preventing toxins and luminal antigens from impairing the body's defense mechanism, thereby reducing the severity of intestine inflammation.

The hybrid peptides proposed in this study antagonize the effects of LPS in RAW264.7 cells and in the mouse by binding to the TLR4-MD2 complex. To identify the binding ability of LTA to the TLR4/MD-2 complex, binding assays were performed by flow cytometry and confocal laser-scanning microscopy. The results demonstrated that that LTA competitively blocks LPS binding to the TLR4/MD-2 complex. Consistently, the MD simulation showed that LTA binds to the hydrophobic pocket of MD-2, which partially overlaps with the LPS binding sites on MD-2 (52). This binding mode could be the cause of the LPS-antagonizing effect. Therefore, the present study indicated that LTA confers its anti-inflammatory activity by blocking LPS binding to the TLR4/MD-2 complex.

NF-κB signaling regulates cytokines and cells involved in the inflammatory process (77), and LPS is a strong activator of NF-κB, through its interactions with TLR4. NF-κB is considered to be a crucial initiative factor regulating inflammatory gene expression (78). Thus, we tested the expression of the major proteins involved in the NF-κB pathway to clarify the anti-inflammatory mechanism of LTA in intestinal inflammation. LTA effectively inhibited the activation of NF-κB signaling by suppressing of phosphorylation of IKK-β, IκB-α, and NF-κB.

CONCLUSION

In this study, a feasible approach for the design of anti-inflammatory peptides by the hybridization of different native anti-inflammatory peptides was proposed (**Figure 13**). The anti-inflammatory potency of the peptides was enhanced while cytotoxicity was reduced. Moreover, the different hybrid peptide combinations may provide a range of opportunities for obtaining a more active anti-inflammatory peptide.

One novel hybrid peptide, LTA, was most effective at reducing the LPS-induced inflammatory response. This peptide, which was identified by molecule docking and *in vitro* experiments, had low cytotoxicity. Our study also confirmed that the anti-inflammatory effects of LTA on the LPS-induced murine intestinal inflammation model may be associated with the neutralization of LPS, the maintenance of the TJ network, the binding activity on the TLR4/MD-2 complex, and the inhibition of the NF-κB signal pathway. Thus, LTA is able to modulate TJ proteins, such as Occludin and ZO-1, and inhibit the production of inflammation mediators, such as TNF-α, IFN-γ, IL-6, and IL-1β. As a result of its broad effects against inflammation, LTA exhibits great potential as a useful tool to study or potentially treat inflammatory disorders.

ETHICS STATEMENT

All of the animal experiments were approved by the Institutional Animal Care and Use Committee of China Agricultural University and were performed in accordance with guidelines set forth by the Care and Use of Laboratory Animals of the Ministry of Science and Technology of China (certificate of the Beijing Laboratory Animal employee, ID: 18086).

AUTHOR CONTRIBUTIONS

LZ, XW, RZ, JP, and DS conceived the project and designed the experiments. LZ, XW, ZL, JC, and MD conducted experiments. LZ and JP wrote the manuscript and analyzed data. All authors read and commented on the manuscript. The authors are in debt to JP for his contribution toward English proficiency.

REFERENCES

1. Song YS, Lee Y, Kwon TR, Kim YH, Kim BJ. Picrasma quassioides inhibits LPS- and IFN-γ-stimulated nitric oxide production and inflammatory response in RAW264.7 macrophage cells. *Biotechnol Bioproc E.* (2014) 19:404–10. doi: 10.1007/s12257-014-0131-4
2. Burrin DG, Stoll B, Guan XF, Cui LW, Chang XY, Holst JJ. Glucagon-like peptide 2 dose-dependently activates intestinal cell survival and proliferation in neonatal piglets. *Endocrinology.* (2005) 146:22–32. doi: 10.1210/en.2004-1119
3. Gillen CD, Walmsley RS, Prior P, Andrews HA, Allan RN. Ulcerative colitis and Crohn's disease: a comparison of the colorectal cancer risk in extensive colitis. *Gut.* (1994) 35:1590–2. doi: 10.1136/gut.35.11.1590
4. Eaden JA, Abrams KR, Mayberry JF. The risk of colorectal cancer in ulcerative colitis: a meta-analysis. *Gut.* (2001) 48:526–35. doi: 10.1136/gut.48.4.526
5. Bernstein CN, Blanchard JF, Kliewer E, Wajda A. Cancer risk in patients with inflammatory bowel disease - a population-based study. *Cancer.* (2001) 91:854–62. doi: 10.1002/1097-0142(20010215)91:4<;854::AID-CNCR1073>3.0.CO;2-Z
6. Sartor RB. Mechanisms of disease: pathogenesis of Crohn's disease and ulcerative colitis. *Nat Clin Pract Gastr.* (2006) 3:390–407. doi: 10.1038/ncpgasthep0528
7. Boumpas DT, Chrousos GP, Wilder RL, Cupps TR, Balow JE. Glucocorticoid therapy for immune-mediated diseases - basic and clinical correlates. *Ann Intern Med.* (1993) 119:1198–208. doi: 10.7326/0003-4819-119-12-199312150-00007
8. Faubion WA, Loftus EV, Harmsen WS, Zinsmeister AR, Sandborn WJ. The natural history of corticosteroid therapy for inflammatory bowel disease: a population-based study. *Gastroenterology.* (2001) 121:255–60. doi: 10.1053/gast.2001.26279
9. Smoak KA, Cidlowski JA. Mechanisms of glucocorticoid receptor signaling during inflammation. *Mech Ageing Dev.* (2004) 125:697–706. doi: 10.1016/j.mad.2004.06.010
10. Anstead GM. Steroids, retinoids, and wound healing. *Adv Wound Care.* (1998) 11:277–85.
11. Stanbury RM, Graham EM. Systemic corticosteroid therapy - side effects and their management. *Brit J Ophthalmol.* (1998) 82:704–8. doi: 10.1136/bjo.82.6.704
12. Heinbockel L, Weindl G, Martinez-de-Tejada G, Correa W, Sanchez-Gomez S, Barcena-Varela S, et al. Inhibition of lipopolysaccharide- and lipoprotein-induced inflammation by antitoxin peptide pep 19-2.5. *Front Immunol.* (2018) 9:1704. doi: 10.3389/fimmu.2018.01704
13. Wu BC, Lee AHY, Hancock REW. Mechanisms of the innate defense regulator peptide-1002 anti-inflammatory activity in a sterile inflammation mouse model. *J Immunol.* (2017) 199:3592–603. doi: 10.4049/jimmunol.1700985
14. Zong X, Hu WY, Song DG, Li Z, Du HH, Lu ZQ, et al. Porcine lactoferrin-derived peptide LFP-20 protects intestinal barrier by maintaining tight junction complex and modulating inflammatory response. *Biochem Pharmacol.* (2016) 104:74–82. doi: 10.1016/j.bcp.2016.01.009
15. Bhunia A, Chua GL, Domadia PN, Warshakoon H, Cromer JR, David SA, et al. Interactions of a designed peptide with lipopolysaccharide: bound

conformation and anti-endotoxic activity. *Biochem Bioph Res Commun.* (2008) 369:853–7. doi: 10.1016/j.bbrc.2008.02.105
16. Mu LX, Zhou L, Yang JJ, Zhuang L, Tang J, Liu T, et al. The first identified cathelicidin from tree frogs possesses anti-inflammatory and partial LPS neutralization activities. *Amino Acids.* (2017) 49:1571–85. doi: 10.1007/s00726-017-2449-7
17. Vandamme D, Landuyt B, Luyten W, Schoofs L. A comprehensive summary of LL-37, the factotum human cathelicidin peptide. *Cell Immunol.* (2012) 280:22–35. doi: 10.1016/j.cellimm.2012.11.009
18. Ishida W, Harada Y, Fukuda K, Fukushima A. Inhibition by the antimicrobial peptide LL37 of lipopolysaccharide-induced innate immune responses in human corneal fibroblasts. *Invest Ophth Vis Sci.* (2016) 57:30–9. doi: 10.1167/ iovs.15-17652
19. van Dijk A, van Eldik M, Veldhuizen EJA, Tjeerdsma-van Bokhoven HLM, de Zoete MR, Bikker FJ, et al. Immunomodulatory and anti-inflammatory activities of chicken cathelicidin-2 derived peptides. *PLoS ONE.* (2016) 11:e0147919. doi: 10.1371/journal.pone.0147919
20. Hou M, Zhang NW, Yang JJ, Meng XY, Yang R, Li J, et al. Antimicrobial peptide LL-37 and IDR-1 ameliorate MRSA pneumonia *in vivo*. *Cell Physiol Biochem.* (2013) 32:614–23. doi: 10.1159/000354465
21. Singh VK, Biswas S, Mathur KB, Haq W, Garg SK, Agarwal SS. Thymopentin and splenopentin as immunomodulators - current status. *Immunol Res.* (1998) 17:345–68. doi: 10.1007/BF02786456
22. Lee HW, Lee JI, Um SH, Ahn SH, Chang HY, Park YK, et al. Combination therapy of thymosin alpha-1 and lamivudine for HBeAg positive chronic hepatitis B: a prospective randomized, comparative pilot study. *J Gastroenterol Hepatol.* (2008) 23:729–35. doi: 10.1111/j.1440-1746.2008.05387.x
23. Low TL, Thurman GB, McAdoo M, McClure J, Rossio JL, Naylor PH, et al. The chemistry and biology of thymosin. I. Isolation, characterization, and biological activities of thymosin alpha1 and polypeptide beta1 from calf thymus. *J Biol Chem.* (1979) 254:981–6.
24. Romani L, Bistoni F, Perruccio K, Montagnoli C, Gaziano R, Bozza S, et al. Thymosin alpha1 activates dendritic cell tryptophan catabolism and establishes a regulatory environment for balance of inflammation and tolerance. *Blood.* (2006) 108:2265–74. doi: 10.1182/blood-2006-02-004762
25. Romani L, Oikonomou V, Moretti S, Iannitti RG, D'Adamo MC, Villella VR, et al. Thymosin α1 represents a potential potent single-molecule-based therapy for cystic fibrosis. *Nat Med.* (2017) 23:590–600. doi: 10.1038/nm.4305
26. Mendling W, Koldovsky U. Investigations by cell-mediated immunologic tests and therapeutic trials with thymopentin in vaginal mycoses. *Infect Dis Obstet Gynecol.* (1996) 4:225–31. doi: 10.1155/S1064744996000439
27. Wang FW, Yu TT, Zheng H, Lao XZ. Thymosin alpha1-fc modulates the immune system and down-regulates the progression of melanoma and breast cancer with a prolonged half-life. *Sci Rep.* (2018) 8:12351. doi: 10.1038/s41598-018-30956-y
28. Zhang P, Chan J, Dragoi AM, Gong X, Ivanov S, Li ZW, et al. Activation of IKK by thymosin alpha 1 requires the TRAF6 signalling pathway. *EMBO Rep.* (2005) 6:531–7. doi: 10.1038/sj.embor.7400433
29. Romani L, Bistoni F, Gaziano R, Bozza S, Montagnoli C, Perruccio K, et al. Thymosin alpha 1 activates dendritic cells for antifungal Th1 resistance through Toll-like receptor signaling. *Blood.* (2004) 103:4232–9. doi: 10.1182/blood-2003-11-4036
30. Romani L, Bistoni F, Montagnoli C, Gaziano R, Bozza S, Bonifazi P, et al. Thymosin alpha1: an endogenous regulator of inflammation, immunity, and tolerance. *Ann N Y Acad Sci.* (2007) 1112:326–38. doi: 10.1196/annals.1415.002
31. Pierluigi B, D'Angelo C, Fallarino F, Moretti S, Zelante T, Bozza S, et al. Thymosin alpha1: the regulator of regulators? *Ann N Y Acad Sci.* (2010) 1194:1–5. doi: 10.1111/j.1749-6632.2010.05465.x
32. Lunin SM, Novoselova TV, Khrenov MO, Glushkova OV, Parfeniuk SB, Smolikhina TI, et al. Immunomodulatory effects of thymopentin under acute and chronic inflammations in mice. *Biofizika.* (2009) 54:182–7. doi: 10.1134/S0006350909020122
33. Goldstein G, Scheid MP, Boyse EA, Schlesinger DH, Vanwauwe J. Synthetic pentapeptide with biological-activity characteristic of the thymic hormone thymopoietin. *Science.* (1979) 204:1309–10. doi: 10.1126/science.451537
34. Goldstein AL, Goldsten AL. From lab to bedside: emerging clinical applications of thymosin alpha(1). *Expert Opin Biol Ther.* (2009) 9:593–608. doi: 10.1517/14712590902911412
35. Anders E, Dahl S, Svensson D, Nilsson BO. LL-37-induced human osteoblast cytotoxicity and permeability occurs independently of cellular LL-37 uptake through clathrin-mediated endocytosis. *Biochem Bioph Res Commun.* (2018) 501:280–5. doi: 10.1016/j.bbrc.2018.04.235
36. Haney EF, Mansour SC, Hilchie AL, de la Fuente-Nunez C, Hancock REW. High throughput screening methods for assessing antibiofilm and immunomodulatory activities of synthetic peptides. *Peptides.* (2015) 71:276–85. doi: 10.1016/j.peptides.2015.03.015
37. Li YQ, Smith C, Wu HF, Teng P, Shi Y, Padhee S, et al. Short antimicrobial lipo-α/γ-AA hybrid peptides. *Chembiochem.* (2014) 15:2275–80. doi: 10.1002/cbic.201402264
38. Nell MJ, Tjabringa GS, Wafelman AR, Verrijk R, Hiemstra PS, Drijfhout JW, et al. Development of novel LL-37 derived antimicrobial peptides with LPS and LTA neutralizing and antimicrobial activities for therapeutic application. *Peptides.* (2006) 27:649–60. doi: 10.1016/j.peptides.2005.09.016
39. Nan YH, Bang JK, Jacob B, Park IS, Shin SY. Prokaryotic selectivity and LPS-neutralizing activity of short antimicrobial peptides designed from the human antimicrobial peptide LL-37. *Peptides.* (2012) 35:239–47. doi: 10.1016/j.peptides.2012.04.004
40. Grottesi A, Sette M, Palamara AT, Rotilio G, Garaci E, Paci M. The conformation of peptide thymosin alpha 1 in solution and in a membrane-like environment by circular dichroism and NMR spectroscopy. A possible model for its interaction with the lymphocyte membrane. *Peptides.* (1998) 19:1731–8. doi: 10.1016/S0196-9781(98)00132-6
41. Mandaliti W, Nepravishta R, Vallebona PS, Pica F, Garaci E, Paci M. Thymosin α1 interacts with exposed phosphatidylserine in membrane models and in cells and uses serum albumin as a carrier. *Biochemistry.* (2016) 55:1462–72. doi: 10.1021/acs.biochem.5b01345
42. Guo ST, Huang YY, Zhang WD, Wang WW, Wei T, Lin DS, et al. Ternary complexes of amphiphilic polycaprolactone-graft-poly (N,N-dimethylaminoethyl methaaylate), DNA and polyglutamic acid-graft-poly (ethylene glycol) for gene delivery. *Biomaterials.* (2011) 32:4283–92. doi: 10.1016/j.biomaterials.2011.02.034
43. Chiu CJ, Scott HJ, Gurd FN. Intestinal mucosal lesion in low-flow states. 2. protective effect of intraluminal glucose as energy substrate. *Arch Surg.* (1970) 101:484–8. doi: 10.1001/archsurg.1970.01340280036010
44. Chen H, Hu YH, Fang Y, Djukic Z, Yamamoto M, Shaheen NJ, et al. Nrf2 deficiency impairs the barrier function of mouse oesophageal epithelium. *Gut.* (2014) 63:711–9. doi: 10.1136/gutjnl-2012-303731
45. Zong X, Song DG, Wang TH, Xia X, Hu WY, Han FF, et al. LFP-20, a porcine lactoferrin peptide, ameliorates LPS-induced inflammation via the MyD88/NF-kappa B and MyD88/MAPK signaling pathways. *Dev Comp Immunol.* (2015) 52:123–31. doi: 10.1016/j.dci.2015.05.006
46. Sastry GM, Adzhigirey M, Day T, Annabhimoju R, Sherman W. Protein and ligand preparation: parameters, protocols, and influence on virtual screening enrichments. *J Comput Aid Mol Des.* (2013) 27:221–34. doi: 10.1007/s10822-013-9644-8
47. Duan Y, Wu C, Chowdhury S, Lee MC, Xiong GM, Zhang W, et al. A point-charge force field for molecular mechanics simulations of proteins based on condensed-phase quantum mechanical calculations. *J Comput Chem.* (2003) 24:1999–2012. doi: 10.1002/jcc.10349
48. Wang JM, Wolf RM, Caldwell JW, Kollman PA, Case DA. Development and testing of a general amber force field. *J Comput Chem.* (2004) 25:1157–74. doi: 10.1002/jcc.20035
49. Darden T, York D, Pedersen L. Particle mesh Ewald - an N.Log(N) method for Ewald sums in large systems. *J Chem Phys.* (1993) 98:10089–92. doi: 10.1063/1.464397
50. Massova I, Kollman PA. Combined molecular mechanical and continuum solvent approach (MM-PBSA/GBSA) to predict ligand binding. *Perspect Drug Discov.* (2000) 18:113–35. doi: 10.1023/A:1008763014207
51. Semple F, MacPherson H, Webb S, Cox SL, Mallin LJ, Tyrrell C, et al. Human β-defensin 3 affects the activity of pro-inflammatory pathways associated with MyD88 and TRIF. *Eur J Immunol.* (2011) 41:3291–300. doi: 10.1002/eji.201141648
52. Garate JA, Oostenbrink C. Lipid a from lipopolysaccharide recognition: Structure, dynamics and cooperativity by molecular dynamics simulations. *Proteins.* (2013) 81:658–74. doi: 10.1002/prot.24223

53. Gibson PR. Increased gut permeability in Crohn's disease: is TNF the link? *Gut.* (2004) 53:1724–5. doi: 10.1136/gut.2004.047092
54. Matricon J. Immunopathogenesis of inflammatory bowel disease. *Med Sci.* (2010) 26:405–10. doi: 10.1051/medsci/2010264405
55. Spiegelman BM, Flier JS. Obesity and the regulation of energy balance. *Cell.* (2001) 104:531–43. doi: 10.1016/S0092-8674(01)00240-9
56. Saleh M, Trinchieri G. Innate immune mechanisms of colitis and colitis-associated colorectal cancer. *Nat Rev Immunol.* (2011) 11:9–20. doi: 10.1038/nri2891
57. DeGraw JI, Almquist RG, Hiebert CK, Colwell WT, Crase J, Hayano T, et al. Stabilized analogs of thymopentin. 1. 4,5-ketomethylene pseudopeptides. *J Med Chem.* (1997) 40:2386–97. doi: 10.1021/jm950803a
58. Liu YF, Xia X, Xu L, Wang YZ. Design of hybrid β-hairpin peptides with enhanced cell specificity and potent anti-inflammatory activity. *Biomaterials.* (2013) 34:237–50. doi: 10.1016/j.biomaterials.2012.09.032
59. Ma Z, Wei DD, Yan P, Zhu X, Shan AS, Bi ZP. Characterization of cell selectivity, physiological stability and endotoxin neutralization capabilities of α-helix-based peptide amphiphiles. *Biomaterials.* (2015) 52:517–30. doi: 10.1016/j.biomaterials.2015.02.063
60. Gangloff M, Gay NJ. MD-2: the Toll 'gatekeeper' in endotoxin signalling. *Trends Biochem Sci.* (2004) 29:294–300. doi: 10.1016/j.tibs.2004.04.008
61. Ohto U, Fukase K, Miyake K, Satow Y. Crystal structures of human MD-2 and its complex with antiendotoxic lipid IVa. *Science.* (2007) 316:1632–4. doi: 10.1126/science.1139111
62. Roh E, Lee HS, Kwak JA, Hong JT, Nam SY, Jung SH, et al. MD-2 as the target of nonlipid chalcone in the inhibition of endotoxin LPS-induced TLR4 activity. *J Infect Dis.* (2011) 203:1012–20. doi: 10.1093/infdis/jiq155
63. Park BS, Song DH, Kim HM, Choi BS, Lee H, Lee JO. The structural basis of lipopolysaccharide recognition by the TLR4-MD-2 complex. *Nature.* (2009) 458:1191–5. doi: 10.1038/nature07830
64. Peri F, Piazza M. Therapeutic targeting of innate immunity with Toll-like receptor 4 (TLR4) antagonists. *Biotechnol Adv.* (2012) 30:251–60. doi: 10.1016/j.biotechadv.2011.05.014
65. Podolsky DK. Inflammatory bowel disease. *N Engl J Med.* (2002) 347:417–29. doi: 10.1056/NEJMra020831
66. Buell MG, Berin MC. Neutrophil-independence of the initiation of colonic injury - comparison of results from 3 models of experimental colitis in the rat. *Digest Dis Sci.* (1994) 39:2575–88. doi: 10.1007/BF02087693
67. Zhang Y, Zhu JL, Guo L, Zou Y, Wang F, Shao H, et al. Cholecystokinin protects mouse liver against ischemia and reperfusion injury. *Int Immunopharmacol.* (2017) 48:180–6. doi: 10.1016/j.intimp.2017.03.028
68. Han FF, Zhang HW, Xia X, Xiong HT, Song DG, Zong X, et al. Porcine β-defensin 2 attenuates inflammation and mucosal lesions in dextran sodium sulfate-induced colitis. *J Immunol.* (2015) 194:1882–93. doi: 10.4049/jimmunol.1402300
69. Raetz CRH, Whitfield C. Lipopolysaccharide endotoxins. *Annu Rev Biochem.* (2002) 71:635–700. doi: 10.1146/annurev.biochem.71.110601.135414
70. Fessler MB, Malcolm KC, Duncan MW, Worthen GS. A genomic and proteomic analysis of activation of the human neutrophil by lipopolysaccharide and its mediation by p38 mitogen-activated protein kinase. *J Biol Chem.* (2002) 277:31291–302. doi: 10.1074/jbc.M200755200
71. Mu XW, Pan C, Zheng SY, Alhamdi Y, Sun BW, Shi QK, et al. Protective effects of carbon monoxide-releasing molecule-2 on the barrier function of intestinal epithelial cells. *PLoS ONE.* (2014) 9:e104032. doi: 10.1371/journal.pone.0104032
72. Park EJ, Thomson ABR, Clandinin MT. Protection of intestinal occludin tight junction protein by dietary gangliosides in lipopolysaccharide-induced acute inflammation. *J Pediatr Gastr Nutr.* (2010) 50:321–8. doi: 10.1097/MPG.0b013e3181ae2ba0
73. Salim SY, Soderholm JD. Importance of disrupted intestinal barrier in inflammatory bowel diseases. *Inflamm Bowel Dis.* (2011) 17:362–81. doi: 10.1002/ibd.21403
74. Turner JR. Intestinal mucosal barrier function in health and disease. *Nat Rev Immunol.* (2009) 9:799–809. doi: 10.1038/nri2653
75. McCall IC, Betanzos A, Weber DA, Nava P, Miller GW, Parkos CA. Effects of phenol on barrier function of a human intestinal epithelial cell line correlate with altered tight junction protein localization. *Toxicol Appl Pharm.* (2009) 241:61–70. doi: 10.1016/j.taap.2009.08.002
76. Qin HL, Zhang ZW, Hang XM, Jiang YQ. L. plantarum prevents enteroinvasive Escherichia coli-induced tight junction proteins changes in intestinal epithelial cells. *BMC Microbiol.* (2009) 9:63. doi: 10.1186/1471-2180-9-63
77. Zhang D, Cheng L, Huang X, Shi W, Xiang J, Gan H. Tetrandrine ameliorates dextran-sulfate-sodium-induced colitis in mice through inhibition of nuclear factor-kappa B activation. *Int J Colorectal Dis.* (2009) 24:5–12. doi: 10.1007/s00384-008-0544-7
78. Hayden MS, Ghosh S. Signaling to NF-kappa B. *Genes Dev.* (2004) 18:2195–224. doi: 10.1101/gad.1228704

12

A Specific *IL6* Polymorphic Genotype Modulates the Risk of *Trypanosoma cruzi* Parasitemia While *IL18, IL17A* and *IL1B* Variant Profiles and HIV Infection Protect Against Cardiomyopathy in Chagas Disease

Alexandra Gomes dos Santos[1†], Elieser Hitoshi Watanabe[2†], Daiane Tomomi Ferreira[3], Jamille Oliveira[1], Érika Shimoda Nakanishi[3], Claudia Silva Oliveira[1], Edimar Bocchi[4], Cristina Terra Gallafrio Novaes[5], Fatima Cruz[4], Noemia Barbosa Carvalho[5], Paula Keiko Sato[3], Edite Hatsumi Yamashiro-Kanashiro[3,6], Alessandra Pontillo[7], Vera Lucia Teixeira de Freitas[1,3], Luiz Fernando Onuchic[2] and Maria Aparecida Shikanai-Yasuda[1,3*]*

[1] Department of Infectious and Parasitic Diseases, Faculdade de Medicina, University of São Paulo, São Paulo, Brazil, [2] Department of Medicine, Divisions of Molecular Medicine and Nephrology, Faculdade de Medicina, University of São Paulo, São Paulo, Brazil, [3] Laboratory of Immunology (LIM 48), Hospital das Clínicas, Faculdade de Medicina, University of São Paulo, São Paulo, Brazil, [4] Heart Institute, Hospital das Clínicas, Faculdade de Medicina, University of São Paulo, São Paulo, Brazil, [5] Division of Infectious Diseases, Hospital das Clinicas, Faculdade de Medicina, University of São Paulo, São Paulo, Brazil, [6] Instituto de Medicina Tropical, University of São Paulo, São Paulo, Brazil, [7] Departament of Immunology, Instituto de Ciências Biomédicas (ICB), University of São Paulo, São Paulo, Brazil

***Correspondence:**
Luiz Fernando Onuchic
lonuchic@usp.br
Maria Aparecida Shikanai-Yasuda
masyasuda@yahoo.com.br

[†]These authors have contributed equally to this work

Background: Chagas disease caused by *Trypanosoma cruzi* (*T. cruzi*) affects approximately six million individuals worldwide. Clinical manifestations are expected to occur due to the parasite persistence and host immune response. Herein we investigated potential associations between *IL1B*, *IL6*, *IL17A*, or *IL18* polymorphism profiles and cardiomyopathy or *T. cruzi* parasitemia, as well as the impact of HIV infection on cardiopathy.

Methods: Two hundred twenty-six patients and 90 control individuals were analyzed. *IL1B* rs1143627 T>C, *IL6* rs1800795 C>G, *IL17A* rs2275913 G>A, *IL18* rs187238 C>G, and *IL18* rs1946518 C>A SNVs were analyzed by real-time PCR and *T. cruzi* parasitemia by PCR.

Results: Our data revealed association between a cytokine gene polymorphism and parasitemia never previously reported. The *IL6* rs1800795 CG genotype lowered the risk of positive parasitemia (OR = 0.45, 95% CI 0.24–0.86, P = 0.015). Original findings included associations between *IL17A* rs2275913 AA and *IL18* s1946518 AA genotypes with decreased risk of developing cardiomyopathy (OR = 0.27, 95% CI 0.07–0.97, P = 0.044; and OR = 0.35, 95% CI 0.14–0.87, P = 0.023, respectively). *IL18* rs1946518 AA and *IL1B* rs1143627 TC were associated with reduced risk for cardiomyopathy severity, including NYHA (New York Heart Association) class ≥ 2 (OR = 0.21, 95% CI 0.06–0.68, P = 0.009; and OR = 0.48, 95% CI 0.24–0.95, P = 0.036, respectively) and LVEF (left ventricular ejection fraction) <45% for *IL18* rs1946518 AA (OR = 0.22, 95% CI 0.05–0.89, P = 0.034). A novel, unexpected protective effect of HIV infection against development/progression of cardiomyopathy was identified, based on a lower risk of developing cardiopathy (OR = 0.48, 95% CI 0.23–0.96, P = 0.039), NYHA class ≥ 2 (OR = 0.15, 95% CI 0.06–0.39, P < 0.001), and LVEF < 45% (OR = 0.03, 95% CI 0.00–0.25, P = 0.001). Digestive involvement was negatively associated with NYHA ≥ 2 and LVEF < 45% (OR = 0.20, 95% CI 0.09–0.47, P < 0.001; and OR = 0.24, 95% CI 0.09–0.62, P = 0.004, respectively).

Conclusions: Our data support a protective role of *IL17A* AA, *IL18* AA, and *IL1B* TC genotypes against development/progression of cardiomyopathy and a modulatory effect of the *IL6* CG genotype on the risk of parasitemia in Chagas disease. Notably, HIV infection was shown to protect against development/progression of cardiopathy, potentially associated with a synergistic effect of HIV and highly active antiretroviral therapy (HAART), attenuating a Th1-mediated response in the myocardium. This proposed hypothesis requires confirmation, however, in larger and more comprehensive future studies.

Keywords: *T. cruzi* parasitemia, cardiomyopathy, Chagas disease, HIV, *IL1 B*, *IL6*, *IL17 A* and *IL18* polymorphisms

INTRODUCTION

Chagas disease, a potentially life-threatening illness caused by the protozoan *Trypanosoma cruzi* (*T. cruzi*) and endemic in Latin America, affects approximately 6 million individuals worldwide. The natural course of the infection comprises acute and chronic phases. A clinically relevant acute form is observed in only 1/30 infected people, including fever, adenopathy, palpebral or legs edema and/or hepatosplenomegaly and, less often, myocarditis and meningoencephalitis. In the chronic phase, on the other hand, ~30% of the patients develop the cardiac form, expressed as arrhythmia, heart failure, and/or thromboembolic events. The chronic phase also includes a digestive form, which comprises dysphagia and/or constipation in 10–15% of the cases and, in ~5% of them, a cardio-digestive form. The indeterminate form, in turn, represented by asymptomatic patients with normal electrocardiogram and thorax and digestive tract X-rays, constitutes the most frequent chronic form, affecting 60–70% of the referred group (1, 2).

Chagas cardiopathy is a major cause of cardiovascular-related mortality within the 30–50-year age range in Latin American endemic areas (1, 3). Previous studies have recognized the fundamental role of host features in Chagas disease pathophysiology, revealing different immunological profiles in patients affected and not affected by cardiopathy (4). While the development of cardiopathy has been linked to a Thl response in heart tissue associated with mononuclear cell infiltrate, cardiomyocyte damage, and fibrosis, a Th2 response predominates in the indeterminate form (5, 6). Reports of higher levels/expression of IL-6, IL1β, TNFα, and IFNγ in the cardiac form (7, 8) and IL6 and/IL1β or C-reactive protein in the cardiac and/or cardio-digestive forms (9, 10) support a potential role for such cytokines in the adaptative immune response at heart tissue damaging process. IL6 and IL1β could be considered, therefore, a marker of cardiac lesion. In contrast, the finding of higher plasma levels of IL17A directly associated with better systolic function in the indeterminate form suggests a protective role for this cytokine against the development of clinically relevant chronic Chagas cardiopathy, despite inverse association with diastolic performance indices (11, 12).

Previous studies in patients with indeterminate and cardiac forms suggested a role for T reg cells in the modulation of inflammatory immune responses associated with the cardiac form (6, 13). Increased number of Foxp3+, CD25+, CD4+ T cells, T reg cells that stimulate secretion of IL-17 A, IL-10, and granzyme B, was observed in the indeterminate form, in association with less inflammation and better myocardium function. In contrast, more pronounced immune responses to the parasite, associated with higher levels of inflammatory cytokines and myocardial lesion, correlated with higher densities of IL6+, IFNγ+, TNFα+, CTLA4+ T reg cells. Such findings suggest a role for T reg cells in controlling the exacerbated immune response and morbidity as well as mortality in *T. cruzi* infection, likely by stimulating Th17 cells and modulating killing effector cells (14).

An important role in the control of cardiac inflammatory lesions and remodeling has been proposed for IL18 (15, 16). This cytokine stimulates IFNγ expression independently of IL12, allowing an IL18-IFNγ cross-talk at the myocardium level during *T. cruzi* infection (17). IL18 upregulation and correlation between IL18 messenger RNA (mRNA) and IFNγ expression have in fact been reported in human Chagas heart tissue (6, 18).

T. cruzi parasitemia is another major factor implicated in the progression of chronic Chagas cardiopathy, even if intermittent and low at this disease stage (19–22). Available reports, however, are controversial on this point (23–25). Cytokines have also been shown to control *T. cruzi* parasitic burden and myocardial inflammatory lesions in both chronic and acute phases of murine infection. In chronic infection induced with the Colombian strain in *IL18*-KO mice, a significant reduction in the myocardium parasitic load was observed (26). Acute infections of *IL17A*-KO mice, on the other hand, were associated with lack of activation of immune-related cells that are critical for the killing of *T. cruzi* (27) and with increased mortality and higher-degree myocarditis. Variable parasitic loads were detected, however, depending on the mouse line and the parasite strain (27, 28). This finding unraveled a protective effect of IL17 A, evinced by the association between better cardiac function and higher plasma levels of IL17A in patients without cardiomyopathy (11, 12). In addition, in acute murine infection IL6 was shown to drive the survival of *T. cruzi* infected cardiomyocytes. IL6-KO mice lack the innate immunity crucial for host survival and rapidly die with high levels of IL1 β and inflammatory products, a process reverted by adding recombinant IL6 (29). This finding suggests a critical role for IL6 in modulating inflammatory lesions. Due to the modulating effect of IL6 on Chagas disease cardiomyopathy, the data on human disease likely represent a less severe degree of this inflammation (7, 10).

In immunosupressed patients with HIV infection, elevated IL18 serum concentrations have been reported to influence both Aids and the course of associated infections (30). Interestingly, whereas Chagas disease reactivation does not occur in immunocompetent subjects, this illness natural history is changed in HIV infected patients, being associated with increased morbidity and mortality (31).

As part of the genetic assessment of cytokine roles in Chagas disease, single nucleotide variants (SNVs) associated with various cytokine genes have been previously analyzed in *T. cruzi* infection and cardiopathy progression. No significant association involving the *IL6* SNV rs1800795 −174 C>G was identified in Colombia (32), in a context where the G allele has been associated with higher IL6 levels (33, 34) and patients with heart Chagas disease have been found to present higher IL6 levels (7, 10). Positive findings, in turn, included association between increased risk of cardiomyopathy and the CT haplotype for the *IL1B* −31 T>C and +3954 C>T (rs1143634, synonymous coding sequence variant) polymorphisms in Colombia (35). The possible proinflammatory nature of this haplotype (35) is unclear, since the *IL1B* −31 T allele has been associated with increased IL1β secretion (36), and other haplotype TCT, for *IL1B* −511 C>T, *IL1B* −31 T>C, and *IL1B* +3954 C>T, in turn, has been considered a proinflammatory haplotype, with a predominant role of *ILB* −511 C>T (37). Moreover, association between cardiomyopathy and the *IL1B* +5810 G>A (rs1143633, intronic SNV) G allele and GG genotype was also identified, despite no established effect of this allele or genotype on IL1β production (35). It is possible, however, that other biological effects or linkage disequilibrium with other polymorphisms related to functional significance may exist. By comparing seronegative individuals with seropositive cardiac patients in Colombia, a study suggested protection against *T. cruzi* infection and development of cardiopathy for patients that carry the C allele of *IL17A* rs8193036 C>T (promoter SNV) (38). These data were *a priori* not expected, since the C allele has been associated with lower IL17A mRNA expression (39) and previous reports revealed a role of IL17A in resistance to *T. cruzi* in infected mice (27) and higher IL17A levels in patients with no cardiopathy (11, 12). It should be noted, however, that this study conducted with Colombian patients shows that the *IL17A* rs8193036 SNV is probably in linkage disequilibrium with some causative variant that modulates IL17A production (38). This investigation also found no association between the *IL17A* rs7747909 G>A 3' UTR SNV and Chagas cardiopathy and between two other *IL17A* promoter SNVs (rs4711998 and rs3819024) or *IL17A* rs2275913 and heart disease, in a context where the latter A allele is associated with increased IL17 A levels (40, 41). A previous study, in turn, reported association of the *IL17A* rs2275913 G>A (promoter SNV) A allele and AA genotype with chronic cardiomyopathy in Brazil (42). This observation disagrees with previous studies that detected association between higher IL17A levels and absence of cardiomyopathy (11, 12) and are not in line with the often reported association between the A allele and increased IL17A levels (40, 41). Associations between *T. cruzi* infection and the *IL18* rs187238 C>A (promoter SNV) C, rs360719 A>G (promoter SNV) G, rs2043055 A>G (intronic SNV) A, and rs1946518 C>A (promoter SNV) A alleles were also found in Colombia, a finding mainly driven by the rs360719 G allele (43). Of note, this observation was confirmed in a larger cohort in Latin America (44). Importantly, another study detected association between the rs360719 G carrier status and higher serum IL18 mRNA expression in healthy individuals (45) while an additional report revealed increased IL18 mRNA expression at the myocardium level in Chagas disease cardiomyopathy (18). In addition, the *IL18* rs2043055 G allele was found to associate with absence of cardiomyopathy in Colombia (44). In Brazil the *IL18* rs2043055 AG genotype was more frequent in patients with a moderate than a severe cardiac phenotype. This study also suggested that it is possibly that this intronic SNV is in linkage disequilibrium with another variant functionally relevant (46). This SNV, however, has not yet been shown to affect IL18 production.

While meaningful progress has been made in linking cytokine gene polymorphisms to Chagas disease mechanisms, associations between cytokine-related SNVs with different clinical scenarios of this disease remain largely limited. Establishing their consequences in the corresponding cytokine circulating and local levels, moreover, as well as their implications on specific biological pathways at the host environment, comprise even more complexes problems to be addressed. In spite of such challenges, thoughtful and well supported hypotheses can be made to progressively add pieces to this ongoing puzzle. In this context, association studies involving appropriate cytokine-related SNVs and strategic immune-affected medical conditions, in one side, and key Chagas phenotypes, on the other side, should be encouraged as potentially significant contributors to the comprehension of this disease pathogenesis.

Facing the biological and clinical scenarios just described, in the current study we investigated potential associations between SNVs linked to *IL1B*, *IL6*, *IL17A*, or *IL18* and the risks of positive *T. cruzi* parasitemia or development/progression of cardiomyopathy. With the assumption that immunocompromised conditions frequently associated with Chagas disease could potentially bring key mechanistic and clinical insights to the understanding of this illness, we also analyzed possible associations involving HIV infection and Chagas disease phenotypes. Surprisingly, our data revealed that positiveness for HIV protected against the development and/or progression of cardiomyopathy. We also describe novel associations between specific *IL18*, *IL17A*, and *IL1B* variant profiles and the risk of cardiomyopathy as well as between a specific *IL6* polymorphic genotype and the risk of positive *T. cruzi* parasitemia.

PATIENTS, MATERIALS, AND METHODS

Study Subjects

Our cohort included 206 patients with Chagas disease: 78 from the Heart Institute of Hospital das Clínicas da Faculdade de Medicina, University of São Paulo (HCFMUSP), and 129 from the Infectious Diseases Division of HCFMUSP, 49 of whom with HIV co-infection. These 49 cases were followed at Serviço de Extensão e Atendimento aos Paciente com Infecção por HIV/Aids of the same Division. All participants were adults. The diagnosis of trypanosomiasis was based on the 2nd Brazilian Guidelines for Chagas Diseases (1). Two positive tests of the following ones, therefore, were used to establish the diagnosis: ELISA—enzyme linked immunosorbent assay, indirect immunofluorescence, and hemagglutination (47). All patients from the Infectious Diseases Division with positive epidemiology were sent to the HIV/Aids Clinic, where HIV infection was confirmed by ELISA and immunoblot (31). Patients from the Heart Institute were tested for HIV as previously described (31). When included in the current protocol, 26 of the 49 HIV patients were not on regular HAART therapy or had therapeutic failure due to antiretroviral resistance (three patients). In 23 of them, the median viral load was 14,000 (2,618–100,000, 25th–75th percentiles) DNA viral copies/µl while the median CD4 count was 340 (93–510) cells/mm^3. Data from 23 patients under HAART for 1 to >5 years showed a median viral load of 0.0 (0.0–0.0) DNA viral copies/µl. In these 23 patients, the median CD4 count was 631 (439–715) cells/mm^3.

The patients underwent electrocardiography, echocardiography, and thorax, esophagus, and colon radiological examinations, being then classified within one of the clinical forms of Chagas disease (1). Individuals without signs and symptoms and with no alteration in the mentioned tests were classified as having the indeterminate form (n = 51), patients with abnormalities suggestive of Chagas disease on electrocardiography or on dynamic electrocardiography and without digestive involvement as with the cardiac form (n = 96), the cases with abnormal findings on esophagus and/or colon without Chagas cardiac manifestation as presenting the digestive form (n = 32). Twenty-seven patients presented both digestive and cardiac alterations, constituting the cardio-digestive group. Cardiac involvement was detected in 123 patients (cardiac and cardiac/digestive forms) while heart disease was not identified in 83 patients, a group composed of individuals with the indeterminate and digestive forms.

Patients with cardiomyopathy were evaluated for heart failure according to the New York Heart Association (NYHA) classification (48), which includes the following criteria: class 1. Patients with cardiac disease without limitation of physical activity; class 2. Patients with cardiac disease with mild limitation of physical activity and symptomatic in routine physical activity; class 3. Patients with cardiac disease with marked limitation of physical activity and symptomatic in less than ordinary physical activity; and class 4. Patients with cardiac disease and unable to carry any physical activity without discomfort, symptoms may be present even at rest. For the purposes of our study, however, Chagas patients were classified according to two different scenarios related to their cardiac status, being divided in two groups in each of the cases: A) based on the NYHA classification/absence of cardiopathy—group 1: patients without cardiopathy (no CA) and with mild cardiopathy (NYHA 1), and group 2: patients with more severe cardiopathy (NYHA ≥ 2); and B) Based on the left ventricular ejection fraction (LVEF) yielded by echocardiography—group 1: patients with LVEF ≥ 45%, and group 2: patients with LVEF < 45%.

The control group for the SNV analyses consisted of 90 healthy individuals with negative serological tests for *T. cruzi* antigens. Controls and patients comprised a total population of 296 individuals, including 149 females and 147 males: 215 white and 73 non-white. This classification was not available for eight control individuals. Among the 206 patients included in this study, 135 were classified within these groups according to self-declaration; 71 of them, in turn, following a distinct institutional policy, were classified according to their government-issued identification document or by the hospital employee who processed their hospital registration.

Ethics Statement

The present study was approved by the Ethics Committee for Research Project Analysis of Hospital das Clínicas da Faculdade de Medicina da Universidade de São Paulo (HCFMUSP), São Paulo, Brazil (CAPPesq 0174/11). All subjects gave written informed consent in accordance with the Declaration of Helsinki.

Evaluation of Parasitemia

Patients' peripheral blood samples were collected in EDTA (ethylenediaminetetraacetic acid) tubes. DNA extraction was performed using the QIAmp DNA Mini Kit (Qiagen). DNA concentration and purity were analyzed with a spectrophotometer. The parasitemia status was determined employing a qualitative polymerase chain reaction (PCR) performed with the S35/S36 primers designed to the kinetoplastic DNA of *T. cruzi* (Invitrogen, Thermo Fisher Scientific, Carlsbad, CA, USA), as previously described (49).

DNA Extraction and Genotyping

In most patients genomic DNA was extracted from peripheral blood samples using the QIAampTM DNA Mini Kit (Qiagen, Hilden, Germany). For the cases the DNA concentration was inappropriately low, an additional extraction was carried out using the salt precipitation method (DTAB/CTAB; Sigma-Aldrich, Merck, St. Louis, MO, USA) (50). The DNA samples underwent spectrophotometric evaluation to assess yield and purity. SNVs were investigated by real-time PCR with the TaqMan® Genotyping Master Mix assay and the corresponding SNV-specific primers in the StepOnePlus platform (Applied Biosystems, Thermo Fisher Scientific, Foster City, CA, USA). The investigated SNPs included *IL1B* −31 rs1143627 T>C, *IL6* −174 rs1800795 C>G, *IL17A* −152 rs2275913 G>A, *IL18* −137 rs187238 C>G, and *IL18* −607 rs1946518 C>A.

Serum IL-18 Quantification

IL-18 levels were measured using commercial ELISA Kits (R&D Systems, Minneapolis, MN, USA) according to the manufacturer's instructions. Sera from 43 patients, 15 HIV-infected and 28 non-infected, were stored at −70°C. Twenty-four of such patients had cardiac disease. At the time of blood collection, the median viral load in the 15 HIV-infected patients was 0.0 DNA copies/µl. In 14 of them the median of CD4 count was 873.5 (769.8–974.0) cells/mm^3. Three of the 15 HIV-infected patients were not on regular antiretroviral therapy. Two had detectable viremia, with one of them displaying a CD4 count below 350 cells/mm^3. The third is an HIV-1-infected patient with an undetectable viral load and high CD4 level despite the absence of HAART therapy, belonging to the rare group named as "elite suppressor" (51).

Statistical Analyses

The calculations of Hardy-Weinberg equilibrium (HWE) were performed using chi square tests in MS Excel 365 (Microsoft Corporation, Redmond, WA). Multiple contingency analyses were performed to investigate potential associations among elected dependent variables and covariates. Fisher's exact test was used for 2x2 contingency tables; otherwise the chi-square test was applied. When chi square test was used and was applicable, we performed a *post-hoc* test using standardized and adjusted residues with the Bonferroni correction. The P values obtained with single association tests (Fisher exact test or Pearson chi square test) were used as triage to elect candidate variables for multivariable analyses. We included in the logistic regression all variables that reached $P < 0.2$ in the single variable association test with the dependent variable. In the genetic models, when more than one model reached $P < 0.2$, we assumed the model with lower P value as the best-fit model and included it in the logistic regression analysis. To increase the modeling performance, continuous variables were categorized using a ROC (receiving operator characteristic) curve and clinical/biological criteria. Some variables presented missing values in 1–20% of cases and displayed a non-monotone missing pattern. In such cases, we performed multiple imputations including 100 imputed values for each missing one (52). This step was accomplished using MCMC (Markov chain-Monte Carlo simulation) for value imputation. The genotypes were clustered according to four possible models of genetic effects: additive (each genotype was analyzed separately), dominant (the presence of at least one SNV allele is associated with the effect), heterozygous (the heterozygous genotype is associated with the effect on phenotype), and recessive (the presence of SNV homozygosity is associated with the effect on phenotype). We adopted the best-fit model in the chi-square/Pearson exact test analyses, defined by the most significant P-value.

Since rs1946518 and rs187238 are just 470 bp apart from each other in the *IL18* promoter, we investigated linkage disequilibrium between these two SNVs using the Haploview software (53) and evaluated potential associations involving the haplotypes.

Chagas cardiopathy, NYHA (New York Heart Association) score, LVEF, and parasitemia were selected upfront as dependent variables for the multiple logistic regressions. Since there was potential interference of the clinical form in the analyzed endpoints, we considered the digestive form as an independent variable in addition to traditional potential confounding factors. To address this point, such a variable was included in the triage as a potential predictor in the model applied to the logistic regression analysis.

Continuous variables were tested for normality with the Shapiro-Wilk test. Continuous parametric variables were analyzed using *t* test to compare two groups, with the Welch correction if the Levine test pointed to unequal variance between the groups. Continuous non-parametric variables were analyzed using the Mann-Whitney U test when comparing two groups, or Kruskal-Wallis test when comparing more than two groups, followed by *post-hoc* analysis with the Bonferroni correction. Categorical variables were compared using the chi-square or Fisher exact test. Categorical variables are expressed as the number of cases and percentages while continuous variables as mean ± standard deviation when parametric, and median (25–75% range) when non-parametric. We accepted an α risk of 5% in this exploratory research. The statistical analyses were run in SPSS 24.

RESULTS

Single Nucleotide Variant Genotype and Allele Distribution in the Analyzed Patient Population and Potential Implications

The studied Chagas disease patient population presented a balanced gender composition, predominance of whites and a median age of 50 (42-60) years (**Table 1**). Notably, 49 patients

TABLE 1 | Patient distribution according to demographic features, HIV status, parasitemia, cardiac phenotypes, and single nucleotide variant (SNV) genotypes.

Patient characteristics	n/median	%/25–75%
Age (years)	50.62	42.0–60.0
Age Range		
<35	23	11.2
35–50	88	42.7
>50	95	46.1
Skin color		
White	152	73.8
Non-white	54	26.2
Sex		
Female	103	50
Male	103	50
HIV		
HIV infection	49	23.8
No HIV infection	157	76.2
Parasitemia		
Positive	90	43.7
Negative	112	54.4
Missing	4	1.9
Chagas cardiopathy		
No	83	40.3
Yes	123	59.7
Clinical forms		
Indeterminate form	51	24.8
Cardiac form	96	46.6
Digestive form	32	15,5
Cardio-digestive form	27	13.1
NYHA		
NYHA < 2/no CA	79	38.3
NYHA ≥ 2	112	54.4
Missing	15	7.3
LVEF (%)	60	28–67
LVEF < 45%		
Negative	115	55.8
Positive	69	33.5
Missing	22	10.7
IL1B −31 rs1143627 T>C		
TT	68	33.0
TC	92	44.7
CC	46	22.3
IL6 −174 rs1800795 C>G		
CC	12	5.8
CG	65	31.6
GG	129	62.6
IL17A −152 rs2275913 G>A		
GG	131	63.6
GA	62	30.1
AA	13	6.3
IL18 −607 rs1946518 C>A		
CC	74	35.9
CA	93	45.1
AA	39	18.9
IL18 −137 rs187238 C>G		
CC	111	53.9
CG	77	37.4
GG	18	8.7

HIV, human immunodeficiency virus; LVEF, left ventricular ejection fraction; NYHA, New York Heart Association score; no CA, without cardiopathy. n = 206 patients, except of IL18 levels (n = 43). When missing values were not shown those values are zero.

(23.8%) had HIV co-infection. The distribution of SNV-related genotypes, additional clinical features and the Brazilian state of birth are shown in **Supplementary Table 1**.

The entire study population was in Hardy-Weinberg equilibrium (HWE) (**Supplementary Table 2**). The genotype frequencies were also in HWE in whites and non-whites (**Supplementary Table 2**). Interestingly, HWE equilibrium was not present in some disease conditions. We detected HWE violation in *IL6* −174 rs1800795 C>G in patients with detectable *T. cruzi* DNA in peripheric blood; in patients without cardiopathy (*IL17* rs2275913 G>A and *IL18* −137 rs187238 C>G) and in patients with cardiopathy (*IL1B* rs1143627 T>C); in individuals with NYHA < 2 (NYHA 1) or without heart failure (*IL17* rs2275913 G>A and *IL18* −607 rs1946518 C>A); and in subjects with NYHA ≥ 2 (*IL1B* rs1143627 T>C) (**Supplementary Table 2**). Those data suggest that the mentioned disease conditions could be influenced by the allelic composition in the selected *loci*.

We analyzed self-declared/documented ancestry as a potential confounding factor for all dependent variables. The P values are mentioned in **Supplementary Table 3** and the comparisons can be appreciated in **Supplementary Table 4**, which comprises the frequencies of self-declared/documented ancestry for each of the dependent variables. The P values show that there was no significant interference of self-declared/documented ancestry in the analyzed comparisons carried out in this study.

IL1B, IL17A, and *IL18* Polymorphic Genotypes Decrease the Risk or Attenuate Progression of Cardiomyopathy in Chagas Disease

Preliminary univariate analyses showed potential associations between cardiomyopathy and sex (P = 0.023), *IL18* −607 rs1946518 C>T applying the recessive model (P = 0.011), *IL18* −137 rs187238 C>G using the recessive model (P = 0.078), *IL17* rs2275913 G>A based on the recessive model (P = 0.039), and digestive involvement (P = 0.012) (**Supplementary Table 3**).

These initial analyses also predicted potential associations between NYHA score ≥ 2 and gender (p = 0.019), *IL1B* rs1143627 T>C using the heterozygous model (P = 0.008), *IL18* −607 rs1946518 C>A applying the recessive model (P = 0.009), *IL18* −137 rs187238 C>G applying the recessive model (P = 0.194), and digestive involvement (P = 0.001) (**Supplementary Table 3**). LVEF-based analyses, in turn, showed potential associations between LVEF < 45% and sex (P = 0.128), *IL18* −607 rs1946518 C>A applying the recessive model (P = 0.003), *IL18* −137 rs187238 C>G applying the recessive model (P = 0.052), *IL1B* rs1143627 T>C using the heterozygous model (P = 0.033), *IL6* rs 1800795 C>G applying the recessive model (P = 0.028), *IL17* rs2275913 G>A using the recessive model (P = 0.157), and digestive involvement (P < 0.001) (**Supplementary Table 3**).

As for Parasitemia, potential associations were shown with LVEF < 45% (P = 0.031), NYHA score ≥ 2 (P = 0.180), and *IL6* rs1800795 heterozygous model (P = 0.023) (**Supplementary Table 3**).

In this scenario, we performed multiple logistic regression analyses for each of the elected dependent variables. This assessment revealed that males with Chagas disease had an OR of 2.22 (P = 0.011, 95% CI 1.20–4.09) to develop cardiomyopathy

(**Table 2**). Interestingly, homozygosity for the *IL17* rs2275913 A allele carried a heart protective effect, being associated with an OR of 0.27 (P = 0.044, 95% CI 0.07–0.97) (**Table 2**). A similar effect was detected for homozygosity of the *IL18* −607 rs1946518 A allele (OR = 0.35; P = 0.023, 95% CI 0.14–0.87).

Our analyses also established a positive association between NYHA score ≥ 2 and male gender (OR = 2.62, P = 0.007, 95% CI 1.30–5.27) and a negative association between this NYHA score range and the *IL18* −607 rs1946518 AA genotype (OR = 0.21, P = 0.009, 95% CI 0.06–0.68) and *IL1B* rs1143627 T>C using the heterozygous model (OR = 0.48, P = 0.036, 95% CI 0.24–0.95) and digestive involvement (OR = 0.20, P < 0.001, 95% CI 0.09–0.47) (**Table 3**). A similar effect was observed for the *IL18* −607 rs1946518 AA genotype with respect to LVEF < 45% (OR = 0.22, P = 0.034, CI 0.05–0.89), and digestive involvement (OR = 0.24, P = 0.004, 95% CI 0.09–0.62) (**Table 4**).

TABLE 2 | Multiple logistic regression for cardiopathy.

	OR	95% CI	P
Sex (male)	2.22	1.20–4.09	**0.011**
HIV	0.48	0.23–0.96	**0.039**
IL17A −152 rs2275913 G>A recessive	0.27	0.07–0.97	**0.044**
IL18 −607 rs1946518 C>A recessive	0.35	0.14–0.87	**0.023**
IL18 −137 rs187238 C>G recessive	1.04	0.29–3.71	0.953
Digestive Involvement	0.55	0.28–1.05	0.069

95% CI, 95% confidence interval; HIV, human immunodeficiency virus; OR, odds ratio; P values ≤ 0.05 in bold.

TABLE 3 | Multiple logistic regression for New York Heart Association (NYHA) ≥ 2.

	OR	95% CI	P
Sex (male)	2.620	1.30–5.27	**0.007**
HIV	0.153	0.06–0.39	**<0.001**
IL1B −31 rs1143627 T>C heterozygous	0.476	0.24–0.95	**0.036**
IL18 −607 rs1946518 C>A recessive	0.208	0.06–0.68	**0.009**
IL18 −137 rs187238 C>G recessive	2.567	0.52–12.76	0.249
Parasitemia	0.801	0.39–1.63	0.539
Digestive Involvement	0.204	0.09–0.47	**<0.001**

95%, CI 95% confidence interval; HIV, human immunodeficiency virus; NYHA, New York Heart Association score; OR, odds ratio; P values ≤ 0.05 in bold.

TABLE 4 | Multiple logistic regressions for left ventricular ejection fraction (LVEF) < 45%.

	OR	95% CI	P
Sex (male)	1.967	0.82–4.70	0.128
HIV	0.033	0.00–0.25	**0.001**
IL1B −31 rs1143627 T>C heterozygous	0.631	0.29–1.35	0.237
IL6 −174 rs1800795 C>G recessive	13.082	0.40–431.30	0.149
IL17A −152 rs2275913 G>A recessive	0.578	0.05–7.41	0.673
IL18 −607 rs1946518 C>A recessive	0.221	0.05–0.89	**0.034**
IL18 −137 rs187238 C>G recessive	2.213	0.28–17.40	0.450
Parasitemia	0.581	0.26–1.30	0.186
Digestive involvement	0.235	0.09–0.62	**0.004**

95% CI, 95% confidence interval; HIV, human immunodeficiency virus; LVEF, left ventricular ejection fraction; OR, odds ratio; P values ≤ 0.05 in bold.

When investigating linkage disequilibrium between rs1946518 and rs187238, we found D\` of 0.89 and r^2 of 0.43, indicating strong linkage disequilibrium between the two *loci*. Our analysis also revealed that the haplotype *IL18* −607 C/*IL18* −137 C was associated with Chagas cardiopathy (P = 0.0186) and LVEF < 45% (P = 0.0149) (**Supplementary Table 5**). This same haplotype also reached a marginal P value for association with NYHA ≥ 2 (P = 0.0554). No haplotype involving these two SNVs showed significant association with the parasitemia status.

A Specific *IL6* Polymorphism Profile Modulates the Risk of *Trypanosoma cruzi* Parasitemia

Based on univariate analyses, potential associations were predicted to occur between positive *T. cruzi* parasitemia and *IL6* rs1800795 C>G applying the heterozygous model (P = 0.023), NYHA ≥ 2 (P = 0.180) and HIV infection (P = 0.008) (**Supplementary Table 3**).

Notably, multiple logistic regression analyses uncovered a negative association between parasitemia and the *IL6* rs1800795 CG genotype (OR = 0.45, P = 0.015, 95% CI 0.24 −0.86) and a positive association between parasitemia and HIV infection (OR = 2.18, P = 0.039, 95% CI 1.04–4.58) (**Table 5**).

HIV Infection Is Protective Against Development and Progression of Cardiomyopathy in Chagas Disease

Our preliminary univariate analyses suggested a protective cardiac effect of HIV infection in patients with Chagas disease, based on the development of cardiomyopathy (P = 0.045), the NYHA score (P < 0.001), and the LVEF values (P < 0.001) (**Supplementary Table 3**).

To evaluate the potential effect of HIV infection on the cardiac form of Chagas disease, we initially compared the HIV population with the non-HIV patients with respect to potentially interfering parameters (**Table 6**). This analysis showed no differences in age, sex, groups (white x non white), and the SNV genotypes analyzed in the current study.

Remarkably, multiple logistic regression analyses revealed a protective effect of HIV infection against the development of cardiomyopathy, displaying an OR of 0.48 (P = 0.039, 95% CI 0.23–0.96) (**Table 2**). In the same line, negative associations were shown for NYHA score ≥ 2 and HIV infection (OR = 0.15, P < 0.001, 95% CI 0.06–0.39) (**Table 3**) as well as for LVEF < 45%

TABLE 5 | Multiple logistic regressions for parasitemia.

	OR	95% CI	P
HIV	2.18	1.04–4.58	**0.039**
IL6 −174 rs1800795 C>G heterozygous model	0.45	0.24–0.86	**0.015**
NYHA ≥ 2	1.06	0.43–2.58	0.900
LVEF < 45%	0.65	0.24–1.72	0.385

95% CI, 95% confidence interval; HIV, human immunodeficiency virus; LVEF, left ventricular ejection fraction; NYHA, New York Heart Association score; OR, odds ratio; P values ≤ 0.05 in bold.

TABLE 6 | Comparisons between Chagas disease patients with and without HIV infection.

	HIV n(%)/median (25–75%)	Non-HIV n(%)/median (25–75%)	P
Age[a]	49 (39–60.5)	50 (42–60)	0.379
Age range[b]			0.062
<35	10 (20.4)	13 (8.3)	
35-50	19 (38.8)	69 (43.9)	
>50	20 (40.8)	75 (47.8)	
Sex[c]			0.326
Male	28 (57.1)	75 (47.8)	
Female	21 (42.9)	82 (52.2)	
White[c]	37 (75.5)	115(73.2)	0.853
Non-white	12 (24.5)	42 (26.8)	
Chagas cardiopathy[c]			**0.045**
No	26 (53.1)	57 (36.3)	
Yes	23 (46.9)	100 (63.7)	
NYHA ≥ 2[c]			**<0.001**
No			
Yes	8 (16.3)	71 (50.0)	
Missing	0	15	
Left ventricular ejection fraction[a]	0.67 (0.62–0.71)	0.43 (0.25–0.65)	**<0.001**
Ejection fraction ≥ 45%[c]	45 (97.8)	70 (50.7)	**<0.001**
Ejection fraction < 45%	1 (2.2)	68 (49.3)	
Missing	3	19	
Parasitemia: negative[c]	18 (38.3)	94 (60.6)	**0.008**
Parasitemia: positive	29 (61.7)	61 (39.4)	
Missing	2	2	
Clinical form[b]			**0.001**
Indeterminate form	20 (40.8)	31 (19.7)	
Cardiac form	11 (22.4)	85 (54.1)	
Digestive form	8 (16.3)	24 (15.3)	
Cardio-digestive form	10 (20.4)	17 (10.8)	
Genotypes			
IL1B −31 rs1143627 T>C[b]			0.168
TT	11 (22.4)	57 (36.3)	
TC	24 (49.0)	68 (43.3)	
CC	14 (28.6)	32 (20.4)	
IL6 −174 rs1800795 C>G[b]			0.984
CC	3 (25.0)	9 (5.7)	
CG	15 (6.1)	50 (31.8)	
GG	31 (63.3)	98 (62.4)	
IL17A −152 rs2275913 G>A[b]			0.559
GG	33 (67.3)	98 (62.4)	
GA	12 (24.5)	50 (31.8)	
AA	4 (8.2)	9 (5.7)	
IL18 −607 rs1946518 C>A[b]			0.814
CC	16 (32.7)	58 (36.9)	
CA	24 (49.0)	69 (43.9)	
AA	9 (18.4)	30 (19.1)	
IL18 −137 rs187238 C>G[b]			0.180
CC	22 (44.9)	89 (56.7.)	
CG	20 (40.8)	57 (36.3)	
GG	7 (14.3)	11 (7.0)	

NYHA, New York Heart Association score. HIV patients, (n = 49), non-HIV patients, (n = 157). Comparisons: [a]Student t test, [b]Pearson chi square test, [c]Fisher exact test. Percentual distributions considered only valid cases. When missing values were not shown those values are zero. P values ≤ 0.05 in bold.

and positive HIV status (OR = 0.03, P < 0.001, 95% CI 0.00–0.25) (**Table 4**).

IL18 Levels, Cardiopathy, New York Heart Association, Left Ventricular Ejection Fraction, and HIV

IL18 levels were analyzed in 43 patients and assessed with respect to the genotypes/alleles and the presence of cardiopathy, HIV infection, NYHA score, and LVEF (**Table 7**). The IL18 levels did not significantly vary among *IL18* −607 or *IL18* −137 SNV genotypes/alleles. No significant differences in this interleukin levels were detected either between patients with and without cardiopathy or HIV infection as well as among the different NYHA score or LVEF-related groups. Three patients without HAART therapy displayed serum levels of 737.49, 739.87, and 744.29 pg/ml. These last two were viremic and only one had a CD4 count below 350 cells/mm^3. The 13 aviremic individuals under HAART therapy presented a median value of 308.24 pg/ml and all of them had CD4 cells higher than 350 cell/mm^3.

TABLE 7 | IL18 serum levels in Chagas disease patients according to the HIV status, cardiac phenotypes, parasitemia, and *IL 18* -607 and *IL 18* −137 genotypes.

	N	Serum level IL-18 (pg/ml)Median (25–75%)	P
HIV[a]			0.212
Negative	28	268.0 (190.3–736.0)	
Positive	15	736.6 (194.7–747.2)	
Cardiopathy[a]			0.903
No	22	301.3 (215.7–737.4)	
Yes	21	308.2 (176.4–753.4)	
NYHA[a]			0.508
NYHA <2/no CA	28	311.2 (215.0–753.2)	
NYHA ≥ 2	15	250.8 (176.7–739.5)	
LVEF[a]			0.782
LVEF ≥ 45%	28	298.3 (199.7–743.2)	
LVEF < 45%	14	284.9 (174.5–740.6)	
Missing	1		
Parasitemia[a]			0.131
Negative	20	247.2 (183.4–732.2)	
Positive	22	722.4 (214.209.7–751.5)	
Missing	1		
IL18 −607 rs1946518 C>A[b]			0.897
CC	17	314,1 (185.6–740.9)	
CA	16	313.7 (221.0–742.3)	
AA	10	275.2 (182.4–741.8)	
IL18 −607 rs1946518 C>A[a]			0.944
CC+CA	33	275.2 (182.4–741.8)	
AA	10	314.2 (204.7–740.8)	
IL18 −137 rs187238 C>G[b]			0.878
CC	24	316.6 (185.3–742.6)	
CG	15	308.2 (216.1–744.0)	
GG	4	275.2 (206.6–623.8)	
IL18 −137 rs187238 C>G[a]			0.702
CC+CG	39	314.2 (194.7–744.0)	
GG	4	275.2 (206.6–623.8)	

HIV, human immunodeficiency virus; LVEF, left ventricular ejection fraction; NYHA, New York Heart Association score; no CA, without cardiopathy. Tests: [a]Mann Whitney U test, [b]Kruskal Wallis test. Total number of patients = 43. Percentual distributions considered only valid cases. When missing values were not shown those values are zero.

DISCUSSION

IL6, IL1B, IL17A, and *IL18* Single Nucleotide Variants and Parasitemia in Chagas Disease

In a still largely unclear scenario relating cytokines and pathogenesis of Chagas disease, our study seeked for potential associations between strategic cytokine-related SNVs and key Chagas phenotypes restricted to the disease or combined with immune dysregulation.

T. cruzi parasitemia has been recognized as an element that accelerates chronic Chagas cardiopathy (19, 20, 22), although some reports question this effect (23–25). PCR-based *T. cruzi* detection in human biopsies supports that parasite persistence in the heart favors the progression of cardiomyopathy (19, 21). Identification of *T. cruzi* DNA in human blood, moreover, has been associated with a higher risk of development and deterioration of cardiomyopathy (20, 22).

IL6 is a key cytokine in mouse-induced *T. cruzi* myocarditis, triggering protection mechanisms in cardiomyocytes but favoring a higher parasite load (29). Acute *T. cruzi* experimental infection in mice with high inoculum, in fact, was followed by increased IL-6, high parasite load in tissue and marked inflammation (54, 55) while *IL6*-KO mice developed different levels of parasite load in the blood and myocardium depending on the *T. cruzi* strain (29, 54). These animals, however, presented increased mortality (29, 54). Such findings suggest that avoidance of high IL6 levels may play a role in lowering the parasite load whereas a certain tissue level of IL6 must be reached to allow a protective response against the parasite-induced lesion. A balanced level of IL6, therefore, is expected to reduce tissue damage and cardiomyocyte death, mitigating the disease. Of note, our data revealed that *IL6* −174 CG heterozygosity is protective against *T. cruzi* parasitemia. This original finding raises an enticing mechanistic hypothesis for the relationship between IL6 and parasitemia. This SNV is located in the *IL6* promoter, having the G allele been associated with higher IL6 blood levels than the C allele (33, 34, 56, 57). It is likely, therefore, that the low IL6 levels associated with the CC genotype lead to a lack of immune-mediated protection against parasitemia, while the high IL6 levels observed in GG individuals create a relatively severe inflammatory background that also favors *T. cruzi* replication. On the other hand, a balanced scenario of protection and controlled inflammation, displayed by heterozygous patients, would provide the best setting to fight parasitemia.

Facing the possible role of IL18 in reducing parasitic load in *IL18*-KO mice (26), we investigated the influence of *IL18* SNVs on *T. cruzi* parasitemia. The *IL18* human gene harbors several SNVs in its promoter. *IL18* −607 C>A and *IL18* −137 C>G are located in nuclear factor binding sites for CREB (cyclic AMP-responsive element binding protein) and H4TF-1 (human histone H4 gene specific transcription fator-1), respectively. Variants of these two sites can not only affect *IL18* transcription but also IFNγ expression (58). The −607 A allele and AA genotype have been associated with lower *IL18* transcriptional rate and/or protein levels than the C allele and CC genotype in different clinical and physiological settings (59–63), whereas the haplotype C-607/G-137 is associated with higher expression of IL18. Our analyses, however, did not identify a significant impact of *IL18* −607 or *IL18* −137 alleles/genotypes on the *T. cruzi* parasitemic status.

The observation of increased parasitemia in *IL17A*-KO mice infected by *Leishmania infantum* supports a role of IL17A in controlling parasitemia (64). IL17A and IFNγ activate macrophages to phagocyte *T. cruzi* for further killing in the endosomal/lysosomal compartment (65). This finding is not a surprise, since association between higher levels of IL17A and resistance to *Leishmania donovani* had been previously reported (66).

The *IL17A* −152 G>A SNV is a critical regulator of the *IL17A* promoter, being located within a binding motif for NFAT (nuclear factor activated T cells) (67). The A allele is more often associated with higher IL17A serum levels (40, 41, 67). Despite these observations, our analysis did not show association between *IL17A* −152 G>A and *T. cruzi* parasitemia, not supporting a protective role of the A allele against parasitemia in human Chagas disease.

Effects of *IL1B, IL17A, IL18, and IL6* Single Nucleotide Variants on Cardiomyopathy in Chagas Disease

Previous studies showed direct correlation between IL-6 serum levels and cardiomyopathy (7–9) and an inverse correlation between IL-6 levels and LVEF in the setting of cardiopathy (7). Based on these observations and the association of *IL6* −174 C with lower IL6 levels (33, 34, 56, 57), we hypothesized that this allele might be protective. Our findings, however, did not reveal such an impact, corroborating results from Colombia and Peru obtained in an ethnically distinct population affected by different parasite lineages (32, 68). It is possible, therefore, that other factors may also play a role in determining IL6 levels that modulate the cardiac phenotype in Chagas disease.

IL1β triggers an inflammation cascade, leads to generation of reactive free radicals, and may promote IFNγ production (69) and facilitate the differentiation of pro-inflammatory cells such as human Th17 (70). The assessed *IL1B* −31 T>C transition causes disruption of a TATA-box, potentially changing the binding site affinity to regulatory proteins (36). We showed association between the *IL1B* −31 TC genotype and lower NYHA in Chagas disease. It is known that IL1β promotes inflammatory activity in acute experimental myocarditis induced by *T. cruzi* (71) and induces hypertrophy in primary cultures of cardiomyocytes infected by this parasite (72). Based on these data and because the *IL1B* −31 T allele is associated with increased *IL1B* transcription (36), heterozygosity may attenuate inflammation and cardiomyocyte hypertrophy in Chagas myocarditis, still allowing enough IL1β to fight *T. cruzi* infection. This balanced response likely explains the observed protective effect of the *IL1B* −31 TC genotype against cardiac disease severity. Interestingly, the CT haplotype for *IL1B* −31 T>C and +3,954 C>T was more prevalent in patients with Chagas cardiomyopathy in a Colombian population (35).

Higher frequencies of CD4+ IL-17A+ T-cells, lower levels of IL10 and IL10, and higher levels of IFNγ and TNFα are observed in individuals with more severe cardiomyopathy (6, 7). These findings are in agreement with the observation of lower lymphocyte IL17A expression in chronic Chagas cardiomyopathy than in seronegative individuals and patients with the indeterminate form (6). In addition, high IL17A levels were also associated with better heart function in Chagas disease (11). Based on these observations, IL17A was expected to potentially modulate inflammation in cardiac tissue and protect against *T. cruzi* infection (27, 28). A study in Brazil, however, unexpectedly revealed associations between the *IL17A* −152 A allele and the AA genotype with chronic cardiomyopathy (42). In contrast, another study in a Colombian cohort reported a protective effect of the C Allele of *IL17A* rs 8193036 C>T in seronegative individuals in comparison with cardiac seropositive patients (38), in a context of previously established association between the C allele and lower IL 17A mRNA expression (39). These data were *a priori* not expected, since previous reports showed a role for IL17A in mouse resistance to *T. cruzi* infection (27) and/or higher IL17A levels in patients without cardiopathy (11, 12). This study also found no association between the *IL17A* G>A 3' UTR rs7747909 SNV, other two *IL17A* promoter SNVs (rs4711998 and rs3819024) or *IL17A* rs2275913 and Chagas cardiopathy.

In agreement with the expected role of IL17A, but in contrast to most clinical results, we found association between *IL17A* rs2275913 G>A and cardiac protection following a recessive model. Indeed, carriers of the A allele and the AA genotype were found to have a lower risk to develop cardiomyopathy. Since A allele has been found in association with higher IL17A serum levels (40, 41, 67), our data are in accordance with reports that show association between better cardiac function and higher IL17 A levels (11, 12). Our findings suggest that IL17A modulates the host inflammatory response to parasites in the myocardium, impacting the risk of developing cardiac dysfunction. Additional studies are necessary, however, to establish the effect of the AA genotype on IL17A serum levels in Chagas disease patients. It must be pointed out that our study differs from the previous ones (38, 42) with respect to patient geographical origin, ethnicity, classification, sample size, subgroup design, and possibly parasite lineage (68). Given the significant ethnical differences among Brazilian, Colombian, and Bolivian populations, genetic background may be a major determinant for the different results.

Since IL18 induces pathological cardiac remodeling (16), cardiomyocyte hypertrophy (73) and increased fibronectin expression (74), high levels of IL18 are expected to lead to cardiac hypertrophy and fibrosis, with a deleterious impact on heart function. IL18 is expressed in myocardium early in the course of experimental myocarditis induced by *T. cruzi* (15), leading to production of IFNγ. IL18 upregulation and correlation between IL18 mRNA and IFNγ expression have been shown in human Chagas heart tissue (18). Standing as a novel observation, we showed association between the *IL18* −607 AA genotype and decreased risk of developing cardiomyopathy, progressing to NYHA ≥ 2, and progressing to LVEF < 45%. These data are in accordance to previously reported association between this AA genotype and low IL18 production in the presence and in the absence of mitogen stimuli (60–66). Unlike these studies, however, our data did not reveal significant associations between IL18 levels and any of the *IL18* −607 or *IL18* −137 genotypes/alleles. Such differences may rely on the nature and size of the studied populations (55–101 patients), including other diseases, and/or the nature the biological samples and/or experimental conditions, including plasma and mucosal biopsies and peripheral blood cells under mitogen stimuli (58–63). The lack of association between IL18 serum levels and *IL18* −607 C>A or *IL18* −137 C>G genotypes/alleles observed in our study does not allow a straight association between the mentioned cardiac findings and IL18 serum levels. This finding raises the hypothesis that IL18 serum levels may not significantly correlate with IL18 heart tissue levels in Chagas disease. However, since our study did not reproduce the association between IL18 levels and the *IL18* −607 SNV in other contexts, more representative patient samples should be evaluated under different conditions to more conclusively investigate this relationship in this disease. It must be noted that a previous study conducted in Colombian and Latin American Chagas patients did not detect significant frequency differences of *IL18* −607 A allele and AA genotype between asymptomatic patients and ones with cardiac dysfunction (43, 44). Data from an Argentinian population, on the other hand, display a trend similar to our study (44). Our data strengthens the potential benefit of targeting IL18 as a therapy in Chagas cardiomyopathy. IL18 levels have indeed been associated with increased mortality and are inversely correlated with LVEF in heart failure (75). Moreover, neutralization of IL18 has been proposed in heart failure (76), Fabry cardiomyopathy (77) and sepsis-induced cardiac dysfunction (78). Our data also revealed association of the *IL18* −607 C/*IL18* −137 C haplotype with Chagas cardiopathy and LVEF < 45%. Our results on *IL18* −137, however, do not support an additive susceptibility status linking such SNVs.

Our study revealed that men have higher risks for cardiopathy and NYHA ≥ 2. These findings are in line with previous data that report male gender as one of the six independent variables that constitute risk factors for death in Chagas heart disease (3, 79). Male sex, therefore, appears as a robust risk factor for worse prognosis in Chagas cardiomyopathy. As a novel finding, digestive involvement associated negatively with NYHA ≥ 2 and LVEF < 45%, suggesting that such patients may develop a milder cardiopathy than affected individuals without digestive disease. This observation has never been reported (1, 31, 80). Alternative explanations for this finding may comprise a potential inclusion of more severely affected cardiac patients in our study and a potentially smaller than real proportion of patients with the indeterminate form due to underdiagnosis and/or loss of follow-up, raising the cardiac form/indeterminate form ratio. The relatively high proportion of cardio-digestive cases previously reported (1, 31), however, adds further support to the influence of digestive involvement in NYHA and LVEF.

Impact of HIV Infection on Development and Progression of Cardiomyopathy in Chagas Disease

In immunosuppressed patients with HIV infection, elevated IL18 serum concentrations have been shown to favor the development of Aids and associated infections (30). In addition, Chagas disease reactivation does not occur in immunocompetent subjects, while in HIV-infected patients this illness has been associated with increased morbidity and mortality (31). Based on a severe combined immunodeficient (SCID) animal model (81), this observation may be explained by dissociation between a high parasite load and lower tissue inflammation, which is associated with decreased IFNγ levels and early mortality. Interestingly, *T. cruzi* inhibits HIV replication in macrophage-derived monocyte culture (82). In our study the HIV infected and non-infected groups did not differ with respect to the evaluated SNV profiles, age or gender. In the HIV-infected group, 53.1% of the patients were not on HAART therapy. Our findings revealed higher parasitemia in HIV-infected Chagas individuals, confirming previous data (83). Of note, in *T. cruzi*/HIV coinfection a Th2 response likely contributes to the impairment of parasite control (84). Altogether, our data suggest that antiretroviral therapy interferes positively in the host-HIV-*T. cruzi* interaction.

To our surprise, our analyses revealed a previously not described finding: HIV infection exerts a strong protective effect on Chagas disease cardiomyopathy. HIV infection was associated with lower risks to develop cardiopathy and to progress to NYHA ≥ 2 and LVEF < 45%. This *a priori* unexpected effect may be based on actions of the HAART regimens, reported to decrease the prevalence of HIV-associated cardiomyopathy in about 30% of the HIV-infected patients (85). In contrast, HAART failure was associated with continued IL18 elevation (86).

IL18 contributes to Aids pathogenesis by increasing viral replication, death of endothelial cells, and cardiomyocyte proliferation (30). A previous study from our service showed that Chagas reactivation occurred only in patients not in HAART therapy, and progression to a more severe chronic disease and death were observed in 35 and 30% of them, respectively (31). Moreover, progression to severe chronic forms was verified in less than 10% of patients on HAART. In those under HAART therapy, we detected high levels of IL18 (>700 pg/ml) in two of viremic cases and a median of 308.24 pg/ml in 13 aviremic individuals. The small number of analyzed patients, however, did not allow statistical evaluation with respect to IL18 levels and viral load, and no differences in IL18 levels were detected between HIV and non-HIV patients. A previous report did not find difference between 32 HIV viremic and 15 aviremic patients either (87). While our data suggest that IL18 serum levels may not correlate with IL18 levels in cardiac tissue in Chagas disease, a larger future study should address a still possible IL18-reducing effect of HAART on Chagas cardiomyopathy.

Another potential explanation for this positive impact of HIV infection on Chagas disease could be a growth-reduction effect of antiretroviral drugs on *T. cruzi*. HIV protease inhibitors have in fact been reported to restrain epimastigote, trypomastigote, and amastigote growth (88–90). Pretreatment of trypomastigotes with nelfinavir and lopinavir inhibited their association with LLC-MK_2 epithelial cells and RAW macrophages and decreased the number of intracellular amastigotes (88). In addition, interaction of ritonavir, lopinavir and nelfinavir and *T. cruzi* epimastigotes showed potent anti-proliferative effects and led to changes in differentiation (89).

Nelfinavir and lopinavir target vital cellular structures of trypomastigotes, leading to irreversible, lethal metabolic injuries in the size and structure (90). A trypanocidal effect of HIV proteinase inhibitors on the *T. cruzi* aspartyl peptidase intracellular target was also reported using a docking simulation model (91), showing a great affinity of ritonavir and lopinavir to bind to this active enzyme intracellular site. In this setting, saquinavir has been integrated to the computer-guided drug repositioning as a potentially new treatment for Chagas disease (92).

A synergistic interaction between a Th2 predominant response in *T. cruzi*-HIV infected patients and HAART could also potentially lead to reduction in IL18 levels (30). This combined effect might decrease the predominant Th1 response in myocardium (5) and reduce inflammatory cardiac lesions. Other cardiovascular actions of antiretrovirals are unlikely to contribute to the cardioprotective effect, since HAART has been linked to increased risk of cardiovascular illness (30).

While the scientific relevance and possible clinical applications raised by the HIV-related cardioprotective effect on Chagas cardiomyopathy are potentially remarkable, its underlying mechanisms remain unclear. Future studies with larger and more diverse coinfected patient populations, expansion of cardiac function/lesion markers, detailed characterization of the cardiac microenvironment associated this coinfection, and deep characterization of cardiac tissue response to HAART should bring significant contributions to this elucidation.

Our study brought novel and meaningful data to field of Chagas disease, but it also carries some limitations. Such limitations comprise the inclusion of a single center, Brazilian heterogeneous ethnicity, limited analyses of interleukin levels and respective functional impact, and lack of data integration involving the use of HAART, CD4+ count, HIV load, and molecular genetics assessment. The appropriate statistical model employed for small samples and the level of significance detected in key analyses, however, strongly support our conclusions and provide a robust platform for sequential future studies.

In conclusion, our findings revealed a novel association between the *IL6* −174 C>G SNV and parasitemia in Chagas disease, expressed as a decreased risk of its detection in patients with the CG genotype. As additional original findings, our data showed that the *IL17A* −152 AA and the *IL18* −607 AA genotypes are associated with a reduced risk of developing cardiomyopathy in individuals affected by this illness. The *IL18* −607 AA and *IL1B* TC genotypes were also found to associate with a lower risk of manifesting severe cardiac dysfunction. Most of our findings are consistent with previously reported clinical data on Chagas disease and data on cytokine expression. Unexpectedly, our results uncovered a novel protective effect of HIV infection in Chagas disease patients, translated into a decreased risk of developing cardiomyopathy. Available information suggests that a synergistic effect of HIV and HAART may mitigate a Th1-mediated response in the myocardium. The findings revealed by this report not only expand the understanding of Chagas disease pathogenesis and its relationship with other clinical scenarios but also add pieces of information to the field that can be potentially employed in the development of therapeutic interventions.

AUTHOR CONTRIBUTIONS

MS-Y, VF, LO: conception and design. AG, EW, DF, JO, EN, CO, EB, AP, CN, FC, NC, PS, EY-K, VF, LO, MS-Y: analysis and interpretation. AG, EW, LO, MS-Y: drafting the manuscript for important intellectual content. All authors contributed to the article and approved the submitted version.

ACKNOWLEDGMENTS

The authors acknowledge Expedito Luna for revising the epidemiological design of this manuscript.

REFERENCES

1. Dias JC, Ramos ANJr, Gontijo ED, Luquetti A, Shikanai-Yasuda MA, Coura JR, et al. 2nd Brazilian Consensus on Chagas Disease, 2015. *Rev Soc Bras Med Trop* (2016) 49:3–60. doi: 10.1590/0037-8682-0505-2016
2. Bocchi EA, Bestetti RB, Scanavacca MI, Cunha Neto E, Issa VS. Chronic Chagas Heart Disease Management: From Etiology to Cardiomyopathy Treatment. *J Am Coll Cardiol* (2017) 70:1510–24. doi: 10.1016/j.jacc.2017.08.004
3. Rassi AJr, Rassi A, Little WC, Xavier SS, Rassi SG, Rassi AG, et al. Development and validation of a risk score for predicting death in Chagas' heart disease. *N Engl J Med* (2006) 355:799–808. doi: 10.1056/NEJMoa053241
4. Dutra WO, Gollob KJ. Current concepts in immunoregulation and pathology of human Chagas disease. *Curr Opin Infect Dis* (2008) 21:287–92. doi: 10.1097/QCO.0b013e3282f88b80
5. Abel LC, Rizzo LV, Ianni B, Albuquerque F, Bacal F, Carrara D, et al. Chronic Chagas' disease cardiomyopathy patients display an increased IFN-gamma response to *Trypanosoma cruzi* infection. *J Autoimmun* (2001) 17:99–107. doi: 10.1006/jaut.2001.0523
6. de Araújo FF, Corrêa-Oliveira R, Rocha MO, Chaves AT, Fiuza JA, Fares RC, et al. Foxp3+CD25 (high) CD4+ regulatory T cells from indeterminate patients with Chagas disease can suppress the effector cells and cytokines and reveal altered correlations with disease severity. *Immunobiology* (2012) 217:768–77. doi: 10.1016/j.imbio.2012.04.008
7. Sousa GR, Gomes JA, Fares RC, Damásio MP, Chaves AT, Ferreira KS, et al. Plasma cytokine expression is associated with cardiac morbidity in Chagas disease. *PloS One* (2014) 9:e87082. doi: 10.1371/journal.pone.0087082
8. Reis MM, Higuchi M de L, Benvenuti LA, Aiello VD, Gutierrez PS, Bellotti G, et al. An *in situ* quantitative immunohistochemical study of cytokines and IL-2R+ in chronic human chagasic myocarditis: correlation with the presence of myocardial *Trypanosoma cruzi* antigens. *Clin Immunol Immunopathol* (1997) 83(2):165–72. doi: 10.1006/clin.1997.4335
9. Keating SM, Deng X, Fernandes F, Cunha-Neto E, Ribeiro AL, Adesina B, et al. NHLBI Retrovirus Epidemiology Donor Study-II (REDS-II), International Component. Inflammatory and cardiac biomarkers are differentially expressed in clinical stages of Chagas disease. *Int J Cardiol* (2015) 199:451–9. doi: 10.1016/j.ijcard.2015.07.040
10. López L, Arai K, Giménez E, Jiménez M, Pascuzo C, Rodríguez-Bonfante C, et al. C-reactive protein and interleukin-6 serum levels increase as Chagas disease progresses towards cardiac failure. *Rev Esp Cardiol* (2006) 59:50–6. doi: 10.1016/S1885-5857(06)60048-0
11. Magalhaes LM, Villani FN, Nunes M do C, Gollob KJ, Rocha MO, Dutra WO. High interleukin 17 expression is correlated with better cardiac function in human Chagas disease. *J Infect Dis* (2013) 207:661–5.9. doi: 10.1371/journal.ppat.1005902
12. Sousa GR, Gomes JA, Damasio MP, Nunes MC, Costa HS, Medeiros NI, et al. The role of interleukin 17-mediated immune response in Chagas disease: High level is correlated with better left ventricular function. *PloS One* (2017) 12: e0172833. doi: 10.1371/journal.pone.0172833
13. Guedes PM, Gutierrez FR, Silva GK, Dellalibera-Joviliano R, Rodrigues GJ, Bendhack LM, et al. Deficient regulatory T cell activity and low frequency of IL-17 - producing T cells correlate with the extent of cardiomyopathy in human Chagas' disease. *PloS Negl Trop Dis* (2012) 6:e1630. doi: 10.1371/journal.pntd.0001630
14. Cai CW, Blase JR, Zhang X, Eickhoff CS, Hoft DF. Th17 Cells Are More Protective Than Th1 Cells Against the Intracellular Parasite *Trypanosoma cruzi*. *PloS Pathog* (2016) 12(10):e1005902. doi: 10.1371/journal.ppat.1005902
15. Muller U, Kohler G, Mossmann H, Schaub GA, Alber G, Di Santo JP, et al. IL-12- Independent IFN-gamma production by T cells in experimental Chagas' disease is mediated by IL-18. *J Immunol* (2001) 167(6):3346–53. doi: 10.4049/jimmunol.167.6.3346
16. Xiao H, Li H, Wang JJ, Zhang JS, Shen J, An XB, et al. IL-18 cleavage triggers cardiac inflammation and fibrosis upon β-adrenergic insult. *Eur Heart J* (2018) 39:60–9. doi: 10.1093/eurheartj/ehx261
17. Meyer Zum Büschenfelde C, Cramer S, Trumpfheller C, Fleischer B, Frosch S. *Trypanosoma cruzi* induces strong *IL-12* and *IL-18* gene expression in vivo: correlation with interferon-gamma (IFN-gamma) production. *Clin Exp Immunol* (1997) 110:378–85. doi: 10.1046/j.1365-2249.1997.4471463.x
18. Nogueira LG, Santos RH, Fiorelli AI, Mairena EC, Benvenuti LA, Bocchi EA, et al. Myocardial gene expression of T-bet, GATA-3, Ror-γt, FoxP3, and hallmark cytokines in chronic Chagas disease cardiomyopathy: an essentially unopposed TH1-type response. *Mediators Inflamm* (2014) 2014(914326):9. doi: 10.1155/2014/914326
19. Zhang L, Tarleton RL. Parasite persistence correlates with disease severity and localization in chronic Chagas' disease. *J Infect Dis* (1999) 180:480–6. doi: 10.1016/j.micinf.2014.03.007
20. Basquiera AL, Sembaj A, Aguerri AM, Omelianiuk M, Guzman S, Moreno Barral J, et al. Risk progression to chronic Chagas cardiomyopathy: influence of male sex and of parasitaemia detected by polymerase chain reaction. *Heart* (2003) 89:1186–90. doi: 10.1136/heart.89.10.1186
21. Benvenuti LA, Roggerio A, Freitas HF, Mansur AJ, Fiorelli A, Higuchi ML. Chronic American trypanosomiasis: parasite persistence in endomyocardial biopsies is associated with high-grade myocarditis. *Ann Trop Med Parasitol* (2008) 102:481–7. doi: 10.1179/136485908X311740
22. Sabino EC, Ribeiro AL, Lee TH, Oliveira CL, Carneiro-Proietti AB, Antunes AP, et al. Detection of *Trypanosoma cruzi* DNA in blood by PCR is associated with Chagas cardiomyopathy and disease severity. *Eur J Heart* (2015) 17:416–23. doi: 10.1002/ejhf.220
23. Norman FF, Perez-Ayala A, Perez-Molina JA, Flores-Chavez M, Canavate C, Lopez-Velez R. Lack of association between blood-based detection of *Trypanosoma cruzi* DNA and cardiac involvement in a non-endemic area. *Ann Trop Med Parasitol* (2011) 105:425–30. doi: 10.1179/1364859411Y.0000000033
24. Apt W, Arribada A, Zulantay I, Saavedra M, Muñoz C, Toro B. Vega, Rodríguez J.Chronic Chagas cardiopathy in Chile. Importance of *Trypanosoma cruzi* burden and clinical evaluation. *Acta Trop* (2016) 162:155–66. doi: 10.1016/j.actatropica.2016.06.025
25. D'Ávila DA, Galvão LMC, Sousa GR, Britto C, Moreira OC, Chiari E. Monitoring the parasite load in chronic Chagas disease patients: comparison between blood culture and quantitative real time PCR. *PloS One* (2018) 13(11):e0208133. doi: 10.1371/journal.pone.0208133
26. Esper L, Utsch L, Soriani FM, Brant F, Esteves Arantes RM, Campos CF, et al. Regulatory effects of IL-18 on cytokine profiles and development of myocarditis during *Trypanosoma cruzi* infection. *Microb Infect* (2014) 16:481–90. doi: 10.1016/j.micinf.2014.03.007
27. Miyazaki Y, Hamano S, Wang S, Shimanoe Y, Iwakura Y, Yoshida H. IL-17 is necessary for host protection against acute-phase *Trypanosoma cruzi* infection. *J Immunol* (2010) 185:1150–7. doi: 10.4049/jimmunol.0900047
28. da Matta Guedes PM, Gutierrez FR, Maia FL, Milanezi CM, Silva GK, Pavanelli WR, et al. IL-17 produced during *Trypanosoma cruzi* infection plays a central role in regulating parasite-induced myocarditis. *PloS Negl Trop Dis* (2010) 4:e604. doi: 10.1371/journal.pntd.0000604
29. Sanmarco LM, Ponce NE, Visconti LM, Eberhardt N, Theumer MG, Minguez Á. R. Aoki MP. L-6 promotes M2 macrophage polarization by modulating purinergic signaling and regulates the lethal release of nitric oxide during *Trypanosoma cruzi* infection. *Biochim Biophys Acta Mol Basis Dis* (2017) 1863:857–69. doi: 10.1016/j.bbadis.2017.01.006
30. Samarani S, Allam O, Sagala P, Aldabah Z, Jenabian MA, Mehraj V, et al. Imbalanced production of IL-18 and its antagonist in human diseases, and its

implications for HIV-1 infection. *Cytokine* (2016) 82:38–51. doi: 10.1016/j.cyto.2016.01.006
31. Sartori AM, Ibrahim KY, Nunes Westphalen EV, Braz LM, Oliveira OCJr, Gakiya E, et al. Manifestations of Chagas disease (American trypanosomiasis) in patients with HIV/AIDS. *Ann Trop Med Parasitol* (2007) 101:31–50. doi: 10.1179/136485907X154629
32. Torres OA, Calzada JE, Beraún Y, Morillo CA, González A, González CI, et al. Lack of association between *IL6*-174G/C gene polymorphism and Chagas disease. *Tissue Antigens* (2010) 76:131–4. doi: 10.1111/j.1399-0039.2010.01478.x
33. Lorente L, Martín MM, Pérez-Cejas A, Barrios Y, Solé-Violán J, Ferreres J, et al. Association between interleukin-6 promoter polymorphism (-174 G/C), serum interleukin-6 levels and mortality in severe septic patients. *Int J Mol Sci* (2016) 17:E1861. doi: 10.3390/ijms17111861
34. Fishman D, Faulds G, Jeffery R, Mohamed-Ali V, Yudkin JS, Humphries S, et al. The effect of novel polymorphisms in the interleukin-6 (IL-6) gene on IL-6 transcription and plasma IL-6 levels, and an association with systemic-onset juvenile chronic arthritis. *J Clin Invest* (1998) 102:1369–76. doi: 10.1172/JCI2629
35. Flórez O, Zafra G, Morillo C, Martín J, González CI. Interleukin-1 gene cluster polymorphism in Chagas disease in a Colombian case-control study. *Hum Immunol* (2006) 67:741–8. doi: 10.1016/j.humimm.2006.06.004
36. El-Omar EM, Carrington M, Chow WH, McColl KE, Bream JH, Young HA, et al. *Interleukin-1* polymorphisms associated with increased risk of gastric cancer. *Nature* (2000) 404:398–402. doi: 10.1038/35006081
37. Hall SK, Perregaux DG, Gabel CA. Correlation of poly-morphic variation in the promoter region of the interleukin-1 β gene with secretion of interleukin-1β protein. *Arthritis Rheum* (2004) 50:1976. 2004. doi: 10.1002/art.20310
38. Leon Rodriguez DA, Echeverría LE, González CI, Martin J. Investigation of the role of *IL17A* gene variants in Chagas disease. *Genes Immun* (2015) 16:536–40. doi: 10.1038/gene.2015.42
39. Kim SW, Kim ES, Moon CM, Park JJ, Kim TI, Kim WH, et al. Genetic polymorphisms of IL-23R and IL-17A and novel insights into their associations with inflammatory bowel disease. *Gut* (2011) 60:1527–36. doi: 10.1136/gut.2011.238477
40. Zidan HE, Rezk NA, Alnemr AA, Moniem MI. Interleukin-17 and leptin genes polymorphisms and their levels in relation to recurrent pregnancy loss in Egyptian females. *Immunogenetics* (2015) 67:665–73. doi: 10.1007/s00251-015-0876-8
41. Correa JD, Madeira MF, Resende RG, Correia-Silva JF, Gomez RS, Souza DG, et al. Association between polymorphisms in interleukin-17 A and -17 F genes and chronic periodontal disease. *Mediators Inflammation* (2012) 2012:846052. doi: 10.1155/2012/846052
42. Reis PG, Ayo CM, de Mattos LC, Brandão de Mattos CC, Sakita KM, de Moraes AG, et al. Genetic Polymorphisms of *IL17* and Chagas disease in the south and southeast of Brazil. *J Immunol Res* (2017) 2017(1017621):7. doi: 10.1155/2017/1017621
43. Leon Rodriguez DA, Carmona FD, Echeverría LE, González CI, Martin J. IL18 Gene Variants Influence the Susceptibility to Chagas Disease. *PloS Negl Trop Dis* (2016) 10:e0004583. doi: 10.1371/journal.pntd.0004583
44. Strauss M, Acosta-Herrera M, Alcaraz A, Casares-Marfil D, Bosch-Niccolau P, Lo Presti MS, et al. Association of IL18 genetic polymorphisms with Chagas disease in Latin American populations. *PloS Negl Trop Dis* (2019) 13(11): e0007859. doi: 10.1371/journal.pntd.0007859
45. Sanchez E, Palomino-Morales RJ, Ortego-Centeno N, Jimenez-Alonso J, Gonzalez-Gay MA, López-Nevot MA, et al. Identification of a new putative functional IL18 gene variant through an association study in systemic lupus erythematosus. *Hum Mol Genet* (2009) 18:3739–48. doi: 10.1093/hmg/ddp301 PMID: 19584085
46. Nogueira LG, Frade AF, Ianni BM, Laugier L, Pissetti CW, Cabantous S, et al. Functional IL18 polymorphism and susceptibility to chronic Chagas disease. *Cytokine* (2015) 73:79–83. doi: 10.1016/j.cyto.2015.01.037
47. Furuchó CR, Umezawa ES, Almeida I, Freitas VL, Bezerra R, Nunes EV, et al. Inconclusive results in conventional serological screening for Chagas' disease in blood banks: evaluation of cellular and humoral response. *Trop Med Int Health* (2008) 13:1527–33. doi: 10.1111/j.1365-3156.2008.02172.x
48. Bennett JA, Riegel B, Bittner V, Nichols J. Validity and reliability of the NYHA classes for measuring research outcomes in patients with cardiac disease. *Heart Lung* (2002) 31:262–70. doi: 10.1067/mhl.2002.124554
49. Britto C, Cardoso MA, Wincker P, Morel CM. A simple protocol for the physical cleavage of *Trypanosoma cruzi* kinetoplast DNA present in blood samples and its use in polymerase chain reaction (PCR)-based diagnosis of chronic Chagas disease. *Mem Inst Oswaldo Cruz* (1993) 88:171–2. doi: 10.1590/s0074-02761993000100030
50. Gustincich S, Manfioletti G, Del Sal GS, Schneider G, Carninci PA. Fast method for high quality genomic DNA extraction from whole human blood. *Biotechniques* (1991) 11(3):298–300.
51. Sedaghat AR, Rastegar DA, O'Connell KA, Dinoso JB, Claus O, Wilke CO, et al. T Cell dynamics and the response to HAART in a cohort of HIV-1-infected elite suppressors. *Clin Inf Dis* (2009) 49(11):1763–6. doi: 10.1086/648081
52. Collins LM, Schafer JL. Kam CM. A comparison of inclusive and restrictive strategies in modern missing data procedures. *Psychol Methods* (2001) 6 (4):330–51. doi: 10.1037/1082-989X.6.4.330
53. Barrett JC, Fry B, Maller J, Daly MJ. Haploview: analysis and visualization of LD and haplotype maps. *Bioinformatics* (2005) 21(2):263–5. doi: 10.1093/bioinformatics/bth457
54. Borges DC, Araújo NM, Cardoso CR, Lazo Chica JE. Different parasite inocula determine the modulation of the immune response and outcome of experimental *Trypanosoma cruzi* infection. *Immunology* (2013) 138:145–56. doi: 10.1111/imm.12022
55. Gao W, Pereira MA. Interleukin-6 is required for parasite specific response and host resistance to *Trypanosoma cruzi*. *Int J Parasitol* (2002) 32:167–70. doi: 10.1016/s0020-7519(01)00322-8
56. Giannitrapani L, Soresi M, Giacalone A, Campagna ME, Marasà M, Cervello M, et al. IL-6 -174G/C polymorphism and IL-6 serum levels in patients with liver cirrhosis and hepatocellular carcinoma. *OMICS* (2011) 15:183–6. doi: 10.1089/omi.2010.0093
57. Talar-Wojnarowska R, Gasiorowska A, Smolarz B, Romanowicz-Makowska H, Kulig A, Malecka-Panas E. Clinical significance of interleukin-6 (IL-6) gene polymorphism and IL-6 serum level in pancreatic adenocarcinoma and chronic pancreatitis. *Dig Dis Sci* (2009) 54:683–9. doi: 10.1007/s10620-008-0390-z
58. Giedraitis V, He B, Huang W-X, Hillert J. Cloning and mutation analysis of the human IL-18 promoter: a possible role of polymorphisms in expression regulation. *J Neuroimmunol* (2001) 112:146–52. doi: 10.1016/s0165-5728(00)00407-0
59. Hasan FT, Naif HM. Association of Gene Polymorphisms and Serum Levels of IL-18 with the Susceptibility to Infection with Hepatitis B Virus. *J Infect Dis Med* (2017) 2:117. doi: 10.4172/2576-1420.1000117
60. Chen DY, Hsieh CW, Chen KS, Chen YM, Lin FJ, Lan JL. Association of interleukin-18 promoter polymorphisms with WHO pathological classes and serum IL-18 levels in Chinese patients with lupus nephritis. *Lupus* (2009) 18:29–37. doi: 10.1177/0961203308094559
61. Dziedziejko V, Kurzawski M, Paczkowska E, Machalinski B, Pawlik A. The impact of IL-18 gene polymorphism on mRNA levels and interleukin-18 release by peripheral blood mononuclear cells. *Postepy Hig Med Dosw (Online)* (2012) 66:409–14. doi: 10.5604/17322693.1000980
62. Jurecekova J, Babusikova E, Sivonova MK, Drobkova H, Petras M, Kliment J, et al. Association between interleukin-18 variants and prostate cancer in Slovak population. *Neoplasma* (2017) 64:148–55. doi: 10.4149/neo_2017_119. 2017.
63. Sakai K, Kita M, Sawai N, Shiomi S, Sumida Y, Kanemasa K, et al. Levels of interleukin-18 are markedly increased in *Helicobacter pylori*-infected gastric mucosa among patients with specific IL18 genotypes. *J Infect Dis* (2008) 197:1752–61. doi: 10.1086/588196
64. Nascimento MS, Carregaro V, Lima-Junior DS, Costa DL, Ryffel B, Duthie MS, et al. Interleukin 17A Acts Synergistically With Interferon gamma to Promote Protection Against *Leishmania infantum* Infection. *J Infect Dis* (2015) 211:1015–26. doi: 10.1093/infdis/jiu531
65. Erdmann H, Rossnagel C, Bohme J, Iwakura Y, Jacobs T, Schaible UE, et al. IL-17A promotes macrophage effector mechanisms against *Trypanosoma cruzi* by trapping parasites in the endolysosomal compartment. *Immunobiology* (2013) 218:910–23. doi: 10.1016/j.imbio.2012.10.005
66. Pitta MG, Romano A, Cabantous S, Henri S, Hammad A, Kouriba B, et al. IL-17 and IL-22 are associated with protection against human kala azar caused by *Leishmania donovani*. *J Clin Invest* (2009) 119:2379–87. doi: 10.1172/JCI38813

67. Espinoza JL, Takami A, Nakata K, Onizuka M, Kawase T, Akiyama H, et al. A genetic variant in the IL-17 promoter is functionally associated with acute graft-versus host disease after unrelated bone marrow transplantation. *PloS One* (2011) 6:e26229. doi: 10.1371/journal.pone.0026229
68. Zingales B, Miles MA, Campbell DA, Tibayrenc M, Macedo AM, Teixeira MM, et al. The revised *Trypanosoma cruzi* subspecific nomenclature: rationale, epidemiological relevance and research applications. *Infect Genet Evol* (2012) 12:240–53. doi: 10.1016/j.meegid.2011.12.009
69. Luft T, Jefford M, Luetjens P, Hochrein H, Masterman KA, Maliszewski C, et al. IL-1 beta enhances CD40 ligand-mediated cytokine secretion by human dendritic cells (DC): a mechanism for T cell-independent DC activation. *J Immunol* (2002) 168(2):713–22. doi: 10.4049/jimmunol.168.2.713
70. Acosta-Rodriguez EV, Napolitani G, Lanzavecchia A, Sallusto F. Interleukins 1 beta and 6 but not transforming growth factor-beta are essential for the differentiation of interleukin 17-producing human T helper cells. *Nat Immunol* (2007) 8(9):942–9. doi: 10.1038/ni1496
71. Chandrasekar B, Melby PC, Troyer DA, Colston JT, Freeman GL. Temporal expression of pro-inflammatory cytokines and inducible nitric oxide synthase in experimental acute Chagasic cardiomyopathy. *Am J Pathol* (1998) 152 (4):925–34.
72. Petersen CA, Burleigh BA. Role for interleukin-1 beta in *Trypanosoma cruzi*-induced cardiomyocyte hypertrophy. *Infect Immun* (2003) 71:4441–7. doi: 10.1128/IAI.71.8.4441-4447.2003
73. Chandrasekar B, Mummidi S, Claycomb WC, Mestril R. Nemer M.Interleukin-18 is a pro-hypertrophic cytokine that acts through a phosphatidylinositol 3-kinase-phosphoinositide-dependent kinase-1-Akt-GATA4 signaling pathway in cardiomyocytes. *J Biol Chem* (2005) 280 (6):4553–67. doi: 10.1074/jbc.M411787200
74. Reddy VS, Harskamp RE, van Ginkel MW, Calhoon J, Baisden CE, Kim IS, et al. Interleukin-18 stimulates fibronectin expression in primary human cardiac fibroblasts via PI3K. *J Cell Physiol* (2008) 215(3):697–707. doi: 10.1002/jcp.21348
75. Eslick GD, Thampan BV, Nalos M, McLean AS, Sluyter R. Circulating interleukin-18 concentrations and a loss-of-function P2X7 polymorphism in heart failure. *Int J Cardiol* (2009) 137(1):81–3. doi: 10.1016/j.ijcard.2008.05.017
76. O'Brien LC, Mezzaroma E, Van Tassell BW, Marchetti C, Carbone S, Abbate A, et al. Interleukin-18 as a therapeutic target in acute myocardial infarction and heart failure. *Mol Med* (2014) 12:221–9. doi: 10.2119/molmed.2014.00034
77. Chien Y, Chien CS, Chiang HC, Huang WL, Chou SJ, Chang WC, et al. Interleukin-18 deteriorates Fabry cardiomyopathy and contributes to the development of left ventricular hypertrophy in Fabry patients with GLA IVS4 +919 G>A mutation. *Oncotarget* (2016) 7(52):87161–79. doi: 10.18632/oncotarget.13552
78. Okuhara Y, Yokoe S, Iwasaku T, Eguchi A, Nishimura K, Li W, et al. *Interleukin-18* gene deletion protects against sepsis-induced cardiac dysfunction by inhibiting PP2A activity. *Int J Cardiol* (2017) 243:396–403. doi: 10.1016/j.ijcard.2017.04.082
79. Fae KC, Drigo SA, Cunha-Neto E, Ianni B, Mady C, Kalil J, et al. HLA and β-myosin heavy chain do not influence susceptibility to Chagas' disease cardiomyopathy. *Microb Infect* (2000) 2:745–51. doi: 10.1016/s1286-4579(00) 00501-3
80. Matos CS , dos Santos JE Jr., Medeiros FAC, Furtado E, Dias JCP. Current situation and perspectives regarding human Chagas disease in midwestern of the state of Minas Gerais, Brazil. *Mem Inst Osw Cruz* (2014) 109:374–8. doi: 10.1590/0074-0276130385. Rio de Janeiro.
81. Silva JS, Barral-Netto M, Reed SG. Aggravation of both *Trypanosoma cruzi* and murine leukemia virus by concomitant infections. *Amer J Trop Med Hyg* (1997) 49:589–97. doi: 10.4269/ajtmh.1993.49.589
82. Andreani G, Celentano AM, Solana ME, Cazorla S, Malchiodi EL, Martínez Peralta LA, et al. Inhibition of HIV-1 replication in human monocyte-derived macrophages by parasite. *Trypanosoma Cruzi PloS One* (2009) 4(12):e8246. doi: 10.1371/journal.pone.0008246
83. de Freitas VL, da Silva SC, Sartori AM, Bezerra RC, Westphalen EV, Molina TD, et al. Real-time PCR in HIV/*Trypanosoma cruzi* coinfection with and without Chagas disease reactivation: association with HIV viral load and CD4 level. *PloS Negl Trop Dis* (2011) 5(8):e1277. doi: 10.1371/journal.pntd.0001277
84. Rodrigues DBR, Correia D, Marra MD, Giraldo LER, Silva EL, Silva-Vergara ML, et al. Cytokine serum levels in patients infected by human immunodeficiency virus with and without *Trypanosoma cruzi* coinfection. *Rev Soc Bras Med Trop* (2005) 38:483–7. doi: 10.1590/s0037-86822005000600007
85. Barbaro G. Reviewing the cardiovascular complications of HIV infection after the introduction of highly active antiretroviral therapy. *Curr Drug Targets Cardiovasc Haematol Disord* (2005) 5:337–43. doi: 10.2174/15680060 54553444
86. Balagopal A, Gupte N, Shivakoti R, Cox AL, Yang WT, Berendes S, et al. Continued Elevation of Interleukin-18 and Interferon-γ After Initiation of Antiretroviral Therapy and Clinical Failure in a Diverse Multicountry Human Immunodeficiency Virus Cohort. *Open Forum Infect Dis* (2016) 3(3):ofw118. doi: 10.1093/ofid/ofw118
87. Iannello A, Boulassel M-R, Suzanne Samarani S, Tremblay C, Toma E, Routy J-P, et al. HIV-1 Causes an Imbalance in the Production of Interleukin-18 and Its Natural Antagonist in HIV-Infected Individuals: Implications for Enhanced Viral Replication. *J Infect Dis* (2010) 201:608–17. doi: 10.1086/650314
88. Sangenito LS, d'Avila-Levy CM, Branquinha MH, Santos ALS. Nelfinavir and lopinavir impair *Trypanosoma cruzi* trypomastigote infection in mammalian host cells and show anti-amastigote activity. *Int J Antimicrob Agents* (2016) 48 (6):703–11. doi: 10.1016/j.ijantimicag.2016.09.017
89. Sangenito LS, Menna-Barreto RF D, Avila-Levy CM, Santos AL, Branquinha MH. Decoding the anti-*Trypanosoma cruzi* action of HIV peptidase inhibitors using epimastigotes as a model. *PloS One* (2014) 9(12):e113957. doi: 10.1371/journal.pone.0113957
90. Sangenito LS, Menna-Barreto RFS, Oliveira AC, d'Avila-Levy CM, Branquinha MH, Santos ALS. Primary evidence of the mechanisms of action of HIV aspartyl peptidase inhibitors on *Trypanosoma cruzi* trypomastigote forms. *Int J Antimicrob Agents* (2018) 52(2):185–94. doi: 10.1016/j.ijantimicag.2018.03.021
91. Castilho VVS, Gonçalves KCS, Rebello KM, Baptista LPR, Sangenito LS, Santos HLC, et al. Docking simulation between HIV peptidase inhibitors and *Trypanosoma cruzi* aspartyl peptidase. *BMC Res Notes* (2018) 11(1):825. doi: 10.1186/s13104-018-3927-z
92. Bellera CL, Balcazar DE, Vanrell MC, Casassa AF, Palestro PH, Gavernet L, et al. Computer-guided drug repurposing: identification of trypanocidal activity of clofazimine, benidipine and saquinavir. *Eur J Med Chem* (2015) 93:338–48. doi: 10.1016/j.ejmech.2015.01.065

13

Immunomodulation as a Novel Strategy for Prevention and Treatment of *Bordetella* spp. Infections

Monica C. Gestal, Hannah M. Johnson and Eric T. Harvill**

Department of Infectious Diseases, College of Veterinary Sciences, University of Georgia, Athens, GA, United States

***Correspondence:**
Monica C. Gestal
mcarges@gmail.com
Eric T. Harvill
harvill@uga.edu

Well-adapted pathogens have evolved to survive the many challenges of a robust immune response. Defending against all host antimicrobials simultaneously would be exceedingly difficult, if not impossible, so many co-evolved organisms utilize immunomodulatory tools to subvert, distract, and/or evade the host immune response. *Bordetella* spp. present many examples of the diversity of immunomodulators and an exceptional experimental system in which to study them. Recent advances in this experimental system suggest strategies for interventions that tweak immunity to disrupt bacterial immunomodulation, engaging more effective host immunity to better prevent and treat infections. Here we review advances in the understanding of respiratory pathogens, with special focus on *Bordetella* spp., and prospects for the use of immune-stimulatory interventions in the prevention and treatment of infection.

Keywords: immunomodulation, *Bordetella*, Toll-receptors, adjuvants, pertussis

INTRODUCTION TO THE STRATEGY OF IMMUNOMODULATION FOR HEALTH

We are exposed to vast numbers of pathogens during our lifespan, but only a small number manage to cause disease. Invading bacteria face a hostile environment in hosts with arrays of antimicrobial compounds and components of immunity. To persist in such an environment, bacteria must find a way to survive this onslaught of antibacterials. The strategy of resisting them all may be exceedingly challenging or impossible; instead, most of the best-studied pathogens have mechanisms that allow them to evade the full effects of host defenses (1–12). In this review, we will consider examples of novel approaches in vaccine and therapeutic development that have been guided by the better understanding of bacterial immunomodulatory abilities. We will focus on findings with *Bordetella* spp., considering novel adjuvants that enhance host immune response and new immunostimulatory therapies that can augment the most effective aspects of the host immune response. The results highlighted in this review demonstrate that the manipulation and/or disruption of bacterial immunomodulatory properties are providing a highly promising approach that could replace antibiotics in a near future. Understanding the mechanisms that bacteria utilize to manipulate host immune response, as well as the immune signaling pathways that lead to greater protective immunity, can guide the development of targeted interventions that can enhance the host immune response to more effectively kill the bacterial hazard.

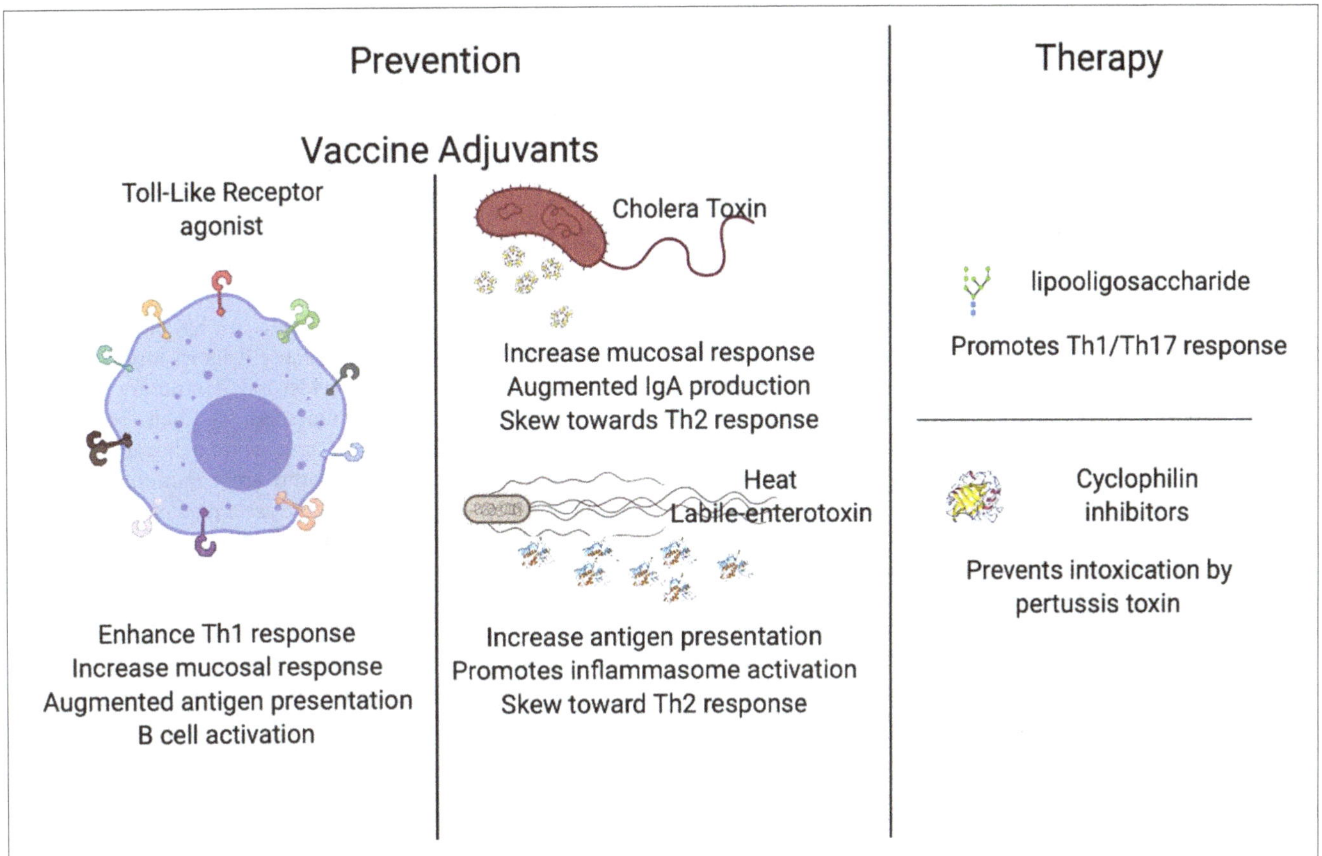

GRAPHICAL ABSTRACT | Areas of investigation focused on the use of immunomodulation in prevention and therapy of infectious diseases. Created with BioRender.

THE BORDETELLAE; BIOLOGY; AND EXPERIMENTAL SYSTEM

Pertussis disease is caused by *B. pertussis*, a highly transmissible human pathogen that causes a respiratory illness also known as the 100-day cough (13). Among the proposed reasons for its resurgence are waning immunity (13), the end of the "honeymoon period" (14), the past vaccination calendar (15), and the failure of the current acellular vaccine to confer sterilizing immunity and long-lasting herd immunity. The increase in the number of cases is associated with more advanced diagnostic tools than ever before, allowing for an increase in the number of identified cases (16–31), but also with increased morbidity and mortality that creates an unambiguous imperative for improved prevention methods.

Vaccination has greatly increased life expectancy by preventing several historically notorious infectious diseases (32–36). However, we are witnessing a rise in several preventable diseases previously thought to be controlled (37), such as pertussis (38). Around 1945, a whole-cell vaccine against *B. pertussis* was introduced, causing an unprecedented decrease in the number of reported pertussis cases. However, due to undesirable adverse effects such as fever, erythema, swelling, drowsiness and others, this was replaced in several industrialized countries by an acellular vaccine that contains between 3 to 5 bacterial proteins (39–44). Despite the fact that both types of vaccines generate antibodies that impede bacterial adhesion and have bactericidal action, these have not been sufficient to halt the increase in the number of cases. In response to this increase a boost was introduced to extend immunological memory, and new vaccination strategies targeted to pregnant women and close family have also been introduced as an attempt to protect highly susceptible newborns (45–48).

As the number of cases continues to increase, the scientific community is working to understand the causes that drive this reemergence (13, 49). Amongst the proposed causes of this increase are, limitation to the protection conferred by the current acellular vaccine. Not only does the acquired anamnestic response wane rapidly (50), but the acellular vaccine still allows for bacterial colonization of the nasal cavity and shedding. Combined, these factors illuminate the fact that the current vaccines used in most industrialized countries still permit transmission of pertussis from host to host (51–54), which has even more significant impacts when considered in tandem with the rise of anti-vaccination movements. Yet another cause for the increase is the differences detected in the immune response triggered by the whole cell vaccine (Th17) vs. the acellular vaccine (Th2) (51, 55–57). It is important to highlight that while neither whole-cell nor acellular vaccines confer long-lasting immunity, and the merits of both responses have been debated in recent years, the general consensus agrees on advantages to skewing T cell response toward Th1/Th17 immunity (58–61).

The "gold standard" of immunity to pertussis is considered to be the classical Th1/Th17 T cell response induced by convalescent immunity (62); however, there is significant cumulative evidence that infection-induced immunity is imperfect and shorter-lived than it could be (50). Current discoveries contribute to better understanding of the immune response to Bordetellae, and the important role that CD4 resident T cells play in a local memory response has been recently demonstrated (63). Another hypothesis is that Bordetellae are evolving, and due to the genome plasticity and adaptability of this pathogen, current isolates of *B. pertussis* have lost some of the antigens included in the acellular vaccine. This phenomenon is referred to as "vaccine driven evolution," which helps justify why immunity is not as robust as it has previously been (64–67).

These are only some of the potential causes that are currently being considered, and it is most likely an uneven combination of all of them that is truly driving this pertussis resurgence. Although the whole-cell vaccine is still used, the trend is shifting toward a safer acellular vaccine, and efforts on improving their performance and the length of protective memory these generate will be discussed in this manuscript.

The current strategy for the development of vaccines is driven by the hypothesis that antibodies provide strong protection. As a consequence, most of the current acellular vaccines are highly safe and generate a rapid antibody response that is protective, albeit limited (68, 69). Importantly, infection triggers a complex and well-orchestrated sequence of responses involving many interacting components of innate and adaptive immunity, directed by several signaling pathways that present numerable known, and probably many more unknown, opportunities to interfere in the succession of events that can skew the resulting immune response.

Bordetellae harbor multiple mechanisms that allow them to modulate the host immune response (1, 70, 71). Some of the proteins that these organisms utilize to manipulate immune cells include adenylate cyclase toxin (ACT), a pore forming protein that leads to the deregulation of cAMP levels within target cells (72, 73); type 3 secretion system (T3SS), a needle-like structure that injects toxins within mammalian cells (74–76); a type 6 secretion system that uses a phage-like mechanism to inject molecules (77); pertussis toxin (PTX), which prevents G proteins from interacting with G protein-coupled receptors on the cell membrane and therefore interfering with intracellular communication (78–80); and filamentous hemagglutinin (FHA), which binds signaling receptors, enables adhesion to epithelial cells and interferes with cytokine production (81, 82). Based on these studies of various immunomodulators we can now begin to adjust the way we design preventative and responsive medications to fight bacterial infections in more effective ways.

A good understanding of the sequential reactions of the immune response (and bacterial manipulation of them) is key to improving the induction and maintenance of robust long-lasting protective immunity. Some of the *Bordetella* spp. virulence factors are already being investigated for treatments, such as PTX for human immunodeficiency virus (HIV) treatment (83–89). Understanding how we can alter bacterial ability to sense and respond to the host to modulate its response can lead to treatments and therapies that focus on the enhancement of more appropriate and effective host immune responses.

IMMUNOTHERAPY IN PREVENTION

Adjuvants

The *Bordetella pertussis* acellular vaccine has not completely blocked the spread of pertussis because it allows for colonization of the nasal cavity (48) and provides only temporary protection (13). Adjuvants are well-documented for their potential to increase vaccine performance, and some adjuvants such as CpG oligodeoxynuceotides or alum are commonly found in vaccine formulations (90, 91). There are a plethora of adjuvants that can potentiate the performance of a vaccine and can be classified into two main groups: Toll-like receptors agonists (92–94) and mucosal adjuvants (58, 95–97). These two distinct classes have been closely considered for their contributions to pertussis vaccines as well as therapeutics (98–103), yielding highly promising enhancing properties.

Toll-Like Receptors Agonists

Toll-Like Receptors (TLRs) are highly sophisticated sentinels that recognize specific pathogen-associated molecular patterns (PAMPs). The differential activation of TLRs is one of the main determinants for an efficient immune response against pathogens. Under this premise, researchers have been working on the addition of TLR agonists to vaccines with the expectation that activating different TLRs will command the type of T cell response produced (104) and will ultimately enhance host protective immunity (105).

One of the best studied Toll-Like Receptors is TLR2, which recognizes a broad spectrum of bacterial cell wall components, including lipopolypeptides, peptidoglycan, and lipochoic acids, that trigger different signals that shape the immune response against the bacterial threat (106). It has been demonstrated that the use of TLR2 agonists as adjuvants to already developed vaccines increases immunity, especially in neonates (93). This feature is highly relevant to the design of vaccines against diseases that primarily affect newborns and young infants (93). Moreover, TLR2 agonists in combination with the BCG vaccine can enhance protection against *Mycobacterium tuberculosis* (107), skewing the cellular response toward Th1 (100), and resulting in a more robust protective memory response, further promoting its use in vaccinology. TLR2 has been also correlated with an efficient response to *B. pertussis* infections (108), and some preliminary data has revealed that the use of these agonists enhances protection against infection by pertussis (58, 100). Altogether, these data suggest that TLR2 agonists may be promising candidates to combine with current or new vaccines to enhance the protective response.

Similarly, TLR4 appears a good candidate for vaccine enhancement because it recognizes lipopolysaccharide (LPS) molecules, which are commonly present on the surface of most bacteria. Agonists of TLR4 enhance the performance of several vaccines including viral, bacterial, and even mycobacterial (109–113). One important aspect is its promotion of mucosal immunity (114–116), which is critical for the generation of protection against certain infections including gut and respiratory diseases like pertussis (117–119), although this increase is achieved via mucosal delivery of the vaccine rather than systemic (120). Molecular evidence has revealed that the addition of a TLR4 ligand to the acellular pertussis vaccine resulted in a shift from a Th2-dominant response to additional induction of Th17 (121, 122). The abundant immunological evidence that highlights the role of TLR4 in the immune response to *B. pertussis* (102, 123–130) indicates that TLR4 agonists are promising candidate for the generation of more robust protective immunity.

TLR5 (131) is also a highly plausible candidate to augment vaccine performance since it recognizes flagella, which are present in a multitude of bacterial species. Previous literature has indicated that ectopic expression of flagella in *Bordetella* spp. leads to faster clearance of the infection (132), and it was later revealed that TLR5 activates antigen-presenting cells, increasing T cell response (133) (*manuscript in preparation*), and may ultimately contribute to the more rapid clearance previously reported. In several other microorganisms, the addition of TLR5 agonists have resulted in an increased performance of the vaccine (134–141). Altogether these data suggest that TLR5 agonists could significantly increase the performance of the current acellular pertussis vaccine.

TLR7 recognizes single-stranded RNA (142–153) and has been demonstrated to be a promising vaccine adjuvant for protection against several microorganisms (154, 155). Similar to TLR2, the TLR7 agonist augments immunity in newborns, the most susceptible population (93, 102, 143, 156, 157). The addition of a TLR7 agonist to an alum-adjuvant of pertussis vaccine skewed the immune response toward Th1/Th17 and significantly decreased colonization (98), providing preliminary data to further pursue this agonist in other animal models.

Lastly, TLR9 recognizes unmethylated CpG oligodeoxynucleotides and promotes IL-6 secretion and consequent B cell activation (158–168). It has been demonstrated that enhancement of TLR9 receptors augment activity of antigen-presenting cells in neonates (93, 102, 169). Addition of a TLR9 agonist to the acellular pertussis vaccine resulted in greater stimulation of B and T cells and a shift to Th1, as well as higher antibody titers (81, 170–174), suggesting that an agonist of TLR9 is also a candidate to add to the current pertussis vaccines. These have the potential to be widely used agonists, as most of the current vaccine's efficacy is measured as an increase in antibody titers.

Altogether, these results demonstrate that TLR agonists are great candidates to be used as vaccine adjuvants to increase protective immunity. Interestingly, some of the TLR agonists substantially augment vaccine performance in newborns and infants, which represent the most susceptible population (93, 169) although there are substantial hurdles to applying this knowledge. Moreover, preliminary data obtained with TLR2, and TLR7 agonists demonstrate the improved performance of the current *B. pertussis* vaccine and indicates that the use of adjuvants can feasibly potentiate and augment the generation of protective immunity (58, 98, 100).

Mucosal Adjuvants

Adjuvants have been used to potentiate, enhance, or accelerate vaccine effects since the 1920s (105) and the field has greatly evolved since. Mucosal adjuvants include cholera toxin, heat-labile enterotoxin, and other compounds have been studied for their particular ability to increase protection on mucosal surfaces (175). These are of extreme importance, not only because of the aforementioned increase in vaccine performance, but also because the delivery method involving intranasal vaccination has a lot of potential for improving the delivery of the vaccine and increasing acceptance among needle-phobic population. In the following paragraphs we will detail the mechanisms of action and the data compiled for some of the most promising mucosal adjuvants.

Cholera toxin (CT) and heat-labile enterotoxin of *Escherichia coli* (LT) are highly antigenic; however, due to their toxicity, they are not ideal candidates for human therapies. Recently, safe forms of these toxins created via genetic manipulation have been utilized as adjuvants to enhance the function of mucosal vaccines (103, 176–181). The mechanism behind this augmented immune response induced by CT is an increase in the permeability of the mucosal epithelium, enhanced antigen presentation, the consequent promotion of dendritic cell maturation, increased IgA response, and finally, the generation of complex stimulatory and inhibitory effects on T cell proliferation and cytokine production such as IL-4, IL-5, IL-6, and IL-10 that skew the response toward a Th2-type (177, 182). CTA1 is the subunit responsible for the immunomodulatory activity in conjunction with ERdj5 in the endoplasmic reticulum, which is the target for CT. In the absence of ERdj5, mice failed to produce inflammatory cytokines, indicating that CT action requires ERdj5 (183). Similarly, the calcium-binding protein S100A4 is required for efficient antigen presentation and enhanced activity of CT, as it is necessary for the humoral and cellular response (184). CT has been tested as an adjuvant for pertussis vaccine and preliminary data suggests that it substantially improves mucosal protection by augmenting IgA levels (183, 185), and it has even been suggested that this adjuvant may be safe for use in humans (186, 187). Some studies have revealed that conjugation of CT with pertussis toxoid added to the current acellular vaccine (188) or Fimbriae (Fim2) (189) are highly promising candidates to improve the generation of protective immunity from these vaccines.

Similar to CT, the heat-labile enterotoxin from *E. coli* (LT) promotes an antigen-specific response inducing IgA antibodies, Th17 response, and the enhancement of long-lasting protective immunity (190) while also being safe for use in humans (191). LT promotes maturation of dendritic cells, antigen-specific IL-17 positive cells, and production of IL-1α, IL-1β, and IL-23 by dendritic cells. Trials in animals have revealed the efficacy of this adjuvant at enhancing mucosal response (192). LT promotes dendritic cell maturation enhancing IL-1β production through activation of caspase-1 and the NLRP3 inflammasome complex. Simultaneously, LT enhances LPS-induced IL-1α and IL-23 expression through activation of ERK MAPK in dendritic cells inducing the development of Th17 T cells (193). Interestingly, LT derivatives LTK63 (non-toxic mutant of LT) and LTR72 (which retains partial enzymatic activity) revealed two distinct phenotypes characterized by stimulation of IL-12 and TNF-α production by macrophages, resulting in enhanced Th1 responses with the LTK63 adjuvants. In contrast, LTR72 suppresses LPS-induced IL-12 production, increases type 2 responses, inhibits Th1 response, and facilitates clearance of bacterial burden (194), demonstrating that both subunits of the toxin have particular activities that can be beneficial for the improvement of the current acellular pertussis vaccine.

Another mucosal adjuvant that is widely investigated is retinoic acid, a powerful immunomodulator that interferes with growth, differentiation, and other aspects of the cell life cycle. Importantly, retinoic acid is also essential in the generation of mucosal immunity, the promotion of tolerogenic effects, the generation of a robust innate and adaptive immune response, and moreover, it also acts as a negative regulator of IgE production (195–197). It has been hypothesized that retinoic acid plays a fundamental role in sustaining mucosal homeostasis by down-regulating IgE levels (197). Its performance as an adjuvant has been studied in several organisms and the plethora of results obtained have revealed that retinoic acid is a promising candidate to use as an adjuvant of mucosal vaccines by itself or encapsulated in nanoparticles (198–203). Unfortunately, its activity in conjunction with the pertussis vaccine has not yet been assessed.

The use of biopolymers in mucosally-administered vaccines has substantially improved the current vaccine formulations and has great potential for the future (204). Some of the presently investigated biopolymers include alginate (205–212) and gellan (213, 214). Although these are still in early stages of study, other biopolymers, such as chitosan (95–97, 215–232), starch (233), and β-glucan (234–241), have already been tested in animal trials with encouraging success. While the use of biopolymers is still rising, this area of investigation is highly promising, especially for enhancement of mucosal protection. Mucosal delivery has been explored for pertussis immunization from different approaches that have resulted in hopeful results in which Th17 response was enhanced and the animals were more robustly protected against challenge (58, 170, 242, 243).

To summarize, several mucosal adjuvants are being investigated, some of which are derived from toxins while still others are derived from biopolymers. Both act to enhance the performance of vaccines, particularly those that can be orally or intranasally delivered, usually in cases in which mucosal protection is a key component of immunity. However, these further demonstrate that different strategies and approaches can be used to improve the performance of the current vaccines to produce and enhance individual and herd immunity.

Novel Vaccination Strategies

The combination of BCG and acellular pertussis vaccination has been shown to reduce the mortality rate of pertussis (244–247). Immunological studies unraveling the underlying mechanism by which protection against pertussis is enhanced are necessary. Some groups have focused on the addition of antigens to the current vaccine in order to improve performance. After demonstrating via *in vitro* experiments that the autotransporter BrkA would be a good candidate to generate antibodies that kill *Bordetella* spp., BrkA has been tested as an adjuvant of the current acellular pertussis vaccine, the results of which revealed robust lung protection against infection with *B. pertussis* (248, 249). Two other autotransporters, Vag8 (250, 251) and SphB1, when added to the current pertussis vaccine resulted in improved protection against *B. pertussis* infection (252). Adenylate cyclase toxin (ACT), when added to a current vaccine formulation significantly decreased inflammation and increased the generation of protective immunity (253, 254). BcfA (colonization factor A) has been used as adjuvant in the current vaccine, and the preliminary data obtained with the murine model reveals that the addition of this adjuvant shifts the T cell response toward Th1/Th17 (255).

Live vaccines have the potential to induce strong mucosal protection, but suffer from concern about their risk. An exciting new vaccine candidate against *B. pertussis* is the live attenuated vaccine, BPZE1, which has been shown to induce a robust local B and T cell response (256–282) despite genetically engineered mutations that render it relatively safe (283, 284). Excitingly, phase I trials demonstrate that the intranasal formulation of the vaccine transiently colonizes the nasal cavity, leading to the generation of stronger immunity (264, 268).

Several groups are currently working on the development of outer membrane vesicles and outer membrane proteins in protection against *B. pertussis* as well as cross-protection against several *Bordetella* spp. and characterizing the immune response as well as protective immunity (285–295). In animal studies, immunization with outer membrane vesicles led to not only better humoral and cellular (Th17) memory, but also to a significant increase in IgA titers, which is one of the major hurdles of current vaccination strategies against this pathogen (296–298). It is important to highlight that the increase in IgA responses upon immunization with outer membrane vesicles is only obtained when these are administrated mucosally (299). The classic delivery for OMV's, which is subcutaneous or intraperitoneal immunization, does not induce IgA responses and this novel delivery method provides a great advance, as it can be administered with more ease and induces an even better immunological response. The increase in mucosal protection has led to efforts toward improved nasal delivery approaches and a thermostable spray containing outer membrane vesicles has been developed. This spray significantly improves delivery and decreases the discomfort other intranasal formulations might cause. Importantly, this delivery method still maintains all the outstanding qualities of the classical delivery of these purified outer membrane vesicles (300).

Finally, another highly promising strategy is focused on the disruption of bacterial ability to manipulate the host immune response. Under the premise that bacteria harbor mechanisms that allow them to sense and respond to host immunity, disrupting these pathways would allow for the generation of more robust protective immunity. A live attenuated vaccine in which immunomodulatory mechanisms are disrupted might confer cross-protection against classical Bordetellae, which are known to share many antigens. Although this is only the first study for this method of vaccine design (*manuscript in revision*), this novel approach has great potential for the generation of new vaccine candidates and possibly therapeutics.

IMMUNOTHERAPY IN TREATMENT

LOS-Derived Oligosaccharide Glycoconjugates

Pertussis toxin (PTX) in an inactivated form (PTd) functions as a major protective antigen, stimulating production of toxin-neutralizing antibodies which can protect against damage caused by the toxin, but do not target the bacteria itself (301, 302); however, it also demonstrates possible partial reversion back to its toxic active form (303, 304), which may be responsible for the reactogenicity seen in a small percentage of vaccine recipients. It is also a secretory protein, which is only loosely associated with the cell and is therefore not an ideal target for bactericidal antibodies. A more effective target is an abundant surface component such as the endotoxin lipooligosaccharide (LOS), an LPS analog with a complete absence of the O-specific polysaccharide chain that is produced by several varieties of Gram-negative bacteria (305). LOS provides significant adjuvant properties via induction of IL-12 and 1L-1β that promote Th1 and Th17 responses, respectively (306, 307). It also displays pyrogenic, mitogenic, and endotoxic activity that necessitate its conjugation or conversion to a less destructive form prior to its use in a vaccine.

LOS conjugated to protein carriers filamentous hemagglutinin, bovine serum albumin, and tetanus toxoid (TTd) successfully induce a strong bactericidal response specific to LOS presented on the surface of *B. pertussis*, leading to complement-mediated destruction of the cell (90, 308, 309). These protein carriers are also surface components, like LOS, and the resulting surface-associated conjugate acts as a strong target for antibody action directed against *B. pertussis*.

Somewhat surprisingly, another conjugate iteration in which an LOS-derived oligosaccharide is covalently linked with the secretory protein PTX yields a uniquely non-toxic and immunogenic glycoconjugate that retains the antigenic properties of PTX while also inducing the production of bactericidal antibodies. The presumed linkage at the fetuin- and glycoprotein-binding sites of PTX inactivates the enzymatic activity of the protomer A and binding properties of oligomer B, demonstrated using *in vitro* assays (310). Although the use of LOS appears to be highly promising, *in vivo* studies still need to be done to assess pharmacological parameters of safety and biodistribution.

Cyclophilin Inhibitors

PTX is internalized in cells via endocytosis and then follows a retrograde transport system to the endoplasmic reticulum. The enzymatically active (A) subunit of PTX, PTS1, detaches from the rest of the toxin in the ER and unfolds due to its thermal instability. It is then transported into the cytosol with the help of cyclophilin (Cyps), an important protein folding helper enzyme that also is required to facilitate membrane translocation from early endosomes into the cytosol of various ADP-ribosylating toxins (311–313). Inhibiting Cyps activity has been shown to in turn inhibit membrane translocation and protect cells from intoxication with PTX and others (311).

Inhibition can be achieved via the approved immunosuppressive drug cyclosporine A (CsA), which specifically inhibits Cyps activity in mammalian cells by binding directly to Cyps and forming a ternary complex. It has been used as the primary agent in immunosuppressive regimens such as grafts and transplants since the 1980s. It is now suggested that CsA might interfere with the translocation of PTS1 from the ER into the cytosol; it may also play a role in reassembling the unfolded PTS1 subunit (311).

In vitro intoxication assays performed on CHO-K1 cells demonstrated that CsA-treated cells were protected from PTX intoxication. Interestingly, up to 50% of CsA is retained intracellularly, even in the absence of extracellular inhibitor, after 18 h (314). Thus, presumably, intracellular Cyps stay inhibited over a longer period of time, explaining the toxin-resistant phenotype. This is also concomitant with the long retention of CsA in different tissues observed after CsA administration in human patients (315, 316). This inhibitor was delivered orally during trials, but its use in a mucosal spray or as a directly injectable vaccine component has yet to be investigated.

FUTURE DIRECTIONS AND CONCLUSION

Since the years of our notoriously premature celebration of victory over infectious disease, there has been seemingly inexorable retaliation. There is now justifiable concern, shifting toward fear, about the combined threats of increasing antibiotic resistance and the failures of current vaccines due to factors including incomplete vaccine uptake, vaccine-driven evolution and other threats. However, recent advances in our understanding of immunology and the tools to manipulate it present hope for more rational targeted interventions that are focused on enhancing the natural host response. Similarly, improved understanding of strategies and mechanisms by which bacteria modulate the immune response provides new targets for treatment and prevention. In the coming years, we will likely witness an expansion in the field of immunotherapy promoted by a better understanding of the finely tuned interactions of bacteria and host.

AUTHOR CONTRIBUTIONS

MG: original idea of the manuscript, writing, and editing. HJ: writing and editing. EH: editing and final approval.

ACKNOWLEDGMENTS

The authors would like to acknowledge the members of the EH Lab for helpful and fruitful discussions and brainstorming.

REFERENCES

1. Gestal MC, Whitesides LT, Harvill ET. Integrated signaling pathways mediate *Bordetella* immunomodulation, persistence, and transmission. *Trends Microbiol.* (2019) 27:118–30. doi: 10.1016/j.tim.2018.09.010
2. Hancock RE, Nijnik A, Philpott DJ. Modulating immunity as a therapy for bacterial infections. *Nat Rev Microbiol.* (2012) 10:243–54. doi: 10.1038/nrmicro2745
3. Liu Y, Islam EA, Jarvis GA, Gray-Owen SD, Russell MW. Neisseria gonorrhoeae selectively suppresses the development of Th1 and Th2 cells, and enhances Th17 cell responses, through TGF-β-dependent mechanisms. *Mucosal Immunol.* (2012) 5:320–31. doi: 10.1038/mi.2012.12
4. Wolfe DN, Karanikas AT, Hester SE, Kennett MJ, Harvill ET. IL-10 induction by *Bordetella parapertussis* limits a protective IFN-gamma response. *J Immunol.* (2010) 184:1392–400. doi: 10.4049/jimmunol.0803045
5. Carbonetti NH. Immunomodulation in the pathogenesis of *Bordetella pertussis* infection and disease. *Curr Opin Pharmacol.* (2007) 7:272–8. doi: 10.1016/j.coph.2006.12.004
6. Tateda K, Ishii Y, Horikawa M, Matsumoto T, Miyairi S, Pechere JC, et al. The *Pseudomonas aeruginosa* autoinducer N-3-oxododecanoyl homoserine lactone accelerates apoptosis in macrophages and neutrophils. *Infect Immun.* (2003) 71:5785–93. doi: 10.1128/IAI.71.10.5785-5793.2003
7. Ritchie AJ, Yam AO, Tanabe KM, Rice SA, Cooley MA. Modification of *in vivo* and *in vitro* T- and B-cell-mediated immune responses by the *Pseudomonas aeruginosa* quorum-sensing molecule N-(3-oxododecanoyl)-L-homoserine lactone. *Infect Immun.* (2003) 71:4421–31. doi: 10.1128/IAI.71.8.4421-4431.2003
8. Sperandio V. Pathogens' adaptation to the human host. *Proc Natl Acad Sci USA.* (2018) 115:9342–3. doi: 10.1073/pnas.1813379115
9. Lustri BC, Sperandio, V, and Moreira, CG. Bacterial chat: intestinal metabolites and signals in host-microbiota-pathogen interactions. *Infect Immun.* (2017) 85:e00476-17. doi: 10.1128/IAI.00476-17
10. Bäumler AJ, Sperandio V. Interactions between the microbiota and pathogenic bacteria in the gut. *Nature.* (2016) 535:85–93. doi: 10.1038/nature18849
11. Kendall MM, Sperandio V. What a dinner party! mechanisms and functions of interkingdom signaling in host-pathogen associations. *MBio.* (2016) 7:e01748. doi: 10.1128/mBio.01748-15
12. Curtis MM, Sperandio V. A complex relationship: the interaction among symbiotic microbes, invading pathogens, and their mammalian host. *Mucosal Immunol.* (2011) 4:133–8. doi: 10.1038/mi.2010.89
13. Kilgore PE, Salim AM, Zervos MJ, and Schmitt HJ. Pertussis: microbiology, disease, treatment, and prevention. *Clin Microbiol Rev.* (2016) 29, 449–486. doi: 10.1128/CMR.00083-15
14. Domenech de Cellès M, Magpantay FM, King AA, and Rohani P. The pertussis enigma: reconciling epidemiology, immunology and evolution. *Proc Biol Sci.* (2016) 283:20152309. doi: 10.1098/rspb.2015.2309
15. Broutin H, Viboud C, Grenfell BT, Miller MA, and Rohani P. Impact of vaccination and birth rate on the epidemiology of pertussis: a comparative study in 64 countries. *Proc Biol Sci.* (2010) 277:3239–45. doi: 10.1098/rspb.2010.0994
16. Miyashita N, Akaike H, Teranishi H, Kawai Y, Ouchi K, Kato T, et al. Diagnostic value of symptoms and laboratory data for pertussis in adolescent and adult patients. *BMC Infect Dis.* (2013) 13:129. doi: 10.1186/1471-2334-13-129
17. Subissi L, Rodeghiero C, Martini H, Litzroth A, Huygen K, Leroux-Roels G, et al. Assessment of IgA anti-PT and IgG anti-ACT reflex testing to improve *Bordetella pertussis* serodiagnosis in recently vaccinated subjects. *Clin Microbiol Infect.* (2019) pii: S1198-743X(19)30528-2. doi: 10.1016/j.cmi.2019.10.001
18. Gil-Prieto R, Walter S, San-Román-Montero J, Marín-García P, González-Escalada A, Gil-de-Miguel A. Paediatric hospitalizations due to whooping cough in Spain (1997-2017). *Vaccine.* (2019) 37:6342–7. doi: 10.1016/j.vaccine.2019.09.017
19. Stefanelli P. Pertussis: identification, prevention and control. *Adv Exp Med Biol.* (2019). doi: 10.1007/5584_2019_408
20. Wu DX, Chen Q, Yao KH, Li L, Shi W, Ke JW, et al. Pertussis detection in children with cough of any duration. *BMC Pediatr.* (2019) 19:236. doi: 10.1186/s12887-019-1615-3
21. Rabi A, Rokni T, Bennaoui F, Rada N, El Idrissi Slitine N, Draiss G, et al. Epidemiology of pertussis in Marrakech and contribution of molecular diagnosis. *Infect Dis.* (2019) 51:703–5. doi: 10.1080/23744235.2019.1637537
22. Fumimoto R, Otsuka N, Kamiya H, Sunagawa T, Tanaka-Taya K, Kamachi K, et al. Seroprevalence of IgA and IgM antibodies to *Bordetella pertussis* in healthy Japanese donors: assessment for the serological diagnosis of pertussis. *PLoS ONE.* (2019) 14:e0219255. doi: 10.1371/journal.pone.0219255
23. Dou M, Macias N, Shen F, Bard JD, Domínguez DC, Li X. Rapid and accurate diagnosis of the respiratory disease pertussis on a point-of-care biochip. *EClinicalMedicine.* (2019) 8:72–7. doi: 10.1016/j.eclinm.2019.02.008
24. Dou M, Sanchez J, Tavakoli H, Gonzalez JE, Sun J, Dien Bard J, et al. A low-cost microfluidic platform for rapid and instrument-free detection of whooping cough. *Anal Chim Acta.* (2019) 1065:71–8. doi: 10.1016/j.aca.2019.03.001
25. Markey K, Douglas-Bardsley A, Asokanathan C, Fry NK, Barkoff AM, Bacci S, et al. Improvement in serological diagnosis of pertussis by external quality assessment. *J Med Microbiol.* (2019) 68:741–7. doi: 10.1099/jmm.0.000926
26. Damouni Shalabi R, Srugo I, Golan-Shany O, Kugelman A, Bamberger E. Respiratory viruses frequently mimic pertussis in young infants. *Pediatr Infect Dis J.* (2019) 38:e107–9. doi: 10.1097/INF.0000000000002223
27. Moosa F, du Plessis M, Wolter N, Carrim M, Cohen C, von Mollendorf C, et al. Challenges and clinical relevance of molecular detection of *Bordetella pertussis* in South Africa. *BMC Infect Dis.* (2019) 19:276. doi: 10.1186/s12879-019-3869-7
28. Tascini C, Carannante N, Sodano G, Tiberio C, Atripaldi L, Di Caprio G, et al. Neonatal pertussis diagnosis: low procalcitonin level and high lymphocyte count are able to discriminate pertussis from bacterial and viral infections. *New Microbiol.* (2019) 42:49–51.
29. Choi GS, Huh DH, Han SB, Ahn DH, Kang KR, Kim JA, et al. Enzyme-linked immunosorbent assay for detecting anti-pertussis toxin antibody in mouse. *Clin Exp Vaccine Res.* (2019) 8:64–9. doi: 10.7774/cevr.2019.8.1.64
30. Saiki-Macedo S, Valverde-Ezeta J, Cornejo-Tapia A, Castillo ME, Petrozzi-Helasvuo V., Aguilar-Luis MA, et al. Identfication of viral and bacterial etiologic agents of the pertussis-like syndrome in children under 5 years old hospitalized. *BMC Infect Dis.* (2019) 19:75. doi: 10.1186/s12879-019-3671-6
31. Di Matola T, Miele C, Coppola M, Fumi M, Pancione Y, Sale S, et al. Utility of peripheral blood smear in rapid diagnosis of Pertussis. *Int J Lab Hematol.* (2019) 41:e41–2. doi: 10.1111/ijlh.12947
32. Wadman M, You J. The vaccine wars. *Science.* (2017) 356:364–5. doi: 10.1126/science.356.6336.364
33. Paff ML, Nuismer SL, Ellington A, Molineux IJ, Bull JJ. Virus wars: using one virus to block the spread of another. *PeerJ.* (2016) 4:e2166. doi: 10.7717/peerj.2166
34. De Gregorio E, Rappuoli R. Vaccines for the future: learning from human immunology. *Microb Biotechnol.* (2012) 5:149–55. doi: 10.1111/j.1751-7915.2011.00276.x
35. Frishman WH. Ten secrets to a long life. *Am J Med.* (2019) 132:564–6. doi: 10.1016/j.amjmed.2018.12.020
36. Roush SW, Murphy TV, and Vaccine-Preventable Disease Table Working Group. Historical comparisons of morbidity and mortality for vaccine-preventable diseases in the United States. *JAMA.* (2007) 298:2155–63. doi: 10.1001/jama.298.18.2155
37. McKee M, Middleton J. Information wars: tackling the threat from disinformation on vaccines. *BMJ.* (2019) 365:l2144. doi: 10.1136/bmj.l2144
38. Rohani P, Drake JM. The decline and resurgence of pertussis in the US. *Epidemics.* (2011) 3:183–8. doi: 10.1016/j.epidem.2011.10.001
39. Goezsy B, Kato L. Sensitizing properties of *B. pertussis* in the mouse and rat. *Rev Can Biol.* (1964) 23:427–37.
40. Morrone G, Nunziata B, Picciotto L. [Immunitary response of the infant vaccinated with quadruple DPT-polio vaccine]. *Riv Ist Sieroter Ital.* (1959) 34:321–9.
41. Chen BL, Chou CT, Huang CT, Wang YT, Ko HH, Huang WC, et al. Studies on diphtheria-pertussis-tetanus combined immunization in children. II. Immune responses after the primary vaccination. *J Immunol.* (1957) 79:39–45.

42. Ipsen J, Bowen HE. Effects of routine immunization of children with triple vaccine (diphtheria-tetanus-pertussis). *Am J Public Health Nations Health.* (1955) 45:312–8. doi: 10.2105/AJPH.45.3.312
43. Albkrt A. Diphtheria-pertussis-tetanus immunizing of infants. *J Maine Med Assoc.* (1954) 45:126.
44. Combined immunization against diphtheria tetanus pertussis. *Squibb Memo.* (1947) 26:4–7.
45. Caboré RN, Maertens K, Dobly A, Leuridan E, Van Damme P, and Huygen K. Influence of maternal vaccination against diphtheria, tetanus, and pertussis on the avidity of infant antibody responses to a pertussis containing vaccine in Belgium. *Virulence.* (2017) 8: 1245–54. doi: 10.1080/21505594.2017.1296998
46. Gaillard ME, Bottero D, Zurita ME, Carriquiriborde F, Martin Aispuro P, Bartel E, et al. Pertussis maternal immunization: narrowing the knowledge gaps on the duration of transferred protective immunity and on vaccination frequency. *Front Immunol.* (2017) 8:1099. doi: 10.3389/fimmu.2017.01099
47. Gkentzi D, Katsakiori P, Marangos M, Hsia Y, Amirthalingam G, Heath PT, et al. Maternal vaccination against pertussis: a systematic review of the recent literature. *Arch Dis Child Fetal Neonatal Ed.* (2017) 102:F456–63. doi: 10.1136/archdischild-2016-312341
48. Warfel JM, Papin JF, Wolf RF, Zimmerman LI, Merkel TJ. Maternal and neonatal vaccination protects newborn baboons from pertussis infection. *J Infect Dis.* (2014) 210:604–10. doi: 10.1093/infdis/jiu090
49. Black RE, Cousens S, Johnson HL, Lawn JE, Rudan I, Bassani DG, et al. Global, regional, and national causes of child mortality in 2008: a systematic analysis. *Lancet.* (2010) 375:1969–87. doi: 10.1016/S0140-6736(10)60549-1
50. Wendelboe AM, Van Rie A, Salmaso S, Englund JA. Duration of immunity against pertussis after natural infection or vaccination. *Pediatr Infect Dis J.* (2005) 24:S58–61. doi: 10.1097/01.inf.0000160914.59160.41
51. Warfel JM, Zimmerman LI, Merkel TJ. Acellular pertussis vaccines protect against disease but fail to prevent infection and transmission in a nonhuman primate model. *Proc Natl Acad Sci USA.* (2014) 111:787–92. doi: 10.1073/pnas.1314688110
52. Zhang X, Weyrich LS, Lavine JS, Karanikas AT, Harvill ET. Lack of cross-protection against *Bordetella holmesii* after pertussis vaccination. *Emerg Infect Dis.* (2012) 18:1771–9. doi: 10.3201/eid1811.111544
53. Lavine J, Broutin H, Harvill ET, Bjørnstad ON. Imperfect vaccine-induced immunity and whooping cough transmission to infants. *Vaccine.* (2010) 29:11–6. doi: 10.1016/j.vaccine.2010.10.029
54. Long GH, Karanikas AT, Harvill ET, Read AF, and Hudson PJ. Acellular pertussis vaccination facilitates *Bordetella parapertussis* infection in a rodent model of bordetellosis. *Proc Biol Sci.* (2010) 277:2017–25. doi: 10.1098/rspb.2010.0010
55. Diavatopoulos DA, and Edwards KM. What is wrong with pertussis vaccine immunity? why immunological memory to pertussis is failing. *Cold Spring Harb Perspect Biol.* (2017) 9:a029553. doi: 10.1101/cshperspect.a0 29553
56. Burdin N, Handy LK, and Plotkin SA. What is wrong with pertussis vaccine immunity? the problem of waning effectiveness of pertussis vaccines. *Cold Spring Harb Perspect Biol.* (2017) 9:a029454. doi: 10.1101/cshperspect.a029454
57. Bancroft T, Dillon MB, da Silva Antunes R, Paul S, Peters B, Crotty S, et al. Th1 versus Th2 T cell polarization by whole-cell and acellular childhood pertussis vaccines persists upon re-immunization in adolescence and adulthood. *Cell Immunol.* (2016) 304–5:35–43. doi: 10.1016/j.cellimm.2016.05.002
58. Allen AC, Wilk MM, Misiak A, Borkner L, Murphy D, and Mills KHG. Sustained protective immunity against *Bordetella pertussis* nasal colonization by intranasal immunization with a vaccine-adjuvant combination that induces IL-17-secreting T_{RM} cells. *Mucosal Immunol.* (2018) 11:1763–76. doi: 10.1038/s41385-018-0080-x
59. Kapil P, Merkel TJ. Pertussis vaccines and protective immunity. *Curr Opin Immunol.* (2019) 59:72–8. doi: 10.1016/j.coi.2019.03.006
60. Lambert EE, Buisman AM, and van Els CACM. Superior *B. pertussis* specific CD4+ T-cell immunity imprinted by natural infection. *Adv Exp Med Biol.* (2019). doi: 10.1007/5584_2019_405
61. Wilk MM, Borkner L, Misiak A, Curham L, Allen AC, and Mills KHG. Immunization with whole cell but not acellular pertussis vaccines primes CD4 T_{RM} cells that sustain protective immunity against nasal colonization with *Bordetella pertussis. Emerg Microbes Infect.* (2019) 8:169–85. doi: 10.1080/22221751.2018.1564630
62. Raeven RH, Brummelman J, Pennings JL, Nijst OE, Kuipers B, Blok LE, et al. Molecular signatures of the evolving immune response in mice following a *Bordetella pertussis* infection. *PLoS ONE.* (2014) 9:e104548. doi: 10.1371/journal.pone.0104548
63. Wilk MM, Misiak A, McManus RM, Allen AC, Lynch MA, and Mills KHG. Lung CD4 Tissue-resident memory t cells mediate adaptive immunity induced by previous infection of mice with *Bordetella pertussis. J Immunol.* (2017) 199:233–43. doi: 10.4049/jimmunol.1602051
64. Bouchez V, Hegerle N, Strati F, Njamkepo E, Guiso N. New data on vaccine antigen deficient *Bordetella pertussis* isolates. *Vaccines.* (2015) 3:751–70. doi: 10.3390/vaccines3030751
65. Azarian T, Ali A, Johnson JA, Mohr D, Prosperi M, Veras NM, et al. Phylodynamic analysis of clinical and environmental *Vibrio cholerae* isolates from Haiti reveals diversification driven by positive selection. *MBio.* (2014) 5:e01824-14. doi: 10.1128/mBio.01824-14
66. Hegerle N, and Guiso N. Antibody-mediated inhibition of *Bordetella pertussis* adenylate cyclase-haemolysin-induced macrophage cytotoxicity is influenced by variations in the bacterial population. *Microbiology.* (2014) 160(Pt 5):962–9. doi: 10.1099/mic.0.074690-0
67. Octavia S, Maharjan RP, Sintchenko V, Stevenson G, Reeves PR, Gilbert GL, et al. Insight into evolution of *Bordetella pertussis* from comparative genomic analysis: evidence of vaccine-driven selection. *Mol Biol Evol.* (2011) 28:707–15. doi: 10.1093/molbev/msq245
68. Kirimanjeswara GS, Mann PB, Harvill ET. Role of antibodies in immunity to *Bordetella* infections. *Infect Immun.* (2003) 71:1719–24. doi: 10.1128/IAI.71.4.1719-1724.2003
69. Wolfe DN, Goebel EM, Bjornstad ON, Restif O, Harvill ET. The O antigen enables *Bordetella parapertussis* to avoid *Bordetella pertussis*-induced immunity. *Infect Immun.* (2007) 75:4972–9. doi: 10.1128/IAI.00763-07
70. Melvin JA, Scheller EV, Miller JF, Cotter PA. *Bordetella pertussis* pathogenesis: current and future challenges. *Nat Rev Microbiol.* (2014) 12:274–88. doi: 10.1038/nrmicro3235
71. Fedele G, Bianco M, Ausiello CM. The virulence factors of *Bordetella pertussis*: talented modulators of host immune response. *Arch Immunol Ther Exp.* (2013) 61:445–57. doi: 10.1007/s00005-013-0242-1
72. Gorgojo J, Scharrig E, Gómez RM, Harvill ET, Rodríguez ME. *Bordetella parapertussis* circumvents neutrophil extracellular bactericidal mechanisms. *PLoS ONE.* (2017) 12:e0169936. doi: 10.1371/journal.pone.0169936
73. Fedele G, Schiavoni I, Adkins I, Klimova N, and Sebo P. Invasion of dendritic cells, macrophages and neutrophils by the *Bordetella* adenylate cyclase toxin: a subversive move to fool host immunity. *Toxins.* (2017) 9:E293. doi: 10.3390/toxins9100293
74. Nicholson TL, Brockmeier SL, Loving CL, Register KB, Kehrli ME, Shore SM. The *Bordetella bronchiseptica* type III secretion system is required for persistence and disease severity but not transmission in swine. *Infect Immun.* (2014) 82:1092–103. doi: 10.1128/IAI.01115-13
75. Fennelly NK, Sisti F, Higgins SC, Ross PJ, van der Heide H, Mooi FR, et al. *Bordetella pertussis* expresses a functional type III secretion system that subverts protective innate and adaptive immune responses. *Infect Immun.* (2008) 76:1257–66. doi: 10.1128/IAI.00836-07
76. Skinner JA, Pilione MR, Shen H, Harvill ET, Yuk MH. *Bordetella* type III secretion modulates dendritic cell migration resulting in immunosuppression and bacterial persistence. *J Immunol.* (2005) 175:4647–52. doi: 10.4049/jimmunol.175.7.4647
77. Coulthurst S. The Type VI secretion system: a versatile bacterial weapon. *Microbiology.* (2019) 165:503–15. doi: 10.1099/mic.0.000789
78. Starost LJ, Karassek S, Sano Y, Kanda T, Kim KS, Dobrindt U, et al. Pertussis Toxin Exploits host cell signaling pathways induced by meningitis-causing *E. coli* K1-RS218 and enhances adherence of monocytic THP-1 cells to human cerebral endothelial cells. *Toxins.* (2016) 8:E291. doi: 10.3390/toxins8100291
79. Suh HW, Sim YB, Park SH, Sharma N, Im HJ, Hong JS. Effect of pertussis toxin pretreated centrally on blood glucose level induced by stress. *Korean J Physiol Pharmacol.* (2016) 20:467–76. doi: 10.4196/kjpp.2016.20.5.467

80. Kirimanjeswara GS, Agosto LM, Kennett MJ, Bjornstad ON, Harvill ET. Pertussis toxin inhibits neutrophil recruitment to delay antibody-mediated clearance of *Bordetella pertussis*. *J Clin Invest.* (2005) 115:3594–601. doi: 10.1172/JCI24609
81. Bakhshaei P, Kazemi MH, Golara M, Abdolmaleki S, Khosravi-Eghbal R, Khoshnoodi J, et al. Investigation of the cellular immune response to recombinant fragments of filamentous hemagglutinin and pertactin of *Bordetella pertussis* in BALB/c mice. *J Interferon Cytokine Res.* (2018) 38:161–70. doi: 10.1089/jir.2017.0060
82. Villarino Romero R, Hasan S, Faé K, Holubova J, Geurtsen J, Schwarzer M, et al. *Bordetella pertussis* filamentous hemagglutinin itself does not trigger anti-inflammatory interleukin-10 production by human dendritic cells. *Int J Med Microbiol.* (2016) 306:38–47. doi: 10.1016/j.ijmm.2015.11.003
83. Rizzi C, Crippa MP, Jeeninga RE, Berkhout B, Blasi F, Poli G, et al. Pertussis toxin B-oligomer suppresses IL-6 induced HIV-1 and chemokine expression in chronically infected U1 cells via inhibition of activator protein 1. *J Immunol.* (2006) 176:999–1006. doi: 10.4049/jimmunol.176.2.999
84. Alfano M, Grivel JC, Ghezzi S, Corti D, Trimarchi M, Poli G, et al. Pertussis toxin B-oligomer dissociates T cell activation and HIV replication in CD4 T cells released from infected lymphoid tissue. *AIDS.* (2005) 19:1007–14. doi: 10.1097/01.aids.0000174446.40379.3b
85. Alfano M, Rizzi C, Corti D, Adduce L, Poli G. Bacterial toxins: potential weapons against HIV infection. *Curr Pharm Des.* (2005) 11:2909–26. doi: 10.2174/1381612054546725
86. Lapenta C, Spada M, Santini SM, Racca S, Dorigatti F, Poli G, et al. Pertussis toxin B-oligomer inhibits HIV infection and replication in hu-PBL-SCID mice. *Int Immunol.* (2005) 17:469–75. doi: 10.1093/intimm/dxh226
87. Alfano M, Vallanti G, Biswas P, Bovolenta C, Vicenzi E, Mantelli B, et al. The binding subunit of pertussis toxin inhibits HIV replication in human macrophages and virus expression in chronically infected promonocytic U1 cells. *J Immunol.* (2001) 166:1863–70. doi: 10.4049/jimmunol.166.3.1863
88. Alfano M, Pushkarsky T, Poli G, Bukrinsky M. The B-oligomer of pertussis toxin inhibits human immunodeficiency virus type 1 replication at multiple stages. *J Virol.* (2000) 74:8767–70. doi: 10.1128/JVI.74.18.8767-8770.2000
89. Alfano M, Schmidtmayerova H, Amella CA, Pushkarsky T, Bukrinsky M. The B-oligomer of pertussis toxin deactivates CC chemokine receptor 5 and blocks entry of M-tropic HIV-1 strains. *J Exp Med.* (1999) 190:597–605. doi: 10.1084/jem.190.5.597
90. Robbins JB, Schneerson R, Kubler-Kielb J, Keith JM, Trollfors B, Vinogradov E, et al. Toward a new vaccine for pertussis. *Proc Natl Acad Sci USA.* (2014) 111:3213–6. doi: 10.1073/pnas.1324149111
91. Coffman RL, Sher A, Seder RA. Vaccine adjuvants: putting innate immunity to work. *Immunity.* (2010) 33:492–503. doi: 10.1016/j.immuni.2010.10.002
92. Kumar S, Sunagar R, Gosselin E. Bacterial protein toll-like-receptor agonists: a novel perspective on vaccine adjuvants. *Front Immunol.* (2019) 10:1144. doi: 10.3389/fimmu.2019.01144
93. Surendran N, Simmons A, Pichichero ME. TLR agonist combinations that stimulate Th type I polarizing responses from human neonates. *Innate Immun.* (2018) 24:240–51. doi: 10.1177/1753425918771178
94. Ignacio BJ, Albin TJ, Esser-Kahn AP, Verdoes M. Toll-like receptor agonist conjugation: a chemical perspective. *Bioconjug Chem.* (2018) 29:587–603. doi: 10.1021/acs.bioconjchem.7b00808
95. Sinani G, Sessevmez M, Gök MK, Özgümüş S, Oya Alpar H, and Cevher E. Modified chitosan-based nanoadjuvants enhance immunogenicity of protein antigens after mucosal vaccination. *Int J Pharm.* (2019) 569:118592. doi: 10.1016/j.ijpharm.2019.118592
96. Mehrabi M, Montazeri H, Mohamadpour Dounighi N, Rashti A, Vakili-Ghartavol R. Chitosan-based nanoparticles in mucosal vaccine delivery. *Arch Razi Inst.* (2018) 73:165–76. doi: 10.22092/ari.2017.109235.1101
97. Moran HBT, Turley JL, Andersson M, Lavelle EC. Immunomodulatory properties of chitosan polymers. *Biomaterials.* (2018) 184:1–9. doi: 10.1016/j.biomaterials.2018.08.054
98. Misiak A, Leuzzi R, Allen AC, Galletti B, Baudner BC, D'Oro U, et al. Addition of a TLR7 agonist to an acellular pertussis vaccine enhances Th1 and Th17 responses and protective immunity in a mouse model. *Vaccine.* (2017) 35:5256–63. doi: 10.1016/j.vaccine.2017.08.009
99. Brummelman J, Wilk MM, Han WG, van Els CA, Mills KH. Roads to the development of improved pertussis vaccines paved by immunology. *Pathog Dis.* (2015) 73:ftv067. doi: 10.1093/femspd/ftv067
100. Dunne A, Mielke LA, Allen AC, Sutton CE, Higgs R, Cunningham CC, et al. A novel TLR2 agonist from *Bordetella pertussis* is a potent adjuvant that promotes protective immunity with an acellular pertussis vaccine. *Mucosal Immunol.* (2015) 8:607–17. doi: 10.1038/mi.2014.93
101. Dunne A, Marshall NA, Mills KH. TLR based therapeutics. *Curr Opin Pharmacol.* (2011) 11:404–11. doi: 10.1016/j.coph.2011.03.004
102. Higgins SC, Mills KH. TLR, NLR Agonists, and other immune modulators as infectious disease vaccine adjuvants. *Curr Infect Dis Rep.* (2010) 12:4–12. doi: 10.1007/s11908-009-0080-9
103. Pizza M, Giuliani MM, Fontana MR, Monaci E, Douce G, Dougan G, et al. Mucosal vaccines: non toxic derivatives of LT and CT as mucosal adjuvants. *Vaccine.* (2001) 19:2534–41. doi: 10.1016/S0264-410X(00)00553-3
104. Walsh KP, Mills KH. Dendritic cells and other innate determinants of T helper cell polarisation. *Trends Immunol.* (2013) 34:521–30. doi: 10.1016/j.it.2013.07.006
105. Di Pasquale A, Preiss SF, Tavares Da Silva, Garçon N. Vaccine adjuvants: from 1920 to 2015 and Beyond. *Vaccines.* (2015) 3:320–43. doi: 10.3390/vaccines3020320
106. Guo X, Wu N, Shang Y, Liu X, Wu T, Zhou Y, et al. The novel toll-like receptor 2 agonist SUP3 enhances antigen presentation and T cell activation by dendritic cells. *Front Immunol.* (2017) 8:158. doi: 10.3389/fimmu.2017.00158
107. Jiang L, Liu G, Ni W, Zhang N, Jie J, Xie F, et al. The combination of MBP and BCG-induced dendritic cell maturation through TLR2/TLR4 promotes Th1 activation *in vitro* and *vivo*. *Mediators Inflamm.* (2017) 2017:1953680. doi: 10.1155/2017/1953680
108. Asgarian-Omran H, Amirzargar AA, Zeerleder S, Mahdavi M, van Mierlo G, Solati S, et al. Interaction of *Bordetella pertussis* filamentous hemagglutinin with human TLR2: identification of the TLR2-binding domain. *APMIS.* (2015) 123:156–62. doi: 10.1111/apm.12332
109. Rostamian M, Bahrami F, Niknam HM. Vaccination with whole-cell killed or recombinant leishmanial protein and toll-like receptor agonists against Leishmania tropica in BALB/c mice. *PLoS ONE.* (2018) 13:e0204491. doi: 10.1371/journal.pone.0204491
110. Rostamian M, Niknam HM. Evaluation of the adjuvant effect of agonists of toll-like receptor 4 and 7/8 in a vaccine against leishmaniasis in BALB/c mice. *Mol Immunol.* (2017) 91:202–8. doi: 10.1016/j.molimm.2017.09.010
111. Lebedeva E, Bagaev A, Pichugin A, Chulkina M, Lysenko A, Tutykhina I, et al. The differences in immunoadjuvant mechanisms of TLR3 and TLR4 agonists on the level of antigen-presenting cells during immunization with recombinant adenovirus vector. *BMC Immunol.* (2018) 19:26. doi: 10.1186/s12865-018-0264-x
112. Goff PH, Hayashi T, He W, Yao S, Cottam HB, Tan GS, et al. Synthetic Toll-like receptor 4 (TLR4) and TLR7 ligands work additively via myd88 to induce protective antiviral immunity in mice. *J Virol.* (2017) 91:e01050-17. doi: 10.1128/JVI.01050-17
113. Su Y, Li D, Xing Y, Wang H, Wang J, Yuan J, et al. Subcutaneous immunization with fusion protein DnaJ-ΔA146Ply without additional adjuvants induces both humoral and cellular immunity against Pneumococcal infection partially depending on TLR4. *Front Immunol.* (2017) 8:686. doi: 10.3389/fimmu.2017.00686
114. Shibata N, Kunisawa J, Hosomi K, Fujimoto Y, Mizote K, Kitayama N, et al. Lymphoid tissue-resident Alcaligenes LPS induces IgA production without excessive inflammatory responses via weak TLR4 agonist activity. *Mucosal Immunol.* (2018) 11:693–702. doi: 10.1038/mi.2017.103
115. Reed SG, Hsu FC, Carter D, Orr MT. The science of vaccine adjuvants: advances in TLR4 ligand adjuvants. *Curr Opin Immunol.* (2016) 41:85–90. doi: 10.1016/j.coi.2016.06.007
116. Zaffaroni L, Peri F. Recent advances on Toll-like receptor 4 modulation: new therapeutic perspectives. *Future Med Chem.* (2018) 10:461–76. doi: 10.4155/fmc-2017-0172
117. Rolin O, Smallridge W, Henry M, Goodfield L, Place D, Harvill ET. Toll-like receptor 4 limits transmission of *Bordetella bronchiseptica*. *PLoS ONE.* (2014) 9:e85229. doi: 10.1371/journal.pone.0085229

118. Dadaglio G, Fayolle C, Zhang X, Ryffel B, Oberkampf M, Felix T, et al. Antigen targeting to CD11b+ dendritic cells in association with TLR4/TRIF signaling promotes strong CD8+ T cell responses. *J Immunol.* (2014) 193:1787–98. doi: 10.4049/jimmunol.1302974
119. Fedele G, Spensieri F, Palazzo R, Nasso M, Cheung GY, Coote JG, et al. *Bordetella pertussis* commits human dendritic cells to promote a Th1/Th17 response through the activity of adenylate cyclase toxin and MAPK-pathways. *PLoS ONE.* (2010) 5:e8734. doi: 10.1371/journal.pone.0008734
120. Boehm DT, Wolf MA, Hall JM, Wong TY, Sen-Kilic E, Basinger HD, et al. Intranasal acellular pertussis vaccine provides mucosal immunity and protects mice from. *NPJ Vaccines.* (2019) 4:40. doi: 10.1038/s41541-019-0136-2
121. Brummelman J, Raeven RH, Helm K, Pennings JL, Metz B, van Eden W, et al. Transcriptome signature for dampened Th2 dominance in acellular pertussis vaccine-induced CD4(+) T cell responses through TLR4 ligation. *Sci Rep.* (2016) 6:25064. doi: 10.1038/srep25064
122. Brummelman J, Helm K, Hamstra HJ, van der Ley P, Boog CJ, Han WG, et al. Modulation of the CD4(+) T cell response after acellular pertussis vaccination in the presence of TLR4 ligation. *Vaccine.* (2015) 33:1483–91. doi: 10.1016/j.vaccine.2015.01.063
123. Wolfe DN, Buboltz AM, Harvill ET. Inefficient Toll-like receptor-4 stimulation enables *Bordetella parapertussis* to avoid host immunity. *PLoS ONE.* (2009) 4:e4280. doi: 10.1371/journal.pone.0004280
124. Fedele G, Nasso M, Spensieri F, Palazzo R, Frasca L, Watanabe M, et al. Lipopolysaccharides from *Bordetella pertussis* and *Bordetella parapertussis* differently modulate human dendritic cell functions resulting in divergent prevalence of Th17-polarized responses. *J Immunol.* (2008) 181:208–16. doi: 10.4049/jimmunol.181.1.208
125. MacArthur I, Mann PB, Harvill ET, Preston A. IEIIS Meeting minireview: *Bordetella* evolution: lipid A and Toll-like receptor 4. *J Endotoxin Res.* (2007) 13:243–7. doi: 10.1177/0968051907082609
126. Kirimanjeswara GS, Mann PB, Pilione M, Kennett MJ, Harvill ET. The complex mechanism of antibody-mediated clearance of *Bordetella* from the lungs requires TLR4. *J Immunol.* (2005) 175:7504–11. doi: 10.4049/jimmunol.175.11.7504
127. Mann PB, Wolfe D, Latz E, Golenbock D, Preston A, Harvill ET. Comparative toll-like receptor 4-mediated innate host defense to *Bordetella* infection. *Infect Immun.* (2005) 73:8144–52. doi: 10.1128/IAI.73.12.8144-8152.2005
128. Mann PB, Elder KD, Kennett MJ, Harvill ET. Toll-like receptor 4-dependent early elicited tumor necrosis factor alpha expression is critical for innate host defense against *Bordetella bronchiseptica*. *Infect Immun.* (2004) 72:6650–8. doi: 10.1128/IAI.72.11.6650-6658.2004
129. McKay PF, King DF, Mann JF, Barinaga G, Carter D, Shattock RJ. TLR4 and TLR7/8 adjuvant combinations generate different vaccine antigen-specific immune outcomes in minipigs when administered via the ID or IN routes. *PLoS ONE.* (2016) 11:e0148984. doi: 10.1371/journal.pone.0148984
130. Mann PB, Kennett MJ, Harvill ET. Toll-like receptor 4 is critical to innate host defense in a murine model of bordetellosis. *J Infect Dis.* (2004) 189:833–6. doi: 10.1086/381898
131. Mizel SB, West AP, Hantgan RR. Identification of a sequence in human toll-like receptor 5 required for the binding of Gram-negative flagellin. *J Biol Chem.* (2003) 278:23624–9. doi: 10.1074/jbc.M303481200
132. Akerley BJ, Cotter PA, Miller JF. Ectopic expression of the flagellar regulon alters development of the *Bordetella*-host interaction. *Cell.* (1995) 80:611–20. doi: 10.1016/0092-8674(95)90515-4
133. Tremblay MM, Bilal MY, Houtman JC. Prior TLR5 induction in human T cells results in a transient potentiation of subsequent TCR-induced cytokine production. *Mol Immunol.* (2014) 57:161–70. doi: 10.1016/j.molimm.2013.09.002
134. Bargieri DY, Rosa DS, Braga CJ, Carvalho BO, Costa FT, Espíndola NM, et al. New malaria vaccine candidates based on the *Plasmodium vivax* merozoite surface protein-1 and the TLR-5 agonist Salmonella Typhimurium FliC flagellin. *Vaccine.* (2008) 26:6132–42. doi: 10.1016/j.vaccine.2008.08.070
135. Honko AN, Sriranganathan N, Lees CJ, Mizel SB. Flagellin is an effective adjuvant for immunization against lethal respiratory challenge with *Yersinia pestis*. *Infect Immun.* (2006) 74:1113–20. doi: 10.1128/IAI.74.2.1113-1120.2006
136. Letran SE, Lee SJ, Atif SM, Uematsu S, Akira S, McSorley SJ. TLR5 functions as an endocytic receptor to enhance flagellin-specific adaptive immunity. *Eur J Immunol.* (2011) 41:29–38. doi: 10.1002/eji.201040717
137. Taylor DN, Treanor JJ, Strout C, Johnson C, Fitzgerald T, Kavita U, et al. Induction of a potent immune response in the elderly using the TLR-5 agonist, flagellin, with a recombinant hemagglutinin influenza-flagellin fusion vaccine (VAX125, STF2.HA1 SI). *Vaccine.* (2011) 29:4897–902. doi: 10.1016/j.vaccine.2011.05.001
138. Kinnebrew MA, Ubeda C, Zenewicz LA, Smith N, Flavell RA, Pamer EG. Bacterial flagellin stimulates Toll-like receptor 5-dependent defense against vancomycin-resistant Enterococcus infection. *J Infect Dis.* (2010) 201:534–43. doi: 10.1086/650203
139. Kim JR, Holbrook BC, Hayward SL, Blevins LK, Jorgensen MJ, Kock ND, et al. Inclusion of flagellin during vaccination against influenza enhances recall responses in nonhuman primate neonates. *J Virol.* (2015) 89:7291–303. doi: 10.1128/JVI.00549-15
140. Song H, Xiong D, Wang J, Zhai X, Liang G. A porcine reproductive and respiratory syndrome virus vaccine candidate based on PRRSV glycoprotein 5 and the Toll-like receptor 5 agonist Salmonella typhimurium flagellin. *J Mol Microbiol Biotechnol.* (2015) 25:56–9. doi: 10.1159/000375496
141. Cunningham AL, Dang KM, Yu JJ, Guentzel MN, Heidner HW, Klose KE, et al. Enhancement of vaccine efficacy by expression of a TLR5 ligand in the defined live attenuated *Francisella tularensis* subsp. novicida strain U112ΔiglB::fljB. *Vaccine.* (2014) 32:5234–40. doi: 10.1016/j.vaccine.2014.07.038
142. Dowling DJ. Recent advances in the discovery and delivery of TLR7/8 agonists as vaccine adjuvants. *Immunohorizons.* (2018) 2:185–97. doi: 10.4049/immunohorizons.1700063
143. Dowling DJ, van Haren SD, Scheid A, Bergelson I, Kim D, Mancuso CJ, et al. TLR7/8 adjuvant overcomes newborn hyporesponsiveness to pneumococcal conjugate vaccine at birth. *JCI Insight.* (2017) 2:e91020. doi: 10.1172/jci.insight.91020
144. van Haren SD, Dowling DJ, Foppen W, Christensen D, Andersen P, Reed SG, et al. Age-specific adjuvant synergy: dual TLR7/8 and mincle activation of human newborn dendritic cells enables Th1 polarization. *J Immunol.* (2016) 197:4413–24. doi: 10.4049/jimmunol.1600282
145. van Haren SD, Ganapathi L, Bergelson I, Dowling DJ, Banks M, Samuels RC, et al. *In vitro* cytokine induction by TLR-activating vaccine adjuvants in human blood varies by age and adjuvant. *Cytokine.* (2016) 83:99–109. doi: 10.1016/j.cyto.2016.04.001
146. Ganapathi L, Van Haren S, Dowling DJ, Bergelson I, Shukla NM, Malladi SS, et al. The imidazoquinoline toll-like receptor-7/8 agonist hybrid-2 potently induces cytokine production by human newborn and adult leukocytes. *PLoS ONE.* (2015) 10:e0134640. doi: 10.1371/journal.pone.0134640
147. Wilkinson A, Lattmann E, Roces CB, Pedersen GK, Christensen D, Perrie Y. Lipid conjugation of TLR7 agonist Resiquimod ensures co-delivery with the liposomal Cationic Adjuvant Formulation 01 (CAF01) but does not enhance immunopotentiation compared to non-conjugated Resiquimod+CAF01. *J Control Release.* (2018) 291:1–10. doi: 10.1016/j.jconrel.2018.10.002
148. Collier MA, Junkins RD, Gallovic MD, Johnson BM, Johnson MM, Macintyre AN, et al. Acetalated dextran microparticles for codelivery of STING and TLR7/8 agonists. *Mol Pharm.* (2018) 15:4933–46. doi: 10.1021/acs.molpharmaceut.8b00579
149. McGowan DC, Herschke F, Khamlichi MD, Rosauro ML, Benedicto SMP, Pauwels F, et al. Design and synthesis of tetrahydropyridopyrimidine based toll-like receptor (TLR) 7/8 dual agonists. *Bioorg Med Chem Lett.* (2018) 28:3216–21. doi: 10.1016/j.bmcl.2018.08.015
150. Gadd AJR, Castelletto V, Kabova E, Shankland K, Perrie Y, Hamley I, et al. High potency of lipid conjugated TLR7 agonist requires nanoparticulate or liposomal formulation. *Eur J Pharm Sci.* (2018) 123:268–76. doi: 10.1016/j.ejps.2018.07.048
151. Vo HTM, Baudner BC, Sammicheli S, Iannacone M, D'Oro U, Piccioli D. Alum/toll-like receptor 7 adjuvant enhances the expansion of memory B cell compartment within the draining lymph node. *Front Immunol.* (2018) 9:641. doi: 10.3389/fimmu.2018.00641

152. Carignan D, Herblot S, Laliberté-Gagné M, Bolduc M, Duval M, Savard P, et al. Activation of innate immunity in primary human cells using a plant virus derived nanoparticle TLR7/8 agonist. *Nanomedicine.* (2018) 14:2317–27. doi: 10.1016/j.nano.2017.10.015
153. Van Hoeven N, Fox CB, Granger B, Evers T, Joshi SW, Nana GI, et al. A formulated TLR7/8 agonist is a flexible, highly potent and effective adjuvant for pandemic influenza vaccines. *Sci Rep.* (2017) 7:46426. doi: 10.1038/srep46426
154. Rubtsova K, Rubtsov AV, Halemano K, Li SX, Kappler JW, Santiago ML, et al. T cell production of IFNγ in response to TLR7/IL-12 stimulates optimal B cell responses to viruses. *PLoS ONE.* (2016) 11:e0166322. doi: 10.1371/journal.pone.0166322
155. Hu Y, Cong X, Chen L, Qi J, Wu X, Zhou M, et al. Synergy of TLR3 and 7 ligands significantly enhances function of DCs to present inactivated PRRSV antigen through TRIF/MyD88-NF-κB signaling pathway. *Sci Rep.* (2016) 6:23977. doi: 10.1038/srep23977
156. Aguado-Martínez A, Basto AP, Tanaka S, Ryser LT, Nunes TP, Ortega-Mora LM, et al. Immunization with a cocktail of antigens fused with OprI reduces Neospora caninum vertical transmission and postnatal mortality in mice. *Vaccine.* (2019) 37:473–83. doi: 10.1016/j.vaccine.2018.11.060
157. Buonsanti C, Balocchi C, Harfouche C, Corrente F, Galli Stampino L, Mancini F, et al. Novel adjuvant Alum-TLR7 significantly potentiates immune response to glycoconjugate vaccines. *Sci Rep.* (2016) 6:29063. doi: 10.1038/srep29063
158. Lu F, Mosley YC, Carmichael B, Brown DD, HogenEsch H. Formulation of aluminum hydroxide adjuvant with TLR agonists poly(I:C) and CpG enhances the magnitude and avidity of the humoral immune response. *Vaccine.* (2019) 37:1945–53. doi: 10.1016/j.vaccine.2019.02.033
159. Li N, Zhang L, Zheng B, Li W, Liu J, Zhang H, et al. RSV recombinant candidate vaccine G1F/M2 with CpG as an adjuvant prevents vaccine-associated lung inflammation, which may be associated with the appropriate types of immune memory in spleens and lungs. *Hum Vaccin Immunother.* (2019) 15:2684–94. doi: 10.1080/21645515.2019.1596710
160. Jin JW, Tang SQ, Rong MZ, Zhang MQ. Synergistic effect of dual targeting vaccine adjuvant with aminated β-glucan and CpG-oligodeoxynucleotides for both humoral and cellular immune responses. *Acta Biomater.* (2018) 78:211–23. doi: 10.1016/j.actbio.2018.08.002
161. Guan X, Chen J, Hu Y, Lin L, Sun P, Tian H, et al. Highly enhanced cancer immunotherapy by combining nanovaccine with hyaluronidase. *Biomaterials.* (2018) 171:198–206. doi: 10.1016/j.biomaterials.2018.04.039
162. Alkie TN, Taha-Abdelaziz K, Barjesteh N, Bavananthasivam J, Hodgins DC, Sharif S. Characterization of innate responses induced by PLGA encapsulated- and soluble TLR ligands *in vitro* and *in vivo* in chickens. *PLoS ONE.* (2017) 12:e0169154. doi: 10.1371/journal.pone.0169154
163. Hawksworth D. Advancing Freund's and addaVax adjuvant regimens using CpG oligodeoxynucleotides. *Monoclon Antib Immunodiagn Immunother.* (2018) 37:195–9. doi: 10.1089/mab.2018.0022
164. Lai CY, Yu GY, Luo Y, Xiang R, Chuang TH. Immunostimulatory activities of CpG-oligodeoxynucleotides in teleosts: toll-like receptors 9 and 21. *Front Immunol.* (2019) 10:179. doi: 10.3389/fimmu.2019.00179
165. Akkaya M, Akkaya B, Miozzo P, Rawat M, Pena M, Sheehan PW, et al. B cells produce type 1 IFNs in response to the TLR9 agonist CpG-A conjugated to cationic lipids. *J Immunol.* (2017) 199:931–40. doi: 10.4049/jimmunol.1700348
166. Ye L, Feng Z, Doycheva D, Malaguit J, Dixon B, Xu N, et al. CpG-ODN exerts a neuroprotective effect via the TLR9/pAMPK signaling pathway by activation of autophagy in a neonatal HIE rat model. *Exp Neurol.* (2018) 301(Pt A):70–80. doi: 10.1016/j.expneurol.2017.12.008
167. Zhang H, Yan T, Xu S, Feng S, Huang D, Fujita M, et al. Graphene oxide-chitosan nanocomposites for intracellular delivery of immunostimulatory CpG oligodeoxynucleotides. *Mater Sci Eng C Mater Biol Appl.* (2017) 73:144–51. doi: 10.1016/j.msec.2016.12.072
168. Zhang P, Dong S, Guo J, Yang Y, Liu C, Li B, et al. CpG-oligodeoxynucleotides improved irradiation-induced injuries by G-CSF and IL-6 up-regulation. *Cell Physiol Biochem.* (2017) 44:2368–77. doi: 10.1159/000486153
169. Ramirez A, Co M, Mathew A. CpG improves influenza vaccine efficacy in young adult but not aged mice. *PLoS ONE.* (2016) 11:e0150425. doi: 10.1371/journal.pone.0150425
170. Asokanathan C, Corbel M, Xing D. A CpG-containing oligodeoxynucleotide adjuvant for acellular pertussis vaccine improves the protective response against *Bordetella pertussis. Hum Vaccin Immunother.* (2013) 9:325–31. doi: 10.4161/hv.22755
171. Knight JB, Huang YY, Halperin SA, Anderson R, Morris A, Macmillan A, et al. Immunogenicity and protective efficacy of a recombinant filamentous haemagglutinin from *Bordetella pertussis. Clin Exp Immunol.* (2006) 144:543–51. doi: 10.1111/j.1365-2249.2006.03097.x
172. Boyd AP, Ross PJ, Conroy H, Mahon N, Lavelle EC, Mills KH. *Bordetella pertussis* adenylate cyclase toxin modulates innate and adaptive immune responses: distinct roles for acylation and enzymatic activity in immunomodulation and cell death. *J Immunol.* (2005) 175:730–8. doi: 10.4049/jimmunol.175.2.730
173. Maletto B, Rópolo A, Morón V, Pistoresi-Palencia MC. CpG-DNA stimulates cellular and humoral immunity and promotes Th1 differentiation in aged BALB/c mice. *J Leukoc Biol.* (2002) 72:447–54.
174. Gracia A, Polewicz M, Halperin SA, Hancock RE, Potter AA, Babiuk LA, et al. Antibody responses in adult and neonatal BALB/c mice to immunization with novel *Bordetella pertussis* vaccine formulations. *Vaccine.* (2011) 29:1595–604. doi: 10.1016/j.vaccine.2010.12.083
175. de Apostólico JS, Lunardelli VA, Coirada FC, Boscardin SB, Rosa DS. Adjuvants: classification, modus operandi, and licensing. *J Immunol Res.* (2016) 2016:1459394. doi: 10.1155/2016/1459394
176. Holmgren J, Adamsson J, Anjuère F, Clemens J, Czerkinsky C, Eriksson K, et al. Mucosal adjuvants and anti-infection and anti-immunopathology vaccines based on cholera toxin, cholera toxin B subunit and CpG DNA. *Immunol Lett.* (2005) 97:181–8. doi: 10.1016/j.imlet.2004.11.009
177. Bromander AK, Kjerrulf M, Holmgren J, Lycke, N. Cholera toxin enhances antigen presentation. *Adv Exp Med Biol.* (1995) 371B:1501–6.
178. Holmgren J, Czerkinsky C, Lycke N, Svennerholm AM. Strategies for the induction of immune responses at mucosal surfaces making use of cholera toxin B subunit as immunogen, carrier, and adjuvant. *Am J Trop Med Hyg.* (1994) 50:42–54.
179. Bromander AK, Kjerrulf M, Holmgren J, Lycke N. Cholera toxin enhances alloantigen presentation by cultured intestinal epithelial cells. *Scand J Immunol.* (1993) 37:452–8. doi: 10.1111/j.1365-3083.1993.tb03318.x
180. Holmgren J, Lycke N, Czerkinsky C. Cholera toxin and cholera B subunit as oral-mucosal adjuvant and antigen vector systems. *Vaccine.* (1993) 11:1179–84. doi: 10.1016/0264-410X(93)90039-Z
181. Holmgren J, Nordqvist S, Blomquist M, Jeverstam F, Lebens M, Raghavan S. Preclinical immunogenicity and protective efficacy of an oral *Helicobacter pylori* inactivated whole cell vaccine and multiple mutant cholera toxin: a novel and non-toxic mucosal adjuvant. *Vaccine.* (2018) 36:6223–30. doi: 10.1016/j.vaccine.2018.07.073
182. Lavelle EC, Jarnicki A, McNeela E, Armstrong ME, Higgins SC, Leavy O, et al. Effects of cholera toxin on innate and adaptive immunity and its application as an immunomodulatory agent. *J Leukoc Biol.* (2004) 75:756–63. doi: 10.1189/jlb.1103534
183. Kim MS, Yi EJ, Kim YI, Kim SH, Jung YS, Kim SR, et al. ERdj5 in innate immune cells is a crucial factor for the mucosal adjuvanticity of cholera toxin. *Front Immunol.* (2019) 10:1249. doi: 10.3389/fimmu.2019.01249
184. Sun JB, Holmgren J, Larena M, Terrinoni M, Fang Y, Bresnick AR, et al. Deficiency in calcium-binding protein S100A4 impairs the adjuvant action of cholera toxin. *Front Immunol.* (2017) 8:1119. doi: 10.3389/fimmu.2017.01119
185. Barati B, Ebrahimi F, Nazarian S. Production of chicken egg yolk antibody (IgY) against recombinant cholera toxin B subunit and evaluation of its prophylaxis potency in mice. *Iran J Immunol.* (2018) 15:47–58.
186. Isaka M, Komiya T, Takahashi M, Yasuda Y, Taniguchi T, Zhao Y, et al. Recombinant cholera toxin B subunit (rCTB) as a mucosal adjuvant enhances induction of diphtheria and tetanus antitoxin antibodies in mice by intranasal administration with diphtheria-pertussis-tetanus (DPT) combination vaccine. *Vaccine.* (2004) 22:3061–8. doi: 10.1016/j.vaccine.2004.02.019
187. Lee SF, Halperin SA, Salloum DF, MacMillan A, Morris A. Mucosal immunization with a genetically engineered pertussis toxin S1 fragment-cholera toxin subunit B chimeric protein. *Infect Immun.* (2003) 71:2272–5. doi: 10.1128/IAI.71.4.2272-2275.2003

188. Isaka M, Yasuda Y, Taniguchi T, Kozuka S, Matano K, Maeyama J, et al. Mucosal and systemic antibody responses against an acellular pertussis vaccine in mice after intranasal co-administration with recombinant cholera toxin B subunit as an adjuvant. *Vaccine.* (2003) 21:1165–73. doi: 10.1016/S0264-410X(02)00516-9
189. Olivera N, Castuma CE, Hozbor D, Gaillard ME, Rumbo M, Gómez RM. Immunization with the recombinant Cholera toxin B fused to Fimbria 2 protein protects against *Bordetella pertussis* infection. *Biomed Res Int.* (2014) 2014:421486. doi: 10.1155/2014/421486
190. Clements JD, Norton EB. The mucosal vaccine adjuvant LT(R192G/L211A) or dmLT. *mSphere.* (2018) 3:e00215-18. doi: 10.1128/mSphere.00215-18
191. Albert MJ, Haridas S, Ebenezer M, Raghupathy R, Khan I. Immunization with a double-mutant (R192G/L211A) of the heat-labile enterotoxin of escherichia coli offers partial protection against campylobacter jejuni in an adult mouse intestinal colonization model. *PLoS ONE.* (2015) 10:e0142090. doi: 10.1371/journal.pone.0142090
192. Chang YC, Chang CY, Tsai PS, Chiou HY, Jeng CR, Pang VF, et al. Efficacy of heat-labile enterotoxin B subunit-adjuvanted parenteral porcine epidemic diarrhea virus trimeric spike subunit vaccine in piglets. *Appl Microbiol Biotechnol.* (2018) 102:7499–507. doi: 10.1007/s00253-018-9110-6
193. Brereton CF, Sutton CE, Ross PJ, Iwakura Y, Pizza M, Rappuoli R, et al. *Escherichia coli* heat-labile enterotoxin promotes protective Th17 responses against infection by driving innate IL-1 and IL-23 production. *J Immunol.* (2011) 186:5896–906. doi: 10.4049/jimmunol.1003789
194. Ryan EJ, McNeela E, Pizza M, Rappuoli R, O'Neill L, Mills KH. Modulation of innate and acquired immune responses by Escherichia coli heat-labile toxin: distinct pro- and anti-inflammatory effects of the nontoxic AB complex and the enzyme activity. *J Immunol.* (2000) 165:5750–9. doi: 10.4049/jimmunol.165.10.5750
195. Coleman MM, Basdeo SA, Coleman AM, Cheallaigh CN, Peral de Castro C, McLaughlin AM, et al. All-trans retinoic acid augments autophagy during intracellular bacterial infection. *Am J Respir Cell Mol Biol.* (2018) 59:548–556. doi: 10.1165/rcmb.2017-0382OC
196. Oliveira LM, Teixeira FME, Sato MN. Impact of retinoic acid on immune cells and inflammatory diseases. *Mediators Inflamm.* (2018) 2018:3067126. doi: 10.1155/2018/3067126
197. Seo GY, Lee JM, Jang YS, Kang SG, Yoon SI, Ko HJ, et al. Mechanism underlying the suppressor activity of retinoic acid on IL4-induced IgE synthesis and its physiological implication. *Cell Immunol.* (2017) 322:49–55. doi: 10.1016/j.cellimm.2017.10.001
198. Bezerra IPS, Costa-Souza BLS, Carneiro G, Ferreira LAM, de Matos Guedes HL, Rossi-Bergmann B. Nanoencapsulated retinoic acid as a safe tolerogenic adjuvant for intranasal vaccination against cutaneous leishmaniasis. *Vaccine.* (2019) 37:3660–7. doi: 10.1016/j.vaccine.2019.05.043
199. Mwanza-Lisulo M, Kelly P. Potential for use of retinoic acid as an oral vaccine adjuvant. *Philos Trans R Soc Lond B Biol Sci.* (2015) 370:20140145. doi: 10.1098/rstb.2014.0145
200. Lisulo MM, Kapulu MC, Banda R, Sinkala E, Kayamba V, Sianongo S, et al. Adjuvant potential of low dose all-trans retinoic acid during oral typhoid vaccination in Zambian men. *Clin Exp Immunol.* (2014) 175:468–75. doi: 10.1111/cei.12238
201. Tan X, Sande JL, Pufnock JS, Blattman JN, Greenberg PD. Retinoic acid as a vaccine adjuvant enhances CD8+ T cell response and mucosal protection from viral challenge. *J Virol.* (2011) 85:8316–27. doi: 10.1128/JVI.00781-11
202. Qiang Y, Xu J, Yan C, Jin H, Xiao T, Yan N, et al. Butyrate and retinoic acid imprint mucosal-like dendritic cell development synergistically from bone marrow cells. *Clin Exp Immunol.* (2017) 189:290–7. doi: 10.1111/cei.12990
203. Raverdeau M, Mills KH. Modulation of T cell and innate immune responses by retinoic acid. *J Immunol.* (2014) 192:2953–8. doi: 10.4049/jimmunol.1303245
204. Torres-Sangiao E, Holban AM, Gestal MC. Advanced nanobiomaterials: vaccines, diagnosis and treatment of infectious diseases. *Molecules.* (2016) 21:E867. doi: 10.3390/molecules21070867
205. Alagpulinsa DA, Cao JJL, Driscoll RK, Sîrbulescu RF, Penson MFE, Sremac M, et al. Alginate-microencapsulation of human stem cell-derived β cells with CXCL12 prolongs their survival and function in immunocompetent mice without systemic immunosuppression. *Am J Transplant.* (2019) 19:1930–40. doi: 10.1111/ajt.15308
206. Ibe MI, Odimegwu DC, Onuigbo EB. Alginate-coated chitosan microparticles encapsulating an oral plasmid-cured live *Salmonella enterica* serovar Gallinarum vaccine cause a higher expression of interferon-gamma in chickens compared to the parenteral live vaccine. *Avian Pathol.* (2019) 48:423–28. doi: 10.1080/03079457.2019.1616673
207. Minakshi P, Ghosh M, Brar B, Kumar R, Lambe UP, Ranjan K, et al. Nano-antimicrobials: a new paradigm for combating mycobacterial resistance. *Curr Pharm Des.* (2019) 25:1554–79. doi: 10.2174/1381612825666190620094041
208. Vaghasiya K, Eram A, Sharma A, Ray E, Adlakha S, Verma RK. Alginate microspheres elicit innate M1-inflammatory response in macrophages leading to bacillary killing. *AAPS PharmSciTech.* (2019) 20:241. doi: 10.1208/s12249-019-1458-0
209. Coelho-Rocha ND, de Castro CP, de Jesus LCL, Leclercq SY, de Cicco Sandes SH, Nunes AC, et al. Microencapsulation of lactic acid bacteria improves the gastrointestinal delivery and *in situ* expression of recombinant fluorescent protein. *Front Microbiol.* (2018) 9:2398. doi: 10.3389/fmicb.2018.02398
210. Kordbacheh E, Nazarian S, Hajizadeh A, Sadeghi D. Entrapment of LTB protein in alginate nanoparticles protects against Enterotoxigenic *Escherichia coli*. *APMIS.* (2018) 126:320–8. doi: 10.1111/apm.12815
211. Lee J, Kim YM, Kim JH, Cho CW, Jeon JW, Park JK, et al. Nasal delivery of chitosan/alginate nanoparticle encapsulated bee (*Apis mellifera*) venom promotes antibody production and viral clearance during porcine reproductive and respiratory syndrome virus infection by modulating T cell related responses. *Vet Immunol Immunopathol.* (2018) 200:40–51. doi: 10.1016/j.vetimm.2018.04.006
212. Yuan J, Guo L, Wang S, Liu D, Qin X, Zheng L, et al. Preparation of self-assembled nanoparticles of ε-polylysine-sodium alginate: a sustained-release carrier for antigen delivery. *Colloids Surf B Biointerfaces.* (2018) 171:406–12. doi: 10.1016/j.colsurfb.2018.07.058
213. Wu H, Bao Y, Wang X, Zhou D, Wu W. Alkyl polyglycoside, a highly promising adjuvant in intranasal split influenza vaccines. *Hum Vaccin Immunother.* (2017) 13:1–9. doi: 10.1080/21645515.2016.1278098
214. Bacon A, Makin J, Sizer PJ, Jabbal-Gill I, Hinchcliffe M, Illum L, et al. Carbohydrate biopolymers enhance antibody responses to mucosally delivered vaccine antigens. *Infect Immun.* (2000) 68:5764–70. doi: 10.1128/IAI.68.10.5764-5770.2000
215. Bagheripour MJ, Ebrahimi F, Hajizade A, Nazarian S. Immunogenicity evaluation of rBoNT/E nanovaccine after mucosal administration. *Iran J Basic Med Sci.* (2019) 22:353–9.
216. Díaz AG, Quinteros DA, Paolicchi FA, Rivero MA, Palma SD, Pardo RP, et al. Mucosal immunization with polymeric antigen BLSOmp31 using alternative delivery systems against *Brucella ovis* in rams. *Vet Immunol Immunopathol.* (2019) 209:70–7. doi: 10.1016/j.vetimm.2019.02.005
217. Ghaffari Marandi BH, Zolfaghari MR, Kazemi R, Motamedi MJ, Amani J. Immunization against *Vibrio cholerae*, ETEC, and EHEC with chitosan nanoparticle containing LSC chimeric protein. *Microb Pathog.* (2019) 134:103600. doi: 10.1016/j.micpath.2019.103600
218. Kole S, Qadiri SSN, Shin SM, Kim WS, Lee J, Jung SJ. Nanoencapsulation of inactivated-viral vaccine using chitosan nanoparticles: evaluation of its protective efficacy and immune modulatory effects in olive flounder (*Paralichthys olivaceus*) against viral haemorrhagic septicaemia virus (VHSV) infection. *Fish Shellfish Immunol.* (2019) 91:136–47. doi: 10.1016/j.fsi.2019.05.017
219. Korupalli C, Pan WY, Yeh CY, Chen PM, Mi FL, Tsai HW, et al. Single-injecting, bioinspired nanocomposite hydrogel that can recruit host immune cells *in situ* to elicit potent and long-lasting humoral immune responses. *Biomaterials.* (2019) 216:119268. doi: 10.1016/j.biomaterials.2019.119268
220. Muralidharan A, Russell MS, Larocque L, Gravel C, Sauvé S, Chen Z, et al. Chitosan alters inactivated respiratory syncytial virus vaccine elicited immune responses without affecting lung histopathology in mice. *Vaccine.* (2019) 37:4031–9. doi: 10.1016/j.vaccine.2019.06.003
221. Senevirathne A, Hewawaduge C, Hajam IA, Lalsiamthara J, Lee JH. Intranasally administered anti-Brucella subunit vaccine formulation induces protective immune responses against nasal Brucella challenge. *Vet Microbiol.* (2019) 228:112–8. doi: 10.1016/j.vetmic.2018.11.022
222. Singh A, Nisaa K, Bhattacharyya S, Mallick AI. Immunogenicity and protective efficacy of mucosal delivery of recombinant hcp of *Campylobacter*

jejuni type VI secretion system (T6SS) in chickens. *Mol Immunol.* (2019) 111:182–97. doi: 10.1016/j.molimm.2019.04.016
223. Soh SH, Shim S, Im YB, Park HT, Cho CS, Yoo HS. Induction of Th2-related immune responses and production of systemic IgA in mice intranasally immunized with *Brucella abortus* malate dehydrogenase loaded chitosan nanoparticles. *Vaccine.* (2019) 37:1554–64. doi: 10.1016/j.vaccine.2019.02.005
224. Zhang J, Fu X, Zhang Y, Zhu W, Zhou Y, Yuan G, et al. Chitosan and anisodamine improve the immune efficacy of inactivated infectious spleen and kidney necrosis virus vaccine in Siniperca chuatsi. *Fish Shellfish Immunol.* (2019) 89:52–60. doi: 10.1016/j.fsi.2019.03.040
225. Hojatizade M, Soleymani M, Tafaghodi M, Badiee A, Chavoshian O, Jaafari MR. Chitosan nanoparticles loaded with whole and soluble leishmania antigens, and evaluation of their immunogenecity in a mouse model of leishmaniasis. *Iran J Immunol.* (2018) 15:281–93. doi: 10.22034/IJI.2018.39397
226. Huang T, Song X, Jing J, Zhao K, Shen Y, Zhang X, et al. Chitosan-DNA nanoparticles enhanced the immunogenicity of multivalent DNA vaccination on mice against *Trueperella pyogenes* infection. *J Nanobiotechnol.* (2018) 16:8. doi: 10.1186/s12951-018-0337-2
227. Malik A, Gupta M, Mani R, Gogoi H, Bhatnagar R. Trimethyl chitosan nanoparticles encapsulated protective antigen protects the mice against anthrax. *Front Immunol.* (2018) 9:562. doi: 10.3389/fimmu.2018.00562
228. Sun B, Yu S, Zhao D, Guo S, Wang X, Zhao K. Polysaccharides as vaccine adjuvants. *Vaccine.* (2018) 36:5226–34. doi: 10.1016/j.vaccine.2018.07.040
229. Lebre F, Bento D, Ribeiro J, Colaço M, Borchard G, de Lima MCP, et al. Association of chitosan and aluminium as a new adjuvant strategy for improved vaccination. *Int J Pharm.* (2017) 527:103–14. doi: 10.1016/j.ijpharm.2017.05.028
230. Spinner JL, Oberoi HS, Yorgensen YM, Poirier DS, Burkhart DJ, Plante M, et al. Methylglycol chitosan and a synthetic TLR4 agonist enhance immune responses to influenza vaccine administered sublingually. *Vaccine.* (2015) 33:5845–53. doi: 10.1016/j.vaccine.2015.08.086
231. Torlak E, Sert D. Antibacterial effectiveness of chitosan-propolis coated polypropylene films against foodborne pathogens. *Int J Biol Macromol.* (2013) 60:52–5. doi: 10.1016/j.ijbiomac.2013.05.013
232. Kang ML, Kang SG, Jiang HL, Guo DD, Lee DY, Rayamahji N, et al. Chitosan microspheres containing *Bordetella bronchiseptica* antigens as novel vaccine against atrophic rhinitis in pigs. *J Microbiol Biotechnol.* (2008) 18:1179–85.
233. de Paula Oliveira Santos B, Trentini MM, Machado RB, Rúbia Nunes Celes M, Kipnis A, Petrovsky N, et al. Advax4 delta inulin combination adjuvant together with ECMX, a fusion construct of four protective mTB antigens, induces a potent Th1 immune response and protects mice against *Mycobacterium tuberculosis* infection. *Hum Vaccin Immunother.* (2017) 13:2967–76. doi: 10.1080/21645515.2017.1368598
234. Horst G, Levine R, Chick R, Hofacre C. Effects of beta-1,3-glucan (AletaTM) on vaccination response in broiler chickens. *Poult Sci.* (2019) 98:1643–7. doi: 10.3382/ps/pey523
235. Wang H, Yang B, Wang Y, Liu F, Fernández-Tejada A, Dong S. β-Glucan as an immune activator and a carrier in the construction of a synthetic MUC1 vaccine. *Chem Commun.* (2018) 55:253–6. doi: 10.1039/C8CC07691J
236. Whelan AO, Flick-Smith HC, Homan J, Shen ZT, Carpenter Z, Khoshkenar P, et al. Protection induced by a Francisella tularensis subunit vaccine delivered by glucan particles. *PLoS ONE.* (2018) 13:e0200213. doi: 10.1371/journal.pone.0200213
237. Hung CY, Zhang H, Castro-Lopez N, Ostroff GR, Khoshlenar P, Abraham A, et al. Glucan-chitin particles enhance Th17 response and improve protective efficacy of a multivalent antigen (rCpa1) against pulmonary *Coccidioides posadasii* infection. *Infect Immun.* (2018) 86:e00070-18. doi: 10.1128/IAI.00070-18
238. Bundle DR, Paszkiewicz E, Elsaidi HRH, Mandal SS, Sarkar S. A three component synthetic vaccine containing a β-mannan T-cell peptide epitope and a β-glucan dendritic cell ligand. *Molecules.* (2018) 23:E1961. doi: 10.3390/molecules23081961
239. Ferreira LG, Endrighi M, Lisenko KG, de Oliveira MRD, Damasceno MR, Claudino JA, et al. Oat beta-glucan as a dietary supplement for dogs. *PLoS ONE.* (2018) 13:e0201133. doi: 10.1371/journal.pone.0201133
240. Deepe GS, Buesing WR, Ostroff GR, Abraham A, Specht CA, Huang H, et al. Vaccination with an alkaline extract of Histoplasma capsulatum packaged in glucan particles confers protective immunity in mice. *Vaccine.* (2018) 36:3359–67. doi: 10.1016/j.vaccine.2018.04.047
241. Jin Y, Li P, Wang F. β-glucans as potential immunoadjuvants: a review on the adjuvanticity, structure-activity relationship and receptor recognition properties. *Vaccine.* (2018) 36:5235–44. doi: 10.1016/j.vaccine.2018.07.038
242. Li P, Asokanathan C, Liu F, Khaing KK, Kmiec D, Wei X, et al. PLGA nano/micro particles encapsulated with pertussis toxoid (PTd) enhances Th1/Th17 immune response in a murine model. *Int J Pharm.* (2016) 513:183–90. doi: 10.1016/j.ijpharm.2016.08.059
243. Shi W, Kou Y, Jiang H, Gao F, Kong W, Su W, et al. Novel intranasal pertussis vaccine based on bacterium-like particles as a mucosal adjuvant. *Immunol Lett.* (2018) 198:26–32. doi: 10.1016/j.imlet.2018.03.012
244. Claesson MH. Immunological links to nonspecific effects of DTwP and BCG vaccines on infant mortality. *J Trop Med.* (2011) 2011:706304. doi: 10.1155/2011/706304
245. Nascimento IP, Dias WO, Quintilio W, Hsu T, Jacobs WR, Leite LC. Construction of an unmarked recombinant BCG expressing a pertussis antigen by auxotrophic complementation: protection against *Bordetella pertussis* challenge in neonates. *Vaccine.* (2009) 27:7346–51. doi: 10.1016/j.vaccine.2009.09.043
246. Nascimento IP, Dias WO, Quintilio W, Christ AP, Moraes JF, Vancetto MD, et al. Neonatal immunization with a single dose of recombinant BCG expressing subunit S1 from pertussis toxin induces complete protection against *Bordetella pertussis* intracerebral challenge. *Microbes Infect.* (2008) 10:198–202. doi: 10.1016/j.micinf.2007.10.010
247. Nascimento IP, Dias WO, Mazzantini RP, Miyaji EN, Gamberini M, Quintilio W, et al. Recombinant *Mycobacterium bovis* BCG expressing pertussis toxin subunit S1 induces protection against an intracerebral challenge with live *Bordetella pertussis* in mice. *Infect Immun.* (2000) 68:4877–83. doi: 10.1128/IAI.68.9.4877-4883.2000
248. Cainelli Gebara VC, Risoléo L, Lopes AP, Ferreira VR, Quintilio W, Lépine F, et al. Adjuvant and immunogenic activities of the 73kDa N-terminal alpha-domain of BrkA autotransporter and Cpn60/60kDa chaperonin of *Bordetella pertussis. Vaccine.* (2007) 25:621–9. doi: 10.1016/j.vaccine.2006.08.033
249. Oliver DC, Fernandez RC. Antibodies to BrkA augment killing of *Bordetella pertussis. Vaccine.* (2001) 20:235–41. doi: 10.1016/S0264-410X(01)00269-9
250. Marr N, Shah NR, Lee R, Kim EJ, Fernandez RC. *Bordetella pertussis* autotransporter Vag8 binds human C1 esterase inhibitor and confers serum resistance. *PLoS ONE.* (2011) 6:e20585. doi: 10.1371/journal.pone.0020585
251. Finn TM, Amsbaugh DF. Vag8, a *Bordetella pertussis* bvg-regulated protein. *Infect Immun.* (1998) 66:3985–9.
252. Suzuki K, Shinzawa N, Ishigaki K, Nakamura K, Abe H, Fukui-Miyazaki A, et al. Protective effects of *in vivo*-expressed autotransporters against *Bordetella pertussis* infection. *Microbiol Immunol.* (2017) 61:371–9. doi: 10.1111/1348-0421.12504
253. Boehm DT, Hall JM, Wong TY, DiVenere AM, Sen-Kilic E, Bevere JR, et al. Evaluation of adenylate cyclase toxoid antigen in acellular pertussis vaccines by using a *Bordetella pertussis* challenge model in mice. *Infect Immun.* (2018) 86:e00857-17. doi: 10.1128/IAI.00857-17
254. Wang X, Gray MC, Hewlett EL, Maynard JA. The *Bordetella* adenylate cyclase repeat-in-toxin (RTX) domain is immunodominant and elicits neutralizing antibodies. *J Biol Chem.* (2015) 290:23025. doi: 10.1074/jbc.A114.585281
255. Jennings-Gee J, Quataert S, Ganguly T, D'Agostino R, Deora R, Dubey P. The adjuvant *Bordetella* colonization factor A attenuates alum-induced Th2 responses and enhances *Bordetella pertussis* clearance from mouse lungs. *Infect Immun.* (2018) 86:e00935-17. doi: 10.1128/IAI.00935-17
256. Scanlon KM, Skerry C, Carbonetti NH. Novel therapies for the treatment of pertussis disease. *Pathog Dis.* (2015) 73:ftv074. doi: 10.1093/femspd/ftv074
257. Skerry CM, Mahon BP. A live, attenuated *Bordetella pertussis* vaccine provides long-term protection against virulent challenge in a murine model. *Clin Vaccine Immunol.* (2011) 18:187–93. doi: 10.1128/CVI.00371-10
258. Skerry CM, Cassidy JP, English K, Feunou-Feunou P, Locht C, Mahon BP. A live attenuated *Bordetella pertussis* candidate vaccine does not cause

disseminating infection in gamma interferon receptor knockout mice. *Clin Vaccine Immunol.* (2009) 16:1344–51. doi: 10.1128/CVI.00082-09
259. Brennan MJ. A new whooping cough vaccine that may prevent colonization and transmission. *Vaccines.* (2017) 5:E43. doi: 10.3390/vaccines5040043
260. Locht C, Papin JF, Lecher S, Debrie AS, Thalen M, Solovay K, et al. Live attenuated pertussis vaccine BPZE1 protects baboons against *Bordetella pertussis* disease and infection. *J Infect Dis.* (2017) 216:117–24. doi: 10.1093/infdis/jix254
261. Locht C. Live pertussis vaccines will they protect against carriage and spread of pertussis? *Clin Microbiol Infect.* (2016) 22(Suppl. 5):S96–102. doi: 10.1016/j.cmi.2016.05.029
262. Locht C. Pertussis: where did we go wrong and what can we do about it? *J Infect.* (2016) 72(Suppl.): S34–40. doi: 10.1016/j.jinf.2016.04.020
263. Feunou PF, Kammoun H, Debrie AS, Locht C. Heterologous prime-boost immunization with live attenuated *B. pertussis* BPZE1 followed by acellular pertussis vaccine in mice. *Vaccine.* (2014) 32:4281–8. doi: 10.1016/j.vaccine.2014.06.019
264. Jahnmatz M, Amu S, Ljungman M, Wehlin L, Chiodi F, Mielcarek N, et al. B-cell responses after intranasal vaccination with the novel attenuated *Bordetella pertussis* vaccine strain BPZE1 in a randomized phase I clinical trial. *Vaccine.* (2014) 32:3350–6. doi: 10.1016/j.vaccine.2014.04.048
265. Lim A, Ng JK, Locht C, Alonso S. Protective role of adenylate cyclase in the context of a live pertussis vaccine candidate. *Microbes Infect.* (2014) 16:51–60. doi: 10.1016/j.micinf.2013.10.002
266. Schiavoni I, Fedele G, Quattrini A, Bianco M, Schnoeller C, Openshaw PJ, et al. Live attenuated *B. pertussis* BPZE1 rescues the immune functions of Respiratory Syncytial virus infected human dendritic cells by promoting Th1/Th17 responses. *PLoS ONE.* (2014) 9:e100166. doi: 10.1371/journal.pone.0100166
267. Schnoeller C, Roux X, Sawant D, Raze D, Olszewska W, Locht C, et al. Attenuated *Bordetella pertussis* vaccine protects against respiratory syncytial virus disease via an IL-17-dependent mechanism. *Am J Respir Crit Care Med.* (2014) 189:194–202. doi: 10.1164/rccm.201307-1227OC
268. Thorstensson R, Trollfors B, Al-Tawil N, Jahnmatz M, Bergström J, Ljungman M, et al. A phase I clinical study of a live attenuated *Bordetella pertussis* vaccine–BPZE1; a single centre, double-blind, placebo-controlled, dose-escalating study of BPZE1 given intranasally to healthy adult male volunteers. *PLoS ONE.* (2014) 9:e83449. doi: 10.1371/journal.pone.0083449
269. Kammoun H, Roux X, Raze D, Debrie AS, De Filette M, Ysenbaert T, et al. Immunogenicity of live attenuated *B. pertussis* BPZE1 producing the universal influenza vaccine candidate M2e. *PLoS ONE.* (2013) 8:e59198. doi: 10.1371/journal.pone.0059198
270. Kammoun H, Feunou PF, Foligne B, Debrie AS, Raze D, Mielcarek N, et al. Dual mechanism of protection by live attenuated *Bordetella pertussis* BPZE1 against *Bordetella bronchiseptica* in mice. *Vaccine.* (2012) 30:5864–70. doi: 10.1016/j.vaccine.2012.07.005
271. Li R, Cheng C, Chong SZ, Lim AR, Goh YF, Locht C, et al. Attenuated *Bordetella pertussis* BPZE1 protects against allergic airway inflammation and contact dermatitis in mouse models. *Allergy.* (2012) 67:1250–8. doi: 10.1111/j.1398-9995.2012.02884.x
272. Fedele G, Bianco M, Debrie AS, Locht C, Ausiello CM. Attenuated *Bordetella pertussis* vaccine candidate BPZE1 promotes human dendritic cell CCL21-induced migration and drives a Th1/Th17 response. *J Immunol.* (2011) 186:5388–96. doi: 10.4049/jimmunol.1003765
273. Li R, Lim A, Alonso S. Attenuated *Bordetella pertussis* BPZE1 as a live vehicle for heterologous vaccine antigens delivery through the nasal route. *Bioeng Bugs.* (2011) 2:315–9. doi: 10.4161/bbug.2.6.18167
274. Li R, Lim A, Ow ST, Phoon MC, Locht C, Chow VT, et al. Development of live attenuated *Bordetella pertussis* strains expressing the universal influenza vaccine candidate M2e. *Vaccine.* (2011) 29:5502–11. doi: 10.1016/j.vaccine.2011.05.052
275. Feunou PF, Bertout J, Locht C. T- and B-cell-mediated protection induced by novel, live attenuated pertussis vaccine in mice. Cross protection against parapertussis. *PLoS ONE.* (2010) 5:e10178. doi: 10.1371/journal.pone.0010178
276. Feunou PF, Kammoun H, Debrie AS, Mielcarek N, Locht C. Long-term immunity against pertussis induced by a single nasal administration of live attenuated *B. pertussis* BPZE1. *Vaccine.* (2010) 28:7047–53. doi: 10.1016/j.vaccine.2010.08.017
277. Kavanagh H, Noone C, Cahill E, English K, Locht C, Mahon BP. Attenuated *Bordetella pertussis* vaccine strain BPZE1 modulates allergen-induced immunity and prevents allergic pulmonary pathology in a murine model. *Clin Exp Allergy.* (2010) 40:933–41. doi: 10.1111/j.1365-2222.2010.03459.x
278. Li R, Lim A, Phoon MC, Narasaraju T, Ng JK, Poh WP, et al. Attenuated *Bordetella pertussis* protects against highly pathogenic influenza A viruses by dampening the cytokine storm. *J Virol.* (2010) 84:7105–13. doi: 10.1128/JVI.02542-09
279. Mielcarek N, Debrie AS, Mahieux S, Locht C. Dose response of attenuated *Bordetella pertussis* BPZE1-induced protection in mice. *Clin Vaccine Immunol.* (2010) 17:317–24. doi: 10.1128/CVI.00322-09
280. Feunou PF, Ismaili J, Debrie AS, Huot L, Hot D, Raze D, et al. Genetic stability of the live attenuated *Bordetella pertussis* vaccine candidate BPZE1. *Vaccine.* (2008) 26:5722–7. doi: 10.1016/j.vaccine.2008.08.018
281. Ho SY, Chua SQ, Foo DG, Locht C, Chow VT, Poh CL, et al. Highly attenuated *Bordetella pertussis* strain BPZE1 as a potential live vehicle for delivery of heterologous vaccine candidates. *Infect Immun.* (2008) 76:111–9. doi: 10.1128/IAI.00795-07
282. Mielcarek N, Debrie AS, Raze D, Bertout J, Rouanet C, Younes AB, et al. Live attenuated B. *pertussis* as a single-dose nasal vaccine against whooping cough. *PLoS Pathog.* (2006) 2:e65. doi: 10.1371/journal.ppat.0020065
283. Debrie AS, Coutte L, Raze D, Mooi F, Alexander F, Gorringe A, et al. Construction and evaluation of *Bordetella pertussis* live attenuated vaccine strain BPZE1 producing Fim3. *Vaccine.* (2018) 36:1345–52. doi: 10.1016/j.vaccine.2018.02.017
284. Solans L, Debrie AS, Borkner L, Aguiló N, Thiriard A, Coutte L, et al. IL-17-dependent SIgA-mediated protection against nasal *Bordetella pertussis* infection by live attenuated BPZE1 vaccine. *Mucosal Immunol.* (2018) 11:1753–62. doi: 10.1038/s41385-018-0073-9
285. Gasperini G, Biagini M, Arato V, Gianfaldoni C, Vadi A, Norais N, et al. Outer Membrane Vesicles (OMV)-based and proteomics-driven antigen selection identifies novel factors contributing to epithelial cells. *Mol Cell Proteomics.* (2018) 17:205–15. doi: 10.1074/mcp.RA117.000045
286. Gasperini G, Biagini M, Arato V, Gianfaldoni C, Vadi A, Norais N, et al. Outer Membrane Vesicles (OMV)-based and proteomics-driven antigen selection identifies novel factors contributing to *Bordetella pertussis* adhesion to epithelial cells. *Mol Cell Proteomics.* (2017) 17:205–15.
287. Saito M, Odanaka K, Otsuka N, Kamachi K, Watanabe M. Development of vaccines against pertussis caused by *Bordetella holmesii* using a mouse intranasal challenge model. *Microbiol Immunol.* (2016) 60:599–608. doi: 10.1111/1348-0421.12409
288. Bottero D, Zurita ME, Gaillard ME, Bartel E, Vercellini C, Hozbor D. Membrane vesicles derived from *Bordetella bronchiseptica*: active constituent of a new vaccine against infections caused by this pathogen. *Appl Environ Microbiol.* (2018) 84:e01877-17. doi: 10.1128/AEM.01877-17
289. Bottero D, Zurita ME, Gaillard ME, Bartel E, Vercellini C, Hozbor D. Membrane vesicles derived from *Bordetella bronchiseptica*: active constituent of a new vaccine against infections caused by this pathogen. *Appl Environ Microbiol.* (2017) 84:e01877-17.
290. Bottero D, Gaillard ME, Zurita E, Moreno G, Martinez DS, Bartel E, et al. Characterization of the immune response induced by pertussis OMVs-based vaccine. *Vaccine.* (2016) 34:3303–9. doi: 10.1016/j.vaccine.2016.04.079
291. Gaillard ME, Bottero D, Errea A, Ormazábal M, Zurita ME, Moreno G, et al. Acellular pertussis vaccine based on outer membrane vesicles capable of conferring both long-lasting immunity and protection against different strain genotypes. *Vaccine.* (2014) 32:931–7. doi: 10.1016/j.vaccine.2013.12.048
292. Ormazábal M, Bartel E, Gaillard ME, Bottero D, Errea A, Zurita ME, et al. Characterization of the key antigenic components of pertussis vaccine based on outer membrane vesicles. *Vaccine.* (2014) 32:6084–90. doi: 10.1016/j.vaccine.2014.08.084
293. Bottero D, Gaillard ME, Errea A, Moreno G, Zurita E, Pianciola L, et al. Outer membrane vesicles derived from *Bordetella parapertussis* as an acellular vaccine against *Bordetella parapertussis* and *Bordetella pertussis* infection. *Vaccine.* (2013) 31:5262–8. doi: 10.1016/j.vaccine.2013.08.059

294. Gaillard ME, Bottero D, Castuma CE, Basile LA, Hozbor D. Laboratory adaptation of *Bordetella pertussis* is associated with the loss of type three secretion system functionality. *Infect Immun.* (2011) 79:3677–82. doi: 10.1128/IAI.00136-11
295. Roberts R, Moreno G, Bottero D, Gaillard ME, Fingermann M, Graieb A, et al. Outer membrane vesicles as acellular vaccine against pertussis. *Vaccine.* (2008) 26:4639–46. doi: 10.1016/j.vaccine.2008.07.004
296. Raeven RH, Brummelman J, Pennings JLA, van der Maas L, Helm K, Tilstra WA, et al. Molecular and cellular signatures underlying superior immunity against *Bordetella pertussis* upon pulmonary vaccination. *Mucosal Immunol.* (2018) 11:979–93. doi: 10.1038/mi.2017.81
297. Raeven RH, van der Maas L, Tilstra W, Uittenbogaard JP, Bindels TH, Kuipers BA, et al. Immunoproteomic profiling of *Bordetella pertussis* outer membrane vesicle vaccine reveals broad and balanced humoral immunogenicity. *J Proteome Res.* (2015) 14:2929–42. doi: 10.1021/acs.jproteome.5b00258
298. Raeven RH, Brummelman J, Pennings JL, van der Maas L, Tilstra W, Helm K, et al. *Bordetella pertussis* outer membrane vesicle vaccine confers equal efficacy in mice with milder inflammatory responses compared to a whole-cell vaccine. *Sci Rep.* (2016) 6:38240. doi: 10.1038/srep38240
299. Raeven RHM, Brummelman J, Pennings JLA, van der Maas L, Helm K, Tilstra WA, et al. Molecular and cellular signatures underlying superior immunity against *Bordetella pertussis* upon pulmonary vaccination. *Mucosal Immunol.* (2018) 11:979–93. doi: 10.1038/mi.2017.110
300. Kanojia G, Raeven RHM, van der Maas L, Bindels THE, van Riet E, Metz B, et al. Development of a thermostable spray dried outer membrane vesicle pertussis vaccine for pulmonary immunization. *J Control Release.* (2018) 286:167–78. doi: 10.1016/j.jconrel.2018.07.035
301. Weiss AA, Patton AK, Millen SH, Chang SJ, Ward JI, Bernstein DI. Acellular pertussis vaccines and complement killing of *Bordetella pertussis. Infect Immun.* (2004) 72:7346–51. doi: 10.1128/IAI.72.12.7346-7351.2004
302. Coutte L, Locht C. Investigating pertussis toxin and its impact on vaccination. *Future Microbiol.* (2015) 10:241–54. doi: 10.2217/fmb.14.123
303. Isbrucker RA, Bliu A, Prior F. Modified binding assay for improved sensitivity and specificity in the detection of residual pertussis toxin in vaccine preparations. *Vaccine.* (2010) 28:2687–92. doi: 10.1016/j.vaccine.2010.01.040
304. Quentin-Millet MJ, Arminjon F, Danve B, Cadoz M, Armand J. Acellular pertussis vaccines: evaluation of reversion in a nude mouse model. *J Biol Stand.* (1988) 16:99–108. doi: 10.1016/0092-1157(88)90037-6
305. Kilár A, Dörnyei Á, Kocsis B. Structural characterization of bacterial lipopolysaccharides with mass spectrometry and on- and off-line separation techniques. *Mass Spectrom Rev.* (2013) 32:90–117. doi: 10.1002/mas.21352
306. Higgs R, Higgins SC, Ross PJ, Mills KH. Immunity to the respiratory pathogen *Bordetella pertussis. Mucosal Immunol.* (2012) 5:485–500. doi: 10.1038/mi.2012.54
307. Mahon BP, Ryan MS, Griffin F, Mills KH. Interleukin-12 is produced by macrophages in response to live or killed *Bordetella pertussis* and enhances the efficacy of an acellular pertussis vaccine by promoting induction of Th1 cells. *Infect Immun.* (1996) 64:5295–301.
308. Kubler-Kielb J, Vinogradov E, Lagergård T, Ginzberg A, King JD, Preston A, et al. Oligosaccharide conjugates of *Bordetella pertussis* and bronchiseptica induce bactericidal antibodies, an addition to pertussis vaccine. *Proc Natl Acad Sci USA.* (2011) 108:4087–92. doi: 10.1073/pnas.1100782108
309. Niedziela T, Letowska I, Lukasiewicz J, Kaszowska M, Czarnecka A, Kenne L, et al. Epitope of the vaccine-type *Bordetella pertussis* strain 186 lipooligosaccharide and antiendotoxin activity of antibodies directed against the terminal pentasaccharide-tetanus toxoid conjugate. *Infect Immun.* (2005) 73:7381–9. doi: 10.1128/IAI.73.11.7381-7389.2005
310. Koj S, Ługowski C, Niedziela T. [*Bordetella pertussis* lipooligosaccharide-derived neoglycoconjugates - new components of pertussis vaccine]. *Postepy Hig Med Dosw (Online)* (2015) 69:1013–30.
311. Ernst K, Eberhardt N, Mittler AK, Sonnabend M, Anastasia A, Freisinger S, et al. Pharmacological cyclophilin inhibitors prevent intoxication of mammalian cells with *Bordetella pertussis* toxin. *Toxins.* (2018) 10:E181. doi: 10.3390/toxins10050181
312. Kaiser E, Pust S, Kroll C, Barth H. Cyclophilin A facilitates translocation of the *Clostridium botulinum* C2 toxin across membranes of acidified endosomes into the cytosol of mammalian cells. *Cell Microbiol.* (2009) 11:780–95. doi: 10.1111/j.1462-5822.2009.01291.x
313. Lang AE, Ernst K, Lee H, Papatheodorou P, Schwan C, Barth H, et al. The chaperone Hsp90 and PPIases of the cyclophilin and FKBP families facilitate membrane translocation of *Photorhabdus luminescens* ADP-ribosyltransferases. *Cell Microbiol.* (2014) 16:490–503. doi: 10.1111/cmi.12228
314. Shitara Y, Takeuchi K, Nagamatsu Y, Wada S, Sugiyama Y, Horie T. Long-lasting inhibitory effects of cyclosporin A, but not tacrolimus, on OATP1B1- and OATP1B3-mediated uptake. *Drug Metab Pharmacokinet.* (2012) 27:368–78. doi: 10.2133/dmpk.DMPK-11-RG-096
315. Fabre I, Fabre G, Lena N, Cano JP. Kinetics of uptake and intracellular binding of Cyclosporine A in RAJI cells, *in vitro. Biochem Pharmacol.* (1986) 35:4261–6. doi: 10.1016/0006-2952(86)9 0704-5
316. Bertault-Pérès P, Maraninchi D, Carcassonne Y, Cano JP, Barbet J. Clinical pharmacokinetics of ciclosporin A in bone marrow transplantation patients. *Cancer Chemother Pharmacol.* (1985) 15:76–81. doi: 10.1007/BF00 257300

14

Polymorphisms in Genes Affecting Interferon-γ Production and Th1 T Cell Differentiation are Associated with Progression to Chagas Disease Cardiomyopathy

Amanda Farage Frade-Barros [1,2,3,4,5], Barbara Maria Ianni [1], Sandrine Cabantous [3], Cristina Wide Pissetti [6], Bruno Saba [7], Hui Tzu Lin-Wang [7], Paula Buck [1], José Antonio Marin-Neto [8], André Schmidt [8], Fabrício Dias [8], Mario Hiroyuki Hirata [9], Marcelo Sampaio [7], Abílio Fragata [7], Alexandre Costa Pereira [1], Eduardo Donadi [8], Virmondes Rodrigues [6], Jorge Kalil [1,2,5], Christophe Chevillard [10†] and Edecio Cunha-Neto [1,2,4†]*

[1] Heart Institute (InCor), University of São Paulo School of Medicine (FMUSP), São Paulo, Brazil, [2] Institute for Investigation in Immunology (iii), INCT, São Paulo, Brazil, [3] Aix-Marseille Université, INSERM, GIMP UMR_S906, Marseille, France, [4] Division of Clinical Immunology and Allergy, University of São Paulo School of Medicine, São Paulo, Brazil, [5] Bioengineering Program, Instituto Tecnológico, Universidade Brasil, São Paulo, Brazil, [6] Laboratory of Immunology, Universidade Federal Do Triângulo Mineiro (UFTM), Uberaba, Brazil, [7] Laboratório de Investigação Molecular em Cardiologia, Instituto de Cardiologia Dante Pazzanese (IDPC), São Paulo, Brazil, [8] School of Medicine of Ribeirão Preto (FMRP), University of São Paulo, Ribeirão Preto, Brazil, [9] Department of Clinical and Toxicological Analyses, Faculty of Pharmaceutical Sciences, University of São Paulo (USP), São Paulo, Brazil, [10] Aix Marseille Université, INSERM, TAGC Theories and Approaches of Genomic Complexity, UMR_1090, Marseille, France

***Correspondence:**
Amanda Farage Frade-Barros
amanda.frade@universidadebrasil.edu.br

† These authors have contributed equally to this work

Background: Chagas disease, caused by the protozoan *Trypanosoma cruzi*, is endemic in Latin America. Thirty percent of infected individuals develop chronic Chagas cardiomyopathy (CCC), an inflammatory dilated cardiomyopathy that is the most important clinical consequence of *T. cruzi* infection, while the others remain asymptomatic (ASY). IFN-γ and IFN-γ-producing Th1-type T cells are increased in peripheral blood and CCC myocardium as compared to ASY patients, while the Th1-antagonizing cytokine IL-10 is more expressed in ASY patients. Importantly IFN-γ-producing Th1-type T cells are the most frequent cytokine-producing T cell subset in CCC myocardium, while expression of Th1-antagonizing cytokines IL-10 and IL-4 is unaltered. The control of IFN-γ production by Th1-type T cells may be a key event for progression toward CCC. A genetic component to disease progression was suggested by the familial aggregation of cases and the association of gene polymorphisms with CCC development. We here investigate the role of gene polymorphisms (SNPs) in several genes involved in the control of IFN-γ production and Th1 T cell differentiation in CCC development.

Methods: We studied a Brazilian population including 315 CCC cases and 118 ASY subjects. We assessed 35 Tag SNPs designed to represent all the genetic information contained in the *IL12B, IL10, IFNG*, and *IL4* genes.

Results: We found 2 *IL12* SNPs (rs2546893, rs919766) and a trend of association for a *IL10* SNP (rs3024496) to be significantly associated with the ASY group. these associations were confirmed by multivariate analysis and allele tests. The rs919766C,

12rs2546893G, and rs3024496C alleles were associated to an increase risk to CCC development.

Conclusions: Our data show that novel polymorphisms affecting *IL12B* and *IL10*, but not *IFNG* or *IL4* genes play a role in genetic susceptibility to CCC development. This might indicate that the increased Th1 differentiation and IFN-γ production associated with CCC is genetically controlled.

Keywords: Chagas disease, cardiomyopathy, susceptibility, IL12, IL 10, IFN, IL4

INTRODUCTION

Chagas disease (American trypanosomiasis) is caused by the protozoan *Trypanosoma cruzi* (*T. cruzi*) and mainly transmitted by the reduviid arthropod vector. It is endemic in Latin America, where an estimated 8 million people are infected (https://www.cdc.gov/parasites/chagas/index.html). Imported disease is increasingly recognized as an emerging problem in the USA and Europe due to immigration from Latin America (https://www.who.int/chagas/disease/en/). Decades after acute infection, 20–30% of the patients develop chronic Chagas disease cardiomyopathy (CCC), where heart tissue inflammation and remodeling, fibrosis, electrical and structural abnormalities often lead to life-threatening heart failure and arrhythmia (1). Five to 10% of infected individuals develop digestive disease, with denervation and dilation of the digestive tract. The remaining two-thirds of infected individuals remain asymptomatic (ASY) and free from symptomatic disease for life (2). Heart failure due to CCC has a worse prognosis, with 50% shorter survival when compared to like ischemic, idiopathic and hypertensive cardiomyopathies (3, 4). The pathogenic determinants of differential disease progression have not yet been completely elucidated.

The finding that 30% of Chagas disease patients develop CCC suggested the participation of genetics in differential disease progression. In addition, familial aggregation of CCC cases has been described (5), and a significant number of genetic polymorphisms has been associated with CCC development. A recent literature search found ca. 150 case-control genetic association studies addressing polymorphisms in 76 genes, which disclosed 62 SNPs from 44 genes to be associated with CCC, mostly related to immunology and inflammation. From those, a much smaller number of SNPs were associated with CCC severity (ventricular dysfunction) (6–8).

Many of these SNPs are related to pathogen resistance and disease tolerance genes—those related to direct control of parasitism or to reduction of tissue damage, respectively (7). Chagas disease is associated with increased production of inflammatory cytokines; IFN-γ is a major pathogen resistance gene and plays a major role in the disease; *T. cruzi* infection of mice genetically deficient of IFNG leads to uncontrolled parasitism and 100% mortality (9, 10). While it is a key player in pathogen protection, excessive levels lead to increased inflammation and tissue damage during the acute phase as well as CCC (7). During acute infection, *T. cruzi* pathogen-associated molecular patterns (PAMPs) trigger innate immunity (3, 11, 12) leading to the release of proinflammatory cytokines and chemokines, including IL-12 and IL-18, the major drivers of differentiation of IFN-γ-producing *T. cruzi*–specific Th1 T cells which migrate to sites of *T. cruzi*-induced inflammation (13, 14). IFNγ is then produced at high levels, inducing production of microbicidal and potentially tissue-damaging reactive oxygen and nitrogen species that kill intracellular *T. cruzi*. This leads to the control—but not complete elimination—of parasitism, establishing a low-grade chronic persistent infection by *T. cruzi*. On the other hand, cytokines that are able to modulate excessive IFN-γ production/Th1 T cell differentiation can modulate tissue damage in the acute phase of infection. Mice genetically deficient in disease tolerance genes IL10 (15), IL4 (16) and IL27b/Ebi3 (17), factors known to limit Th1 T cell differentiation and IFNγ production (17–20) display increased inflammation and may die early. Animals who keep a balance between inflammatory Th1 and anti-inflammatory cytokines may survive and progress to the chronic phase. As a result of persistent infection, both CCC and ASY chronic Chagas disease patients produce higher levels of IFNγ than seronegative controls (21, 22), but those who develop Chagas cardiomyopathy display a particularly strong Th1-type immune response with increased numbers of IFN-γ-producing Th1 cells in peripheral blood mononuclear cells (PBMC) (19, 20, 22, 23) and decreased IFNγ -modulating factors IL-10, IL-27b/Ebi3, and Treg cells (17–20). Accordingly, CCC patients displayed increased plasma levels of IFNγ while levels of IL-10 are reduced when compared to ASY individuals (24–26). These data suggest that the cytokine balance can modulate progression to CCC development. Indeed, CCC hearts display a prominent IFNγ -producing T-cell dependent myocarditis. IFNγ is the most highly expressed cytokine in CCC myocardium (27), and mononuclear cells producing this cytokine are abundant in CCC heart (12, 14, 22). mRNA expression IL-10 and other Th1-antagonizing cytokines and cell types (Treg and Th2) was low or undetectable in CCC heart tissue. This indicates that the Th1 infiltrate in CCC myocardium is essentially unopposed by regulatory cells or cytokines, and subject to little regulation (27). The failure to regulate Th1 responses and IFNγ production may thus be one key immune defect of patients who progress to CCC. This creates a paradox, in that IFNγ is essential for control of parasitism in acute and chronic Chagas disease, but at the same time causes tissue damage (7).

Cytokine gene polymorphisms may contribute to the control of Th1 T cell differentiation/IFN-γ production. Previous studies have assessed the association of SNPs in cytokines important for regulation of IFN-γ responses with CCC. For *IFNG*, no

SNP was found to be associated with CCC when compared to ASY after comparison for multiple testing (28). Likewise, *IL4* SNP case-control studies between CCC and ASY failed to show associations, but may have been underpowered, with only110 and 260 total Chagasic patients, respectively (29, 30). A promoter polymorphism in *IL12B* +1188 (rs3212227) was found to be associated with CCC in an Colombian population (31). The SNP IL10-1082 (rs1800896) was shown to be functional (32) and was associated to CCC in a Brazilian population comparing ASY individuals vs. CCC (33). On a Brazilian population, the frequency of the polymorphic rs1800896A allele (associated with lower expression of IL-10) was higher in the asymptomatic group than in the cardiac group. On the other hand, Florez et al. compared CCC ($n = 130$) to ASY ($n = 130$) cases in a Colombian population. Florez et al. failed to show associations in the genotypes and allele frequencies neither in *IL10* SNPs *IL10*-1082 (rs1800896) nor in the additional SNPs *IL10*-819 (rs1800871) and *IL10*-592 (rs1800872). It is possible that this lack of association in our study is was due to a small sample size or to epistasis between IL-10 and MHC.

Since the previous studies had some limitations, i.e., focused on selected polymorphisms, failed to be replicated in other populations, or lacked appropriate statistical power, we here comprehensively assessed the role of polymorphisms in these genes on CCC progression. For that matter we here performed a thorough genetic study focusing on 35 polymorphisms of *IL4, IL12B, IL10*, and *IFNG* using the Tag SNP approach, which represent all the genetic information contained in the mentioned genes, in a larger cohort ($n = 433$) of Brazilian Chagas disease patients, including CCC patients with or without ventricular dysfunction as well as asymptomatic patients. With the tag SNP approach, we could both replicate the study of previously investigated SNPs as well as novel polymorphisms. This way, we could perform a more sensitive assessment of the contribution of genetic variants in prognosis to CCC either confirming or finding additional associated SNPs in the mentioned genes. In addition, our experimental design allowed the study of possible interactions between polymorphisms in different cytokines.

METHODS

Ethical Standard

Written informed consent was obtained from all the patients, in accordance with the guidelines of the various internal review boards of all the involved institutions. The protocol was also approved by the INSERM Internal Review Board and the Brazilian National Ethics in Research Commission (CONEP). All the patients enrolled in this study were over 21 years old. Investigations were conformed to the principles outlined in the declaration of Helsinki.

Diagnostic Criteria

The diagnostic criteria for Chagas disease included the detection of antibodies against *T. cruzi* in at least two of three independent serological tests (EIA [Hemobio Chagas; Embrabio São Paulo], indirect immunofluorescence assays [IFA-immunocruzi; Biolab Merieux], and indirect hemagglutination tests [Biolab Merieux]) (34). All Chagas disease patients underwent standard electrocardiography and echocardiography. Echocardiography was performed at the hospital, with a Sequoia model 512 echocardiograph with a broad-band transducer. Left ventricular dimensions and regional and global function, including the recording of left ventricular ejection fraction (LVEF), were evaluated with a two-dimensional, M-mode approach, in accordance with the recommendations of the American Society of Echocardiography. ASY subjects had no electrocardiography and echocardiography changes. CCC patients presented typical conduction abnormalities (right bundle branch block and/or left anterior division hemiblock) (35). CCC patients with significant left ventricular systolic dysfunction (LVEF $< 40\%$) were classified as having severe CCC, whereas those with no significant ventricular dysfunction (LVEF $\geq 40\%$) were classified as having moderate CCC. We selected 40% as arbitrary cutoff value that has been previously used to define significant ventricular dysfunction by our group and others (36–38).

Study Population for Polymorphism Analysis

The CCC and ASY patients were born and raised in rural areas of Sao Paulo, Minas Gerais and Bahia states and enrolled in one of the study centers (Incor, FMUSP, FMRP, UFTM, IDPC). Patients with digestive forms were excluded of this study. Patients were classified as ASY ($n = 118$) or as having CCC ($n = 315$). ASY individuals were used as the control subjects for this study because they were from the same areas of endemicity as the patients with CCC, had encountered the parasite and had tested seropositive for T. cruzi infection, but the infection had not progressed to CCC. Here, the Case/Control ratio, which is 0.375, illustrate the difficulty to enroll real ASY subjects. For our association study, if we are fixing the significant level to 0.05, the disease prevalence to 30%, the disease allele Frequency to 0.2 and the genotype relative risk to 1.5, the expected power of our association study reaches 0.895.

Of 315 patients with CCC, 106 (42 men [39.6%] and 64 women [60.4%]) showed no significant ventricular dysfunction (LVEF $\geq 40\%$) and were thus classified as having moderate CCC, whereas 199 (144 men [72.4%] and 55 women [27.6%]) had severe ventricular dysfunction (LVEF $< 40\%$) and were classified as having severe CCC. Data for left ventricular ejection fraction were missing for 10 patients with CCC. So, when we compared moderate patients to severe patients, these 10 individuals were excluded from the analysis. Regarding progression of the ASY cases to CCC, the yearly progression rate –regardless of age group- is ca. 1–2%/year. The average age of Subjects with asymptomatic form was above 55 years. Taking into account that they were all born in endemic areas before vector transmission was interrupted, it is likely that in most if not all cases vector-borne infection occurred in early childhood. The odds that a significant number of such mature patients convert to CCC, and that this thwarts our statistical calculation is rather low; however, this is a pitfall of all cross sectional studies on diseases that display progression.

Blood Samples and DNA Preparation

For each subject, 5–15 ml of blood were collected in EDTA tubes. Genomic DNA was isolated on a silica-membrane according to the manufacturer's protocol (QIAamp DNA Blood Max Kit, Qiagen, Hilden, Germany).

SNP Selection

Tag single nucleotide polymorphisms (SNPs) were selected on the basis on Ensembl Release GRCh38 for the Caucasian and Yoruba reference populations. Tag SNPs were selected within a region extending 5 kb on either side of the candidate gene. The minor allele frequency (MAF) cut off value was arbitrarily set at 20% (so the markers characterized by a MAF <20% were excluded from the analysis by lack of power). In each reference population, the markers with MAF > 20% are included in different blocks of correlation (based on the r^2 values). For each correlation block in the gene, one marker was selected and considered as a Tag SNP. Indeed, markers located in the same block of correlation yielded the same genetic information in association studies. Tag SNPs characterized by a MAF over 20% on at least one reference population were selected. These Tag SNPs were thus defined to gather all the genetic information from each candidate gene. we selected a total of 35 Tag SNPs: sixteen tag SNPs for *IL12B*, six tag SNPs for *IL10*, six for *IFNG* and seven tag SNPs for *IL4*.

SNP Genotyping

Most of the genotyping was done with the Golden Gate genotyping assay (Illumina, San Diego, USA). In some cases, genotyping assays were performed with the *Taq*Man system (Applied Biosystems, Foster City, USA) according to the manufacturer's instructions. Genotyes are available on request.

Statistical Analysis

SPSS Statistics software v. 17.0 (IBM, Armonk, USA) was used for statistical analyses. We performed stepwise binary logistic regression analysis on the whole population, to analyse the relationship between the probability of an individual to develop chronic Chagas cardiomyopathy and the main covariates (sex and polymorphisms). Sex was considered as a binary covariate. In our stepwise binary logistic regression analysis, genotypes were considered as binary covariates. Indeed, for each polymorphism we had two alleles (A frequent one; a rare one). So, we obtained three genotypes (AA, Aa, and aa). In our stepwise binary logistic regression analysis, genotypes were considered as binary covariates. So, we performed three different analyses (Analysis 1: AA vs. Aa + aa (we supposed that the a allele is dominant); Analysis 2: AA + aa vs. Aa (we supposed that the heterozygote carriers are different from the homozygote ones); Analysis 3: AA + Aa vs. aa (we supposed that the A allele is dominant).

In multivariate analyses, several polymorphisms and gender were included as covariates. All the covariates are analyzed in the same time. In a stepwise approach, the worse associated covariate (non-significant) is removed and the analysis is run again up to keep only significant associated covariates.

An investigation of a candidate gene should test many SNPs individually for association. However, such multiple testing will increase the false-positive (type I error) rate under nominal significance thresholds ($\alpha = 0.05$). So, we applied the Holm-Bonferroni sequential correction for multiple testing (39).

RESULTS

We conducted a study focusing on the *IL12B, IL10, IFNG*, and *IL4* genes. 35 Tag SNPs were selected (**Supplementary Table 1**). 97.8% markers were genotyped successfully on our cohort including ASY subjects ($n = 118$) and CCC patients ($n = 315$). The genotype distribution of each SNP is summarized in **Supplementary Table 2**. All the SNPs were in Hardy-Weinberg equilibrium on the ASY individuals considered as control subjects. Of the 118 ASY subjects, 45.3% were male, whereas in the CCC patients group, this percentage reaches 61.3%. The difference in sex distribution between the groups was significant ($p = 1.21E\text{-}4$; OR = 2.126; 95%CI: 1.450–3.12). It is well-known that male patients infected with T. cruzi have a higher risk of progression to CCC than female patients. Of 315 patients with CCC, 106 (42 men [39.6%] and 64 women [60.4%]) showed no significant ventricular dysfunction and were thus classified as having moderate CCC, whereas 199 (144 men [72.4%] and 55 women [27.6%]) had severe ventricular dysfunction and were classified as having severe CCC.

Polymorphisms rs2546893G/A, rs919766A/C in and Around the *IL12B* Gene Are Associated to an Increased Risk of CCC

Fourteen on sixteen tag SNPs for the IL12B gene were genotyped successfully. *IL-12B* genotype data are shown in **Tables 1**, **2**. All these markers are located in intronic region of IL12B gene. In the CCC subjects group, 269 (86.8%) subjects carried the rs2546893G/G or G/A genotypes whereas 79 (73.8%) of the ASY carried these genotypes ($p = 0.002$; OR = 1.548; 95%CI: 1.176–2.037 (see **Table 1**). These data suggest that rs2546893G/G or G/A genotypes are associated to an increased susceptibility to CCC.

For the rs919766A/C polymorphism, 107 (34.7%) CCC subjects carried the C/C or A/C genotypes vs. 17 (15.9%) for the ASY group ($p = 0.001$; OR = 1.653; 95%CI: 1.241–2.198). For the rs1003199C/T polymorphism, 276 (88.7%) CCC subjects carried the C/C or C/T genotypes vs. 285 (78.7%) for the ASY group. This difference was significant ($p = 0.005$; OR = 1.522; 95%CI: 1.134–2.045). For the rs11574790C/T polymorphism, 95 (30.5%) CCC subjects carried the C/T or T/T genotypes vs. 17 (15.7%) for the ASY group ($p = 0.006$; OR = 1.497; 95%CI: 1.124–1.996). For the rs2569253T/C polymorphism, 256 (87.46%) CCC subjects carried the T/T or T/C genotypes vs. 81 (79.4%) for the ASY ($p = 0.039$; OR = 1.371; 95%CI: 1.015–1.852). After performing a correction for multiple testing using the Bonferroni methods, the two main polymorphisms (rs919766 and rs25466893) remain significant (corrected p-values were 0.014 and 0.026, respectively).

In a multivariate analysis, including these five polymorphisms and gender as covariates, the gender ($p = 0.004$; OR = 2.036; 95% CI: 1.249–3.318) and two markers (rs2546893: $p = 0.005$;

TABLE 1 | Association studies between CCC and ASY including as covariates the gender and the polymorphisms (genotype associations and allelic tests).

GENE	Tag SNP	Genotype groups	Association test
IL12B	rs2546890	GG vs. GA + AA	$p = 0.103$; OR = 1.231; 95%CI: 0.959–1.579
		MAF	ASY MAF(A) = 46.6%; CCC MAF(A) = 40.9%
		Allelic test	Chi-square = 2.11 and $p = 0.15$
	rs730691	GG vs. GA	$p = 0.441$; OR = 1.274; 95%CI: 0.688–2.358
		MAF	ASY MAF(A) = 9.1%; CCC MAF(A) = 11.1%
		Allelic test	Chi-square = 0.56 and $p = 0.46$
	rs2546893	GG + GA vs. AA	$p = 0.002$; OR = 1.548; 95%CI: 1.176–2.037
		MAF	ASY MAF(A) = 45.8%; CCC MAF(A) = 35.0%
		Allelic test	Chi-square = 7.89 and $p = 0.005$
	rs1003199	CC + CT vs. TT	$p = 0.005$; OR = 1.522; 95%CI: 1.134–2.045
		MAF	ASY MAF(T) = 43.1%; CCC MAF(T) = 35.9%
		Allelic test	Chi-square = 3.54 and $p = 0.06$
	rs3181216	TT vs. TA + AA	$p = 0.702$; OR = 1.047; 95%CI: 0.829–1.321
		MAF	ASY MAF(A) = 21.6%; CCC MAF(A) = 21.8%
		Allelic test	Chi-square = 0.001 and $p = 0.97$
	rs2569253	TT + TC vs. CC	$p = 0.039$; OR = 1.371; 95%CI: 1.015–1.852
		MAF	ASY MAF(C) = 40.7%; CCC MAF(C) = 35.3%
		Allelic test	Chi-square = 1.87 and $p = 0.17$
	rs2853694	AA vs. AC + CC	$p = 0.382$; OR = 1.105; 95%CI: 0.884–1.381
		MAF	ASY MAF(C) = 34.7%; CCC MAF(C) = 32.7%
		Allelic test	Chi-square = 0.28 and $p = 0.60$
	rs919766	AA vs. AC + CC	$p = 0.001$; OR = 1.653; 95%CI: 1.241–2.198
		MAF	ASY MAF(C) = 8.9%; CCC MAF(C) = 19.3%
		Allelic test	Chi-square = 36.67 and $p < 0.00001$
	rs2853696	GG vs. GA + AA	$p = 0.981$; OR = 1.003; 95%CI: 0.759–1.328
		MAF	ASY MAF(A) = 10.6%; CCC MAF(A) = 10.6%
		Allelic test	Chi-square = 0.002 and $p = 0.097$
	rs11574790	CC vs. CT + TT	$p = 0.006$; OR = 1.497; 95%CI: 1.124–1.996
		MAF	ASY MAF(T) = 8.3%; CCC MAF(T) = 16.6%
		Allelic test	Chi-square = 8.78 and $p = 0.03$
	rs3212227	AA vs. AC + CC	$p = 0.973$; OR = 1.004; 95%CI: 0.803–1.254
		MAF	ASY MAF(C) = 31.1%; CCC MAF(C) = 31.0%
		Allelic test	Chi-square = 0.001 and $p = 0.97$
	rs1368439	TT vs. TG + GG	$p = 0.735$; OR = 1.048; 95%CI: 0.800–1.373
		MAF	ASY MAF(G) = 11.2%; CCC MAF(G) = 10.5%
		Allelic test	Chi-square = 0.073 and $p = 0.79$
	rs6870828	AA vs. AG + GG	$p = 0.754$; OR = 1.040; 95%CI: 0.814–1.328
		MAF	ASY MAF(G) = 39.4%; CCC MAF(G) = 40.6%
		Allelic test	Chi-square = 0.086 and $p = 0.77$
	rs6859018	CC vs. CT + TT	$p = 0.603$; OR = 1.093; 95%CI: 0.782–1.527
		MAF	ASY MAF(T) = 33.0%; CCC MAF(T) = 32.5%
		Allelic test	Chi-square = 0.018 and $p = 0.89$
IL10	rs1800890	TT vs. TA + AA	$p = 0.636$; OR = 1.055; 95%CI: 0.845–1.318
		MAF	ASY MAF(A) = 26.4%; CCC MAF(A) = 24.7%
		Allelic test	Chi-square = 0.25 and $p = 0.62$
	rs1800896	AA + AG vs. GG	$p = 0.013$; OR = 1.527; 95%CI: 1.092–2.137
		MAF	ASY MAF(G) = 36.9%; CCC MAF(G) = 32.7%
		Allelic test	Chi-square = 1.24 and $p = 0.27$
	rs1800871	CC + TT vs. CT	$p = 0.059$; OR = 1.246; 95%CI: 0.992–1.566
		MAF	ASY MAF(T) = 35.3%; CCC MAF(T) = 35.3%
		Allelic test	Chi-square = 0.0001 and $p = 0.99$

(Continued)

TABLE 1 | Continued

GENE	Tag SNP	Genotype groups	Association test
	rs1518111	GG + AA vs. GA	$p = 0.104$; OR = 1.208; 95%CI: 0.962–1.516
		MAF	ASY MAF(A) = 32.4%; CCC MAF(A) = 34.2%
		Allelic test	Chi-square = 0.24 and $p = 0.62$
	rs3024496	TT + TC vs. CC	$p = 0.031$; OR = 1.437; 95%CI: 1.033–2.000
		MAF	ASY MAF(C) = 40.3%; CCC MAF(C) = 35.0%
		Allelic test	Chi-square = 1.89 and $p = 0.17$
	rs6673928	CC vs. CA	$p = 0.329$; OR = 2.141; 95%CI: 0.464–9.885
		MAF	ASY MAF(A) = 1.3%; CCC MAF(A) = 0.6%
		Allelic test	Chi-square = 0.95 and $p = 0.33$
IFNG	rs2069705	TT vs. TC + CC	$p = 0.337$; OR = 1.12; 95%CI: 0.89–1.41
		MAF	ASY MAF(C) = 39.6%; CCC MAF(C) = 37.9%
		Allelic test	Chi-square = 0.20 and $p = 0.66$
	rs1861494	AA vs. AG + GG	$p = 0.057$; OR = 1.24; 95%CI: 0.99–1.55
		MAF	ASY MAF(G) = 24.3%; CCC MAF(G) = 18.8%
		Allelic test	Chi-square = 3.21 and $p = 0.07$
	rs2069718	CC + CT vs. TT	$p = 0.183$; OR = 1.18; 95%CI: 0.92–1.52
		MAF	ASY MAF(C) = 48.2%; CCC MAF(C) = 52.4%
		Allelic test	Chi-square = 1.16 and $p = 0.28$
	rs2069727	AA + AG vs. GG	$p = 0.232$; OR = 1.22; 95%CI: 0.88–1.70
		MAF	ASY MAF(G) = 36.4%; CCC MAF(G) = 38.9%
		Allelic test	Chi-square = 0.45 and $p = 0.50$
	rs3181035	GG vs. GA + AA	$p = 0.371$; OR = 1.12; 95%CI: 0.88–1.42
		MAF	ASY MAF(A) = 17.0%; CCC MAF(A) = 13.7%
		Allelic test	Chi-square = 1.38 and $p = 0.24$
IL4	rs2070874	CC vs. CT + TT	$p = 0.481$; OR = 1.08; 95%CI: 0.87–1.34
		MAF	ASY MAF(T) = 27.0%; CCC MAF(T) = 27.9%
		Allelic test	Chi-square = 0.07 and $p = 0.79$
	rs2227284	AA + AC vs. CC	$p = 0.268$; OR = 1.15; 95%CI: 0.90–1.46
		MAF	ASY MAF(C) = 53.2%; CCC MAF(C) = 48.2%
		Allelic test	Chi-square = 1.62 and $p = 0.20$
	rs2243261	GG vs. GT + TT	$p = 0.651$; OR = 1.10; 95%CI: 0.74–1.63
		MAF	ASY MAF(T) = 3.8%; CCC MAF(T) = 4.6%
		Allelic test	Chi-square = 0.26 and $p = 0.61$
	rs2243268	AA vs. AC + CC	$p = 0.467$; OR = 1.08; 95%CI: 0.86–1.38
		MAF	ASY MAF(C) = 20.0%; CCC MAF(C) = 21.2%
		Allelic test	Chi-square = 0.15 and $p = 0.70$
	rs2243274	GG + GA vs. AA	$p = 0.423$; OR = 1.15; 95%CI: 0.82–1.60
		MAF	ASY MAF(A) = 31.2%; CCC MAF(A) = 35.8%
		Allelic test	Chi-square = 1.53 and $p = 0.22$
	rs2243290	CC + CA vs. AA	$p = 0.352$; OR = 1.21; 95%CI: 0.81–1.82
		MAF	ASY MAF(A) = 23.7%; CCC MAF(A) = 24.8%
		Allelic test	Chi-square = 0.12 and $p = 0.73$
	rs2406539	AA vs. AT + TT	$p = 0.570$; OR = 1.19; 95%CI: 0.65–2.17
		MAF	ASY MAF(T) = 7.5%; CCC MAF(T) = 9.2%
		Allelic test	Chi-square = 0.60 and $p = 0.44$

MAF, Minor Allelic frequency.

OR = 1.536; 95% CI: 1.139–2.070; rs919766: $p = 0.014$; OR = 1.477; 95% CI: 1.081–2.020) remained significantly associated. The three other markers were excluded from the best model. Allelic tests confirmed the association of these two IL12 markers. The rs919766C allele ($p < 0.00001$) and the rs2546893G allele ($p = 0.005$) were associated to an increase risk to CCC development.

The same analysis was performed between the ASY subjects and severe CCC patients. The same polymorphisms were

TABLE 2 | Association studies between CCC with a left ventricular ejection fraction value under 0.4% and ASY including as covariates the gender and the polymorphism one by one.

GENE	Tag SNP		Association tests
IL12B	rs2546890	GG vs. GA + AA	p = 0.121; OR = 1.23; 95%CI: 0.95–1.61
		MAF	ASY MAF(A) = 46.6%; SEV CCC MAF(A) = 378%
		Allelic test	Chi-square = 4.30 and p = 0.04
	rs730691	GG vs. GA	p = 0.407; OR = 1.33; 95%CI: 0.68–2.58
		MAF	ASY MAF(A) = 9.1%; SEV CCC MAF(A) = 12.0%
		Allelic test	Chi-square = 0.91 and p = 0.34
	rs2546893	GG + GA vs. AA	p = 0.001; OR = 1.69; 95%CI: 1.23–2.34
		MAF	ASY MAF(A) = 45.8%; SEV CCC MAF(A) = 32.8%
		Allelic test	Chi-square = 9.84 and p = 0.002
	rs1003199	CC + CT vs. TT	p = 0.013; OR = 1.52; 95%CI: 1.09–2.13
		MAF	ASY MAF(T) = 43.123.7%; SEV CCC MAF(T) = 34.8%
		Allelic test	Chi-square = 3.98 and p = 0.05
	rs3181216	TT vs. TA + AA	p = 0.430; OR = 1.11; 95%CI: 0.86–1.43
		MAF	ASY MAF(A) = 23.7%; SEV CCC MAF(A) = 24.8%
		Allelic test	Chi-square = 0.80 and p = 0.37
	rs2569253	TT + CC vs. TC	p = 0.036; OR = 1.45; 95%CI: 1.02–2.05
		MAF	ASY MAF(C) = 40.7%; SEV CCC MAF(C) = 34.3%
		Allelic test	Chi-square = 2.33 and p = 0.13
	rs2853694	AA vs. AC + CC	p = 0.360; OR = 1.12; 95%CI: 0.88–1.43
		MAF	ASY MAF(C) = 34.7%; SEV CCC MAF(C) = 30.2%
		Allelic test	Chi-square = 1.34 and p = 0.25
	rs919766	AA vs. AC + CC	p = 0.007; OR = 1.49; 95%CI: 1.11–1.98
		MAF	ASY MAF(C) = 8.9%; SEV CCC MAF(C) = 20.7%
		Allelic test	Chi-square = 13.91 and p = 0.0002
	rs2853696	GG vs. GA + AA	p = 0.649; OR = 1.27; 95%CI: 0.45–3.56
		MAF	ASY MAF(A) = 10.6%; SEV CCC MAF(A) = 9.5%
		Allelic test	Chi-square = 0.21 and p = 0.64
	rs11574790	CC vs. CT + TT	p = 0.026; OR = 1.39; 95%CI: 1.04–1.86
		MAF	ASY MAF(T) = 8.3%; SEV CCC MAF(T) = 18.3%
		Allelic test	Chi-square = 10.98 and p = 0.0009
	rs3212227	AA vs. AC + CC	p = 0.631; OR = 1.06; 95%CI: 0.83–1.35
		MAF	ASY MAF(C) = 31.1%; SEV CCC MAF(C) = 31.9%
		Allelic test	Chi-square = 0.04 and p = 0.84
	rs1368439	TT vs. TG + GG	p = 0.547; OR = 1.09; 95%CI: 0.82–1.47
		MAF	ASY MAF(G) = 11.2%; SEV CCC MAF(G) = 9.9%
		Allelic test	Chi-square = 0.24 and p = 0.62
	rs6870828	AA + AG vs. GG	p = 0.181; OR = 1.28; 95%CI: 0.89–1.82
		MAF	ASY MAF(G) = 39.4%; SEV CCC MAF(G) = 42.4%
		Allelic test	Chi-square = 0.48 and p = 0.49
	rs6859018	CC vs. CT + TT	P = 0.898; OR = 1.02; 95%CI: 0.80–1.29
		MAF	ASY MAF(T) = 33.0%; SEV CCC MAF(T) = 34.3%
		Allelic test	Chi-square = 0.10 and p = 0.75
IL10	rs1800890	TT vs. TA + AA	p = 0.181; OR = 1.22; 95%CI: 0.91–1.63
		MAF	ASY MAF(A) = 26.4%; SEV CCC MAF(A) = 24.0%
		Allelic test	Chi-square = 0.44 and p = 0.51
	rs1800896	AA + AG vs. GG	p = 0.097; OR = 1.38; 95%CI: 0.94–2.01
		MAF	ASY MAF(G) = 36.9%; SEV CCC MAF(G) = 33.4%
		Allelic test	Chi-square = 0.74 and p = 0.39
	rs1800871	CC + TT vs. CT	p = 0.041; OR = 1.30; 95%CI: 1.01–1.66
		MAF	ASY MAF(T) = 35.3%; SEV CCC MAF(T) = 34.1%
		Allelic test	Chi-square = 6.18 and p = 0.01

(Continued)

TABLE 2 | Continued

GENE	Tag SNP		Association tests
	rs1518111	GG + AA vs. GA	$p = 0.067$; OR = 1.26; 95%CI: 0.98–1.61
		MAF	ASY MAF(A) = 32.4%; SEV CCC MAF(A) = 32.6%
		Allelic test	Chi-square = 0.001 and $p = 0.97$
	rs3024496	TT + TC vs. CC	$p = 0.036$; OR = 1.49; 95%CI: 1.03–2.16
		MAF	ASY MAF(C) = 40.3%; SEV CCC MAF(C) = 35.2%
		Allelic test	Chi-square = 1.55 and $p = 0.21$
	rs6673928	CC vs. CA	$p = 0.432$; OR = 2.12; 95%CI: 0.33–13.83
		MAF	ASY MAF(A) = 1.3%; SEV CCC MAF(A) = 0.5%
		Allelic test	Chi-square = 1.12 and $p = 0.29$
IFNG	rs2069705	TT vs. TC + CC	$p = 0.333$; OR = 1.13; 95%CI: 0.88–1.46
		MAF	ASY MAF(C) = 39.6%; SEV CCC MAF(C) = 37.1%
		Allelic test	Chi-square = 0.38 and $p = 0.54$
	rs1861494	AA vs. AG + GG	$p = 0.067$; OR = 1.26; 95%CI: 0.98–1.61
		MAF	ASY MAF(G) = 24.3%; SEV CCC MAF(G) = 17.0%
		Allelic test	Chi-square=4.88 and p=0.03
	rs2069718	CC + CT vs. TT	$p = 0.147$; OR = 1.23; 95%CI: 0.93–1.63
		MAF	ASY MAF(T) = 51.8%; SEV CCC MAF(T) = 46.7%
		Allelic test	Chi-square = 1.47 and $p = 0.22$
	rs2069727	AA + AG vs. GG	$p = 0.254$; OR = 1.23; 95%CI: 0.86–1.75
		MAF	ASY MAF(G) = 36.4%; SEV CCC MAF(G) = 39.5%
		Allelic test	Chi-square = 0.60 and $p = 0.44$
	rs3181035	GG vs. GA + AA	$p = 0.440$; OR = 1.11; 95%CI: 0.85–1.45
		MAF	ASY MAF(A) = 17.0%; SEV CCC MAF(A) = 13.4%
		Allelic test	Chi-square = 1.46 and $p = 0.23$
IL4	rs2070874	CC vs. CT + TT	$p = 0.274$; OR = 1.14; 95%CI: 0.90–1.45
		MAF	ASY MAF(T) = 27.0%; SEV CCC MAF(T) = 30.8%
		Allelic test	Chi-square = 1.07 and $p = 0.30$
	rs2227284	AA + AC vs. CC	$p = 0.059$; OR = 1.30; 95%CI: 0.99–1.72
		MAF	ASY MAF(C) = 53.2%; SEV CCC MAF(C) = 43.3%
		Allelic test	Chi-square = 5.48 and $p = 0.02$
	rs2243261	GG vs. GT + TT	$p = 0.841$; OR = 1.05; 95%CI: 0.68–1.62
		MAF	ASY MAF(T) = 3.8%; SEV CCC MAF(T) = 4.8%
		Allelic test	Chi-square = 0.34 and $p = 0.56$
	rs2243268	AA vs. AC + CC	$p = 0.159$; OR = 1.20; 95%CI: 0.93–1.55
		MAF	ASY MAF(C) = 20.0%; SEV CCC MAF(C) = 23.8%
		Allelic test	Chi-square = 1.20 and $p = 0.27$
	rs2243274	GG + GA vs. AA	$p = 0.225$; OR = 1.25; 95%CI: 0.87–1.80
		MAF	ASY MAF(A) = 31.2%; SEV CCC MAF(A) = 38.4%
		Allelic test	Chi-square = 3.16 and $p = 0.08$
	rs2243290	CC + CA vs. AA	$p = 0.842$; OR = 1.04; 95%CI: 0.68–1.61
		MAF	ASY MAF(A) = 23.7%; SEV CCC MAF(A) = 27.2%
		Allelic test	Chi-square = 0.91 and $p = 0.34$
	rs2406539	AA vs. AT + TT	$p = 0.538$; OR = 1.23; 95%CI: 0.64–2.35
		MAF	ASY MAF(T) = 7.5%; SEV CCC MAF(T) = 10.0%
		Allelic test	Chi-square = 1.05 and $p = 0.30$

These association tests are genotype association and allelic tests.
SEV CCC, Severe CCC.

associated, in univariate analysis, to an increased risk to develop severe chronic cardiomyopathy (rs2546893G/A: $p = 0.001$; OR = 1.706; 95%CI: 1.236–2.353; rs919766A/C: $p = 0.001$; OR = 1.672; 95%CI: 1.231–2.267; rs1003199C/T: $p = 0.013$; OR = 1.531; 95%CI: 1.236–2.353; rs2569253T/C: $p = 0.037$; OR = 1.445; 95%CI: 1.022–2.041; rs11574790C/T: $p = 0.004$; OR =

1.562; 95%CI: 1.151–2.123) (see **Table 2**). After correction for multiple testing the polymorphism rs2546893 remains significant (corrected p-value = 0.014) and the polymorphism rs919766 is borderline (corrected p-value = 0.091). In a multivariate analysis, the gender and the two polymorphisms remained significantly associated (rs2546893G/A: p = 0.005; OR = 1.667; 95% CI: 1.170–2.375; rs919766A/C: p = 0.024; OR = 1.471; 95%CI: 1.051–2.058; gender: $p = 2.25 \times 10^{-5}$; OR = 3.261; 95% CI: 1.888–5.632). the allelic tests confirmed that the rs2546893G allele ($p <$ 0.002) and the rs919766C allele (p = 0.0002) were associated to an increase risk to severe CCC. None of the studied *IL12B* markers discriminated moderate from severe CCC patient groups.

Polymorphism rs3024496T/C Around the *IL10* Gene Is Showing a Trend of Association to CCC

Six tag SNPs were genotyped for the *IL10* gene. **Table 1** shows comparison between CCC and ASY, while **Table 2** shows comparison of severe CCC and ASY. For the rs1800896A/G polymorphism, 282 (91.9%) CCC subjects carried the A/A or A/G genotypes vs. 90 (84.1%) for the ASY (p = 0.013; OR = 1.527; 95%CI: 1.092–2.137). The same result was obtained when the analysis was restricted to severe CCC vs. ASY (p = 0.028; OR = 1.536; 95%CI: 1.047–2.252) (see **Table 2**). For the rs3024496T/C polymorphism, 284 (91.3%) CCC subjects carried the T/T or T/C genotypes vs. 92 (84.3%) for the ASY (p = 0.031; OR = 1.437; 95%CI: 1.033–2.000) (see **Table 1**). The same result was obtained when the analysis was restricted to severe CCC vs. ASY (p = 0.049; OR = 1.462; 95%CI: 1.002–2.132) (see **Table 2**). For the rs1800871 marker, we found a significant association when severe CCC patients were compared the ASY subjects (p = 0.035; OR = 1.311; 95%CI: 1.019–1.686). No association was found for this last marker in the comparison between ASY and the whole CCC group (see **Table 1**). After correction for multiple testing, the polymorphism rs1800896A/G and rs3024496T/C has shown only trends of association (rs1800896A/G: corrected p-value = 0.078). The allelic tests reach the same trends of association (rs3024496C p = 0.17 and rs1800896G p = 0.27).

Based on the results of the multivariate analysis, we had an association between CCC and ASY with two SNPs located in the IL12B gene (rs2546893 and rs919766) and one polymorphism in the IL10 gene (rs3024496). Subjects carrying the three susceptibility genotypes [rs2546893(GG or GA) + rs919766(CC or AC) + rs3024496(TT or TC)] have a higher risk (OR = 2.68) to develop CCC. In contrast, subjects carrying the resistant genotypes (rs2546893AA + r919766AA + rs3024496CC) have a lower risk [OR = 4.48 (1/0.223)] to develop CCC (**Table 3**).

No Clear Evidence of Association Was Detected for Tag Polymorphisms in the *IFNG* and *IL4* Genes

Six tag SNPs were genotyped for the *IFNG* gene. For the rs1861494 A/G polymorphism, a trend of association was detected. Indeed, 202 (64.7%) CCC subjects carried the A/A genotype vs. 62 (54.9%) for the ASY (p = 0.057; OR = 1.24; 95%CI: 0.99–1.55) (see **Supplementary Table 2**). The same trend appeared on severe cases (p = 0.067; OR = 1.26; 95%CI: 0.98–1.61) (see **Table 2**). Seven tag SNPs into the *IL4* gene were genotyped on our whole study population (see **Supplementary Table 2**). Comparisons between ASY and CCC patients disclosed no significant associations (see **Tables 1**, **2**).

DISCUSSION

Association studies of cytokine gene polymorphisms in Chagas disease frequently include a small number of patients, and are often not replicated in different studies or ethnical groups. The present study was designed to determine whether SNPs in *IL12B, IL10, IFNG* and *IL4,* key genes involved in the promotion and control of Th1 differentiation and IFN-g production to *T. cruzi*, are associated with Chagas disease outcome. For that, we used a larger population and performed a comprehensive assessment of 35 Tag SNPs covering all the genetic information

TABLE 3 | Genotype combination analysis based on the following polymorphisms (rs2546893/rs919766/rs3024496).

Genotype combinations	IL12 rs2546893	IL12 rs919766	IL10 rs3024496	CCC	ASY	Total	% in ASY	% in CCC	Ratio CCC/ASY	p-value	Odds Ratio	95% C.I. for EXP(B)
1 S1 S2 S3	GG + GA	CC + AC	TC + CC	89	14	103	**14%**	**86%**	**6.36**	0.0006	2.677	1.468–4.838
2 S1 S2 R3	GG + GA	CC + AC	CC	9	3	12	**25%**	**75%**	**3.00**	0.6340	1.028	0.2758
3 S1 R2 S3	GG + GA	AA	TC + CC	149	46	195	**24%**	**76%**	**3.24**	0.1963	1.217	0.7777–1.928
4 R1 S2 S3	AA	AC + CC	TC + CC	6	0	6	**0%**	**100%**	**X**	0.1688	X	X
5 S1 R2 R3	GG + GA	AA	CC	13	11	24	**46%**	**54%**	**1.18**	0.0058	0.3483	0.1434–0.7776
6 R1 S2 R3	AA	AC + CC	CC	1	0	1	**0%**	**100%**	**X**	0.7450	X	X
7 R1 R2 S3	AA	AA	TC + CC	29	25	54	**46%**	**54%**	**1.16**	<0.0001	0.3320	0.1834–0.6135
8 R1 R2 R3	AA	AA	CC	2	3	5	**60%**	**40%**	**0.67**	0.1075	0.2230	0.0393–1.110

R, Resistant genotype; S, Susceptibility genotype; SNP 1 = rs2546893/SNP2 = rs919766/SNP3 = rs3024496.
Bold value indicates % ASY, Percentage of ASY subjects carrying the genotype combination; % CCC, Percentage of CCC subjects carrying the genotype combination Ratio; CCC/ASY, Ratio between these two percentage.

of the mentioned genes. We found significant associations of genotypes and alleles of *IL12B* and *IL10* with increased risk to CCC progression.

For the *IL12B* gene region, in a multivariate analysis, two SNPs were significantly associated to disease (rs2546893G/A, rs919766A/C). The rs919766C and rs2546893G alleles were associated to an increase risk to CCC development. Interestingly, these two markers are located 5 to 13 kb away from the rs3212227 polymorphism (*IL12B* 3′UTR region), that was previously associated to Chagas cardiomyopathy (31). Our results are consistent as these 3 markers are in linkage disequilibrium ($D' = 0.99$) on the African (Yoruba) reference population and the markers rs919766 and rs3212227 are in strong linkage disequilibrium ($D' = 0.99$) on the European reference population.

For the *IL10* gene, the rs3024496 polymorphism (located in the 3′UTR region), and rs1800896 polymorphism (located in the promoter region) have shown trends of association to susceptibility to cardiomyopathy. The rs3024496C and rs1800896G alleles were more frequent in patients. Our data are consistent with the previous study that showed that the marker (IL10-1082 known as rs1800896 too) was previously associated with development of CCC (33). Costa et al. have shown that the A allele has been associated with lower IL-10 expression in disease and lower left ventricular ejection fraction values in CCC (33). The two markers (rs3024496 and rs1800896) are in strong linkage disequilibrium on the European reference population ($D' = 1$) and on the Yoruba population ($D' = 0.83$).

Three SNPs in the *IL10* gene (the two rs3024496, rs1800896 mentioned above, plus rs1800871) detected trends of association. A study performed on a Brazilian population infected by *Leishmania braziliensis* has shown that these markers are correlated (r^2 value >0.8) (40). So, from one Brazilian sub population to another one, the associated marker may change (due to light allelic frequency variation) or population stratification. However, the associated marker is coming from the same correlation block.

We did not find any significant association with SNPs from the *IFNG* and *IL4* genes. This is in agreement with Arnez et al. who studied some of these same SNPs (rs2070874, rs2227284, rs2243268, rs2243274, rs2243290 in an Bolivian population (29), and Flórez et al. who studied one SNP not tested by our group (rs2243250) in a Colombian population, failing to find any association (30). Taken together, these results suggest that we do not have evidence that polymorphisms in or within the IFN gene control the expression of this key cytokine for the pathogenic process.

During *T. cruzi* infection, once the inflammatory process starts, IFN-γ will be produced by Th1 cells and act as a prime inflammatory cytokine in different pathways of the immune system, such as upregulating MHC class I and class II molecules, suppressing Th2 immune responses by antagonism of IL-4 production, inducing high levels of antigen presentation and activating macrophages (41). Moreover, CCC patients have an increased peripheral production of IFN-γ and TNF-α when compared to patients with the asymptomatic/indeterminate form. On the other hand, IFN-γ has direct effects on cardiomyocytes and perhaps other cells of the myocardium (34). At this level we can speculate that the existence of functional or pathogenic variants in or within the IFN gene will have a too strong deleterious effect that will be lethal. So, the genetic control of the human susceptibility to cardiomyopathy mainly target genes that are involved in the regulation of this TH1 response, such as *IL12B* and *IL10* genes.

On the other hand, our data confirmed the involvement of *IL12B* and *IL10* in the control of susceptibility to human Chagas cardiomyopathy. The *IL10* polymorphism has been described as a functional polymorphism. It remains to be tested whether the *IL12B* polymorphism and linked SNPs are functional as well. Taking into account the effects of both cytokines on Th1 T cell differentiation and IFNγ production, it can be hypothesized that this is linked to the increased number of IFNγ producing Th1 T cells in the peripheral blood and heart tissue of CCC patients. Our study and others have identified several genes in the control of human susceptibility to chronic disease. However, each gene is characterized by a low odds ratio, implying a small contribution in Chagas disease infection. However, the combination of the several genetic markers increases the protection from disease development, with individual odds ratio around 1.5, to ca. 4.5 in patients carrying all the protection genotypes in all three loci. The identification of more genetic markers for CCC will provide information for pathogenesis as well as therapeutic targets. Identifying early or causal predictive genetic factors for the clinical progression of the disease is essential for clarifying the pathogenesis and defining appropriate treatment modalities.

ETHICS STATEMENT

The studies involving human participants were reviewed and approved by The INSERM Internal Review Board, The Brazilian National Ethics in Research Commission (CONEP). The patients/participants provided their written informed consent to participate in this study.

AUTHOR CONTRIBUTIONS

JK, EC-N, and CC: study design. AF-B and SC: experiments. AF-B, BI, CP, BS, HL-W, PB, JM-N, AS, FD, MH, MS, AF, AP, ED, VR, JK, CC, and EC-N: manuscript preparation. All authors contributed to the article and approved the submitted version.

ACKNOWLEDGMENTS

We are thankful for the access to the genotyping platform (Denis Milan, Cecile Donnadieu, and Frederic Martins).

REFERENCES

1. Bocchi EA, Bestetti RB, Scanavacca MI, Cunha Neto E, Issa VS. Chronic chagas heart disease management: from etiology to cardiomyopathy treatment. *J Am Coll Cardiol.* (2017) 70:1510–24. doi: 10.1016/j.jacc.2017.08.004
2. Coura JR, Borges-Pereira J. Chagas disease. What is known and what should be improved: a systemic review. *Rev Soc Bras Med Trop.* (2012) 45:286–96. doi: 10.1590/S0037-86822012000300002
3. Barbosa AP, Cardinalli Neto A, Otaviano AP, Rocha BF, Bestetti RB. Comparison of outcome between Chagas cardiomyopathy and idiopathic dilated cardiomyopathy. *Arq Bras Cardiol.* (2011) 97:517–25. doi: 10.1590/S0066-782X2011005000112
4. Bestetti RB, Muccillo G. Clinical course of Chagas' heart disease: a comparison with dilated cardiomyopathy. *Int J Cardiol.* (1997) 60:187–93. doi: 10.1016/S0167-5273(97)00083-1
5. Zicker F, Smith PG, Netto JC, Oliveira RM, Zicker EM. Physical activity, opportunity for reinfection, and sibling history of heart disease as risk factors for Chagas' cardiopathy. *Am J Trop Med Hyg.* (1990) 43:498–505. doi: 10.4269/ajtmh.1990.43.498
6. Acosta-Herrera M, Strauss M, Casares-Marfil D, Martin J. Genomic medicine in Chagas disease. *Acta Trop.* (2019) 197:105062. doi: 10.1016/j.actatropica.2019.105062
7. Chevillard C, Nunes JPS, Frade AF, Almeida RR, Pandey RP, Nascimento MS, et al. Disease tolerance and pathogen resistance genes may underlie *Trypanosoma cruzi* persistence and differential progression to chagas disease cardiomsyopathy. *Front Immunol.* (2018) 9:2791. doi: 10.3389/fimmu.2018.02791
8. Strauss M, Acosta-Herrera M, Alcaraz A, Casares-Marfil D, Bosch-Nicolau P, Lo Presti MS, et al. Association of IL18 genetic polymorphisms with Chagas disease in Latin American populations. *PLoS Negl Trop Dis.* (2019) 13:e0007859. doi: 10.1371/journal.pntd.0007859
9. Cunha-Neto E, Chevillard C. Chagas disease cardiomyopathy: immunopathology and genetics. *Mediators Inflamm.* (2014) 2014:683230. doi: 10.1155/2014/683230
10. Michailowsky V, Silva NM, Rocha CD, Vieira LQ, Lannes-Vieira J, Gazzinelli RT. Pivotal role of interleukin-12 and interferon-gamma axis in controlling tissue parasitism and inflammation in the heart and central nervous system during *Trypanosoma cruzi* infection. *Am J Pathol.* (2001) 159:1723–33. doi: 10.1016/S0002-9440(10)63019-2
11. Bilate AM, Cunha-Neto E. Chagas disease cardiomyopathy: current concepts of an old disease. *Rev Inst Med Trop Sao Paulo.* (2008) 50:67–74. doi: 10.1590/S0036-46652008000200001
12. Reis MM, Higuchi Mde L, Benvenuti LA, Aiello VD, Gutierrez PS, Bellotti G, et al. An *in situ* quantitative immunohistochemical study of cytokines and IL-2R+ in chronic human chagasic myocarditis: correlation with the presence of myocardial *Trypanosoma cruzi* antigens. *Clin Immunol Immunopathol.* (1997) 83:165–72. doi: 10.1006/clin.1997.4335
13. Muller U, Kohler G, Mossmann H, Schaub GA, Alber G, Di Santo JP, et al. IL-12-independent IFN-gamma production by T cells in experimental Chagas' disease is mediated by IL-18. *J Immunol.* (2001) 167:3346–53. doi: 10.4049/jimmunol.167.6.3346
14. Rocha Rodrigues DB, dos Reis MA, Romano A, Pereira SA, Teixeira Vde P, Tostes S, et al. *In situ* expression of regulatory cytokines by heart inflammatory cells in Chagas' disease patients with heart failure. *Clin Dev Immunol.* (2012) 2012:361730. doi: 10.1155/2012/361730
15. Holscher C, Mohrs M, Dai WJ, Kohler G, Ryffel B, Schaub GA, et al. Tumor necrosis factor alpha-mediated toxic shock in *Trypanosoma cruzi*-infected interleukin 10-deficient mice. *Infect Immun.* (2000) 68:4075–83. doi: 10.1128/IAI.68.7.4075-4083.2000
16. Soares MP, Gozzelino R, Weis S. Tissue damage control in disease tolerance. *Trends Immunol.* (2014) 35:483–94. doi: 10.1016/j.it.2014.08.001
17. Medina TS, Oliveira GG, Silva MC, David BA, Silva GK, Fonseca DM, et al. Ebi3 prevents *Trypanosoma cruzi*-induced myocarditis by dampening IFN-gamma-driven inflammation. *Front Immunol.* (2017) 8:1213. doi: 10.3389/fimmu.2017.01213
18. Araujo FF, Gomes JA, Rocha MO, Williams-Blangero S, Pinheiro VM, Morato MJ, et al. Potential role of CD4+CD25HIGH regulatory T cells in morbidity in Chagas disease. *Front Biosci.* (2007) 12:2797–806. doi: 10.2741/2273
19. Cunha-Neto E, Kalil J. Heart-infiltrating and peripheral T cells in the pathogenesis of human Chagas' disease cardiomyopathy. *Autoimmunity.* (2001) 34:187–92. doi: 10.3109/08916930109007383
20. Gomes JA, Bahia-Oliveira LM, Rocha MO, Martins-Filho OA, Gazzinelli G, Correa-Oliveira R. Evidence that development of severe cardiomyopathy in human Chagas' disease is due to a Th1-specific immune response. *Infect Immun.* (2003) 71:1185–93. doi: 10.1128/IAI.71.3.1185-1193.2003
21. Ribeirao M, Pereira-Chioccola VL, Renia L, Augusto Fragata Filho A, Schenkman S, Rodrigues MM. Chagasic patients develop a type 1 immune response to Trypanosoma cruzi trans-sialidase. *Parasite Immunol.* (2000) 22:49–53. doi: 10.1046/j.1365-3024.2000.00260.x
22. Abel LC, Rizzo LV, Ianni B, Albuquerque F, Bacal F, Carrara D, et al. Chronic Chagas' disease cardiomyopathy patients display an increased IFN-gamma response to *Trypanosoma cruzi* infection. *J Autoimmun.* (2001) 17:99–107. doi: 10.1006/jaut.2001.0523
23. Gomes JA, Bahia-Oliveira LM, Rocha MO, Busek SC, Teixeira MM, Silva JS, et al. Type 1 chemokine receptor expression in Chagas' disease correlates with morbidity in cardiac patients. *Infect Immun.* (2005) 73:7960–6. doi: 10.1128/IAI.73.12.7960-7966.2005
24. Ferreira RC, Ianni BM, Abel LC, Buck P, Mady C, Kalil J, et al. Increased plasma levels of tumor necrosis factor-alpha in asymptomatic/"indeterminate" and Chagas disease cardiomyopathy patients. *Mem Inst Oswaldo Cruz.* (2003) 98:407–11. doi: 10.1590/S0074-02762003000300021
25. Sousa GR, Gomes JA, Fares RC, Damasio MP, Chaves AT, Ferreira KS, et al. Plasma cytokine expression is associated with cardiac morbidity in chagas disease. *PLoS ONE.* (2014) 9:e87082. doi: 10.1371/journal.pone.0087082
26. Talvani A, Rocha MO, Ribeiro AL, Correa-Oliveira R, Teixeira MM. Chemokine receptor expression on the surface of peripheral blood mononuclear cells in Chagas disease. *J Infect Dis.* (2004) 189:214–20. doi: 10.1086/380803
27. Nogueira LG, Santos RH, Fiorelli AI, Mairena EC, Benvenuti LA, Bocchi EA, et al. Myocardial gene expression of T-bet, GATA-3, Ror-gammat, FoxP3, and hallmark cytokines in chronic Chagas disease cardiomyopathy: an essentially unopposed TH1-type response. *Mediators Inflamm.* (2014) 2014:914326. doi: 10.1155/2014/914326
28. de Alba-Alvarado M, Salazar-Schettino PM, Jimenez-Alvarez L, Cabrera-Bravo M, Garcia-Sancho C, Zenteno E, et al. Th-17 cytokines are associated with severity of *Trypanosoma cruzi* chronic infection in pediatric patients from endemic areas of Mexico. *Acta Trop.* (2018) 178:134–41. doi: 10.1016/j.actatropica.2017.11.009
29. Alvarado Arnez LE, Venegas EN, Ober C, Thompson EE. Sequence variation in the IL4 gene and resistance to *Trypanosoma cruzi* infection in Bolivians. *J Allergy Clin Immunol.* (2011) 127:279–82, 282 e1–3. doi: 10.1016/j.jaci.2010.10.026
30. Florez O, Martin J, Gonzalez CI. Interleukin 4, interleukin 4 receptor-alpha and interleukin 10 gene polymorphisms in Chagas disease. *Parasite Immunol.* (2011) 33:506–11. doi: 10.1111/j.1365-3024.2011.01314.x
31. Zafra G, Morillo C, Martin J, Gonzalez A, Gonzalez CI. Polymorphism in the 3′ UTR of the IL12B gene is associated with Chagas' disease cardiomyopathy. *Microbes Infect.* (2007) 9:1049–52. doi: 10.1016/j.micinf.2007.04.010
32. Turner DM, Williams DM, Sankaran D, Lazarus M, Sinnott PJ, Hutchinson IV. An investigation of polymorphism in the interleukin-10 gene promoter. *Eur J Immunogenet.* (1997) 24:1–8. doi: 10.1111/j.1365-2370.1997.tb00001.x
33. Costa GC, da Costa Rocha MO, Moreira PR, Menezes CA, Silva MR, Gollob KJ, et al. Functional IL-10 gene polymorphism is associated with Chagas disease cardiomyopathy. *J Infect Dis.* (2009) 199:451–4. doi: 10.1086/596061
34. Cunha-Neto E, Dzau VJ, Allen PD, Stamatiou D, Benvenutti L, Higuchi ML, et al. Cardiac gene expression profiling provides evidence for cytokinopathy as a molecular mechanism in Chagas' disease cardiomyopathy. *Am J Pathol.* (2005) 167:305–13. doi: 10.1016/S0002-9440(10)62976-8
35. Jorge MT, Macedo TA, Janones RS, Carizzi DP, Heredia RA, Acha RE. Types of arrhythmia among cases of American trypanosomiasis, compared with those in other cardiology patients. *Ann Trop Med Parasitol.* (2003) 97:139–48. doi: 10.1179/000349803235001561

36. Januzzi JL Jr. Natriuretic peptides, ejection fraction, and prognosis: parsing the phenotypes of heart failure. *J Am Coll Cardiol.* (2013) 61:1507–9. doi: 10.1016/j.jacc.2013.01.039
37. van Veldhuisen DJ, Linssen GC, Jaarsma T, van Gilst WH, Hoes AW, Tijssen JG, et al. B-type natriuretic peptide and prognosis in heart failure patients with preserved and reduced ejection fraction. *J Am Coll Cardiol.* (2013) 61:1498–506. doi: 10.1016/j.jacc.2012.12.044
38. Nogueira LG, Santos RH, Ianni BM, Fiorelli AI, Mairena EC, Benvenuti LA, et al. Myocardial chemokine expression and intensity of myocarditis in Chagas cardiomyopathy are controlled by polymorphisms in CXCL9 and CXCL10. *PLoS Negl Trop Dis.* (2012) 6:e1867. doi: 10.1371/journal.pntd.0001867
39. Holm S. A simple sequentially rejective multiple test procedure. *Scand J Stat.* (1979) 6:65–70.
40. Salhi A, Rodrigues V Jr, Santoro F, Dessein H, Romano A, Roberto Castellano L, et al. Immunological and genetic evidence for a crucial role of IL-10 in cutaneous lesions in humans infected with Leishmania braziliensis. *J Immunol.* (2008) 180:6139–48. doi: 10.4049/jimmunol.180.9.6139
41. Schroder K, Hertzog PJ, Ravasi T, Hume DA. Interferon-gamma: an overview of signals, mechanisms and functions. *J Leukoc Biol.* (2004) 75:163–89. doi: 10.1189/jlb.0603252

15

Association of IL-10 Gene Polymorphism with IL-10 Secretion by CD4 and T Regulatory Cells in Human Leprosy

Mohammad Tarique[1†], Huma Naz[2†], Chaman Saini[1], Mohd Suhail[3,4], Hari Shankar[5], Neena Khanna[6] and Alpana Sharma[1]*

[1] Department of Biochemistry, All India Institute of Medical Sciences (AIIMS), New Delhi, India, [2] Centre for Interdisciplinary Research in Basic Sciences, Jamia Millia Islamia, New Delhi, India, [3] King Fahd Medical Research Center, King Abdulaziz University, Jeddah, Saudi Arabia, [4] Department of Medical Laboratory Technology, Faculty of Applied Medical Sciences, King Abdulaziz University, Jeddah, Saudi Arabia, [5] Parasite-Host Biology Group, ICMR – National Institute of Malaria Research, New Delhi, India, [6] Department of Dermatovenerology, All India Institute of Medical Sciences (AIIMS), New Delhi, India

***Correspondence:**
Alpana Sharma
dralpanasharma@gmail.com

†Present address:
Mohammad Tarique, Department of Surgery, University of Miami, Miami, FL, United States
Huma Naz, Department of Anesthesiology, University of Miami, Miami, FL, United States

Leprosy is a chronic bacterial disease caused by *Mycobacterium leprae*. Cytokines are known to play vital role as a peacekeeper during inflammatory and other immunocompromised conditions such as leprosy. This study has tried to bridge the gap of information on cytokine gene polymorphisms and its potential role in the pathogenesis of leprosy. Interleukin-10 (IL-10) is an immunosuppressive cytokine, found to be elevated in leprosy that accounted for the suppression of host's immune system by regulating the functions of other immune cells. T helper cells and T regulatory (Tregs) cells are the major source of IL-10 in lepromatous leprosy patients. In this study, we have documented the association of IL-10 cytokine gene polymorphism with the disease progression. A total of 132 lepromatous leprosy patients and 120 healthy controls were analyzed for IL-10 cytokine gene polymorphisms using PCR-SSP assay and flow cytometry was used to analyze IL-10 secretion by CD4 and Tregs in various genotype of leprosy patients. The frequencies of IL-10 (-819) TT and IL-10 (-1082) GG genotypes were significantly higher in leprosy patients as compared to healthy controls. This observation advocates that these genotypes were associated with the susceptibility and development of the disease. In addition, flow cytometry analysis demonstrated an increased number of IL-10 producing CD4 and Treg cells in IL-10 (819) TT genotype compared to CT and CC genotypes. These observations were further supported by immunohistochemical studies. Therefore, we can conclude that IL-10 cytokine gene polymorphisms by affecting its production can determine the predilection and progression of leprosy in the study population.

Keywords: cytokines, gene polymorphisms, leprosy, interleukin-10, regulatory T-cells, helper T-cells

INTRODUCTION

Leprosy is a bacterial disease caused by *Mycobacterium leprae* (*M. leprae*), which mainly affects macrophages and Schwann cells from the peripheral nerves. It offers an ideal model to study the host pathogen interaction and immune dysregulation in human because each clinical form of the disease is accompanied with the diverse levels of immunological alterations during

M. leprae infection (1). Leprosy disease is mainly classified into two forms, paucibacillary (PB) and multibacillary (MB). PB pole is associated with a strong cell-mediated immunity (CMI), and it is relatively resistant to the pathogens and localized infections. While, MB pole is characterized by the defective cell-mediated immune response comprising foamy macrophages in the dermis due to very high number of bacilli accompanied with the lesions all over the body parts. In between two poles of the disease, borderline forms of tuberculoid and lepromatous disease are laid which are immunologically unstable (2–4).

Cytokines play a vital role in activating host-pathogen interaction and in the immunopathogenesis of leprosy (2). PB form of the disease commencement correlates with Th1 (IL-2, IL-12, TNF-α, IFN-γ) cytokines with a localized infection but vigorous cell mediated immune response; whereas, MB form is associated with a Th2 and Th3 cytokine (IL-10, TGF-β, IL-4) response, presence of local skin lesions, prominent antibody production, but very weak CMI response (5). IL-10 and TGF-β appeared as the sole factor puts forth an anti-proliferative effect on Th1 and Th2 cells by perturbing the differentiation of either Th1 or Th2 cells and inhibition of pro-inflammatory cytokine production, that eventually result into the progression of Th3 immune response (6, 7). Our laboratory have previously reported the association of increased levels of IL-10 in lepromatous leprosy patients with high bacterial load of *M. leprae* and suppressed immune system of the host (2, 6). Furthermore, an increased frequency of IL-35 producing Tregs was observed in lepromatous leprosy patients, which is associated with the disease severity (8). Treg cells plays vital role in leprosy pathogenesis and fate of these cells also depends on cytokine milieu. This is supported from our previous study that explored the changes in the plasticity of Tregs under the influence of IL-12 and IL-23 treatment (9). Besides Tregs, another immunosuppressive population of γδ T cells plays an important role in the pathogenesis of leprosy (10, 11). IL-10, secreted by monocytes/macrophage, T cell subsets (Th2, Tregs) and B regulatory cells shows immune regulatory effects in case of human leprosy (12). IL-10-producing regulatory B cells transformed T effector cells into Tregs, thus enhanced regulatory T cells functions in human leprosy. Also, high levels of IL-10 are reported in lepromatous polar form compared with tuberculoid polar form and a low TNF-α/IL-10 ratio was found associated with disease progression (13). Single nucleotide polymorphisms (SNPs) are thought to be one of the most abundant causes of genomic variation in humans. The presence of SNPs in a gene can create differences in the structure and functions of a coded protein (14). Some SNPs are vital for the susceptibility and outcome of leprosy (13). Studies on IL-10 gene polymorphisms at −819 and −1082 positions within the promoter region have shown disease susceptibility and resistance between populations (15–17). Reports suggests that polymorphisms of the IL-10 promoters at positions −1082 (G/A), −819 (C/T), and −592 (C/A) are associated with the resistance against leprosy in Brazilian (18), Indian groups (15) and Columbian population (19).

Although cytokine gene polymorphism is associated with the susceptibility and resistance of a disease, but its association with cytokine production is not well studied. Therefore, the goal of current study is to investigate the association of IL-10 cytokine gene polymorphisms with Th and Treg cells mediated production of IL-10 and its association with the susceptibility and progression of leprosy in Indian population.

MATERIALS AND METHODS

Patients and Controls

A total of 132 leprosy patients (71 males, 61 females) with bacteriological index (BI) 2–6 and 120 healthy controls were recruited from Department of Dermatovenerology, AIIMS, New Delhi, India (**Table 1**). The study was approved by the Institute Ethics Committee, All India Institute of Medical Sciences (AIIMS), New Delhi. Patients and age matched healthy volunteers were recruited after obtaining their informed consent. All patients were without any history of mycobacterial, HIV or any other infection and belonging to the same geographical region as the patients were included and healthy controls.

Genotyping of SNPs for Cytokine Genes

Ten milliliters blood from each leprosy patients and healthy control was collected. 5 mL of blood in heparinized vials were subjected to DNA isolation and PCR-SSP assay, while and another 5 ml collected for IL-10 ELISA and flowcytometry. DNA was extracted by using phenol–chloroform method and stored at −80°C till further use. DNA was quantified by NanoDrop1000 spectrophotometer (Thermo Scientific NanoDrop 1000; NanoDrop Technologies, Wilmington, DE, United States) and samples having 260/280 ratio in the range of 1.82–1.86 were used for the PCR-SSP analysis. Subsequently, DNA was subjected to PCR amplification using Cytokine CTS-PCR-SSP Tray Kit (Heidelberg, Germany, United Kingdom) according to manufacturer's instructions and data was analyzed as described in earlier report (16) (**Supplementary Figure S1**).

ELISA

IL-10 cytokine level was quantified by ELISA (Ready Set Go, eBioscience, San Diego, CA, United States) as per manufacturer's instructions. Serum samples were tested in duplicates in a 96-wells plate (Nunc, Rochester, NY, United States) precoated with biotin conjugated anti-human antibodies IL-10. Protocol was followed according to the manufacturer's instructions and optical density of each well was measured at 450 nm.

TABLE 1 | Characteristics of the study population.

	Leprosy patients (*n* = 132)	Controls (*n* = 120)
Age (years)	***n* (%)**	***n* (%)**
Mean	38.4 ± 15.3	32.2 ± 13.1
Gender		
Male	71 (53.8)	74 (61.7)
Female	61 (46.2)	46 (38.3)

Leprosy patients were classified according to Ridley–Jopling classification.

PBMCs Isolation and Flow Cytometry

Blood samples were layered on ficoll-hypaque (Sigma Aldrich, United States), and mononuclear cells were isolated by centrifugation at 1,500 rpm for 25 min. Cells were washed thrice in sterile phosphate buffer saline (PBS) by centrifugation at 1,500 rpm for 10 min. Washed cells were resuspended in RPMI 1640 along with 10% fetal calf serum (Gibco, CA, United States) and cell viability and enumeration were estimated by 0.2% trypan blue using hemocytometer. 1×10^6 cells/ml were stimulated with *M. leprae* sonicated antigen (10 μg/ml) kindly provided by Dr. P. J. Brennan of Colorado State University. All the cultures were stimulated with IL-2, anti-CD3/CD28. After stimulation, cultures were incubated in 5% CO_2 incubator at 37°C for 48 h. After 48 h, cultured cells were harvested and stained with surface antibodies Alexa Fluor 488 Mouse Anti-Human CD4 (RPA-T4), APC-Cy7 Mouse Anti-Human CD25 (Clone: M-A251) for 60 min at 4°C in the dark. After surface staining, cells were incubated with intracellular staining buffer for 15 min at room temperature; cells were washed twice and permeabilized with 1X permeabilization buffer (eBioscience, United States) 30 min at room temperature. The cells were washed twice, resuspended in staining buffer, and incubated with PE Rat Anti-Human IL-10 (Clone: JES3-19F1). Staining was performed according to the specifications of the manufacturer. All the antibodies were obtained from BD Biosciences, San Diego, CA, United States. The cells were fixed in 400 μl of 2% paraformaldehyde and stored at 4°C. For intracellular staining, cultures were incubated with Protein Transport Inhibitor containing Monensin (BD Golgi Stop) for 4 h prior to harvest to block the secretion of cytokines. The data were collected using FACS Canto flow cytometer (BD Biosciences, United States) and analyzed cytometry along with isotype controls of phycoerythrin (PE mouse IgG1), Alexa Fluor 488 (mouse IgG1), APC Cy7 (mouse IgG1) using FlowJo software. Details of gating strategy are provided in **Supplementary Figure S2**.

Immunohistochemistry (IHC)

Five micrometer thick formalin fixed paraffin embedded tissues were cut by rotary microtome (Leica Biosystems Nussloch, Germany, United Kingdom). The sections were picked-up on poly L-lysine (Sigma Aldrich, St. Louis, MO, United States) coated glass slides and stored at room temperature. Rabbit anti human IL-10 antibody (Abcam, CA, United Kingdom) was used in the dilution of 1:100. Briefly, sections were first deparaffinized, followed by rehydration and blocking of endogenous peroxidase activity by 3% H_2O_2 and antigen-retrieval with Tris-EDTA (pH-9.0) buffer. The sections were incubated with 1% albumin for 1 h for blocking. After three washes with PBS, sections were incubated with anti-human IL-10 overnight at 4°C in humidified chamber. The sections were again subjected to three washes of PBS followed by incubation with secondary antibody anti rabbit IgG (VECTASTAIN® ABC-HRP Kit) for 30 min. Color was developed using diaminobenzidine (DAB1) chromogen system. Positive and negative stained cells were counted under the microscope using Image Pro express 6.0 software (Media cybernetics, United States) and percentage calculated from multiple fields.

Statistical Analysis

Genotype frequencies were obtained through direct counting. Data was analyzed using statistical software Graph-Pad Prism (San Diego, CA, United States). All categorical variables were expressed in n (%) and continuous variables were expressed in Mean ± SD. ANOVA was applied to compare the continuous variables between multiple groups; whereas t-test was applied to compare the two groups. Proportions of categorical variables among groups were compared using chi-Square test. Logistic regression analysis was used to calculate the Odds Ratio (OR). A p-value of <0.05 was considered to be statistically significant.

RESULTS

Association Between IL-10 (-819) CT/TT Genotypes With Leprosy Susceptibility

Mutations occurred more often in the IL-10 (anti-inflammatory cytokine) promoter gene than in the TNF-α (pro-inflammatory) promoter gene in all leprosy groups (18). Genotype distribution for IL-10 −819 (*C/T at −819: rs1800871*) are shown in **Table 2**. A significantly higher frequency of −819 TT genotype was observed in leprosy patients (59.8%) as compared to healthy controls (27.5%) ($p < 0.0001$, OR = 0.25, 95% CI 0.149–0.432). Contrasting to this, leprosy patients (7.6%) had significantly lower frequency of −819 CC genotype than the control subjects (20.8%) ($p = 0.002$, OR = 3.21, 95% CI 1.47–7.01). Genotype distribution analysis also revealed that 32.6% of leprosy patients and 51.7% of control subjects had −819 CT genotype ($p = 0.002$, OR = 2.21, 95% CI 1.31–3.68). These results demonstrate that substitution of C allele by T allele make the individuals susceptible toward the leprosy disease. As shown in **Table 2**, TT genotype has higher bacteriological index (BI: 4.2-6) as compared to the CC genotype (BI: 3-4). These data corelates BI with TT genotypes and pointing out that TT genotypes are susceptible and CC genotypes are resistance toward the *M. leprae* infection.

TABLE 2 | Distribution of IL-10 (*C/T at −819: rs1800871*) genotypes in leprosy patients and control subjects.

SNPs	Genotype	Controls	Patients	BI	OR (*P*-value)	CI
IL10-^{819}	CC	25 (20.8)	10 (7.6)	3.0–4.0	3.21 (0.002**)	1.470–7.011
	CT	62 (51.7)	43 (32.6)	2.5–4.5	2.21 (0.002**)	1.328–3.687
	TT	33 (27.5)	79 (59.8)	4.5–6.0	0.25 (<0.0001****)	0.149–0.432

*χ^2 test with contingency table for genotype between leprosy patients and control subjects, bacteriological index (BI), odds ratio (OR), p** > 0.005; p**** > 0.0005 and confidence interval (CI).*

TABLE 3 | Distribution of IL-10 (*G/A at −1082: rs1800896*) genotypes in leprosy patients and control subjects.

SNPs	Genotype	Controls	Patients	BI	OR (*P*-value)	CI
IL10-^{1082}	GG	11 (9.2)	34 (25.8)	4.8–6.0	0.29 (0.0006***)	0.140–0.605
	GA	49 (40.8)	50 (37.9)	3.0–4.5	1.13 (0.6987)	0.682–1.878
	AA	60 (50.0)	48 (36.5)	2.0–3.2	1.75 (<0.0289*)	1.057–2.897

*χ^2 test with contingency table for genotype between leprosy patients and control subjects, bacteriological index (BI), odds ratio (OR), *p < 0.05; ***p < 0.0005 and confidence interval (CI).*

Association Between IL-10 (-1082) GA/GG Genotypes and Leprosy Susceptibility and Resistance

Notably, a significantly higher frequency of the homozygous −1082 GG (*G/A at −1082: rs1800896*) genotype was observed when leprosy patients were compared with control subjects (25.8 vs. 9.2%) ($p = 0.0006$, OR = 0.29, 95% CI 0.139–0.605). Moreover, frequency of homozygous GA genotype was lower compared between leprosy patients and healthy controls at −1082GA position. We found a lower frequency in patient group (37.9%) compared to control group (40.8%) ($p = 0.698$, OR = 1.13, 95% CI 0.682–1.88). When leprosy patients (36.5%) were compared with controls (50%) at −1082AA position, significant difference was observed ($p = 0.03$, OR = 1.75, 95% CI 1.05–2.89) (**Table 3**). Higher bacteriological index (4.8–6) in GG genotype as compared to AA genotype (2–3.2) indicates its susceptibility toward leprosy as compared to AA genotype that showed resistance.

819TT Genotypes Are Higher Producer of T Helper Cells (CD4$^+$IL-10$^+$) IL-10 in Leprosy Patients

IL-10 is an anti-inflammatory cytokine produced by several immune cells like monocytes and macrophages, T cells, Treg cells as well as Breg cells (20). To find out the association of cytokine gene polymorphism with IL-10 production by T helper cells, we performed flowcytometry using CD4 and IL-10 antibodies. As shown in **Figures 1C,D**, IL-10 production by CD4$^+$ was affected by cytokine gene polymorphism at −819 position. IL-10 levels produced by CD4 cells were significantly higher in TT genotype as compared to CC genotype. CT genotype was also higher producer of IL-10 as compared to CC genotype, but lower than the TT genotype. These results suggest that the substitution of C by T allele does affect the IL-10 production by CD4 cells in leprosy patients. Increased IL-10 levels in serum of TT bearing genotype at IL-10^{-819} position as compared to CC genotype in leprosy patients further complemented these results (**Figures 1A,B**).

Increased Production of IL-10 in −819TT Genotypes by T Regulatory Cells (CD4$^+$CD25$^+$IL-10$^+$) in Leprosy Patients

To identify the frequency of Treg cells in various (CC, CT, TT) genotypes at −819 position in leprosy patients, immunophenotyping was done by using CD4, CD25 markers (**Figure 2A**) in PBMCs isolated from leprosy patients. Treg cells was profoundly augmented in TT genotype as compared to CC and CT genotypes in leprosy patients (**Figures 2A,B**). Increased Treg population in TT genotype patients suggested their important role in the host immune suppression observed in TT genotypes. To evaluate the functional enrichment of Treg cells in various genotypes (CC, CT and TT) in leprosy patients, we measured intracellular IL-10 production by flow cytometry (**Figure 2C**), using PBMCs derived from leprosy patients. Percentage of IL-10 producing Treg cells (CD4 + CD25 +) was significantly higher among TT genotypes in leprosy patients (**Figures 2C,D**) compared to that of CC and CT genotypes of leprosy patients ($P = 0.0003$). The augmentation of IL-10 producing Treg cells in TT genotypes directs their suppressive role by releasing IL-10. We also observed the simmiler pattern of IL-10 production by CD4$^+$CD25$^-$ cells in various genotypes (CC, CT and TT) of leprosy patients (**Figures 2E,F**).

Higher Expression of IL-10 in the Skin of IL-10 (-819) TT Genotype of Leprosy Patients

Expression of the IL-10 also measured in skin of leprosy patients bearing TT and CC genotypes at −819 position. The expression of the IL-10, was also significantly higher in the TT genotypes of leprosy patients as compared to CC genotype (**Figures 3A,B**). This again highlights that IL-10 producing immune cells are possibly recruited at the lesioned sites (which is more in TT genotype) of leprosy patients, where they facilitate their characteristic suppressive action. These results suggested that cytokine gene polymorphism at −819 position are associated with IL-10 production in leprosy patients and makes more susceptible toward leprosy.

DISCUSSION

During leprosy, there is a full-blown systemic activation of immune responses. As a result, leprosy is escorted by altered immune and imbalanced cytokine responses, which ultimately leads to excessive inflammation. Cytokines modulates the immune response of a host but cytokine gene polymorphism affects the cytokine production. This is the underlying reason to the distinct individual-specific immune responses. The idea behind studying the cytokine polymorphism in leprosy patients was: hypothetically a change either in regulatory region (promoter) or coding region is expected to modulate the expression of cytokines. A specific genotype either may result in low or high production of respective cytokine, which in turn could eventually alter the direction of immune response.

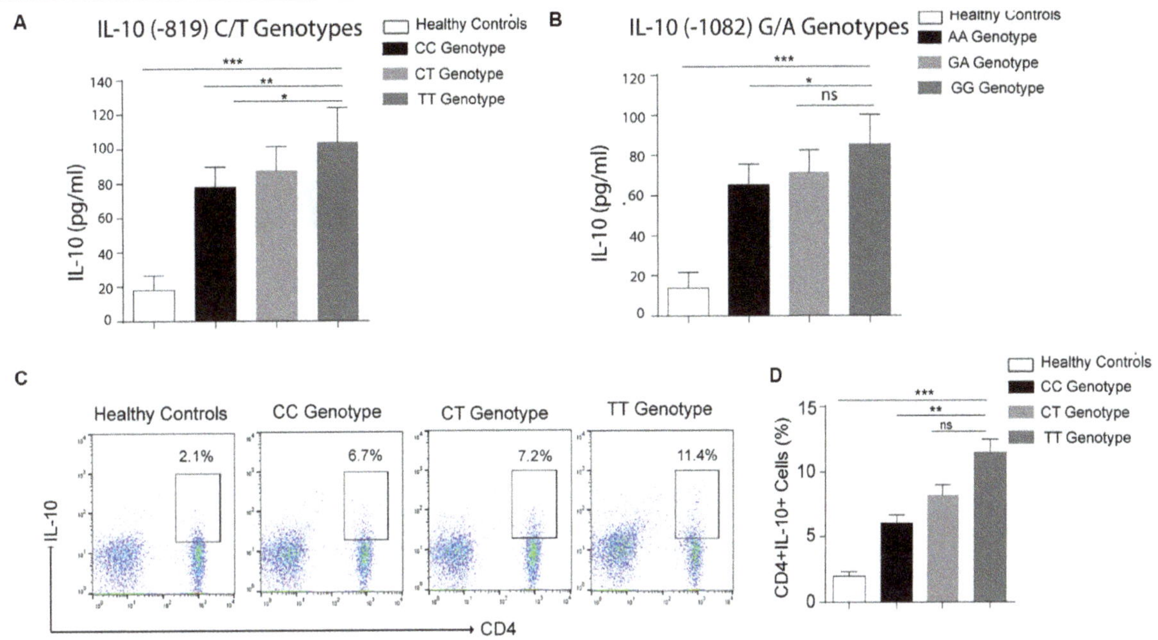

FIGURE 1 | Graph plot is showing IL-10 level in the serum of leprosy patients produced by various genotypes **(A)** Healthy controls (HCs), −819 CC, CT and TT genotypes **(B)** Healthy controls (HCs), 1082 AA, GA, and GG genotypes. **(C)** Representative FACS plot showing enumeration of T helper cell producing IL-10 ($CD4^+IL\text{-}10^+$) frequency in peripheral blood mononuclear cells isolated from leprosy patients with various genotypes (-819CC, CT and TT) and healthy controls (HCs) cultured with *M. leprae* sonicated antigen for 48 h. **(D)** Graph Plots are showing total interleukin-10 (IL-10) producing $CD4^+$ cells by various genotype (-819CC, CT and TT) in leprosy patients ($n = 10$) and healthy controls (HCs),Mean ± SD values are shown in each set while p value <0.05 was considered significant. 100,000 cells were acquired and analyzed by flow cytometry. Data analysis was performed with flowjo software. Statistical analysis was done using ANOVA test ($^*p < 0.05$; $^{**}p < 0.005$; $^{***}p < 0.0005$).

Increased IL-10 production has been observed in leprosy patients and up-regulation of IL-10 is a vital mechanism in the suppression of T cell-driven immune response (21). SNPs in IL-10 in the distal and the proximal regions are formed of haplotypes in the promoter gene, and such haplotypes were found to be associated with differential secretion of IL-10 cytokine (22). Our present data demonstrates that IL-10 −819 TT genotype frequency was greater among the leprosy patients than the control subjects. Frequency of GG genotype at IL-10 −1082 position was also higher in the leprosy patients as compared to healthy control. These results corroborate with our previous findings (16) and it has also been reported that the individuals in Brazilian population bearing IL10 −819 CC genotype were resistant to leprosy (18). Our results are further confirming the results of earlier findings that −819T allele and −819TT genotype were associated with leprosy susceptibility (17) in Indian population. These findings suggested that substitution of C by T at −819 in IL-10 promotor may be involved in differential cell mediated immune response in leprosy patients. It may also influence on the production of IL-10 levels as well as makes the individual susceptible toward leprosy. Moreover, a study by Malhotra et al. (17) suggested that −819TT and −1082GG are the most frequent genotype associated with susceptibility of leprosy. In our study, homozygous IL-10 −1082 GG genotype was significantly higher in leprosy patients compared to the controls, due to the predominance of G allele suggesting an impact for allele G in leprosy susceptibility. Similar findings have been observed by other groups, where they found that the extended genotype 1082GG, 819TT was associated with leprosy susceptibility (15). Moreover, another study by Pereira et al. demonstrated that −1082G/G genotype reinforced the results, indicating that the combination carrying −819TT and −1082G/G was associated with leprosy susceptibility (23).

To evaluate the association of cytokine gene polymorphism on its function, we tested leprosy patients and quantified IL-10 levels in various genotype −819 C/T and −1082 G/A. We observed elevated levels of IL-10 in −819TT and −1082GG genotypes in the serum of leprosy patients as compared to other genotypes. Thus, −819TT and −1082GG bearing genotypes were high IL-10 producers. These findings brought up a new direction to understand the pathogenesis of leprosy. These sustained high levels of IL-10 are necessary to lead leprosy to a chronic and T cells unresponsive state. Leprosy patient presents a state where genetic mosaicism is associated with cytokine production that dictates various immune reactions, resulting to ambiguous interpretations linked with the different clinical outcomes. IL-10 produced by various immune cells such as Tregs, Th2, Bregs and other cells suppresses the immune system of host and responsible for T cell anergy in leprosy patients (24–26). We want to address the source of IL-10 production by various genotypes in leprosy patients. To answer this, we have evaluated the expression of IL-10 in T helper and Treg cells of leprosy patients. Remarkably, IL-10 −819 TT and IL-10 −1082 GG genotypes were

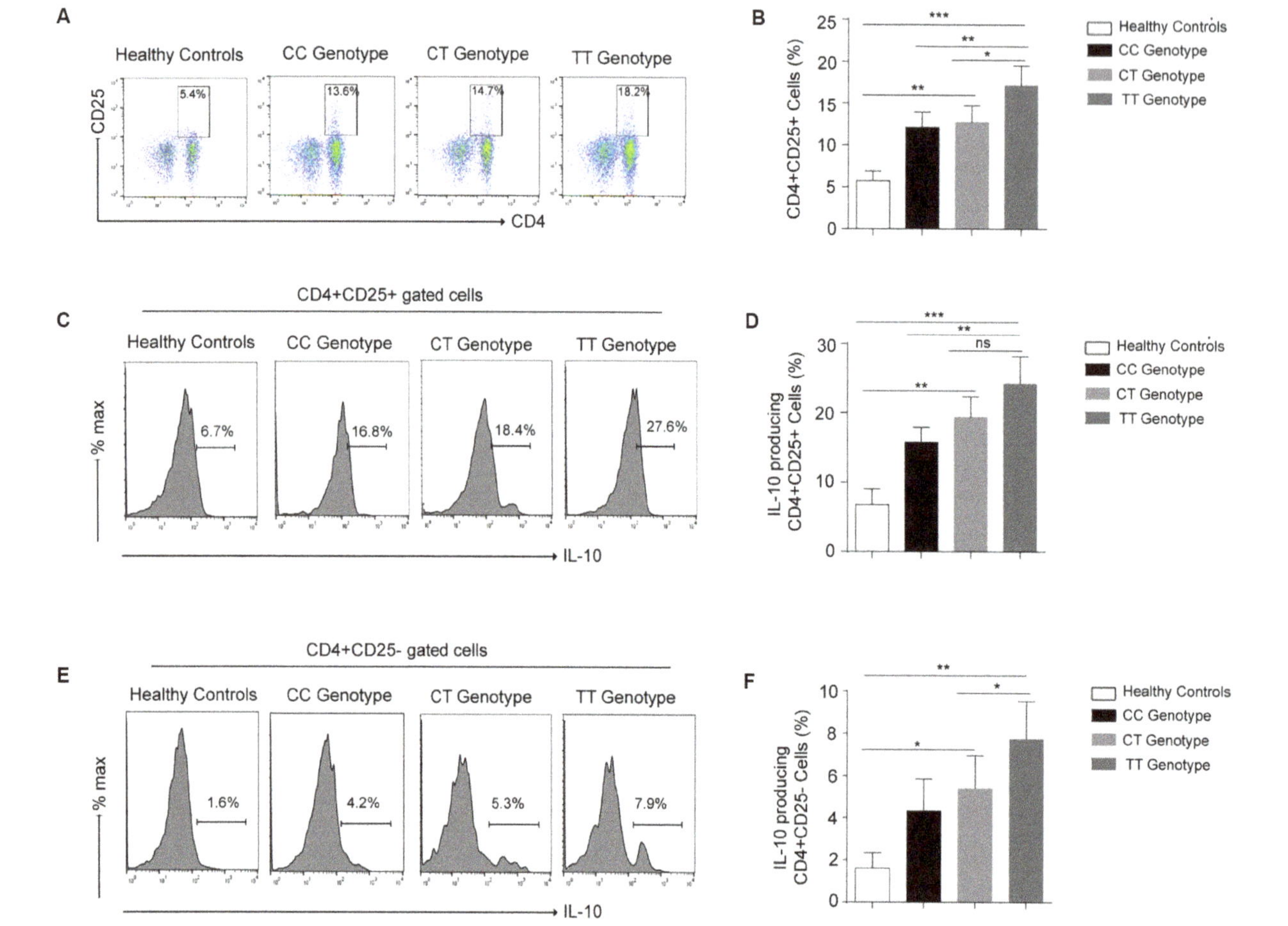

FIGURE 2 | (A) Representative cartoon showing T regulatory cells ($CD4^+CD25^+$) cells in peripheral blood mononuclear cells (PBMCs) isolated from peripheral blood of various genotypes (-819CC, CT and TT) of leprosy patient (n = 10) and healthy controls (HCs). **(B)** Graph plot is showing the percentage of T regulatory cells ($CD4^+CD25^+$) in various genotypes (-819CC, CT and TT) in leprosy patients and healthy controls (HCs). **(C)** Representative histogram showing expression of IL-10 in Treg ($CD4^+CD25^+$) cells in PBMCs isolated from peripheral blood of various genotypes of leprosy patient and healthy controls (HCs). **(D)** Graph plot is showing expression of IL-10 in Tregs in leprosy patients by various genotype and healthy controls (HCs). **(E)** Representative histogram showing secreation of IL-10 by ($CD4^+CD25^-$) cells in PBMCs isolated from peripheral blood of various genotypes of leprosy patient and healthy controls (HCs). **(F)** Graph plot is showing production of IL-10 by ($CD4^+CD25^-$) cells in leprosy patients by various genotype and healthy controls (HCs). Mean ± SD values are shown in each set while p value <0.05 was considered significant. 100,000 cells were acquired and analyzed by flow cytometry. Data analysis was performed with flowjo software. Statistical analysis was done using ANOVA test ($^*p < 0.05$; $^{**}p < 0.005$; $^{***}p < 0.0005$).

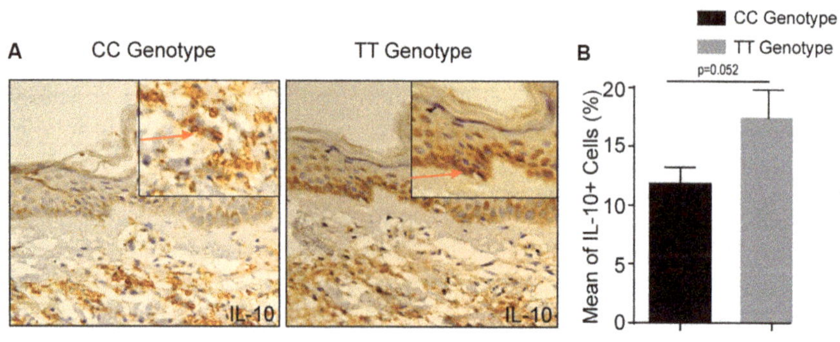

FIGURE 3 | (A) Increased IL-10 + cells in −819TT genotype in leprosy skin lesions. Immunohistochemistry on representative skin lesions from CC and TT genotypes of leprosy patients (n = 5). **(B)** Graph diagram showing increase of cells with $IL\text{-}10^+$ in TT genotype of leprosy patients as compared to CC genotype at −819 position. Bars indicate Mean ± SD of positive cells of 1,000 total cells. Statistical analysis was done using Student's t-test for unpaired samples ($^*p < 0.05$).

appeared as high producer of IL-10 by T helper as well as T regulatory cells. Increased level of IL-10 was found to be logical and supported our previous reports (12, 16). This data designates that high amount of IL-10 in the microenvironment suppresses the host immune system, that eventually may help in expansion of *M. leprae* continually in leprosy patients, as high bacteriological index correlates with high level of IL-10 in −819TT and −1082 GG genotypes. Therefore, it can be inferred here that the patients with −819TT and −1082 GG genotypes are bearing higher risks of the growth of *M. leprae.*

Since leprosy is a chronic inflammatory disease and its severity is associated to the host immune response, and the level of IL-10 production can be vital to define disease outcome. Our data point-outs the conclusive association of the −819TT and −1082 GG genotypes with the susceptibility of leprosy and suggests that these polymorphisms have remarkable role in higher production of IL-10 by T helper and T regulatory cells.

ETHICS STATEMENT

The studies involving human participants were reviewed and approved by The Institute Ethics Committee, All India Institute of Medical Sciences (AIIMS), New Delhi, India (IESC/T-417/01.11.2013). The patients/participants provided their written informed consent to participate in this study.

AUTHOR CONTRIBUTIONS

MT, HN, and CS designed experiments. MT, HS, and CS performed experiments and analyzed the data. MT, HN, and MS wrote the manuscript. NK contributed to clinical diagnosis. AS, HS, and CS critically reviewed the manuscript. All authors discussed the results and contributed to the final manuscript and reviewed manuscript.

REFERENCES

1. Ridley DS, Jopling WH. Classification of leprosy according to immunity. A five-group system. *Int J Lepr Other Mycobact Dis.* (1966) 34:255–73.
2. Tarique M, Saini C, Naz H, Naqvi RA, Khan FI, Sharma A. Fate of T cells and their secretory proteins during the progression of leprosy. *Curr Protein Pept Sci.* (2018) 19:889–99. doi: 10.2174/1389203718666170829120729
3. Saini C, Tarique M, Rai R, Siddiqui A, Khanna N, Sharma A. T helper cells in leprosy: an update. *Immunol Lett.* (2017) 184:61–6. doi: 10.1016/j.imlet.2017.02.013
4. Yamamura M, Uyemura K, Deans RJ, Weinberg K, Rea TH, Bloom BR, et al. Defining protective responses to pathogens: cytokine profiles in leprosy lesions. *Science.* (1991) 254:277–9. doi: 10.1126/science.1925582
5. Alcais A, Mira M, Casanova JL, Schurr E, Abel L. Genetic dissection of immunity in leprosy. *Curr Opin Immunol.* (2005) 17:44–8. doi: 10.1016/j.coi.2004.11.006
6. Kumar S, Naqvi RA, Khanna N, Pathak P, Rao DN. Th3 immune responses in the progression of leprosy via molecular cross-talks of TGF-beta. CTLA-4 and Cbl-b. *Clin Immunol.* (2011) 141:133–42. doi: 10.1016/j.clim.2011.06.007
7. Saini C, Ramesh V, Nath I. Increase in TGF-beta secreting CD4(+)CD25(+) FOXP3(+) T regulatory cells in anergic lepromatous leprosy patients. *PLoS Negl Trop Dis.* (2014) 8:e2639. doi: 10.1371/journal.pntd.0002639
8. Tarique M, Saini C, Naqvi RA, Khanna N, Rao DN. Increased IL-35 producing Tregs and CD19(+)IL-35(+) cells are associated with disease progression in leprosy patients. *Cytokine.* (2017) 91:82–8. doi: 10.1016/j.cyto.2016.12.011
9. Tarique M, Saini C, Naqvi RA, Khanna N, Sharma A, Rao DN. IL-12 and IL-23 modulate plasticity of FoxP3(+) regulatory T cells in human Leprosy. *Mol Immunol.* (2017) 83:72–81. doi: 10.1016/j.molimm.2017.01.008
10. Saini C, Tarique M, Ramesh V, Khanna N, Sharma A. Gammadelta T cells are associated with inflammation and immunopathogenesis of leprosy reactions. *Immunol Lett.* (2018) 200:55–65. doi: 10.1016/j.imlet.2018.07.005
11. Tarique M, Naqvi RA, Ali R, Khanna N, Rao DN. CD4(+) TCRgammadelta(+) FoxP3(+) cells: an unidentified population of immunosuppressive cells towards disease progression leprosy patients. *Exp Dermatol.* (2017) 26:946–8. doi: 10.1111/exd.13302
12. Tarique M, Naz H, Kurra SV, Chaman S, Raza AN, Reeta R, et al. Interleukin-10 producing regulatory B cells transformed CD4(+)CD25(-) into tregs and enhanced regulatory T Cells function in human leprosy. *Front Immunol.* (2018) 9:1636. doi: 10.3389/fimmu.2018.01636
13. Cardoso CC, Pereira AC, De Sales Marques C, Moraes MO. Leprosy susceptibility: genetic variations regulate innate and adaptive immunity, and disease outcome. *Future Microbiol.* (2011) 6:533–49. doi: 10.2217/fmb.11.39
14. Suh Y, Vijg J. SNP discovery in associating genetic variation with human disease phenotypes. *Mutat Res.* (2005) 573:41–53. doi: 10.1016/j.mrfmmm.2005.01.005
15. Moraes MO, Pacheco AG, Schonkeren JJ, Vanderborght PR, Nery JAC, Santos AR, et al. Interleukin-10 promoter single-nucleotide polymorphisms as markers for disease susceptibility and disease severity in leprosy. *Genes Immun.* (2004) 5:592–5. doi: 10.1038/sj.gene.6364122
16. Tarique M, Naqvi RA, Santosh KV, Kamal VK, Khanna N, Rao DN. Association of TNF-alpha-(308(GG)), IL-10(-819(TT)), IL-10(-1082(GG)) and IL-1R1(+1970(CC)) genotypes with the susceptibility and progression of leprosy in North Indian population. *Cytokine.* (2015) 73:61–5. doi: 10.1016/j.cyto.2015.01.014
17. Malhotra D, Darvishi K, Sood S, Swarkar S, Chander G, Vineet R, et al. IL-10 promoter single nucleotide polymorphisms are significantly associated with resistance to leprosy. *Hum Genet.* (2005) 118:295–300. doi: 10.1007/s00439-005-0042-8
18. Santos AR, Suffys PN, Vanderborght PR, Milton OM, Leila MMV, Pedro HC, et al. Role of tumor necrosis factor-alpha and interleukin-10 promoter gene polymorphisms in leprosy. *J Infect Dis.* (2002) 186:1687–91. doi: 10.1086/345366
19. Cardona-Castro N, Sanchez-Jimenez M, Rojas W, Bedoya-Berrio G. IL-10 gene promoter polymorphisms and leprosy in a Colombian population sample. *Biomedica.* (2012) 32:71–6. doi: 10.7705/biomedica.v32i1.386
20. Okeke EB, Uzonna JE. The pivotal role of regulatory T cells in the regulation of innate immune cells. *Front Immunol.* (2019) 10:680. doi: 10.3389/fimmu.2019.00680
21. Misra N, Selvakumar M, Singh S, Bharadwaj M, Ramesh V, Misra RS, et al. Monocyte derived IL 10 and PGE2 are associated with the absence of Th 1 cells and in vitro T cell suppression in lepromatous leprosy. *Immunol Lett.* (1995) 48:123–8. doi: 10.1016/0165-2478(95)02455-7
22. Gibson AW, Edberg JC, Wu J, Westendorp RG, Huizinga TW, Kimberly RP. Novel single nucleotide polymorphisms in the distal IL-10 promoter affect IL-10 production and enhance the risk of systemic lupus erythematosus. *J Immunol.* (2001) 166:3915–22. doi: 10.4049/jimmunol.166.6.3915
23. Pereira AC, Brito-de-Souza VN, Cardoso CC, Dias-Baptista IMF, Parelli FPC, Venturini J, et al. Genetic, epidemiological and biological analysis of interleukin-10 promoter single-nucleotide polymorphisms suggests a definitive role for −819C/T in leprosy susceptibility. *Genes Immun.* (2009) 10:174–80. doi: 10.1038/gene.2008.97
24. Stewart CA, Metheny H, Iida N, Loretta S, Miranda H, Folkert S, et al. Interferon-dependent IL-10 production by Tregs limits tumor Th17 inflammation. *J Clin Invest.* (2013) 123:4859–74. doi: 10.1172/JCI65180

16

Recombinant Influenza Vaccines: Saviors to Overcome Immunodominance

*Nimitha R. Mathew and Davide Angeletti**

Department of Microbiology and Immunology, Institute of Biomedicine, University of Gothenburg, Gothenburg, Sweden

***Correspondence:**
Davide Angeletti
davide.angeletti@gu.se

It has been almost a decade since the 2009 influenza A virus pandemic hit the globe causing significant morbidity and mortality. Nonetheless, annual influenza vaccination, which elicits antibodies mainly against the head region of influenza hemagglutinin (HA), remains as the mainstay to combat and reduce symptoms of influenza infection. Influenza HA is highly antigenically variable, thus limiting vaccine efficacy. In addition, the variable HA head occupies the upper strata of the immunodominance hierarchy, thereby clouding the antibody response toward subdominant epitopes, which are usually conserved across different influenza strains. Isolation of monoclonal antibodies from individuals recognizing such epitopes has facilitated the development of recombinant vaccines that focus the adaptive immune response toward conserved, protective targets. Here, we review some significant leaps in recombinant vaccine development, which could possibly help to overcome B cell and antibody immunodominance and provide heterosubtypic immunity to influenza A virus.

Keywords: influenza A virus, immunodominance, vaccines, B cells, antibodies

INTRODUCTION

Influenza viruses belong to the family of Orthomyxoviridae and consists of A, B, C, and D types. Types A and B are currently circulating among humans (1–4). Influenza causes significant morbidity (30–50 million cases yearly) and mortality, with infection-associated respiratory deaths in the range of 4–8.8 per 100,000 individuals, posing heavy socioeconomic burden to society (5). Annual vaccination remains as the mainstay to prevent influenza infection, but, according to Centers for Disease Control and Prevention, it is effective only in 20–70% of the population, depending on season (6). Based on antigenic and phylogenetic properties of influenza surface glycoproteins, hemagglutinin (HA), and neuraminidase (NA), there are 18 HA (H1–H18), and 11 NA (N1–N11) Influenza A virus (IAV) serotypes and two influenza B of B/Victoria and B/Yamagata lineages (7, 8). HA is further divided into two phylogenetic groups. The current seasonal flu vaccines are either trivalent or quadrivalent containing HA from circulating H1N1, H3N2, and B/Victoria lineage or both influenza B lineages (9). IAV possess an error prone RNA polymerase, which results in mutations in surface antigens, leading to antigenic drift and antibodies being no longer effective. Therefore, it is necessary to update and administer vaccines every year by forecasting the drifted strains. In addition, the annual vaccination becomes ineffective during pandemic outbreaks, in which a new viral strain of zoonotic origin acquires the ability to replicate in humans (10, 11).

HA is the most abundant glycoprotein on the influenza virion surface and is crucial for host viral entry by binding to the terminal sialic acid residues on epithelial cells, resulting in fusion of viral and host cell membranes. HA is a trimer consisting of a globular head, harboring the receptor binding site, and an elongated stem region (12). Even though stem-specific B cells and antibodies are generated during infection and vaccination, the HA head is the main target of neutralizing antibodies. However, possibly due to its immunodominance (13), the head is subjected to higher rate of evolution (2.2–4.4 times) than the stem (14, 15). Intriguingly, while in animals, at least 12 mutations are necessary to drive full escape from immune sera (16), in humans, it appears that the polyclonal response can be extremely focused on one antigenic site (17–19). For example, in a circulating span of 35 years in humans, a single amino acid substitution at only seven sites in HA head beside the receptor binding site (RBS) was enough to drive major antigenic change in H3N2 (17, 20). HA stem, as a target for universal influenza vaccine, has gained enormous traction in recent years. One could argue that the stem region is inaccessible to B cells and antibodies (21). However, a study using a broad neutralizing antibody showed that nearly 75% of the HA on pandemic H1N1 is bound by a stem-specific mAb (22). There is an urgent need to introduce universal vaccines, targeting conserved regions and providing lifelong protection. This review focuses on possible strategies for developing universal influenza vaccines, mainly based on HA. Such strategies are summarized in **Figure 1**.

HEMAGGLUTININ STEM—A PROMISING UNIVERSAL VACCINE TARGET

HA stem has been an important candidate for development of universal vaccines because the stalk region is relatively conserved and evolves much slower and accommodate less amino acid substitutions as compared to the head domain. This could be due to minimal antibody pressure from low amount of circulating anti-stem antibodies (23, 24) and low tolerance to mutations in the stalk domain, which can lead to loss of viral fitness (25, 26), even though partial escape mutations in the stem can be generated (27). However, amino acid substitutions in the stalk have been reported to minimally affect the neutralization capacity of human cross-reactive, anti-stalk monoclonal antibodies (14, 28).

HA stem antibodies protect by (i) preventing viral entry by blocking the fusion of host cell membrane and viral membrane (29), (ii) reducing viral egress by blocking neuraminidase activity through steric hindrance (30–32), and (iii) FcR-mediated induction of antibody-dependent cellular cytotoxicity (ADCC), antibody-dependent cellular phagocytosis and reactive oxygen species production (33–35). Several human-derived broadly neutralizing anti-stem antibodies have been identified against either influenza group 1 (36–39) or group 2 (38, 40–42) or both groups (40, 43–50) or even against both influenza A and B subtypes (51). The identification of these antibodies was an incentive to develop vaccines, which are discussed below.

HEMAGGLUTININ STEM—HUMAN IMMUNE RESPONSES

In humans, memory B cells (Bmem), and antibodies against HA stem are subdominant and present in low levels. Analysis of serum samples from 202 healthy individuals collected between 2004 and 2010 revealed that anti-stem antibodies of group 1 specificity is found in 84% of the population (52); however, their level, as measured in human Intravenous Immunoglobulin preparations, is very low (23).

Ellebedy and colleagues (53) found that immunization with H5N1, which is not currently circulating in humans, boosted cross-reactive antibody response toward HA stem, when compared to seasonal vaccines. Because of the existence of lower levels of H5 head-specific Bmem as compared to stem-specific Bmem, H5N1 vaccination led to recruitment of stem-specific Bmem, their expansion, and antibody production. On the contrary, boosting with the same HA favors anti-head responses (53). Another study found that nearly 6 out of 10 individuals have Bmem specific between group 1 and 2 HA (50). Indeed, it appears that baseline levels of H5-H1 cross-reactive Bmem and H1-specific Bmem are no more than 2-fold different (54). However, after priming with an H5 DNA plasmid vaccine and boosting with A/Indonesia/05/2005 monovalent-inactivated virus, both head and stem Bmem were expanded but only head-specific Bmem persisted, while stem-specific Bmem expanded and contracted rapidly (50, 54). Finally, Andrews et al. observed that immunization with group 1 virus (H5N1) elicited anti-stem memory responses exclusively against group 1, while group 2 (H7N9) induced high levels of cross-protective anti-stem memory B cell responses with diverse repertoire despite a lower overall response. This study in humans suggests the potential of group 2 based vaccines to provide a broader protection as compared to group 1 (55). While all these studies highlight the ability of individuals to generate stem-specific Bmem and plasmablasts, they all note a rapid contraction of stem-specific cells. This disconnect between cell numbers, longevity, and serum antibodies highlight the complexity of B-cell fate decision. Understanding how antigen specificity can influence cell differentiation is a crucial challenge for next generation vaccines.

SITES OF VULNERABILITY IN HEMAGGLUTININ HEAD

Although HA stem is an excellent candidate for the development of universal vaccines, anti-HA stem titers in human correlates only with reduced viral shedding but do not predict the severity of influenza infection (56, 57). A recent study in humans indicated that a 2-fold increase in hemagglutination inhibition titer gave a 23.4% reduction in H1N1 infection risk, while the same increase in HA-stem-specific antibodies conferred only 14.2% reduction (58).

The globular head of the HA is target for most of the neutralizing antibodies, which prevents the viral entry by

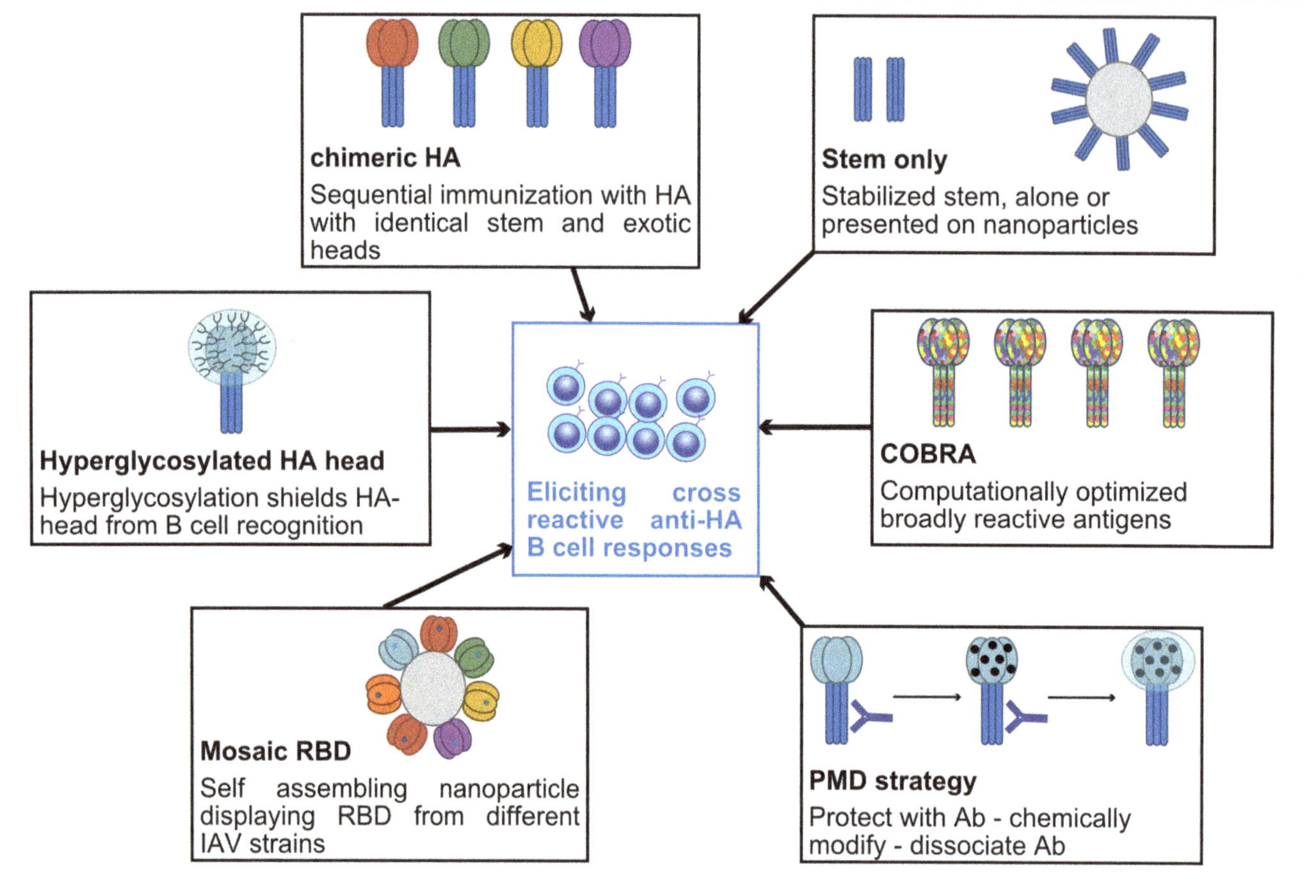

FIGURE 1 | Summary of some promising strategies currently used to elicit broadly cross-reactive anti-HA B-cell responses.

blocking the binding of RBS to sialic acid residues on host cell membrane (59). RBS is a shallow depression on HA head and consists of 130 loop, 150 loop, 190 helix, which are relatively conserved, and 220 loop, which is diverse among IAV subtypes (60, 61). Amino acid substitutions in the RBS determine host tropism, and specific substitutions are connected to altered receptor binding within subtype (62). Some RBS binding, broadly neutralizing antibodies have been identified, such as C05, S139/1, and F045-092, which neutralize within groups; CH65, 5J8, 2G1, and H5.3, which neutralize within subtype (63–71); and C12G6 and CR8033, which neutralize both influenza B lineages (51, 72).

Apart from RBS, broadly neutralizing antibodies have been identified against other conserved sites on HA head (73). An antibody (F005-126) which neutralizes 12 H3N2 subtypes by occupying the cleft formed by two HA head monomers and cross-linking them is known to prevent viral entry by blocking pH-induced HA conformational change (74). Bajic et al. found that subdominant antibodies can target an occluded epitope located on the lateral surface on HA head between two monomers using an H3 immunogen, hyperglycosylated on dominant epitopes. These antibodies protected against H3N2 challenge in an Fc-dependent manner (75). Similarly, two independent studies identified broadly neutralizing antibody, which bind hidden epitopes at HA trimer interface. These antibodies do not neutralize the virus but are suspected to disrupt the HA trimer integrity. Passive transfer experiments revealed that they protect mice from groups 1 and 2 viruses by preventing cell-to-cell viral spread or by FcγR or complement mediated effector mechanism (76, 77). HA exhibits "breathing" phenomenon at neutral or low pH where reversible separation of HA monomers exposes hidden epitopes to these specific antibodies (78–80). Vestigeal esterase domain is another possible HA target; it is located at the base of the HA head and can be target of broadly protective antibodies, which protect within subtypes (81, 82) and both lineages of influenza B virus (83). Like stem-directed antibodies, they protect through various mechanisms such as blocking viral egress, fusion, or by ADCC.

For most of the epitopes described above, we are just at the first step of the reverse vaccinology pipeline. However, there is hope that using some advanced *de novo* protein design tools, we will be able to create effective immune-focusing antigens (84, 85).

BIOENGINEERING ANTIGENS TO REFOCUS IMMUNE RESPONSES

Headless Hemagglutinins

One of the obvious ways to increase the anti-stem antibody response is to remove HA head to circumvent its immunodominance (13, 86). Even though this sounds simple, removing the head and the transmembrane domain may cause conformational changes in the stem leading to loss of recognition by anti-stem antibodies (87). One of many successful attempts was achieved by creating stable trimeric mini-HA from H1N1, which retained similar binding affinity to two broadly neutralizing antibodies, CR9114 and CR6261, as that of full-length HA. When used to immunize non-human primates, the elicited antibodies competed with CR9114, induced ADCC, and neutralized H5N1 virus (88). Another study used H1HA10-Foldon and H3HA10-Foldon mini-HA, which generated neutralizing antibodies cross-reactive to both groups 1 and 2 IAV *in vitro* but with limited cross-group protection *in vivo* (89, 90). In contrast to these mini-HAs, an H5-based mini-HA produced and purified from *Escherichia coli* elicited anti-stem antibody responses and protection against both IAV subtypes (91). Pre-existing immunity plays a role in subsequent immune response to viral infection and vaccination (92). When tested in non-human primates who have been exposed to flu infection, mini-HA were shown to induce higher cross-protective antibody response as compared to seasonal trivalent inactivated vaccine, indicating their potential as a universal vaccine (93).

Ferritin is an iron storage protein which self-assembles into a nanoparticle consisting of 24 repetitive polypeptides, which can induce strong immune response and antigen presentation (94). Based on this, Yassine et al. engineered a nanoparticle containing intact HA stem from H1 (H1-ss-np), which generated anti-stem response almost 2-fold higher than that of trivalent inactivated vaccine. When immunized with H1-ss-np, mice and ferrets elicited broad antibody response against group 1 IAV as well as group 2 IAV, demonstrating heterosubtypic protection (95). Based on this, influenza H1 stabilized stem ferritin vaccine (H1ssF_3928) has entered a phase I ongoing clinical trial to evaluate its tolerability and immunogenicity in healthy adults. However, a thermostable and immunogenic nanoparticle vaccine containing group 2 H3 and H7 stem conferred only protection against homosubtypic viral challenge. Given the fact that these stem immunogens activates IgM BCR of unmutated common ancestor of the cross-reactive human anti-stem antibodies, the authors speculate that the lack of cross-group protection *in vivo* might be due to difference in BCR repertoire in mice and human (96).

Chimeric Hemagglutinin

Chimeric HAs (cHA) are full-length HA with stem derived from human viruses and globular head from distinct, exotic HAs. Based on this concept, repeated immunization with cHA with head from different flu subtype and same H1 HA stem induced high titers of stem-reactive antibodies against homologous and heterologous viruses (97). Several such cHA constructs, which confer protection by eliciting stem Abs, have been developed for group 1, group 2, and Influenza B viruses, with some inducing long-lasting antibodies (98–105). An interim report on a clinical trial using a cHA prime boost strategy was recently released (106). In this study, healthy volunteers, with measurable baseline H1-stalk antibody levels, were boosted with cHAs. The sharpest stem-antibody level increase was obtained when challenging with cH8/1N1 in AS03 adjuvant intramuscularly. However, further immunization with other cHA did not additionally boost stem responses. To build upon these promising findings, more studies are needed to assess the longevity of these responses and their stability upon natural infection or seasonal immunization.

Immune-Focusing Strategies

N-linked glycosylation on HA has been known to stabilize HA and shield virus from host immune response (107). Creating monoglycosylated HA or unmasking HA-stem of N-glycans could induce cross-strain neutralizing anti-stem antibodies (108, 109). Conversely, hyperglycosylating the HA head can also refocus response on stem (110). A recent study used "protect, modify, and deprotect" method to focus antibody response toward a stem epitope. In this strategy, after masking target epitope on stem with a monoclonal antibody, the surrounding undesired epitopes are chemically modified to reduce their antigenicity (111). On the other hand, other residues, outside stem, can also influence the neutralizing sensitivity to anti-stem antibodies by affecting HA-stalk stability and antibody access to stem epitopes (112).

Vaccine Engineering for Cross-Protection

Kanekiyo et al. used a ferritin nanoparticle displaying a repetitive array of HA hyper variable receptor binding domains (RBD from different H1N1 strains). Using this, they could subvert B cell response from strain-specific immunodominant epitopes to conserved, shared epitopes. Since cross-reactive B cells can recognize conserved epitope from an heterogenous array of RBD, these cells get preferentially activated due to avidity advantage and could selectively activate pre-existing cross-reactive Bmem. One of the antibodies generated after immunization, 441D6, binds to a conserved epitope, which lies opposite to RBS and protects against H1N1 strains spanning from 1977 to 2009 (113, 114). Anderson et al. generated cross-reactive antibody responses by injecting a mix of DNA vaccines containing HA genes from six members of group 1 IAV, which was further enhanced by inclusion of an antigen presenting cell targeting unit specific for MHCII, thus favoring BCR cross-linking (115). Another strategy to elicit broadly reactive antibodies within IAV subtypes is to use computationally optimized broadly reactive antigens (COBRA), which are displayed on virus like particles or expressed in live attenuated influenza vaccine. This approach uses multiple rounds of consensus generation to aggregate HA epitopes of IAV from different time periods. Such vaccines elicit polyclonal B cell responses and was shown to protect within subtypes (116–123). Combining several COBRA vaccines could confer heterosubtypic protection.

M2e-Based Vaccines

M2 is an ion channel with its ectodomain (M2e) exposed on virion and infected cell surfaces (124). M2e is quite

TABLE 1 | Characteristics of antibody responses to current universal vaccine targets and ability of seasonal vaccination to recall memory B cells and specific antibodies.

	Antibodies			Seasonal vaccination	
	Broadly cross reactive	**Neutralizing**	**Act via effector functions**	**Recall memory B cells**	**Elicit antibodies**
HA head	–	+	– (33)	+	+
HA head conserved targets	+	+/–[a]	+/–[b]	?[c] (73, 143)	?[d] (143)
HA stem	+	+	+ (33)	–/+[e] (21, 144)	–/+[e] (21)
NA	+	+/–[f] (141)	+ (145)	–[g] (136)	+/–[g] (146, 147)
M2e	+	– (148)	+ (149)	–	–

[a]*HA head conserved targets comprise lot of different targets. Neutralization ability depends on the target.*
[b]*See in the body of this review for references, depending on the target.*
[c]*Not many studies address this question. It appears that vaccination with newly introduced viruses might recall these B cells.*
[d]*Not many studies are addressing this issue, which is probably dependent on the target.*
[e]*Stem-specific memory B cells are mainly recalled and antibodies induced when new viruses are introduced (for example with H1N1/pdm2009).*
[f]*NA antibodies usually have NA-inhibition activity, which correlates well with plaque reduction but are not neutralizing, by definition.*
[g]*NA-B cells and antibodies are most likely not properly boosted, after seasonal vaccination, due to poor vaccine formulation, with variable/low NA amount.*

conserved across IAV; therefore, it has historically been considered as an ideal universal vaccine candidate (125). The mechanism of M2e-mediated protection is debated with both antibodies and T cells being important players (126–128). Several approaches have been undertaken to increase M2e immunogenicity, using VLP or different adjuvants (129–131). Of note, it appears that M2e antibodies act via effector functions and thus are infection permissive, making M2e vaccines more suitable when used in combination with others.

NEURAMINIDASE—THE EMERGING PLAYER

IAV NA as vaccine target has been neglected for decades, despite early discovery of potent anti-viral activity of NA antibodies (132). Even more surprisingly, NA amount in licensed vaccines varies enormously and is not checked by manufactures or regulatory authorities (133). Exciting new studies strongly point to a major role for anti-NA antibodies in protecting from disease and as the best correlates of protection (56, 134, 135). Critically, Chen et al. identified a number of human NA antibodies that cross-protected mice in therapeutic and prophylactic setting (136). Even more promising, several broadly neutralizing anti-NA mAbs have been isolated from an infected patient. These mAbs, directed to NA active site, demonstrated an unusual breadth in binding several IAV and IBV NA and mediating cross-neutralization and cross-protection *in vivo* (137). Still, despite some early studies, we do not know enough about NA antigenicity and the immunodominance of its antigenic sites (138–141). By applying some of the methods that allowed us to study in detail anti-HA responses, we should be able to break down anti-NA responses and identify promising universal vaccine candidates.

CONCLUSIONS—KNOW WHAT WE DO NOT KNOW

Bioengineering and design of epitope-focused immunogens is proceeding at an incredible speed in influenza and other fields. Several promising immunogens are now in clinical trials and, hopefully, will be available to the public soon, as long-lasting universal vaccines. It is, however, crucial to understand more about the basics of B cell responses to interpret results and inform on vaccination policies.

Introduction of pandemic H1N1 2009 virus showed that most individuals, with low serological anti-stem antibodies, were able to mount a stem-directed response, but repeated vaccinations skewed the immune response back to the immunodominant head (21). It will be critical to understand when, in which order and how often give universal vaccines to appropriately boost stem response. Andrews et al. demonstrated that novel B cells specific for variable epitopes have a different phenotype compared to reactivated Bmem specific for stem (142). To maximize success, efforts will need to be put in understanding how B-cell specificity can influence their programming and differentiation. Furthermore, it is still unclear how much of stem-specific antibodies are required for optimal protection from a drifted or heterologous virus. **Table 1** summarizes what we know about antibody responses to the major targets on IAV and how seasonal vaccination is able to boost those responses.

Finally, but not less important, new vaccines platforms are constantly being tested. RNA-based vaccines have shown exciting results when expressing influenza proteins, at least in animals [reviewed in (150)]. Some of the engineered vaccines discussed in this review could be delivered as RNA vaccines, alone or in combination, possibly avoiding clearance from pre-existing antibodies. Other novel, slow-release, vaccine formulations could help refocusing immune responses to subdominant targets (151–153).

We are just entering an exciting season of clinical trials, and while expectations are really high, we should not be discouraged if some of the early attempts fail but rather persevere in the quest for a universal and long-lasting vaccine.

REFERENCES

1. Paules C, Subbarao K. Influenza. *Lancet.* (2017) 390:697–708. doi: 10.1016/S0140-6736(17)30129-0
2. Hause BM, Ducatez M, Collin EA, Ran Z, Liu R, Sheng Z, et al. Isolation of a novel swine influenza virus from Oklahoma in 2011 which is distantly related to human influenza C viruses. *PLoS Pathog.* (2013) 9:e1003176. doi: 10.1371/journal.ppat.1003176
3. Collin EA, Sheng Z, Lang Y, Ma W, Hause BM, Li F. Cocirculation of two distinct genetic and antigenic lineages of proposed influenza D virus in cattle. *J Virol.* (2015) 89:1036–42. doi: 10.1128/JVI.02718-14
4. Jackson D, Elderfield RA, Barclay WS. Molecular studies of influenza B virus in the reverse genetics era. *J Gen Virol.* (2011) 92(Pt 1):1–17. doi: 10.1099/vir.0.026187-0
5. Iuliano AD, Roguski KM, Chang HH, Muscatello DJ, Palekar R, Tempia S, et al. Estimates of global seasonal influenza-associated respiratory mortality:a modelling study. *Lancet.* (2018) 391:1285–300. doi: 10.1016/S0140-6736(17)33293-2
6. Belongia EA, Skowronski DM, McLean HQ, Chambers C, Sundaram ME, De Serres G. Repeated annual influenza vaccination and vaccine effectiveness:review of evidence. *Exp Rev Vaccines.* (2017) 16:1–14. doi: 10.1080/14760584.2017.1334554
7. Hutchinson EC. Influenza Virus. *Trends Microbiol.* (2018) 26:809–810. doi: 10.1016/j.tim.2018.05.013
8. Rota PA, Wallis TR, Harmon MW, Rota JS, Kendal AP, Nerome K. Cocirculation of two distinct evolutionary lineages of influenza type B virus since 1983. *Virology.* (1990) 175:59–68. doi: 10.1016/0042-6822(90)90186-U
9. Grohskopf LA, Alyanak E, Broder KR, Walter EB, Fry AM, Jernigan DB. Prevention and control of seasonal influenza with vaccines:recommendations of the advisory committee on immunization practices - United States, 2019–20 influenza season. *MMWR Recomm Rep.* (2019) 68:1–21. doi: 10.15585/mmwr.rr6803a1
10. Krammer F, Palese P. Advances in the development of influenza virus vaccines. *Nat Rev Drug Discov.* (2015) 14:167–82. doi: 10.1038/nrd4529
11. Past Pandemics. *Centers for Disease Control and Prevention, National Center for Immunization and Respiratory Diseases (NCIRD).* (2018). Available online at: https://www.cdc.gov/flu/pandemic-resources/basics/past-pandemics.html
12. Gaymard A, Le Briand N, Frobert E, Lina B, Escuret V. Functional balance between neuraminidase and haemagglutinin in influenza viruses. *Clin Microbiol Infect.* (2016) 22:975–83. doi: 10.1016/j.cmi.2016.07.007
13. Angeletti D, Gibbs JS, Angel M, Kosik I, Hickman HD, Frank GM, et al. Defining B cell immunodominance to viruses. *Nat Immunol.* (2017) 18:456–63. doi: 10.1038/ni.3680
14. Kirkpatrick E, Qiu X, Wilson PC, Bahl J, Krammer F. The influenza virus hemagglutinin head evolves faster than the stalk domain. *Sci Rep.* (2018) 8:10432. doi: 10.1038/s41598-018-28706-1
15. Angeletti D, Yewdell JW. Understanding and manipulating viral immunity:antibody immunodominance enters center stage. *Trends Immunol.* (2018) 39:549–61. doi: 10.1016/j.it.2018.04.008
16. Das SR, Hensley SE, Ince WL, Brooke CB, Subba A, Delboy MG, et al. Defining influenza A virus hemagglutinin antigenic drift by sequential monoclonal antibody selection. *Cell Host Microbe.* (2013) 13:314–23. doi: 10.1016/j.chom.2013.02.008
17. Chambers BS, Parkhouse K, Ross TM, Alby K, Hensley SE. Identification of hemagglutinin residues responsible for H3N2 antigenic drift during the 2014–2015 influenza season. *Cell Rep.* (2015) 12:1-6. doi: 10.1016/j.celrep.2015.06.005

AUTHOR CONTRIBUTIONS

NM and DA researched the literature and wrote the manuscript.

18. Huang KY, Rijal P, Schimanski L, Powell TJ, Lin TY, McCauley JW, et al. Focused antibody response to influenza linked to antigenic drift. *J Clin Invest.* (2015) 125:2631–45. doi: 10.1172/JCI81104
19. Lee JM, Eguia R, Zost SJ, Choudhary S, Wilson PC, Bedford T, et al. Mapping person-to-person variation in viral mutations that escape polyclonal serum targeting influenza hemagglutinin. *Elife.* (2019) 8:e49324. doi: 10.7554/eLife.49324
20. Koel BF, Burke DF, Bestebroer TM, van der Vliet S, Zondag GC, Vervaet G, et al. Substitutions near the receptor binding site determine major antigenic change during influenza virus evolution. *Science.* (2013) 342:976–9. doi: 10.1126/science.1244730
21. Andrews SF, Huang Y, Kaur K, Popova LI, Ho IY, Pauli NT, et al. Immune history profoundly affects broadly protective B cell responses to influenza. *Sci Transl Med.* (2015) 7:316ra192. doi: 10.1126/scitranslmed.aad0522
22. Harris AK, Meyerson JR, Matsuoka Y, Kuybeda O, Moran A, Bliss D, et al. Structure and accessibility of HA trimers on intact 2009 H1N1 pandemic influenza virus to stem region-specific neutralizing antibodies. *Proc Natl Acad Sci USA.* (2013) 110:4592-7. doi: 10.1073/pnas.12149 13110
23. Sui J, Sheehan J, Hwang WC, Bankston LA, Burchett SK, Huang CY, et al. Wide prevalence of heterosubtypic broadly neutralizing human anti-influenza A antibodies. *Clin Infect Dis.* (2011) 52:1003–9. doi: 10.1093/cid/cir121
24. Hoa LNM, Mai LQ, Bryant JE, Thai PQ, Hang NLK, Yen NTT, et al. Association between Hemagglutinin Stem-Reactive Antibodies and Influenza A/H1N1 Virus Infection during the 2009 Pandemic. *J Virol.* (2016) 90:6549–56. doi: 10.1128/JVI.00093-16
25. Doud MB, Bloom JD, Accurate measurement of the effects of all amino-acid mutations on influenza hemagglutinin. *Viruses.* (2016) 8:155. doi: 10.3390/v8060155
26. Heaton NS, Sachs D, Chen CJ, Hai R, Palese P. Genome-wide mutagenesis of influenza virus reveals unique plasticity of the hemagglutinin and NS1 proteins. *Proc Natl Acad Sci USA.* (2013) 110:20248–53. doi: 10.1073/pnas.1320524110
27. Anderson CS, Ortega S, Chaves FA, Clark AM, Yang H, Topham DJ, et al. Publisher correction:natural and directed antigenic drift of the H1 influenza virus hemagglutinin stalk domain. *Sci Rep.* (2018) 8:276. doi: 10.1038/s41598-017-17926-6
28. Shafieyan Y, Hinz B, Doud MB, Lee JM, Bloom JD. How single mutations affect viral escape from broad and narrow antibodies to H1 influenza hemagglutinin. *Nat Commun.* (2018) 9:1386. doi: 10.1038/s41467-018-03665-3
29. Vareckovà E, Mucha V, Wharton SA, Kostolanský F. Inhibition of fusion activity of influenza A haemagglutinin mediated by HA2-specific monoclonal antibodies. *Arch Virol.* (2003) 148:469–86. doi: 10.1007/s00705-002-0932-1
30. Chen YQ, Lan LY, Huang M, Henry C, Wilson PC. Hemagglutinin stalk-reactive antibodies interfere with influenza virus neuraminidase activity by steric hindrance. *J Virol.* (2019) 93:e01526-18. doi: 10.1128/JVI.01 526-18
31. Kosik I, Angeletti D, Gibbs JS, Angel M, Takeda K, Kosikova M, et al. Neuraminidase inhibition contributes to influenza A virus neutralization by anti-hemagglutinin stem antibodies. *J Exp Med.* (2019) 216:304–16. doi: 10.1084/jem.20181624
32. Wohlbold TJ, Chromikova V, Tan GS, Meade P, Amanat F, Comella P, et al. Hemagglutinin stalk- and neuraminidase-specific monoclonal antibodies protect against Lethal H10N8 influenza virus infection in mice. *J Virol.* (2016) 90:851–61. doi: 10.1128/JVI.02275-15

33. DiLillo DJ, Tan GS, Palese P, Ravetch JV. Broadly neutralizing hemagglutinin stalk-specific antibodies require FcgammaR interactions for protection against influenza virus *in vivo*. *Nat Med.* (2014) 20:143–51. doi: 10.1038/nm.3443
34. DiLillo DJ, Palese P, Wilson PC, Ravetch JV, DiLillo DJ. Broadly neutralizing anti-influenza antibodies require Fc receptor engagement for in vivo protection. *J Clin Invest.* (2016) 126:605–10. doi: 10.1172/JCI84428
35. Mullarkey CE, Bailey MJ, Golubeva DA, Tan GS, Nachbagauer R, He W, et al. Broadly neutralizing hemagglutinin stalk-specific antibodies induce potent phagocytosis of immune complexes by neutrophils in an Fc-dependent manner. *MBio.* (2016) 7:e01624-16. doi: 10.1128/mBio.01624-16
36. Sui J, Hwang WC, Perez S, Wei G, Aird D, Chen LM, et al. Structural and functional bases for broad-spectrum neutralization of avian and human influenza A viruses. *Nat Struct Mol Biol.* (2009) 16:265–73. doi: 10.1038/nsmb.1566
37. Ekiert DC, Bhabha G, Elsliger MA, Friesen RH, Jongeneelen M, Throsby M, et al. Antibody recognition of a highly conserved influenza virus epitope. *Science.* (2009) 324:246–51. doi: 10.1126/science.1171491
38. Nachbagauer R, Shore D, Yang H, Johnson SK, Gabbard JD, Tompkins SM, et al. Broadly reactive human monoclonal antibodies elicited following pandemic H1N1 influenza virus exposure protect mice against highly pathogenic H5N1 challenge. *J Virol.* (2018) 92:e00949-18. doi: 10.1128/JVI.00949-18
39. De Marco D, Clementi N, Mancini N, Solforosi L, Moreno GJ, Sun X, et al. A non-VH1-69 heterosubtypic neutralizing human monoclonal antibody protects mice against H1N1 and H5N1 viruses. *PLoS ONE.* (2012) 7:e34415. doi: 10.1371/journal.pone.0034415
40. Henry Dunand CJ, Leon PE, Kaur K, Tan GS, Zheng NY, Andrews S, et al. Preexisting human antibodies neutralize recently emerged H7N9 influenza strains. *J Clin Invest.* (2015) 125:1255–68. doi: 10.1172/JCI74374
41. Ekiert DC, Friesen RH, Bhabha G, Kwaks T, Jongeneelen M, Yu W, et al. A highly conserved neutralizing epitope on group 2 influenza A viruses. *Science.* (2011) 333:843–50. doi: 10.1126/science.1204839
42. Friesen RH, Lee PS, Stoop EJ, Hoffman RM, Ekiert DC, Bhabha G, et al. A common solution to group 2 influenza virus neutralization. *Proc Natl Acad Sci USA.* (2014) 111:445–50. doi: 10.1073/pnas.1319058110
43. Sakabe S, Iwatsuki-Horimoto K, Horimoto T, Nidom CA, Le Mt, Takano R, et al. A cross-reactive neutralizing monoclonal antibody protects mice from H5N1 and pandemic (H1N1) 2009 virus infection. *Antiviral Res.* (2010) 88:249–55. doi: 10.1016/j.antiviral.2010.09.007
44. Kallewaard NL, Corti D, Collins PJ, Neu U, McAuliffe JM, Benjamin E, et al. Structure and function analysis of an antibody recognizing all influenza A subtypes. *Cell.* (2016) 166:596–608. doi: 10.1016/j.cell.2016.05.073
45. Fu Y, Zhang Z, Sheehan J, Avnir Y, Ridenour C, Sachnik T, et al. A broadly neutralizing anti-influenza antibody reveals ongoing capacity of haemagglutinin-specific memory B cells to evolve. *Nat Commun.* (2016) 7:12780. doi: 10.1038/ncomms12780
46. Tharakaraman K, Subramanian V, Viswanathan K, Sloan S, Yen HL, Barnard DL, et al. A broadly neutralizing human monoclonal antibody is effective against H7N9. *Proc Natl Acad Sci USA.* (2015) 112:10890–5. doi: 10.1073/pnas.1502374112
47. Marjuki H, Mishin VP, Chai N, Tan MW, Newton EM, Tegeris J, et al. Human monoclonal antibody 81.39a effectively neutralizes emerging influenza A viruses of group 1 and 2 hemagglutinins. *J Virol.* (2016) 90:10446–58. doi: 10.1128/JVI.01284-16
48. Wyrzucki A, Bianchi M, Kohler I, Steck M, Hangartner L, et al. Heterosubtypic antibodies to influenza A virus have limited activity against cell-bound virus but are not impaired by strain-specific serum antibodies. *J Virol.* (2015) 89:3136–44. doi: 10.1128/JVI.03069-14
49. Clementi N, De Marco D, Mancini N, Solforosi L, Moreno GJ, Gubareva LV, et al. A human monoclonal antibody with neutralizing activity against highly divergent influenza subtypes. *PLoS ONE.* (2011) 6:e28001. doi: 10.1371/journal.pone.0028001
50. Joyce MG, Wheatley AK, Thomas PV, Chuang GY, Soto C, Bailer RT, et al. Vaccine-induced antibodies that neutralize group 1 and group 2 influenza A viruses. *Cell.* (2016) 166:609–23. doi: 10.1016/j.cell.2016.06.043
51. Dreyfus C, Laursen NS, Kwaks T, Zuijdgeest D, Khayat R, Ekiert DC, et al. Highly conserved protective epitopes on influenza B viruses. *Science.* (2012) 337:1343–8. doi: 10.1126/science.1222908
52. Yassine HM, McTamney PM, Boyington JC, Ruckwardt TJ, Crank MC, Smatti MK, et al. Use of hemagglutinin stem probes demonstrate prevalence of broadly reactive group 1 influenza antibodies in human sera. *Sci Rep.* (2018) 8:8628. doi: 10.1038/s41598-018-26538-7
53. Ellebedy AH, Krammer F, Li GM, Miller MS, Chiu C, Wrammert J, et al. Induction of broadly cross-reactive antibody responses to the influenza HA stem region following H5N1 vaccination in humans. *Proc Natl Acad Sci USA.* (2014) 111:13133–8. doi: 10.1073/pnas.1414070111
54. Wheatley AK, Whittle JR, Lingwood D, Kanekiyo M, Yassine HM, Ma SS, et al. H5N1 Vaccine-elicited memory B cells are genetically constrained by the IGHV locus in the recognition of a neutralizing epitope in the hemagglutinin stem. *J Immunol.* (2015) 195:602–10. doi: 10.4049/jimmunol.1402835
55. Andrews SF, Joyce MG, Chambers MJ, Gillespie RA, Kanekiyo M, Leung K, et al. Preferential induction of cross-group influenza A hemagglutinin stem-specific memory B cells after H7N9 immunization in humans. *Sci Immunol.* (2017) 2:eaan2676. doi: 10.1126/sciimmunol.aan2676
56. Park JK, Han A, Czajkowski L, Reed S, Athota R, Bristol T, et al. Evaluation of preexisting anti-hemagglutinin stalk antibody as a correlate of protection in a healthy volunteer challenge with influenza A/H1N1pdm virus. *MBio.* (2018) 9:e02284-17. doi: 10.1128/mBio.02284-17
57. Memoli MJ, Shaw PA, Han A, Czajkowski L, Reed S, Athota R, et al. Evaluation of antihemagglutinin and antineuraminidase antibodies as correlates of protection in an influenza A/H1N1 virus healthy human challenge model. *MBio.* (2016) 7:e00417-16. doi: 10.1128/mBio.00417-16
58. Christensen SR, Toulmin SA, Griesman T, Lamerato LE, Petrie JG, Martin ET, et al. Assessing the protective potential of H1N1 influenza virus hemagglutinin head and stalk antibodies in humans. *J Virol.* (2019) 93:e02134-18. doi: 10.1128/JVI.02134-18
59. Weis W, Brown JH, Cusack S, Paulson JC, Skehel JJ, Wiley DC. Structure of the influenza virus haemagglutinin complexed with its receptor, sialic acid. *Nature.* (1988) 333:426–31. doi: 10.1038/333426a0
60. Skehel JJ, Wiley DC. Receptor binding and membrane fusion in virus entry:the influenza hemagglutinin. *Annu Rev Biochem.* (2000) 69:531–69. doi: 10.1146/annurev.biochem.69.1.531
61. Wu NC, Xie J, Zheng T, Nycholat CM, Grande G, Paulson JC, et al. Diversity of functionally permissive sequences in the receptor-binding site of influenza hemagglutinin. *Cell Host Microbe.* (2017) 21:742–53.e8. doi: 10.1016/j.chom.2017.05.011
62. Shi Y, Wu Y, Zhang W, Qi J, Gao GF. Enabling the 'host jump':structural determinants of receptor-binding specificity in influenza A viruses. *Nat Rev Microbiol.* (2014) 12:822–31. doi: 10.1038/nrmicro3362
63. Ekiert DC, Kashyap AK, Steel J, Rubrum A, Bhabha G, Khayat R, et al. Cross-neutralization of influenza A viruses mediated by a single antibody loop. *Nature.* (2012) 489:526–32. doi: 10.1038/nature11414
64. Lee PS, Ohshima N, Stanfield RL, Yu W, Iba Y, Okuno Y, et al. Receptor mimicry by antibody F045-092 facilitates universal binding to the H3 subtype of influenza virus. *Nat Commun.* (2014) 5:3614. doi: 10.1038/ncomms4614
65. Whittle JR, Zhang R, Khurana S, King LR, Manischewitz J, Golding H, et al. Broadly neutralizing human antibody that recognizes the receptor-binding pocket of influenza virus hemagglutinin. *Proc Natl Acad Sci USA.* (2011) 108:14216–21. doi: 10.1073/pnas.1111497108
66. Hong M, Lee PS, Hoffman RM, Zhu X, Krause JC, Laursen NS, et al. Antibody recognition of the pandemic H1N1 Influenza virus hemagglutinin receptor binding site. *J Virol.* (2013) 87:12471–80. doi: 10.1128/JVI.01388-13
67. Krause JC, Tsibane T, Tumpey TM, Huffman CJ, Basler CF, Crowe JE. A broadly neutralizing human monoclonal antibody that recognizes a conserved, novel epitope on the globular head of the influenza H1N1 virus hemagglutinin. *J Virol.* (2011) 85:10905–8. doi: 10.1128/JVI.00700-11
68. Lee PS, Yoshida R, Ekiert DC, Sakai N, Suzuki Y, Takada A, et al. Heterosubtypic antibody recognition of the influenza virus hemagglutinin receptor binding site enhanced by avidity. *Proc Natl Acad Sci USA.* (2012) 109:17040–5. doi: 10.1073/pnas.1212371109

69. Yoshida R, Igarashi M, Ozaki H, Kishida N, Tomabechi D, Kida H, et al. Cross-protective potential of a novel monoclonal antibody directed against antigenic site B of the hemagglutinin of influenza A viruses. *PLoS Pathog.* (2009) 5:e1000350. doi: 10.1371/journal.ppat.1000350
70. Krause JC, Tsibane T, Tumpey TM, Huffman CJ, Albrecht R, Blum DL, et al. Human monoclonal antibodies to pandemic 1957 H2N2 and pandemic 1968 H3N2 influenza viruses. *J Virol.* (2012) 86:6334–40. doi: 10.1128/JVI.07158-11
71. Winarski KL, Thornburg NJ, Yu Y, Sapparapu G, Crowe JE, Spiller BW. Vaccine-elicited antibody that neutralizes H5N1 influenza and variants binds the receptor site and polymorphic sites. *Proc Natl Acad Sci USA.* (2015) 112:9346–51. doi: 10.1073/pnas.1502762112
72. Shen C, Chen J, Li R, Zhang M, Wang G, Stegalkina S, et al. A multimechanistic antibody targeting the receptor binding site potently cross-protects against influenza B viruses. *Sci Transl Med.* (2017) 9:eaam5752. doi: 10.1126/scitranslmed.aam5752
73. Raymond DD, Bajic G, Ferdman J, Suphaphiphat P, Settembre EC, Moody MA, et al. Conserved epitope on influenza-virus hemagglutinin head defined by a vaccine-induced antibody. *Proc Natl Acad Sci USA.* (2018) 115:168–73. doi: 10.1073/pnas.1715471115
74. Iba Y, Fujii Y, Ohshima N, Sumida T, Kubota-Koketsu R, Ikeda M, et al. Conserved neutralizing epitope at globular head of hemagglutinin in H3N2 influenza viruses. *J Virol.* (2014) 88:7130–44. doi: 10.1128/JVI.00420-14
75. Bajic G, Maron MJ, Adachi Y, Onodera T, McCarthy KR, McGee CE, et al. Influenza antigen engineering focuses immune responses to a subdominant but broadly protective viral epitope. *Cell Host Microbe.* (2019) 25:827–35.e6. doi: 10.1016/j.chom.2019.04.003
76. Bangaru S, Lang S, Schotsaert M, Vanderven HA, Zhu X, Kose N, et al. A site of vulnerability on the influenza virus hemagglutinin head domain trimer interface. *Cell.* (2019) 177:1136–52.e18. doi: 10.1016/j.cell.2019.04.011
77. Watanabe A, McCarthy KR, Kuraoka M, Schmidt AG, Adachi Y, Onodera T, et al. Antibodies to a conserved influenza head interface epitope protect by an IgG subtype-dependent mechanism. *Cell.* (2019) 177:1124–35.e16. doi: 10.1016/j.cell.2019.03.048
78. Das DK, Govindan R, Nikić-Spiegel I, Krammer F, Lemke EA, Munro JB. Direct visualization of the conformational dynamics of single influenza hemagglutinin trimers. *Cell.* (2018) 174:926–37.e12. doi: 10.1016/j.cell.2018.05.050
79. Adachi Y, Tonouchi K, Nithichanon A, Kuraoka M, Watanabe A, Shinnakasu R, et al. Exposure of an occluded hemagglutinin epitope drives selection of a class of cross-protective influenza antibodies. *Nat Commun.* (2019) 10:3883. doi: 10.1038/s41467-019-11821-6
80. Yewdell JW, Taylor A, Yellen A, Caton A, Gerhard W, Bächi T. et al. Mutations in or near the fusion peptide of the influenza virus hemagglutinin affect an antigenic site in the globular region. *J Virol.* (1993) 67:933–42.
81. Bangaru S, Zhang H, Gilchuk IM, Voss TG, Irving RP, Gilchuk P, et al. A multifunctional human monoclonal neutralizing antibody that targets a unique conserved epitope on influenza. *Nat Commun.* (2018) 9:2669. doi: 10.3410/f.733623822.793548444
82. Paul SS, Mok CK, Mak TM, Ng OW, Aboagye JO, Wohlbold TJ, et al. A cross-clade H5N1 influenza A virus neutralizing monoclonal antibody binds to a novel epitope within the vestigial esterase domain of hemagglutinin. *Antiviral Res.* (2017) 144:299–310. doi: 10.1016/j.antiviral.2017.06.012
83. Chai N, Swem LR, Park S, Nakamura G, Chiang N, Estevez A, et al. A broadly protective therapeutic antibody against influenza B virus with two mechanisms of action. *Nat Commun.* (2017) 8:14234. doi: 10.1038/ncomms14234
84. Sesterhenn F, Bonet J, Correia BE. Structure-based immunogen design-leading the way to the new age of precision vaccines. *Curr Opin Struct Biol.* (2018) 51:163–9. doi: 10.1016/j.sbi.2018.06.002
85. Sesterhenn F, Yang C, Cramer JT, Bonet J, Wen X, Abriata LA, et al. Trivalent cocktail of *de novo* designed immunogens enables the robust induction and focusing of functional antibodies *in vivo*. *bioRxiv.* (2019) 685867. doi: 10.1101/685867
86. Angeletti D, Yewdell JW. Is it possible to develop a "Universal" Influenza virus vaccine? outflanking antibody immunodominance on the road to universal influenza vaccination. *Cold Spring Harb Perspect Biol.* (2018) 10:a028852. doi: 10.1101/cshperspect.a028852
87. Cohen J. Immunology. A once-in-a-lifetime flu shot? *Science.* (2013) 341:1171. doi: 10.1126/science.341.6151.1171
88. Impagliazzo A, Milder F, Kuipers H, Wagner MV, Zhu X, Hoffman RM, et al. A stable trimeric influenza hemagglutinin stem as a broadly protective immunogen. *Science.* (2015) 349:1301–6. doi: 10.1126/science.aac7263
89. Mallajosyula VV, Citron M, Ferrara F, Lu X, Callahan C, Heidecker GJ, et al. Influenza hemagglutinin stem-fragment immunogen elicits broadly neutralizing antibodies and confers heterologous protection. *Proc Natl Acad Sci USA.* (2014) 111:E2514–23. doi: 10.1073/pnas.1402766111
90. Mallajosyula VV, Citron M, Ferrara F, Temperton NJ, Liang X, Flynn JA, et al. Hemagglutinin sequence conservation guided stem immunogen design from influenza A H3 subtype. *Front Immunol.* (2015) 6:329. doi: 10.3389/fimmu.2015.00329
91. Valkenburg SA, Mallajosyula VV, Li OT, Chin AW, Carnell G, Temperton N, et al. Stalking influenza by vaccination with pre-fusion headless HA mini-stem. *Sci Rep.* (2016) 6:22666. doi: 10.1038/srep22666
92. Vatti A, Monsalve DM, Pacheco Y, Chang C, Anaya JM, Gershwin ME. Original antigenic sin: a comprehensive review. *J Autoimmun.* (2017) 83:12–21. doi: 10.1016/j.jaut.2017.04.008
93. van der Lubbe JEM, Huizingh J, Verspuij JWA, Tettero L, Schmit-Tillemans SPR, Mooij P, et al. Mini-hemagglutinin vaccination induces cross-reactive antibodies in pre-exposed NHP that protect mice against lethal influenza challenge. *NPJ Vaccines.* (2018) 3:25. doi: 10.1038/s41541-018-0063-7
94. Lee LA, Wang Q. Adaptations of nanoscale viruses and other protein cages for medical applications. *Nanomedicine.* (2006) 2:137–49. doi: 10.1016/j.nano.2006.07.009
95. Yassine HM, Boyington JC, McTamney PM, Wei CJ, Kanekiyo M, Kong WP, et al. Hemagglutinin-stem nanoparticles generate heterosubtypic influenza protection. *Nat Med.* (2015) 21:1065–70. doi: 10.1038/nm.3927
96. Corbett KS, Moin SM, Yassine HM, Cagigi A, Kanekiyo M, Boyoglu-Barnum S, et al. Design of nanoparticulate group 2 influenza virus hemagglutinin stem antigens that activate unmutated ancestor B cell receptors of broadly neutralizing antibody lineages. *MBio.* (2019) 10:e02810-18. doi: 10.1128/mBio.02810-18
97. Hai R, Krammer F, Tan GS, Pica N, Eggink D, Maamary J, et al. Influenza viruses expressing chimeric hemagglutinins:globular head and stalk domains derived from different subtypes. *J Virol.* (2012) 86:5774–81. doi: 10.1128/JVI.00137-12
98. Krammer F, Pica N, Hai R, Margine I, Palese P. Chimeric hemagglutinin influenza virus vaccine constructs elicit broadly protective stalk-specific antibodies. *J Virol.* (2013) 87:6542–50. doi: 10.1128/JVI.00641-13
99. Nachbagauer R, Miller MS, Hai R, Ryder AB, Rose JK, Palese P, et al. Hemagglutinin stalk immunity reduces influenza virus replication and transmission in ferrets. *J Virol.* (2015) 90:3268–73. doi: 10.1128/JVI.02481-15
100. Nachbagauer R, Kinzler D, Choi A, Hirsh A, Beaulieu E, Lecrenier N, et al. A chimeric haemagglutinin-based influenza split virion vaccine adjuvanted with AS03 induces protective stalk-reactive antibodies in mice. *NPJ Vaccines.* (2016) 1:16015. doi: 10.1038/npjvaccines.2016.15
101. Krammer F, Hai R, Yondola M, Tan GS, Leyva-Grado VH, Ryder AB, et al. Assessment of influenza virus hemagglutinin stalk-based immunity in ferrets. *J Virol.* (2014) 88:3432–42. doi: 10.1128/JVI.03004-13
102. Ryder AB, Nachbagauer R, Buonocore L, Palese P, Krammer F, Rose JK. Vaccination with vesicular stomatitis virus-vectored chimeric hemagglutinins protects mice against divergent influenza virus challenge strains. *J Virol.* (2015) 90:2544–50. doi: 10.1128/JVI.02598-15
103. Margine I, Krammer F, Hai R, Heaton NS, Tan GS, Andrews SA, et al. Hemagglutinin stalk-based universal vaccine constructs protect against group 2 influenza A viruses. *J Virol.* (2013) 87:10435–46. doi: 10.1128/JVI.01715-13
104. Ermler ME, Kirkpatrick E, Sun W, Hai R, Amanat F, Chromikova V, et al. Chimeric hemagglutinin constructs induce broad protection against influenza B virus challenge in the mouse model. *J Virol.* (2017) 91:e00286-17. doi: 10.1128/JVI.00286-17
105. Isakova-Sivak I, Korenkov D, Smolonogina T, Kotomina T, Donina S, Matyushenko V, et al. Broadly protective anti-hemagglutinin stalk antibodies induced by live attenuated influenza vaccine expressing chimeric hemagglutinin. *Virology.* (2018) 518:313–23. doi: 10.1016/j.virol.2018.03.013

106. Bernstein DI, Guptill J, Naficy A, Nachbagauer R, Berlanda-Scorza F, Feser J, et al. Immunogenicity of chimeric haemagglutinin-based, universal influenza virus vaccine candidates:interim results of a randomised, placebo-controlled, phase 1 clinical trial. *Lancet Infect Dis.* 20:80–91 (2020). doi: 10.1016/S1473-3099(19)30393-7.
107. Tate MD, Job ER, Deng YM, Gunalan V, Maurer-Stroh S, Reading PC. Playing hide and seek:how glycosylation of the influenza virus hemagglutinin can modulate the immune response to infection. *Viruses.* (2014) 6:1294–316. doi: 10.3390/v6031294
108. Tseng YC, Wu CY, Liu ML, Chen TH, Chiang WL, Yu YH, et al. Egg-based influenza split virus vaccine with monoglycosylation induces cross-strain protection against influenza virus infections. *Proc Natl Acad Sci USA.* (2019) 116:3935–7. doi: 10.1073/pnas.1819197116
109. Liu WC, Jan JT, Huang YJ, Chen TH, Wu SC. Unmasking Stem-specific neutralizing epitopes by abolishing N-linked glycosylation sites of influenza virus hemagglutinin proteins for vaccine design. *J Virol.* (2016) 90:8496–508. doi: 10.1128/JVI.00880-16
110. Eggink D, Goff PH, Palese P. Guiding the immune response against influenza virus hemagglutinin toward the conserved stalk domain by hyperglycosylation of the globular head domain. *J Virol.* (2014) 88:699–704. doi: 10.1128/JVI.02608-13
111. Weidenbacher PA, Kim PS. Protect, modify, deprotect (PMD):A strategy for creating vaccines to elicit antibodies targeting a specific epitope. *Proc Natl Acad Sci USA.* (2019) 116:9947–52. doi: 10.1073/pnas.1822062116
112. Wang W, Song HS, Keller PW, Alvarado-Facundo E, Vassell R, Weiss CD. Conformational stability of the hemagglutinin of H5N1 influenza a viruses influences susceptibility to broadly neutralizing stem antibodies. *J Virol.* (2018) 92:e00247-18. doi: 10.1128/JVI.00247-18
113. Kanekiyo M, Joyce MG, Gillespie RA, Gallagher JR, Andrews SF, Yassine HM, et al. Mosaic nanoparticle display of diverse influenza virus hemagglutinins elicits broad B cell responses. *Nat Immunol.* (2019) 20:362–72. doi: 10.1038/s41590-018-0305-x
114. Krammer F. Fighting influenza through hemagglutinin diversity. *Nat Immunol.* (2019) 20:246–47. doi: 10.1038/s41590-019-0317-1
115. Anderson AM, Baranowska-Hustad M, Braathen R, Grodeland G, Bogen B. Simultaneous targeting of multiple hemagglutinins to APCs for induction of broad immunity against influenza. *J Immunol.* (2018) 200:2057–66. doi: 10.4049/jimmunol.1701088
116. Carter DM, Darby CA, Lefoley BC, Crevar CJ, Alefantis T, Oomen R, et al. Design and characterization of a computationally optimized broadly reactive hemagglutinin vaccine for H1N1 influenza viruses. *J Virol.* (2016) 90:4720–34. doi: 10.1128/JVI.03152-15
117. Giles BM, Ross TM. Computationally optimized antigens to overcome influenza viral diversity. *Exp Rev Vaccines.* (2012) 11:267–9. doi: 10.1586/erv.12.3
118. Sautto GA, Kirchenbaum GA, Ecker JW, Bebin-Blackwell AG, Pierce SR, Ross TM. Elicitation of broadly protective antibodies following infection with influenza viruses expressing H1N1 computationally optimized broadly reactive hemagglutinin antigens. *Immunohorizons.* (2018) 2:226–37. doi: 10.4049/immunohorizons.1800044
119. Giles BM, Crevar CJ, Carter DM, Bissel SJ, Schultz-Cherry S, Wiley CA, et al. A computationally optimized hemagglutinin virus-like particle vaccine elicits broadly reactive antibodies that protect nonhuman primates from H5N1 infection. *J Infect Dis.* (2012) 205:1562–70. doi: 10.1093/infdis/jis232
120. Giles BM, Ross TM. A computationally optimized broadly reactive antigen (COBRA) based H5N1 VLP vaccine elicits broadly reactive antibodies in mice and ferrets. *Vaccine.* (2011) 29:3043–54. doi: 10.1016/j.vaccine.2011.01.100
121. Wong TM, Allen JD, Bebin-Blackwell AG, Carter DM, Alefantis T, DiNapoli J, et al. Computationally optimized broadly reactive hemagglutinin elicits hemagglutination inhibition antibodies against a panel of H3N2 influenza virus cocirculating variants. *J Virol.* (2017) 91:e01581-17. doi: 10.1128/JVI.01581-17
122. Allen JD, Owino SO, Carter DM, Crevar CJ, Reese VA, Fox CB, et al. Broadened immunity and protective responses with emulsion-adjuvanted H5 COBRA-VLP vaccines. *Vaccine.* (2017) 35:5209–16. doi: 10.1016/j.vaccine.2017.07.107
123. Crevar CJ, Carter DM, Lee KY, Ross TM. Cocktail of H5N1 COBRA HA vaccines elicit protective antibodies against H5N1 viruses from multiple clades. *Hum Vaccin Immunother.* (2015) 11:572–83. doi: 10.1080/21645515.2015.1012013
124. Pinto LH, Lamb RA, The M2 proton channels of influenza A and B viruses. *J Biol Chem.* (2006) 281:8997–9000. doi: 10.1074/jbc.R500020200
125. Neirynck S, Deroo T, Saelens X, Vanlandschoot P, Jou WM, Fiers W. A universal influenza A vaccine based on the extracellular domain of the M2 protein. *Nat Med.* (1999) 5:1157–63. doi: 10.1038/13484
126. De Filette M, Ramne A, Birkett A, Lycke N, Löwenadler B, Min Jou W, et al. The universal influenza vaccine M2e-HBc administered intranasally in combination with the adjuvant CTA1-DD provides complete protection. *Vaccine.* (2006) 24:544–51. doi: 10.1016/j.vaccine.2005.08.061
127. Eliasson DG, Omokanye A, Schön K, Wenzel UA, Bernasconi V, Bemark M, et al. M2e-tetramer-specific memory CD4 T cells are broadly protective against influenza infection. *Mucosal Immunol.* (2018) 11:273–89. doi: 10.1038/mi.2017.14
128. Fu TM, Freed DC, Horton MS, Fan J, Citron MP, Joyce JG, et al. Characterizations of four monoclonal antibodies against M2 protein ectodomain of influenza A virus. *Virology.* (2009) 385:218–26. doi: 10.1016/j.virol.2008.11.035
129. Bernasconi V, Bernocchi B, Ye L, Lê MQ, Omokanye A, Carpentier R, et al. Porous nanoparticles with self-adjuvanting M2e-fusion protein and recombinant hemagglutinin provide strong and broadly protective immunity against influenza virus infections. *Front Immunol.* (2018) 9:2060. doi: 10.3389/fimmu.2018.02060
130. Eliasson DG, El Bakkouri K, Schön K, Ramne A, Festjens E, Löwenadler B, et al. CTA1-M2e-DD:a novel mucosal adjuvant targeted influenza vaccine. *Vaccine.* (2008) 26:1243–52. doi: 10.1016/j.vaccine.2007.12.027
131. McMichael AJ, Picker LJ.Schepens B, De Vlieger D, Saelens X. Vaccine options for influenza:thinking small. *Curr Opin Immunol.* (2018) 53:22–9. doi: 10.1016/j.coi.2018.03.024
132. Kilbourne ED, Laver WG, Schulman JL, Webster RG. Antiviral activity of antiserum specific for an influenza virus neuraminidase. *J Virol.* (1968) 2:281–8.
133. Kosik I, Yewdell JW. Influenza Hemagglutinin and Neuraminidase:Yin(-)Yang proteins coevolving to thwart immunity. *Viruses.* (2019) 11:346. doi: 10.3390/v11040346
134. Maier HE, Nachbagauer R, Kuan G, Ng S, Lopez R, Sanchez N, et al. Pre-existing anti-neuraminidase antibodies are associated with shortened duration of influenza A (H1N1)pdm virus shedding and illness in naturally infected adults. *Clin Infect Dis.* (2019) 2019:ciz639. doi: 10.1093/cid/ciz639
135. Ng S, Nachbagauer R, Balmaseda A, Stadlbauer D, Ojeda S, Patel M, et al. Novel correlates of protection against pandemic H1N1 influenza A virus infection. *Nat Med.* (2019) 25:962–7. doi: 10.1038/s41591-019-0463-x
136. Chen YQ, Wohlbold TJ, Zheng NY, Huang M, Huang Y, Neu KE, et al. Influenza infection in humans induces broadly cross-reactive and protective neuraminidase-reactive antibodies. *Cell.* (2018) 173:417–29.e10. doi: 10.1016/j.cell.2018.03.030
137. Stadlbauer D, Zhu X, McMahon M, Turner JS, Wohlbold TJ, Schmitz AJ, et al. Broadly protective human antibodies that target the active site of influenza virus neuraminidase. *Science.* (2019) 366:499–504. doi: 10.1126/science.aay0678
138. Laver WG, Air GM, Webster RG, Markoff LJ. Amino acid sequence changes in antigenic variants of type A influenza virus N2 neuraminidase. *Virology.* (1982) 122:450–60. doi: 10.1016/0042-6822(82)90244-6
139. Webster RG, Hinshaw VS, Laver WG. Selection and analysis of antigenic variants of the neuraminidase of N2 influenza viruses with monoclonal antibodies. *Virology.* (1982) 117:93–104. doi: 10.1016/0042-6822(82)90510-4
140. Air GM, Els MC, Brown LE, Laver WG, Webster RG. Location of antigenic sites on the three-dimensional structure of the influenza N2 virus neuraminidase. *Virology.* (1985) 145:237–48. doi: 10.1016/0042-6822(85)90157-6
141. Jiang L, Fantoni G, Couzens L, Gao J, Plant E, Ye Z, et al. Comparative efficacy of monoclonal antibodies that bind to different epitopes of the 2009 pandemic H1N1 influenza virus neuraminidase. *J Virol.* (2016) 90:117–28. doi: 10.1128/JVI.01756-15

142. Andrews SF, Chambers MJ, Schramm CA, Plyler J, Raab JE, Kanekiyo M, et al. Activation dynamics and immunoglobulin evolution of pre-existing and newly generated human memory B cell responses to influenza hemagglutinin. *Immunity.* (2019) 51:398–410.e5. doi: 10.1016/j.immuni.2019.06.024

143. Schmidt AG, Therkelsen MD, Stewart S, Kepler TB, Liao HX, Moody MA, et al. Viral receptor-binding site antibodies with diverse germline origins. *Cell.* (2015) 161:1026–34. doi: 10.1016/j.cell.2015.04.028

144. Li GM, Chiu C, Wrammert J, McCausland M, Andrews SF, Zheng NY, et al. Pandemic H1N1 influenza vaccine induces a recall response in humans that favors broadly cross-reactive memory B cells. *Proc Natl Acad Sci USA.* (2012) 109:9047–52. doi: 10.1073/pnas.1118979109

145. Job ER, Ysenbaert T, Smet A, Van Hecke A, Meuris L, Kleanthous H, et al. Fcgamma receptors contribute to the antiviral properties of influenza virus neuraminidase-specific antibodies. *MBio.* (2019) 10:e01667-19. doi: 10.1128/mBio.01667-19

146. Couch RB, Atmar RL, Keitel WA, Quarles JM, Wells J, Arden N, et al. Randomized comparative study of the serum antihemagglutinin and antineuraminidase antibody responses to six licensed trivalent influenza vaccines. *Vaccine.* (2012) 31:190–5. doi: 10.1016/j.vaccine.2012.10.065

147. Laguio-Vila MR, Thompson MG, Reynolds S, Spencer SM, Gaglani M, Naleway A, et al. Comparison of serum hemagglutinin and neuraminidase inhibition antibodies after 2010-2011 trivalent inactivated influenza vaccination in healthcare personnel. *Open Forum Infect Dis.* (2015) 2:ofu115. doi: 10.1093/ofid/ofu115

148. Schotsaert M, Ysenbaert T, Neyt K, Ibañez LI, Bogaert P, Schepens B, et al. Natural and long-lasting cellular immune responses against influenza in the M2e-immune host. *Mucosal Immunol.* (2013) 6:276–87. doi: 10.1038/mi.2012.69

149. El Bakkouri K, Descamps F, De Filette M, Smet A, Festjens E, Birkett A, et al. Universal vaccine based on ectodomain of matrix protein 2 of influenza A:Fc receptors and alveolar macrophages mediate protection. *J Immunol.* (2011) 186:1022–31. doi: 10.4049/jimmunol.0902147

150. Scorza FB, Pardi N. New kids on the block:RNA-based influenza virus vaccines. *Vaccines.* (2018) 6:20. doi: 10.3390/vaccines6020020

151. Angeletti D, Kosik I, Santos JJS, Yewdell WT, Boudreau CM, Mallajosyula VVA, et al. Outflanking immunodominance to target subdominant broadly neutralizing epitopes. *Proc Natl Acad Sci USA.* (2019) 116:13474–9. doi: 10.1073/pnas.1816300116

152. Cirelli KM, Carnathan DG, Nogal B, Martin JT, Rodriguez OL, Upadhyay AA, et al. Slow delivery immunization enhances HIV neutralizing antibody and germinal center responses via modulation of immunodominance. *Cell.* (2019) 177:1153–71.e28. doi: 10.1016/j.cell.2019.04.012

153. Moyer TJ, Zmolek AC, Irvine DJ. Beyond antigens and adjuvants:formulating future vaccines. *J Clin Invest.* (2016) 126:799–808. doi: 10.1172/JCI81083

17

The Immunological Properties of Recombinant Multi-Cystatin-Like Domain Protein from *Trichinella Britovi* Produced in Yeast

Anna Stachyra [1], Anna Zawistowska-Deniziak [1], Katarzyna Basałaj [1], Sylwia Grzelak [1], Michał Gondek [2] and Justyna Bień-Kalinowska [1]**

[1] Witold Stefanski Institute of Parasitology, Polish Academy of Sciences, Warsaw, Poland, [2] Department of Food Hygiene of Animal Origin, Faculty of Veterinary Medicine, University of Life Sciences in Lublin, Lublin, Poland

***Correspondence:**
Anna Stachyra
astachyra@twarda.pan.pl
Justyna Bień-Kalinowska
bien.justyna@hotmail.com

Trichinellosis is a globally-distributed zoonotic parasitic disease caused by nematode worms of the genus *Trichinella*. One of the most common species of *Trichinella* known to affect human health is *T. britovi*; however, it is relatively poorly investigated. A thorough knowledge of the proteins expressed by *Trichinella* is important when developing immunological detection methods and vaccines and studying its interactions with the host. The present study uses the *Pichia pastoris* expression system to produce a soluble TbCLP antigen which induces strong antibody responses in the host during natural infection. Our results demonstrate the feasibility of TbCLP antigen production in yeasts, which are able to carry out post-translational modifications such as glycosylation and disulfide bond formation; they also indicate that the glycosylated TbCLP antigen had immunogenic effects in the tested mice and induced a mixed Th1/Th2 response, and was associated with a reduced larval burden after challenge with *T. britovi*. Subsequent *in vitro* stimulation of mice splenocytes revealed that TbCLP most likely possesses immunomodulatory properties and may play a significant role in the early phase of infection, affecting host immunological responses.

Keywords: ***Trichinella britovi*, cystatin-like protein, *Pichia pastoris*, immunization, immunomodulation**

INTRODUCTION

Trichinellosis is a common food-borne parasitic zoonosis worldwide. Infection occurs through the consumption of raw or inadequately-cooked meat containing *Trichinella* larvae: one of the most widespread intracellular parasitic nematodes affecting vertebrates (1, 2). The entire life cycle of the *Trichinella* parasite takes place in a single host after ingestion of infected muscle tissue. Parasitic infection can be divided into three separate antigenic stages: adult worms (Ad), newborn larvae (NBL), and muscle larvae (ML).

Within the *Trichinella* genus, the most widespread and most widely-investigated species has historically been *T. spiralis*. The parasite mainly occurs in domestic animals, and its circulation is traditionally associated with consumption of pig meat by humans. However, a range of other *Trichinella* species, such as *T. nativa, T. britovi, T. nelsoni, T. murelli*, and *T. pseudospiralis*, also circulate in sylvatic cycles and could also represent an accidental threat for human and domestic animals.

Of these species, *T. britovi* is the most widely distributed (1, 3). It can infect a wide range of mammalian hosts, mostly carnivores such as raccoon dogs, red foxes, and wolves, but is also known to invade various omnivores including wild boars, martens, badgers, and rodents (3–6). Trichinellosis is a widely-known public health hazard, especially in developing countries, but also represents an economic problem in the production of pork products and food safety. In contrast, developed countries tend to have a lower risk of trichinellosis associated with the consumption of pig-based products due to their high biosecurity standards and strict veterinary control in the pig farming and food processing industries. Currently, the most common source of trichinellosis in developed countries is through the consumption of game hunted for recreation: as it is not intended for sale, but only for private consumption, the meat is often not subject to veterinary inspection. Interestingly, while *T. spiralis* was found to predominate in samples of wild boar, a commonly consumed type of meat, *T. britovi* ML were also present in smaller numbers (7, 8). Hence, it is reasonable to assume that some cases of human trichinellosis may be caused by *T. britovi*, and numerous cases have already been confirmed (9–12). Therefore, to better understand the biology of the nematode and the host-parasite relationship, proteomical and immunological studies of *T. britovi* aimed at the identification of active proteins and potent antigens are needed.

Proteomical analysis (13, 14) and immunoscreening of cDNA expression libraries (15, 16) indicate that the multi-cystatin-like domain protein (named MCD or CLP) of *T. spiralis* is a highly antigenic protein. Its expression has been confirmed by RT-PCR in all developmental stages, with the highest level occurring in Ad. The protein was localized in the stichosome of Ad and ML and was also detected as a component of the excretory-secretory antigen (ES) of both Ad and ML (16–18). Hypothetical CLP was also recently detected by immunoblotting of somatic protein extract of *T. britovi* ML (19). Referred studies revealed, that this protein is produced in various stages of the parasite life cycle, after which it accumulates in the stichosome and is later released at specific stages of development as a component of the ES antigen, with its greatest release probably being at the intestinal stage (16).

Cystatins, inhibitors of cysteine proteinases, are a major class of parasitic nematode molecules with immunomodulatory properties that enhance production of the anti-inflammatory IL-10 cytokine and inhibit legumains, thus preventing MHC-II generation (20). Nematode proteinase inhibitors are generally known to play important functions at the host-parasite interface and are targeted by the immunological system. They control their own proteinase activity and that of the host, and weaken the immunological response by influencing antigen processing and presentation, cytokine production, and T-cell proliferation (21, 22).

Interestingly, the *Trichinella* CLP protein most likely has no cysteine protease inhibitory activity, and its function is unknown. The protein is classified within the cystatin superfamily, and demonstrates a similarity to family 3 kininogens: glycosylated and secreted proteins that are of relatively high mass and contain three family 2 cystatin-like domains (23). Robinson et al. (18) report that recombinant TsCLP produced in *E. coli* was not able to inhibit papain *in vitro*; the authors attribute this to the absence of two conserved motifs (QXVXG and PW in each cystatin domain), which are normally present in family 2 cystatins, and which form a structure that blocks the active site of the protease (24, 25). Instead of inhibitory activity, they propose that the protein can undergo self-processing and release single cystatin-like peptides to perform specific functions. Even so, the function of these peptides remains unknown. These low molecular weight isoforms of native CLP were observed in two-dimensional (2-D) analysis of ES antigen; the isoforms were also observed following expression of TsCLP in HeLa cells but not in *E. coli* (14, 16, 18), suggesting that CLP activity requires eukaryotic post-translational modification, such as the formation of disulfide bonds or glycosylation.

Pichia pastoris is a methylotrophic yeast used for expression of recombinant proteins; it is a particularly attractive host for this process due to its potential for methanol-dependent induction, triggered by the tightly-regulated AOX1 promoter (26). The system is useful for both large-scale and laboratory-level production of recombinant proteins, and can produce large amounts of the protein of interest. As a eukaryotic organism, *P. pastoris* ensures that the proteins undergo post-translational modification, and offers very economical handling and propagation. It is therefore an interesting alternative to other expression systems (27). Following eukaryote-specific post-translational modification, the produced recombinant proteins are generally highly similar to native proteins. Their disulfide bonds are correctly formed and preserved (28). The N-glycosylation profile is usually high mannose with no tendency to hyper-glycosylation and the oligosaccharides are often attached at the same positions as in natural glycoproteins (29, 30). A number of pharmacologically-active proteins are commercially produced in this expression system, e.g., hepatitis B vaccine antigen, human serum albumin, human IFNα, anti-RSV antibody and human insulin (source: https://pichia.com/). However, few studies have been published concerning the production of parasitic nematode proteins in this way (31–34), particularly *Trichinella* proteins.

CLP protein was identified as one of the reactive spots in our previous proteomic analysis of *T. britovi* antigens, based on a combination of 2-D immunoblotting of sera from infected pigs followed by LC-MS/MS analysis (19). It was therefore selected as a promising immunoreactive protein for further study, especially that the *T. britovi* homolog of CLP was yet not known. The aim of the present study was to achieve expression of the TbCLP antigen in a eukaryotic system, and to evaluate its potential diagnostic applications and protective efficacy against *T. britovi* infection in a mouse model.

MATERIALS AND METHODS

T. britovi Parasite and Mouse Model

The reference strain of *T. britovi* (ISS002) had been maintained by several passages in male C3H mice at the Institute of Parasitology, PAS. Muscle larvae were used for challenge infection of C3H mice and as a source of genetic material for cloning. The larvae were recovered from the infected mice by HCl-pepsin digestion (35). The animals were housed in a temperature-controlled environment at 24°C with 12-h day-night cycles, and received food and water *ad libitum*.

Sequence Analysis

The amino acid (aa) sequences were aligned using CLUSTALW. The N-glycosylation sites were predicted using NetNGlyc server (http://www.cbs.dtu.dk/services/NetNGlyc/).

Cloning of Recombinant CLP Gene

T. britovi ML were obtained for total RNA isolation using Total RNA mini Plus kit (A&A Biotechnology). The RNA template was then used for cDNA synthesis with the Maxima First Strand cDNA Synthesis Kit for RT-qPCR (Thermo Scientific) according to the manufacturer's protocol. The cDNA coding the TbCLP gene without its signal peptide was amplified by PCR with CLP-specific primers (Forward: 5′-AGGCATCGATACAGATACTTG GTGAAAC-3′, Reverse: 5′-GCTCTAGAGCACATTCAACAG TTGACTTG-3′). Since the nucleotide sequence of *T. britovi* CLP was not known, primers were designed according to the nucleotide sequence of *T. spiralis* CLP (GenBank no. FR694976), whose amino acid sequence is thought to be very similar to the hypothetical sequence of TbCLP (GenBank no. KRY50178). The cDNA coding for TbCLP was sequenced and subcloned into the yeast expression vector pPICZαC with the His-tag sequence at the C-terminus (Invitrogen/Thermo). The correct reading frame of the recombinant plasmid was confirmed by DNA sequencing using vector flanking primers, 5′AOX1 and 3′AOX1.

Expression and Purification of Recombinant CLP in *P. pastoris*

Pichia pastoris cells (X33 strain) were transformed with recombinant plasmids by electroporation. X33 transformant selection was performed using a medium containing Zeocin, and successful integration of the CLP gene into the *P. pastoris* genome was confirmed by PCR. The recombinant TbCLP with C-terminus His-tag was expressed by induction with 0.5% methanol for 24–72 h in 200 ml of Buffered Methanol-complex Medium (BMMY), and then purified by immobilized metal ion affinity chromatography using Protino Ni-NTA agarose (Macherey-Nagel). The protein samples were analyzed qualitatively by SDS PAGE and Western blotting, and their concentration was measured using Pierce BCA Protein Assay Kit (Thermo Scientific).

Enzymatic Deglycosylation

Samples of recombinant protein purified from medium after 24, 48, and 72 h of induction were digested with Endo H (New England Biolabs) in denaturing conditions, according to the manufacturer's instructions. Deglycosylated rTbCLP were analyzed by SDS-PAGE.

SDS-PAGE and Western Blot Analysis

SDS-PAGE was performed in 10% BisTris polyacrylamide gels. After electrophoresis, the gels were either stained with Coomassie brilliant blue or the proteins were transferred to a nitrocellulose membrane (Bio-Rad) for Western blotting. The recombinant protein was detected using monoclonal Anti-polyHistidine–Peroxidase antibody (diluted 1:4,000; Sigma). The proteins were viewed with Super Signal Western Pico Chemiluminescent Substrate (Thermo Scientific). Alternatively, rTbCLP was detected using sera from immunized or infected mice (1:200) and a secondary anti-mouse IgG antibody conjugated with HRP (1:8,000, Abcam).

Determination of Recombinant Antigen Immunoreactivity by ELISA

A panel of *T. britovi* serum samples stored in our collection were used for testing rTbCLP as an antigen in ELISA; the samples had been obtained from pigs experimentally infected with 5000 *T. britovi* ML. Testing was performed on samples were taken at multiple time points post-infection (−4, 3, 6, 9, 13, 15, 17, 20, 24, 29, 36, 41, 45, 51, 55, 59, 62 days post-infection, dpi). ELISA plates were coated with 2 μg/ml of rTbCLP protein and incubated at 4°C overnight.

The pig serum samples were added at 1:100 dilution and the plates were incubated at 37°C for 1 h. Goat anti-pig IgG conjugated with peroxidase (Sigma) at 1:20,000 dilution was used for detection of CLP-specific antibodies. The enzymatic color reaction was generated using TMB substrate (3,3′,5,5′-Tetramethylbenzidine; Sigma), and the absorbance value was measured at 450 nm using a Synergy HT microplate reader (BioTek). The cut-off value of ELISA was evaluated on the basis of the average OD plus three standard deviations (SD) of *Trichinella*-free serum samples of pigs (36).

Immunization and Challenge Infection

Eight-week old male C3H mice were divided into three groups of 12 animals each. The vaccine group was immunized subcutaneously with 25 μg of rTbCLP emulsified with the adjuvant Alhydrogel (InvivoGen) in a total volume of 100 μl (antigen/Alhydrogel = 75/25 v/v). The mice were boosted with the same dose after 1 week. The control groups were injected with PBS or PBS+Alhydrogel using the same regimen. 1 week after the final vaccination, six mice from each group were sacrificed, and their blood and spleens were harvested for immunological tests. The remaining six mice from each group were challenged orally with 500 *T. britovi* ML. 7 weeks (48 days) after infection, all mice were sacrificed, the blood and spleens were harvested, and the *T. britovi* muscle larvae were recovered by HCl-pepsin digestion. Protective immunity was calculated according to the number of ML recovered from the vaccinated group compared with those from the PBS group. Sera from all mouse blood samples were isolated and frozen at −20°C for further analysis.

Determination of Serum-Specific Antibodies

TbCLP-specific antibodies (IgG as well as subclasses IgG1 and IgG2a) in serum samples of vaccinated mice were measured by indirect ELISA, with rTbCLP as coating antigen, at 1 week after final immunization and 7 weeks after challenge infection. ELISA plates were coated with 2 μg/ml of rTbCLP protein and incubated at 4°C overnight. Following this, mouse serum samples at 1:200 dilution were added and incubated at 37°C for 1 h. Then, the plates were incubated with HRP-conjugated antibody goat anti-mouse IgG, IgG1, or IgG2a (1:80,000 or 1:60,000, Abcam) for detection of CLP-specific antibodies. The enzymatic color reaction was generated and the cut-off value of ELISA was evaluated as described in the present study.

Cytokine Analysis

To measure the specific cellular response, the spleens were harvested from vaccinated animals 1 week after final immunization and 7 weeks after challenge infection.

The spleens were pooled into pairs taken from two randomly-selected mice within the same group; following this, the splenocytes were disassociated using a 70 μm cell strainer and then suspended in complete RMPI medium (Biowest). In order to lyse the erythrocytes, the splenocytes were incubated in 5 ml RBC lysis buffer (Thermo Scientific) for 10 min. The cell suspension was centrifuged at 250 × g at room temperature for 7 min. The cell pellets were washed in RPMI medium and then resuspended in complete RPMI medium containing 10% FBS and penicillin/streptomycin (Biowest); following this, the cells were then counted.

For the cytokine stimulation assay, the splenocytes were seeded in a 24-well culture plate (Corning) at 5×10^6 cells per well in 1,000 μl medium. The cells were stimulated with 15 μg/ml rTbCLP and incubated for 72 h at 37°C in a humidified atmosphere of 5% CO_2. Cells stimulated with 5 ug/mL Concavalin A were included as positive controls. Non-stimulated cells were included as negative controls. After 72 h, the cells were pelleted by centrifugation at 1,000 × g for 10 min and the supernatants were collected to measure cytokine production. Samples containing the supernatant were tested for levels of IL-2, IL-4, IL-10, IFN-γ using a Mouse Th1/Th2 uncoated ELISA kit (Invitrogen/Thermo Scientific).

Statistical Analysis

Statistical analysis was performed using Statistica 6 software (StatSoft). Data were expressed as means ± standard deviation (SD). Differences among groups were analyzed by one-way analysis of variance (ANOVA). A value of $p < 0.05$ was considered significant.

RESULTS

Cloning, Expression, and Characterization of Recombinant TbCLP Protein

Since the nucleotide sequence of *T. britovi* CLP was not known, PCR primers were designed according to nucleotide sequence of *T. spiralis* CLP. TsCLP (GenBank no. CBX25716) shares 91.5% identity with the hypothetical sequence of TbCLP (Genbank no. KRY50178) derived from conceptual translation of genomic data (37). As the amino acids in regions including the primers sequences was found to be identical in TbCLP and TsCLP, the DNA sequence for TbCLP without its signal peptide was successfully amplified and subcloned into the expression vector (**Figure 1**). Sequencing revealed full compatibility between the hypothetical and cloned TbCLP, with regard to the amino acid sequence, and the nucleotide sequence was 96.2% identical with

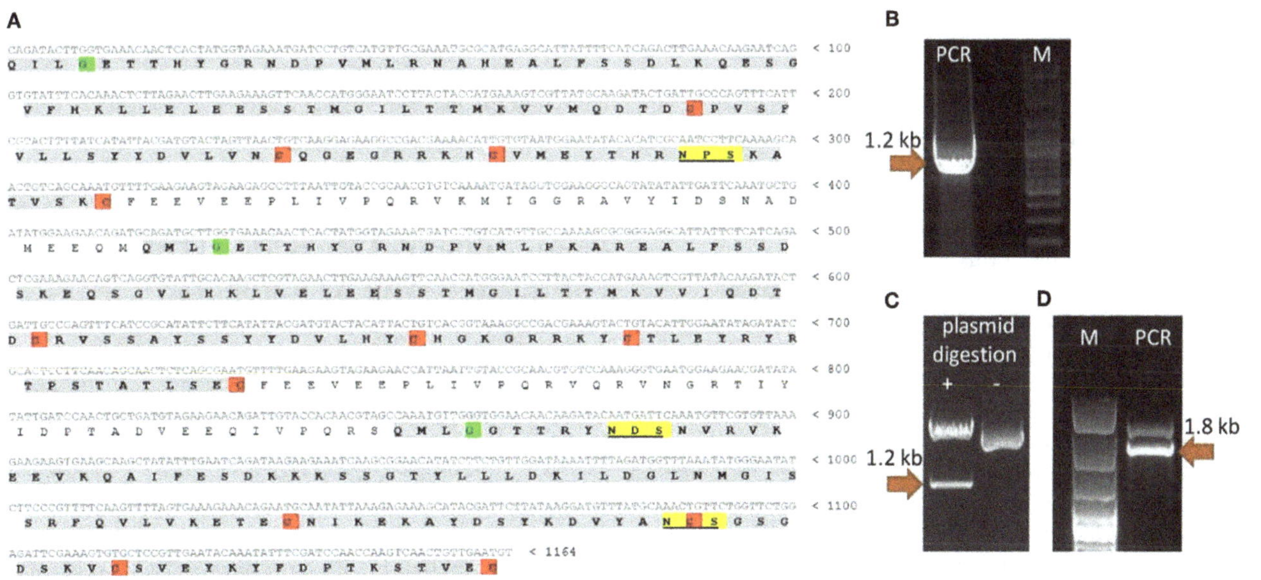

FIGURE 1 | Cloning of TbCLP coding sequence. **(A)** Cloned cDNA sequence and predicted amino acid sequence of TbCLP. Three cystatin-like domains are highlighted in gray [according to Robinson et al. (18)]. Conserved cysteines, that form disulfide bonds are highlighted in red. Conserved glycines are highlighted in green. Predicted N-glycosylation sites are underlined and highlighted in yellow. **(B)** PCR product after amplification of TbCLP cDNA. **(C)** Restriction digestion of recombinant plasmid containing target insert. **(D)** PCR product after screening of *P. pastoris* transformants. Correct DNA fragments are marked with arrows and the molecular mass is indicated.

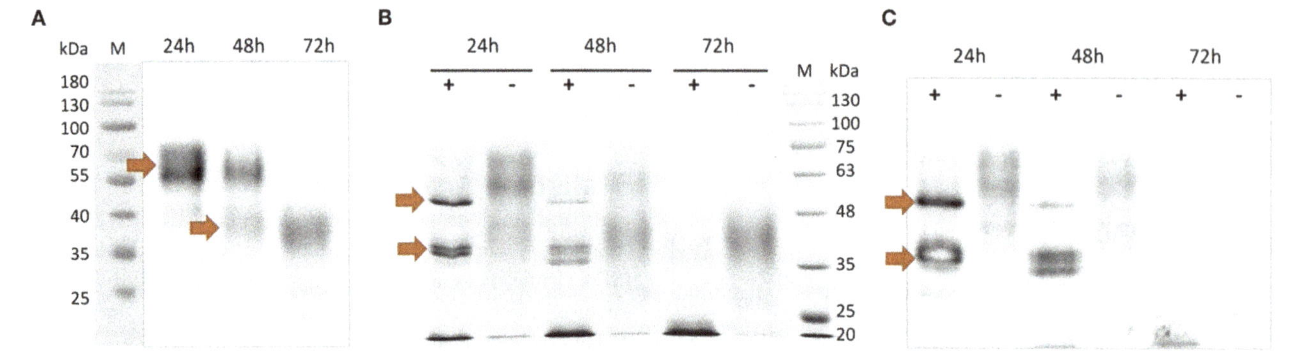

FIGURE 2 | Analysis of purified rTbCLP. **(A)** Anti-His Western blot of protein purified from medium after 24, 48 and 72 h of induction. High molecular weight glycoisoforms (55–70 kDa) and low molecular weight glycoisoforms (35–45 kDa) are marked with arrows. **(B)** SDS PAGE and **(C)** Anti-His Western blot after deglycosylation of rTbCLP with Endo H. Protein samples were incubated with Endo H enzyme (+) or without Endo H (-) in denaturing conditions. Deglycosylated full form rTbCLP (48 kDa) and the shorter isoforms (35–38 kDa) are marked with arrows.

that of the TsCLP gene. The sequence of the cloned TbCLP without the signal peptide is given in **Figure 1A**.

The theoretical molecular weight of the His-tagged TbCLP was predicted as 47.3 kDa, and the molecular weight of a single cystatin-like domain was 12 kDa. NetNGlyc server analysis of the amino acid sequence identified three potential N-glycosylation sites in the protein chain: one in the first cystatin-like domain and another two in the third cystatin-like domain.

CLP gene expression was induced in the X33 *P. pastoris* strain with methanol. In preliminary experiments, 0.5% methanol was added every 24 h until the final time of induction was reached. Further analyses indicated that a single induction with methanol and 24-h cultivation yielded the best rTbCLP level. The recombinant His-tagged protein was purified using affinity chromatography under native conditions.

After purification, the rTbCLP protein appeared to be present as various different glycoisoforms, manifesting as blurred, smear bands with molecular weights of ∼55–70 and 35–45 kDa on Western blot (**Figure 2A**). Interestingly, different protein forms were observed after 24, 48, and 72 h of induction: high molecular weight glycoisoforms were visible after 24 and 48 h of induction, and only low molecular weight glycoisoforms were visible after 72 h of induction. In order to examine the N-glycosylation of recombinant CLP protein, an Endo H digestion procedure was used. Deglycosylation with Endo H reduced the molecular mass of rTbCLP (**Figures 2B,C**) and confirmed that the observed variation in protein masses was caused by changes in glycan content. After the release of N-linked carbohydrates from the protein, the upper band corresponded well with the predicted mass of full length TbCLP (48 kDa), and the lower bands corresponded with the shorter isoforms (35–38 kDa), which may be created by post-translational cleavage events. After 24 and 48 h of induction, the full form of the protein was visible, as well as several shorter forms (**Figures 2B,C**). After 72 h of induction, the full form of protein was no longer visible, and the total amount of protein seemed very low, indicating that the whole pool of rTbCLP expressed in *P. pastoris* had been processed. The protein was taken after 24 h of induction, purified and used in subsequent experiments.

rTbCLP Recognition by Sera From *T. britovi* Infected Pigs

The results in **Figure 3** represent the antibody kinetics in eight pigs that were experimentally infected with 5000 ML *T. britovi* using rTbCLP. The ELISA results demonstrate that seroconversion was detected at 24 days post-infection. The moment of detection was earlier than when using a commercial PrioCHECK® *Trichinella* Antibody ELISA Kit (Thermo Scientific) containing ES *Trichinella* antigen (data not shown). The results confirm the antigenic properties of rTbCLP protein and indicate that rTbCLP is a potential antigen to be used in future experiments for detection of *Trichinella* infection in animals.

Humoral Antibody Response Induced by Immunization of Mice With rTbCLP Formulated With Alhydrogel

Purified rTbCLP was tested for immunogenicity in a mouse model. The total IgG level in serum was first evaluated in immunized and control groups; following this, the humoral antibody responses in the immunized mice were assayed by ELISA, with rTbCLP as a coating antigen (**Figure 4A**).

The results indicate that anti-TbCLP IgG antibodies were elicited by the immunization of mice with rTbCLP+adjuvant. Specific anti-TbCLP IgG were detected in all serum samples from the immunized group; however no anti-TbCLP antibody response was detected in the mice injected with adjuvant or PBS alone. Although anti-TbCLP antibodies were present in sera of all experimental groups after the challenge infection, a significantly higher level of specific anti-TbCLP was observed in the group of mice immunized with rTbCLP+adjuvant than the two control groups.

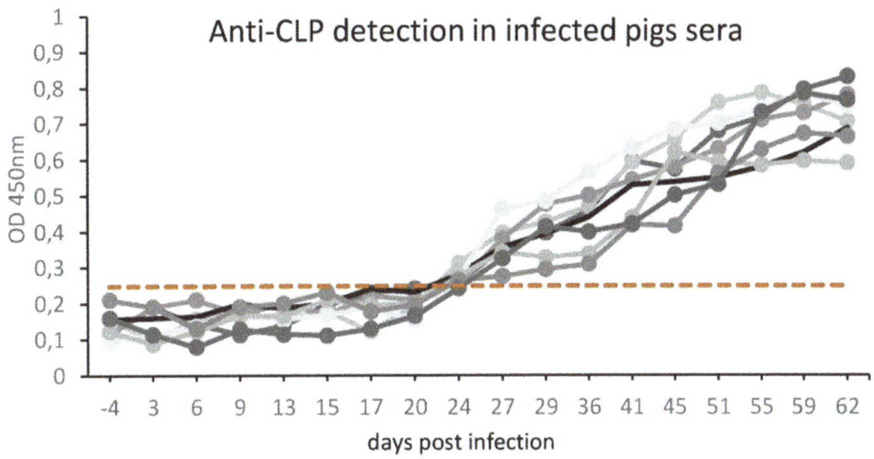

FIGURE 3 | Anti-*Trichinella* IgG levels in pigs infected with *T. britovi* by ELISA with rTbCLP. Pigs ($n = 8$) were experimentally infected with 5,000 ML of *T. britovi* and sera were collected prior to infection (−4 dpi) and 3, 6, 9, 13, 15, 17, 20, 24, 29, 36, 41, 45, 51, 55, 59, 62 dpi. The cut-off value was evaluated on the basis of the average OD plus three SD of *Trichinella*-free serum samples and is marked as a dashed line. All individuals were found positive after 24 days post-infection.

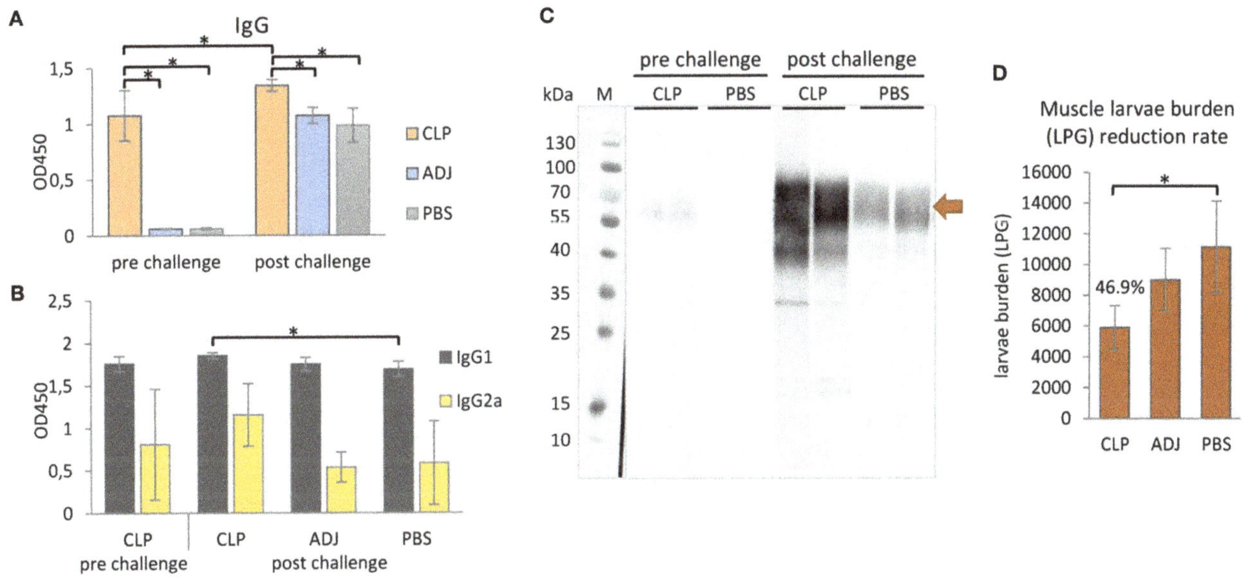

FIGURE 4 | Mouse immune responses to the immunization of rTbCLP. **(A)** Anti-TbCLP total IgG level and **(B)** anti-TbCLP subclasses IgG1 and IgG2a level in sera of immunized mice, measured by ELISA after final immunization and challenge infection, respectively. **(C)** Anti-TbCLP total IgG in sera of experimental mice, detected by Western blot. Two randomly selected sera from each group were used for immunodetection of rTbCLP (3 μg/lane). Specific signal for 55–70 kDa form is marked with arrow. **(D)** Muscle larvae burden reduction rate (%) in three experimental mice groups after challenge infection. Experimental groups: CLP—group injected with rTbCLP+adjuvant, ADJ—group injected with adjuvant, PBS—group injected with PBS. Significant differences are marked with asterisks. Bars represent mean values from six individuals ($n = 6$) ± SD.

A relatively high level of IgG1 and a moderate level of IgG2a were observed following induction by rTbCLP. After the challenge infection with *T. britovi*, all groups demonstrated a high level of IgG1; however, the mice injected with rTbCLP+adjuvant displayed a significantly higher level than the PBS control group. In contrast, moderate levels of anti-TbCLP subclass IgG2a were detected in all tested groups, but no significant differences were detected between groups due to the high level of individual variation (**Figure 4B**). The presence of anti-TbCLP antibodies was also confirmed by Western blot, using sera from the rTbCLP+adjuvant and the PBS control groups after immunization and after challenge infection. Induced IgG were able to give specific signal as showed at **Figure 4C**.

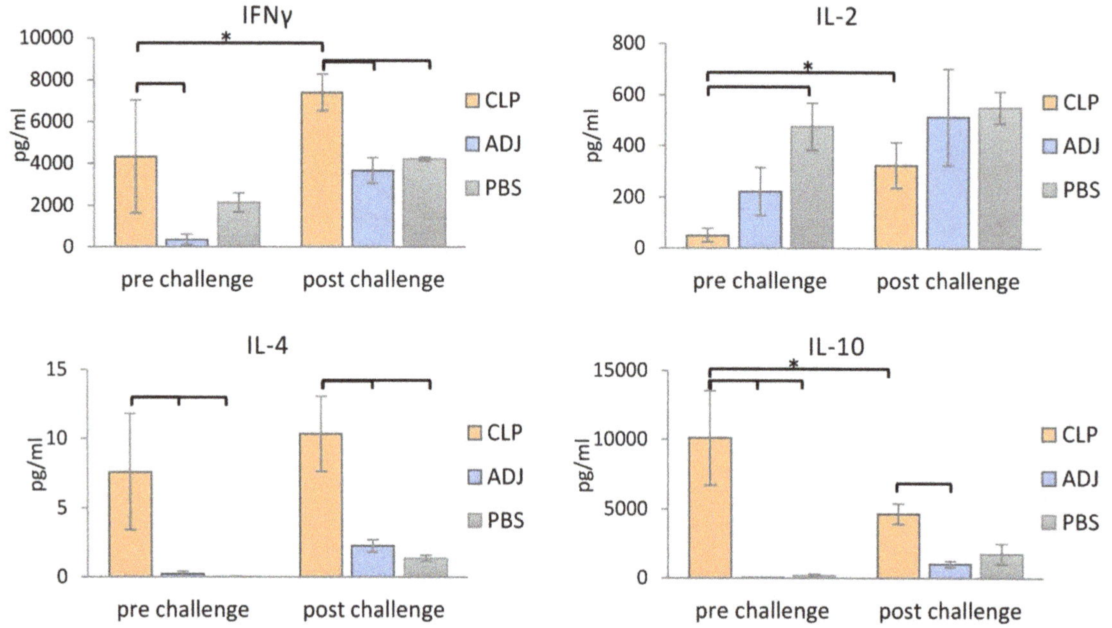

FIGURE 5 | Cytokines detection in supernatants of stimulated splenocytes of the immunized mice. Supernatants harvested after 72 h of incubation were analyzed for detection of secreted cytokines IFNγ, IL-2, IL-4, and IL-10 using Mouse Th1/Th2 uncoated ELISA kit. Experimental groups are indicated as previously described. Immunized groups significantly different from corresponding control groups are marked with empty brackets, while corresponding immunized groups significantly different from each other are marked with asterisks. Bars represent means ± SD from three splenocytes cultures ($n = 3$) each prepared from two pooled spleens from mice from the same group.

Cytokine Profiles of Stimulated Splenocytes From Mice Immunized With rTbCLP

To further confirm that a Th1/Th2 mixed response was induced following rTbCLP vaccination, the levels of selected cytokines (IFNγ, IL-2, IL-4, and IL-10) were measured in the supernatants of stimulated splenocyte cultures. In the case of Th1, higher levels of IFNγ were identified in splenocytes from mice immunized with rTbCLP+adjuvant than controls treated with adjuvant or PBS alone, with significantly lower levels observed in the adjuvant controls. However, after challenge infection with *T. britovi,* significantly higher levels of IFNγ were found in the rTbCLP+adjuvant group than the others (**Figure 5**). In contrast, IL-2 levels were significantly lower in the rTbCLP+adjuvant cultures than the PBS control group. After infection, these levels was still lower in the cultures from immunized mice than controls; however, these differences were not statistically significant.

Clearer differences were visible in case of the Th2 cytokines: the levels of IL-4 and IL-10 were significantly higher in the supernatants of the immunized mice than in the two control groups, in which the cytokine levels were at the limit of detection (**Figure 5**). After infection, the level of IL-4 in the immunized group was at a similar value than before infection, but the level of IL-10 was clearly lower than before infection. These results confirm that immunization with TbCLP triggered a mixed Th1/Th2 response.

Protective Immunity Induced by rTbCLP

The protective response induced by rTbCLP against *T. britovi* infection was investigated in experimental C3H mice. Seven weeks (48 days) after infection, all mice (six per group) were sacrificed and *T. britovi* muscle larvae were recovered from individual mice. The results revealed a significantly different reduction rate (46.9%) between the immunized group and the PBS control group (**Figure 4D**).

DISCUSSION

Multi cystatin-like domain protein (CLP) is promising immunoreactive protein used in studies to control trichinellosis. Although *T. spiralis* CLP has previously been cloned and used for immunization (16, 18, 38), the properties of *T. britovi* CLP are generally unknown, and only genomic data were available of its hypothetical sequence. Our findings indicate a great degree of similarity between the CLP of *T. britovi* and that of *T. spiralis.* Fortunately, the target gene could be successfully amplified by PCR (**Figure 1B**) as the annealing regions in the coding sequences of *T. britovi* and *T. spiralis* were found to share a high degree of similarity. The two nematodes are closely related, and TsCLP and TbCLP share 91.5% identity in their amino acid sequences and 96.2% identity for their nucleotide sequences.

To evaluate the potential of *P. pastoris* as an expression host for production of a recombinant *T. britovi* CLP, the pPICZαC/CLP vector was constructed (**Figures 1C,D**) and expressed in X33 strain cells. The expressed rTbCLP displayed fuzzy, smear bands on Western blot (**Figure 2A**); it was difficult to precisely determine the mass of the detected protein bands and their mass appeared to vary depending on the duration of induction, i.e., 24, 48, or 72 h. It is known that in some cases protein expression in *P. pastoris* demonstrates heterogenic glycosylation, resulting in its protein population displaying diverse structural heterogeneity (30). Within a cell, two molecules of the same protein may present different oligosaccharide profiles, even when they have been exposed to the same glycosylation machinery. Such variation is typically derived from differences in the type, length and identity of the oligosaccharide at a given glycosylation site. The glycoprotein may also vary with regard to site occupancy.

In case of rTbCLP, great variation can be seen in protein subpopulations. Similar results were previously described by Teh et al. (39), where human erythropoietin (EPO) expressed in the *P. pastoris* system also demonstrated broad smear band in Western blot. EPO is a native glycoprotein (40), as is TbCLP and family 3 cystatins. Fractionation of rEPO followed by PNGase F and Endo H treatment found that the observed variations in molecular mass, manifested as the broad smear observed on the membrane, were caused by variations in glycan content: the deglycosylated protein demonstrated a sharp band with the predicted molecular mass. It is important to emphasize that the recombinant EPO was fully functionally active, despite the observed variation in glycosylation. In our study, deglycosylation with Endo H also resulted in the rTbCLP displaying sharp bands, and revealed the presence of high molecular weight and low molecular weight isoforms (**Figures 2B,C**).

A previous study has found recombinant TsCLP to possess different isoforms (18). Two such isoforms were found to be expressed in Hela cells, one of 49 kDa and another of 38 kDa; these were described respectively, as the full-length protein and the shorter isoform. Subsequent incubation at different pH values revealed that a further two low molecular weight isoforms (35 and 38 kDa) were visible in the pH range 4–8, and these bands were most prominent at pH 5. The authors suggest that the CLP undergoes pH-dependent auto-processing, resulting in the release of individual cystatin-like peptides (18).

This conclusion supports our observation that the amount of full length TbCLP decreases during induction in *P. pastoris*, with only low molecular-weight isoforms being observed after 72 h. It is known that in *Pichia* fermentation, the pH decreases while feeding from a carbon source, as the catabolic activity leads to acid production, potentially resulting in greater processing of the secreted rTbCLP into individual peptides. For this reason, only the protein isolated after 24 h of induction was used in the following experiments. In the future, to scale-up protein expression, it will be necessary to optimize the induction conditions, particularly the control of medium pH, to prevent early processing. Nonetheless, it is important to emphasize that in contrast to the rCLP previously produced in bacteria (16, 18), the *P. pastoris* system yielded an active, functional form of rTbCLP: native CLP is most probably secreted as a glycosylated protein containing disulfide bonds, and the initial full length form is further transformed into the shorter forms, these being the single cystatin-like peptides with specific biological functions, due to post-translational modification.

Our previous 2-D immunoblotting and LS-MS/MS analyses revealed some spots that reacted with the sera of *T. britovi* infected pigs; these were identified as a hypothetical protein highly similar to a multi-cystatin-like domain protein precursor from *Trichinella spiralis*. The molecular mass of the spots ranged from 45 to 50 kDa, which corresponded with the expected mass of CLP (19). To confirm this immunological reactivity, ELISA tests were performed to determine the level of anti-rTbCLP IgG in infected pig sera and seroconversion was detected at 24 dpi (**Figure 3**). However, high background values were observed and further optimization of test procedures is needed before the rTbCLP antigen can be used in diagnostics of anti-*Trichinnella* antibodies in serum samples.

Infection with *Trichinella* is initially characterized by the induction of a Th1 response at the beginning of the intestinal phase; however, the extensive dissemination of newborn larvae results in a shift to a Th2 response. The Th2 state is protective and results in parasite expulsion. *Trichinella* worms rapidly develop to maturity and reproduce before the Th2-mediated expulsion eliminates all adult forms from the gut. Thus, during the intestinal phase, the immune response is mixed, i.e., Th1/Th2, with an initial predominance of the Th1 response shifting to that of the Th2 response (41). In the present study an analysis of mouse humoral immune responses revealed high total IgG levels in serum; in addition, while IgG1 levels were clearly higher than those of IgG2a after vaccination with rTbCLP, IgG2a was also elicited, suggesting that the mixed Th1/Th2 immune response was triggered by immunization with rTbCLP (**Figures 4A,B**). The mixed immune response was further verified by the levels of Th1 (IFN-γ, IL-2) and Th2 cytokines (IL-4, IL-10) observed in the spleen cell cultures of immunized mice following stimulation by rTbCLP protein. Although all tested groups of mice displayed unique cytokine profiles, all cytokines in the immunized cultures were significantly elevated compared to controls, while IL-2 was significantly suppressed (**Figure 5**).

IFNγ is a signature cytokine of the adaptive immune response, and the main cytokine associated with Th1. High levels of IFNγ were detected in samples taken from groups after immunization and after challenge infection; however, the level of IFNγ was almost twice as high in the challenged group. This finding suggests that rTbCLP effectively induced the Th1/cellular response, which was then boosted after infection.

IL-2 plays a dual role in immunological system: it is a potent T cell growth factor associated with protective immune responses, but also influences immune tolerance and the downregulation of inflammation. The function of IL-2 *in vivo* is complex, and its influence on the immune response is not only dependent on its presence or absence, but also the level of IL-2 receptor (IL-2R) signaling that takes place (42, 43). The effect of immunization and splenocyte stimulation on IL-2 production *in vitro* is hard to interpret, but it may be related with CLP possessing certain immunomodulatory properties, which are currently unknown; these could affect IL-2R signaling pathways and the cytokine network in immune cells, resulting in inhibited IL-2 secretion and/or possibly augmented IL-2 consumption. Interestingly, our results correspond with those of an immune response analysis of *Trichinella* infection described by Yu et al. (44), where IL-2 level was found to be significantly downregulated in mouse sera during the intestinal and larvae migration phases compared to uninfected controls. Other tested cytokines were elevated or unchanged compared to controls during the respective infection phases, and only IL-2 exhibited downregulation during the early phase of infection. Suppression of IL-2 production may also be partially explained by the release of high amounts of IL-10, since IL-10 can inhibit production of IL-2 (45). Interestingly no other cytokine secretion was inhibited in our experiment, indicating that this phenomenon may be somehow related with the dichotomous role played by IL-2 and IL-2R in self-tolerance and immunity.

IL-4 is closely associated with the humoral (Th2) and anti-helminthic responses (46); as it regulates B-cell immunoglobulin secretion, it was not surprising that it was observed at high levels in cultures following immunization compared to naïve controls. In a similar way to IFNγ, the highest level of IL-4 was observed in the immunized and infected group, demonstrating that vaccination very effectively primed Th2 responses against the *T. britovi* parasite; this response was boosted further after infection, and the findings are in agreement with our IgG level analysis. However, the fact that the amounts of IL-4 found in all experimental supernatants were relatively small might be explained by the fact that IL-4 has a short half-life, and the cells were cultured for 72 h (47).

IL-10 is a well-known anti-inflammatory cytokine, and that during parasite infection, it plays a major role in parasite immunomodulation by suppressing immune responses. More interestingly, the main factor inducing the production of IL-10 by APCs, particularly macrophages, during infection are thought to be nematode cystatins (20, 48). Although the exact mechanism by which these cystatins activate IL-10 production in host cells is unknown, it is most probably independent of protease inhibitory activity, and is likely related to their structural features and receptors engagement. TbCLP was previously assumed to lack protease inhibitory activity; therefore, due to its conserved structure, it may modulate the host immune system by inducing the production of anti-inflammatory IL-10. Indeed, our findings indicate the presence of very high amounts of IL-10 in the supernatants of stimulated splenocytes. The level of IL-10 was the highest in the immunized group; however, these levels were significantly lower in the immunized and infected group, suggesting that impact of recombinant protein alone was very strong, but this influence was balanced by the broad immune response to infection. Interestingly, production of IL-4 and IL-10 by splenocytes was much weaker after *T. britovi* infection than after rTbCLP immunization. This could be possibly explained by the fact that the infection was in its late phase: the splenocytes were harvested 48 dpi, when the parasite is at the convalescent phase of the life cycle.

rTbCLP vaccination resulted in a 46.9% larvae reduction (**Figure 4D**); this was a similar benefit to one reported in a previous study of recombinant CLP in *T. spiralis* (16), where mice vaccinated with rTsCLP exhibited a significant reduction in muscle larvae burden. However, the previous experiment was conducted using Freund's Complete Adjuvant (CFA) and the antigen was administered intraperitoneally. These are very harsh immunization conditions, and CFA is known to cause some concerns in animal usage, due to its toxicity and painful reaction; even so, it is often used in mice (49, 50). In contrast, our present study used an alum adjuvant, which is non-toxic and approved for use in humans (51). It obtained good results, suggesting that yeast-derived antigen is superior to bacteria-derived antigens, as the milder immunization conditions yielded a similar immunoprotective effect. It is important to mention that, as far as we are aware, all recombinant *Trichinella* antigens tested so far have been produced in a bacterial expression system and may not have been fully active (52–56). To better characterize the functions of the proteins of interest, a eukaryotic expression system, such as the yeast expression chosen in this study, should be used.

CONCLUSIONS

Immunization with the active full form of rTbCLP resulted in high immunogenicity in tested mice and a significant reduction of larvae burden after experimental infection. The recombinant protein was produced in *Pichia* cells; this approach ensures that the protein is further processed into individual cystatin-like peptides via post-translational modification. Furthermore, it can be assumed that cytokine profiles of the presented splenocytes are both resultants of the immune response against recombinant TbCLP antigen administered as an experimental vaccine, as well as the product of the immunomodulation of immune cells by this antigen, resulting from its biological function. The molecular events triggered by rTbCLP as an antigen, or as a modulator, could be opposing or synergistic. This dichotomy is manifested in the observed imbalance of IL-2 and IL-10, two cytokines involved in immunosuppression (57). However, it should be remembered that our findings illustrate just a small part of the host response to immunization and infection. Future research on the immunomodulatory properties of TbCLP may allow for a better understanding of its function, and further studies on the usage of TbCLP for the purposes of diagnosis and vaccine development would be also desirable.

ETHICS STATEMENT

The procedures were approved by the First Local Ethical Committee for Scientific Experiments on Animals in Warsaw, Poland (resolution no.: 020/2016, 23 March 2016) and the Second Local Ethical Committee for Scientific Experiments on Animals in Lublin, Poland (resolution no.: 77/2015, 7 July 2015). All efforts were made to minimize suffering. All applicable international, national and/or institutional guidelines for the care and use of animals were followed. In order to collect material from infected and/or immunized mice, the animals were humanely euthanized by cervical dislocation.

AUTHOR CONTRIBUTIONS

AS and JB-K conceived and designed the experiments and analyzed the data. AS, AZ-D, and KB were involved in cloning. AS performed protein expression and analysis and immunological study. AS, J-BK, and SG participated in mice immunization and *in vitro* experiments. MG supplied the pig sera. AS wrote the manuscript. JB-K, AZ-D, and KB participated in reviewing and editing the manuscript. JB-K supervised the manuscript. All of the authors have read and approved the final manuscript.

REFERENCES

1. Gottstein B, Pozio E, Nockler K. Epidemiology, diagnosis, treatment, and control of trichinellosis. *Clin Microbiol Rev.* (2009) 22:127. doi: 10.1128/CMR.00026-08
2. Dupouy-Camet J. Trichinellosis: a worldwide zoonosis. *Vet Parasitol.* (2000) 93:191–200. doi: 10.1016/S0304-4017(00)00341-1
3. Pozio E, Zarlenga DS. New pieces of the *Trichinella* puzzle. *Int J Parasitol.* (2013) 43:983–97. doi: 10.1016/j.ijpara.2013.05.010
4. Pozio E, Rinaldi L, Marucci G, Musella V, Galati F, Cringoli G, et al. Hosts and habitats of *Trichinella spiralis* and *Trichinella britovi* in Europe. *Int J Parasitol.* (2009) 39:71–9. doi: 10.1016/j.ijpara.2008.06.006
5. Moskwa B, Gozdzik K, Bien J, Bogdaszewski M, Cabaj W. Molecular identification of *Trichinella britovi* in martens (*Martes martes)* and badgers (*Meles meles*); new host records in Poland. *Acta Parasitol.* (2012) 57:402–5. doi: 10.2478/s11686-012-0054-1
6. Cybulska A, Kornacka A, Moskwa B. The occurrence and muscle distribution of *Trichinella britovi* in raccoon dogs (*Nyctereutes procyonoides*) in wildlife in the Głeboki Bród Forest District, Poland. *Int J Parasitol Parasites Wildl.* (2019) 9:149–53. doi: 10.1016/j.ijppaw.2019.05.003
7. Moskwa B, Cybulska A, Kornacka A, Cabaj W, Bien J. Wild boars meat as a potential source of human trichinellosis in Poland: current data. *Acta Parasitol.* (2015) 60:530–5. doi: 10.1515/ap-2015-0075
8. Bilska-Zajac E, Rózycki M, Chmurzynska E, Marucci G, Cencek T, Karamon J, et al. *Trichinella* species circulating in wild boar (*Sus scrofa*) populations in Poland. *Int J Parasitol Parasites Wildl.* (2013) 2:211–3. doi: 10.1016/j.ijppaw.2013.05.004
9. Akkoc N, Kuruuzum Z, Akar S, Yuce A, Onen F, Yapar N, et al. A large-scale outbreak of trichinellosis caused by *Trichinella britovi* in Turkey. *Zoonoses Public Health.* (2009) 56:65–70. doi: 10.1111/j.1863-2378.2008.01158.x
10. Fichi G, Stefanelli S, Pagani A, Luchi S, De Gennaro M, Gómez-Morales MA, et al. Trichinellosis outbreak caused by meat from a wild boar hunted in an Italian region considered to be at negligible risk for *Trichinella. Zoonoses Public Health.* (2015) 62:285–91. doi: 10.1111/zph.12148
11. Gomez-Garcia V, Hernandez-Quero J, Rodriguez-Osorio M. Short report: human infection with *Trichinella britovi* in Granada, Spain. *Am J Trop Med Hyg.* (2003) 68:463–4. doi: 10.4269/ajtmh.2003.68.463
12. Messiaen P, Forier A, Vanderschueren S, Theunissen C, Nijs J, Van Esbroeck M. et al. Outbreak of trichinellosis related to eating imported wild boar meat, Belgium, 2014. *Euro Surveil.* (2016) 21:30341. doi: 10.2807/1560-7917.ES.2016.21.37.30341
13. Liu R, Qi X, Sun G, Jiang P, Zhang X, Wang L. Proteomic analysis of *Trichinella spiralis* adult worm excretory-secretory proteins recognized by early infection sera. *Vet Parasitol.* (2016) 231:43–6. doi: 10.1016/j.vetpar.2016.10.008
14. Robinson M, Connolly B. Proteomic analysis of the excretory-secretory proteins of the *Trichinella spiralis* L1 larva, a nematode parasite of skeletal muscle. *Proteomics.* (2005) 5:4525–32. doi: 10.1002/pmic.200402057
15. Wu X, B. Fu, Wang X, Yu L, Yu S, Deng H, et al. Identification of antigenic genes in *Trichinella spiralis* by immunoscreening of cDNA libraries. *Vet Parasitol.* (2009) 159:272–5. doi: 10.1016/j.vetpar.2008.10.035
16. Tang B, Liu M, Wang L, Yu S, Shi H, Boireau P, et al. Characterisation of a high-frequency gene encoding a strongly antigenic cystatin-like protein from *Trichinella spiralis* at its early invasion stage. *Parasit Vectors.* (2015) 8:78. doi: 10.1186/s13071-015-0689-5
17. Liu R, Wang Z, Wang L, Long S, Ren H, Cui J. Analysis of differentially expressed genes of *Trichinella spiralis* larvae activated by bile and cultured with intestinal epithelial cells using real-time PCR. *Parasitol Res.* (2013) 112:4113–20. doi: 10.1007/s00436-013-3602-1
18. Robinson M, Massie D, Connolly B. Secretion and processing of a novel multi-domain cystatin-like protein by intracellular stages of *Trichinella spiralis. Mol Biochem Parasitol.* (2007) 151:9–17. doi: 10.1016/j.molbiopara.2006.09.008
19. Grzelak S, Moskwa B, Bien J. *Trichinella britovi* muscle larvae and adult worms: stage-specific and common antigens detected by two-dimensional gel electrophoresis-based immunoblotting. *Parasit Vectors.* (2018) 11:584. doi: 10.1186/s13071-018-3177-x
20. Hartmann S, Lucius R. Modulation of host immune responses by nematode cystatins. *Int J Parasitol.* (2003) 33:1291–302. doi: 10.1016/S0020-7519(03)00163-2
21. Dzik J. Molecules released by helminth parasites involved in host colonization. *Acta Biochim Pol.* (2006) 53:33–64.
22. Cooper D, Eleftherianos I. Parasitic nematode immunomodulatory strategies: recent advances and perspectives. *Pathogens.* (2016) 5:E58. doi: 10.3390/pathogens5030058
23. Ochieng J, Chaudhuri G. Cystatin superfamily. *J Health Care Poor Underserved.* (2010) 21:51–70. doi: 10.1353/hpu.0.0257
24. Cornwall G, Hsia N. A new subgroup of the family 2 cystatins. *Mol Cell Endocrinol.* (2003) 200:1–8. doi: 10.1016/S0303-7207(02)00408-2
25. Turk V, Bode W. The cystatins - protein inhibitors of cysteine proteinases. *FEBS Lett.* (1991) 285:213–9. doi: 10.1016/0014-5793(91)80804-C
26. Ahmad M, Hirz M, Pichler H, Schwab H. Protein expression in *Pichia pastoris*: recent achievements and perspectives for heterologous protein production. *Appl Microbiol Biotechnol.* (2014) 98:5301–17. doi: 10.1007/s00253-014-5732-5
27. Cereghlno G, Cereghlno J, Ilgen C, Cregg J. Production of recombinant proteins in fermenter cultures of the yeast *Pichia pastoris. Curr Opin Biotechnol.* (2002) 13:329–32. doi: 10.1016/S0958-1669(02)00330-0
28. White C, Kempi N, Komives E. Expression of highly disulfide-bonded proteins in *Pichia pastoris. Structure.* (1994) 2:1003–5. doi: 10.1016/S0969-2126(94)00103-0
29. Grinna L, Tschopp J. Size distribution and general structural features on N-linkedoligosaccharides from the methylotrophic yeast, *Pichia pastoris. Yeast.* (1989) 5:107–15. doi: 10.1002/yea.320050206
30. Daly R, Hearn M. Expression of heterologous proteins in *Pichia pastoris*: a useful experimental tool in protein engineering and production. *J Mol Recogn.* (2005) 18:119–38. doi: 10.1002/jmr.687
31. Gonzalez-Hernandez A, Borloo J, Peelaers I, Casaert S, Leclercq G, Claerebout E. Comparative analysis of the immune responses induced by native versus recombinant versions of the ASP-based vaccine against the bovine intestinal parasite *Cooperia oncophora. Intl J Parasitol.* (2018) 48:41–9. doi: 10.1016/j.ijpara.2017.07.002
32. Holzhausen J, Haake C, Schicht S, Hinse P, Jordan D, Kremmer E. Biological function of *Dictyocaulus viviparus* asparaginyl peptidase legumain-1 and its suitability as a vaccine target. *Parasitology.* (2018) 145:378–92. doi: 10.1017/S0031182017001573
33. Noon J. Schwarz E, Ostroff G, Aroian R. A highly expressed intestinal cysteine protease of Ancylostoma ceylanicum protects vaccinated hamsters from hookworm infection. *PLoS Negl Trop Dis.* (2019) 13:e0007345. doi: 10.1371/journal.pntd.0007345
34. Wei J, Versteeg L, Liu Z, Keegan B, Gazzinelli-Guimaraes A, Fujiwara R, et al. Yeast-expressed recombinant As16 protects mice against *Ascaris suum* infection through induction of a Th2-skewed immune response. *PLoS Negl Trop Dis.* (2017) 11:e0005769. doi: 10.1371/journal.pntd.0005769
35. Kapel C, Gamble H. Infectivity, persistence, and antibody response to domestic and sylvatic *Trichinella* spp. in experimentally infected pigs. *Int J Parasitol.* (2000) 30:215–21. doi: 10.1016/S0020-7519(99)00202-7

36. Pozio E, Sofronic-Milosavljevic L, Morales M, Boireau P, Nockler K. Evaluation of ELISA and western blot analysis using three antigens to detect anti-*Trichinella* IgG in horses. *Vet Parasitol.* (2002) 108:163–78. doi: 10.1016/S0304-4017(02)00185-1
37. Korhonen PK, Pozio E, La Rosa G, Chang BC, Koehler AV, Hoberg EP. Phylogenomic and biogeographic reconstruction of the *Trichinella* complex. *Nat Commun.* (2016) 7:10513. doi: 10.1038/ncomms10513
38. Tang F, Xu L, Yan R, Song X, Li X. Evaluation of the immune response induced by DNA vaccines expressing MIF and MCD-1 genes of *Trichinella spiralis* in BALB/c mice. *J Helminthol.* (2012) 86:430–9. doi: 10.1017/S0022149X11000654
39. Teh S, Fong M, Mohamed Z. Expression and analysis of the glycosylation properties of recombinant human erythropoietin expressed in *Pichia pastoris*. *Genet Mol Biol.* (2011) 34:464–70. doi: 10.1590/S1415-47572011005000022
40. Jelkmann W. Erythropoietin after a century of research: younger than ever. *Eur J Haematol.* (2007) 78:183–205. doi: 10.1111/j.1600-0609.2007.00818.x
41. Ilic N, Gruden-Movsesijan A, Sofronic-Milosavljevic L. *Trichinella spiralis*: shaping the immune response. *Immunol Res.* (2012) 52:111–9. doi: 10.1007/s12026-012-8287-5
42. Nelson BH. IL-2, regulatory T cells, and tolerance. *J Immunol.* (2004) 172:3983–8. doi: 10.4049/jimmunol.172.7.3983
43. Malek T, Castro I. Interleukin-2 receptor signaling: at the interface between tolerance and immunity. *Immunity.* (2010) 33:153–65. doi: 10.1016/j.immuni.2010.08.004
44. Yu YR, Deng MJ, Lu WW, Jia MZ, Wu W, Qi YF. Systemic cytokine profiles and splenic toll-like receptor expression during *Trichinella spiralis* infection. *Exp Parasitol.* (2013)34:92–101. doi: 10.1016/j.exppara.2013.02.014
45. Couper KN, Blount DG, Riley EM. IL-10: the master regulator of immunity to infection. *J Immunol.* (2008) 180:5771–7. doi: 10.4049/jimmunol.180.9.5771
46. Jankovic D, Sher A, Yap G. Th1/Th2 effector choice in parasitic infection: decision making by committee. *Curr Opin Immunol.* (2001) 13:403–9. doi: 10.1016/S0952-7915(00)00234-X
47. Conlon PJ, Tyler S, Grabstein KH, Morrissey P. Interleukin-4 (B-cell stimulatory factor-1) augments the *in vivo* generation of cytotoxic cells in immunosuppressed animals. *Biotechnol Ther.* (1989) 1:31–41.
48. Klotz C, Ziegler T, Daniłowicz-Luebert E, Hartmann S. Cystatins of parasitic organisms. *Adv Exp Med Biol.* (2011) 12:208–21. doi: 10.1007/978-1-4419-8414-2_13
49. Batista-Duharte A, Martinez DT, Carlos IZ. Efficacy and safety of immunological adjuvants. Where is the cut-off? *Biomed Pharmacother.* (2018) 105:616–24. doi: 10.1016/j.biopha.2018.06.026
50. Martinon S, Cisneros A, Villicana S, Hernandez-Miramontes R, Mixcoha E, Calderon-Vargas P. Chemical and immunological characteristics of aluminum-based, oil-water emulsion, and bacterial-origin adjuvants. *J Immunol Res.* (2019) 2019:3974127. doi: 10.1155/2019/3974127
51. Apostolico J, Lunardelli V, Coirada F, Boscardin S, Rosa D. Adjuvants: classification, modus operandi, and licensing. *J Immunol Res.* (2016) 2016:1459394. doi: 10.1155/2016/1459394
52. Bi K, Yang J, Wang L, Gu Y, Zhan B, Zhu X. Partially protective immunity induced by a 20 kDa protein secreted by *Trichinella spiralis* stichocytes. *PLoS ONE.* (2015) 10:e0136189. doi: 10.1371/journal.pone.0136189
53. Li X, Yao JP, Pan AH, Liu W, Hu XC, Wu ZD et al. An antigenic recombinant serine protease from *Trichinella spiralis* induces protective immunity in BALB/c mice. *Parasitol Res.* (2013) 112:3229–38. doi: 10.1007/s00436-013-3500-6
54. Yang Z, Li W, Yang Z, Pan A, Liao W, Zhou X. A novel antigenic cathepsin B protease induces protective immunity in *Trichinella*-infected mice. *Vaccine.* (2018) 36:248–55. doi: 10.1016/j.vaccine.2017.11.048
55. Sun G, Song Y, Jiang P, Ren H, Yan S, Han Y, et al. Characterization of a *Trichinella spiralis* putative serine protease. Study of its potential as sero-diagnostic tool. *PLoS Negl Trop Dis.* (2018) 12:e0006485. doi: 10.1371/journal.pntd.0006485
56. Xu N, Liu X, Tang B, Wang L, Shi H, Boireau P, et al. Recombinant *Trichinella pseudospiralis* serine protease inhibitors alter macrophage polarization *in vitro*. *Front Microbiol.* (2017) 8:1834. doi: 10.3389/fmicb.2017.01834
57. Höfer T, Krichevsky O, Altan-Bonnet G. Competition for IL-2 between regulatory and effector T cells to chisel immune responses. *Front Immunol.* (2012) 3:268. doi: 10.3389/fimmu.2012.00268

18

CCR5 Promoter Polymorphisms Associated with Pulmonary Tuberculosis in a Chinese Han Population

Shuyuan Liu[1†], *Nannan Liu*[1†], *Hui Wang*[2], *Xinwen Zhang*[1], *Yufeng Yao*[1,3*], *Shuqiong Zhang*[2*] and *Li Shi*[1*]

[1] *Institute of Medical Biology, Chinese Academy of Medical Sciences & Peking Union Medical College, Kunming, China,* [2] *The Third People's Hospital of Kunming, Kunming, China,* [3] *Yunnan Key Laboratory of Vaccine Research and Development on Severe Infectious Diseases, Kunming, China*

***Correspondence:**
Yufeng Yao
leoyyf@gmail.com
Shuqiong Zhang
1357626082@qq.com
Li Shi
shili.imb@gmail.com

[†]*These authors have contributed equally to this work*

Background: Tuberculosis (TB), an infectious disease caused by *Mycobacterium tuberculosis*, is a major public health concern. Chemokines and their receptors, such as RANTES, CXCR3, and CCR5, have been reported to play important roles in cell activation and migration in immune responses against TB infection.

Methods: To understand the correlations involving *CCR5* gene variations, *M. tuberculosis* infection, and TB disease progression, a case-control study comprising 450 patients with TB and 306 healthy controls from a Chinese Han population was conducted, along with the detection of polymorphisms in the *CCR5* promoter using a sequencing method.

Results: After adjustment for age and gender, the results of logistic analysis indicated that the frequency of rs2734648-G was significantly higher in the TB patient group (P = 0.002, OR = 1.38, 95% CI: 1.123–1.696); meanwhile, rs2734648-GG showed notable susceptibility to TB (P = 6.32E-06, OR = 2.173, 95% CI: 1.546–3.056 in a recessive model). The genotypic frequency of rs1799987 also varied between the TB and control groups (P = 0.008). In stratified analysis, rs2734648-GG significantly increased susceptibility to pulmonary TB in a recessive model (P < 0.0001, OR = 2.382, 95% CI: 1.663–3.413), and the rs2734648-G allele significantly increased susceptibility to TB recurrence in a dominant model (P = 0.0032, OR = 1.936, 95% CI: 1.221–3.068), whereas rs1799987-AA was associated with susceptibility to pulmonary TB (P = 0.0078, OR = 1.678, 95% CI: 1.141–2.495 in a recessive model) but not with extra-pulmonary TB and TB recurrence. A haplotype constructed with the major alleles of the eight SNPs in the *CCR5* promoter (rs2227010-rs2856758-rs2734648-rs1799987-rs1799988-rs41469351-rs1800023-rs1800024: A-A-G-G-T-C-G-C) exhibited extraordinarily increased risk of susceptibility to TB and pulmonary TB (P = 6.33E-11, OR = 24.887, 95% CI: 6.081–101.841).

Conclusion: In conclusion, *CCR5* promoter polymorphisms were found to be associated with pulmonary TB and TB progression in Chinese Han people.

Keywords: tuberculosis, CCR5, polymorphism, susceptibility, Chinese Han

INTRODUCTION

Tuberculosis (TB) is an infectious disease caused by *Mycobacterium tuberculosis* (*M. tuberculosis*). To date, TB remains a major public health concern since approximately one third of the world's population has been infected with *M. tuberculosis* (1). Approximately 5% of the individuals who become infected with *M. tuberculosis* will develop clinical TB disease within 2 years of infection (2). TB is classified as primary TB or latent TB infection (2). Approximately 5–10% of the individuals with latent TB will develop clinical TB disease during their lifetime (2–4).

It was believed that active TB development was probably caused by the failure of host inflammatory responses against the pathogen (5). However, studies have identified complex interactions involving *M. tuberculosis* and the environment, along with the host genetic background playing a critical role in the outcome of *M. tuberculosis* exposure and TB development (4). A number of immunity-related genes have been reportedly associated with susceptibility to TB among different populations, such as human leukocyte antigen (HLA), low molecular weight polypeptide/transporter with antigen processing, natural resistance-associated macrophage protein 1 (NRAMP1), dendritic cell-specific ICAM-3-grabbing non-integrin (DC-SIGN), Toll-like receptors (TLR) 1 and 2, vitamin D receptor (VDR), TNF, interleukin (IL) -1β, IL-6, IL-8, IL-10, interferon γ (IFN-γ), and nucleotide oligomerization binding domain 2 (NOD2) (2, 4, 6, 7). Chemokines such as chemokine (C-C motif) ligand 2 (CCL-2)/monocyte chemoattractant protein 1 (MCP-1), RANTENS (*CCL5*), and chemokine C-X-C motif ligand 10 (CXCL10) have been found to be relevant in *M. tuberculosis* infection (7).

C-C motif chemokine receptor type 5 (CCR5), a transmembrane G-coupled cell-surface chemokine receptor, binds to different kinds of CC-chemokines, including human macrophage inflammatory protein-1α (MIP-1α), MIP-1β, RANTES (regulated on activation normal T cell expressed and secreted factor), monocyte chemotactic protein 1 (MCP-1), MCP-2, MCP-3, and MCP-4 (8). Previous studies report that *CCR5* is highly expressed during activation of T helper 1 (Th1) cells, which play a critical role in host immune responses against TB (9). Moreover, *CCR5* expression is found to be substantially increased during *M. tuberculosis* infection (10–12). Pokkali et al. found that *CCR5* expression is significantly higher in pulmonary TB patients compared to that in healthy controls (10), and Qiu et al. reported that *CCR5* expression levels in rhesus monkeys with severe TB disease exhibit remarkably up-regulated lymphocytes in the lungs, bronchial lymph nodes, and spleen (11). Additionally, CCR5 and its ligand play important roles in T-cell activation and migration during immune responses against TB infection. Galkina et al. observed that $CCR5^{-/-}$ $CD8^+$ T cells exhibit an approximately 50% reduction in effector $CD8^+$ T cell transmigration from pulmonary vascular compartments into interstitial compartments, as compared with CCR5 wild-type $CD8^+$ T cells (13). CCR5 has also been found to possibly regulate effector $CD8^+$ T cell contraction and memory generation after *M. tuberculosis* infection (14). Furthermore, several studies have suggested that CXCR3, CCR5, and CXCR6 potentially mediate *M. tuberculosis*-specific $CD4^+$T cell migration out of the vascular endothelium, and their entry into the lungs during *M. tuberculosis* infection, which is a critical step in host immune responses against *M. tuberculosis* infection (15). Therefore, CCR5 seems to play an important role in the immune response against *M. tuberculosis* infection.

Although CCR5 is reported to be involved in resistance against *M. tuberculosis* infection, a number of studies have reported the association of *CCR5* gene variants with TB infection and progression. In 2014, Carpenter et al. (16) performed an analysis regarding the possible associations between rs1799987 of *CCR5* and clinically active TB phenotypes in three different populations (Peru, Xhosa, and Colored), but found no significant associations. In this study, we examined genetic polymorphisms in the *CCR5* promoter in the Chinese Han population to investigate the association between *CCR5* promoter polymorphisms and *M. tuberculosis* infection, and TB progression.

METHODS AND MATERIALS

Subjects

A total of 450 patients with TB, including 325 cases of pulmonary TB (PTB) and 125 cases of extrapulmonary TB (EPTB, which was defined as TB influencing extrapulmonary sites such as lymph nodes, abdomen, urinary tract, skin, joints, bones, and meninges, exclusively or in combination with PTB), who were enrolled in the Third People's Hospital of Kunming between 2018–2019, were selected as a TB patient group for this study. All subjects were genetically unrelated and belonged to the Chinese Han population from Yunnan province (southwest China).

Diagnoses of TB were based on clinical case definition guidelines for TB issued by the World Health Organization (WHO) (17), Diagnosis for Pulmonary Tuberculosis (WS 288-2017) (18) and Classification of Tuberculosis (WS 196-2017) (19) from the Health Industry Standard of the People's Republic of China. The diagnostic criteria were as follows: (1) *M. tuberculosis* positively confirmed by sputum smear culture bacteriological assessment; (2) clinical symptoms such as cough, fever and weight loss over two weeks, and chest X-ray consistent with TB disease. Usually, Tuberculin skin test (TST) and interferon-γ release assay (IGRA) are also positive. Patients with immunodeficiency, autoimmune diseases, or other acute or chronic infections were excluded from this study.

Over the same period, 306 healthy individuals were recruited as a control group. All the controls had negative history for TB disease and were without any acute or chronic pulmonary disorder, or any bacterial or viral infection or other immune-mediated disorders. All the controls were self-reported Han Chinese.

DNA Extraction and Sequencing

Two to 5 ml of peripheral blood was drawn from each participant, and genomic DNA was extracted from peripheral lymphocytes using the QIAamp Blood Mini Kit (Qiagen, Hilden,

Germany) in a Biosafety Level 2 Laboratory of the Third People's Hospital of Kunming. The *CCR5* promoter region was PCR amplified using primers used in a previously published study (20); CCR5P_F: 5'-gacgagaaagctgagggtaaga-3' and CCR5P_R: 5'-taaccgtctgaaactcattcca-3'. The amplified PCR fragment was 1388 bp in length. PCR for each sample was carried out using the TAKARA PrimeSTAR Max DNA polymerase kit (TAKARA, Dalian, China) in 50 μl reaction volumes containing 10 ng genomic DNA, 10 pmol of each primer, 25 μl 2 × PrimeSTAR Max Premix (TAKARA). Amplification consisted of an initial denaturation step of 5 min at 98°C, followed by: 30 cycles of denaturation for 10 s at 98°C, 5 s of annealing at 55°C, extension at 72°C for 90 s, and a final extension for 5 min at 72°C. Purified PCR fragments were subjected to Sanger DNA sequencing to detect the sites of polymorphism using the Big Dye Terminator Reaction Mix (Applied Biosystems Foster City, CA, USA), along with the same primers used for PCR amplification. Sequencing reaction products were purified using the Big Dye Terminator Purification Kit (Applied Biosystems) and run on an ABI 3730XL sequencer. Sequencing data were analyzed using the DNASTAR Lasergene v.7.1 package. All the *CCR5* promoter region sequencing data in this study have been deposited in the Figshare database named "*CCR5* promoter sequences of TB patients and controls" (DOI: 10.6084/m9.figshare.12015624).

Polymorphic Loci in CCR5 Promoter

In our previous study (20), we found that there are nine identified single nucleotide polymorphisms (SNPs) loci located in the *CCR5* gene promoter. Six SNPs, rs2227010 (A>G), rs2734648 (T>G), rs1799987 (G>A), rs1799988 (T>G), rs1800023 (G>A), and rs1800024 (C>T) were found to be polymorphic in the Chinese Han population sample, whereas the three remaining sites, rs2856758 (AA), rs41469351 (CC), and rs41355345 (CC), were monomorphic in this sample. Thus, we analyzed association between alleles and genotypes of these six SNPs with TB.

Statistical Analysis

The distribution of age and sex between the case and control groups was compared *via* Student's *t*-test and χ^2-tests in SPSS (v.19.0; SPSS Inc., Chicago, IL, USA). Basic statistical analyses for allelic and genotypic frequencies of the six SNPs were carried out using PLINK v.1.9 (http://zzz.bwh.harvard.edu/plink/data.shtml) (21), and risks were estimated using odds ratios (OR) with 95% confidence intervals (95% CI). A goodness-of-fit χ^2-test was used to test for Hardy-Weinberg equilibrium (HWE) for each SNP in the control group, with a threshold of 0.05, which was also assessed using PLINK.

The Linkage disequilibrium (LD) and haplotype frequencies (deduced from the phenotype) among eight SNPs (rs2227010-rs2856758-rs2734648-rs1799987-rs1799988-rs41469351-rs1800023-rs1800024) were calculated based on the genotype results using a standard Expectation Maximization (ignoring missing data) algorithm with a partition-ligation approach for blocks by Haploview v.4.2 software (22). Haploview calculates the LD coefficient D', LOD and r^2 between each pair of genetic markers. *D'* values were defined in the range [-1, 1], with a value of 1 representing perfect disequilibrium. A *D'* value over 0.8 indicated there is a strong linkage disequilibrium among SNPs. The lowest frequency threshold for haplotype analysis was 0.01, and hhaplotype with frequency less than this number will not be considered in analysis. The differences in the haplotypes (with frequencies over 0.01) between the TB and control groups, between PTB and control groups, as well as between EPTB and control groups were determined by χ^2-test. And risks were estimated using ORs and 95%CI. OR and 95% CI were used to estimate associations between SNPs and TB disease by adjusting for age and gender using multivariate logistic regression models. The threshold for statistical significance was $P < 0.05$. Bonferroni correction was applied for multiple comparisons among alleles and genotypes, and the *P*-value was adjusted to 0.05/n. Power-analysis was performed using Power and Sample Size Calculations (v.3.1.2) (23).

RESULTS

Characteristics of Subjects

Table 1 presents participant demographic characteristic data, including gender, age, and clinical type of TB. The mean age of the TB group was 43.76 ± 16.01 years, with the sex ratio (male/female) being 249/201, while the mean age of the control group was 44.68 ± 9.26 years, with a sex ratio (male/female) of 154/152. The distributions of age and gender between the TB and control groups showed no statistical differences ($P > 0.05$). The mean ages were 45.31 ± 15.82 years in the PTB group and 39.75 ± 15.86 years in the EPTB group; whereas the sex ratio (male/female) was 190/135 in the PTB group and 59/66 in the EPTB group. For the initial treatment (IT) and retreatment (RT) groups, the mean ages were 43.20 ± 16.35 years and 44.68 ± 15.46 years, respectively, and sex ratios (male/female) were 144/135 in the IT and 105/66 in the RT group ($P = 0.043$).

Comparisons of Allelic and Genotypic Frequencies of CCR5 Promoter SNPs Between TB Patients and Controls

All six *CCR5* promoter SNPs with polymorphism exhibited HWE in the control group ($P > 0.05$). However, in the TB patient group, rs2734648, rs1799987, and rs1800023 were not in HWE. The allelic and genotypic frequencies of the six *CCR5* promoter SNPs were compared between the TB patient and control groups, after adjusting for age and gender based on the logistic regression model (**Table 2**). The results showed that the frequency of rs2734648-G was significantly higher in the TB patient group compared to that in the control group ($P = 0.002$, OR = 1.380, 95% CI: 1.123–1.696); the genotypic distribution of rs2734648 was significantly different between the TB and control groups ($P = 1.07E-05$). Furthermore, we performed inheritance model analysis and found that rs2734648-GG was significantly associated with TB disease, and exhibited 2-fold susceptibility in a recessive inheritance model ($P = 6.32E-06$, OR = 2.173, 95% CI: 1.546–3.056). The genotypic distribution of rs1799987 also showed significant difference between the TB and control groups ($P = 0.008$).

TABLE 1 | Demographic and clinical data for tuberculosis patients and controls.

Study groups		Num.	Sex, M:F	Age (mean ± SD), years
TB		450	249:201	43.76 ± 16.01
	PTB	325	190:135	45.31 ± 15.82
	Infiltration	146	80:66	45.97 ± 16.92
	Secondary	161	106:55	44.50 ± 14.80
	Cavity	18	4:14	47.17 ± 15.99
	EPTB	125	59: 66	39.75 ± 15.86
	Lymph nodes	13	7:6	36.31 ± 13.68
	Genitourinary tract	31	7:24	40.48 ± 14.66
	bone and joint	24	13:11	41.58 ± 15.20
	cutaneous	5	1:4	42.20 ± 21.81
	celiac	14	8:6	41.00 ± 23.29
	Meningitis	8	8:0	34.13 ± 10.87
	Peritoneal	2	1:1	20.50 ± 6.36
	Pleuritis	1	0:1	47.00
	Multi-site concurrency	17	8:9	39.53 ± 13.01
	others	10	6:4	42.60 ± 18.91
	Initial treatment	279	144:135	43.20 ± 16.35
	Retreatment	171	105:66	44.68 ± 15.46
Healthy control		306	154:152	44.68 ± 9.26

Num., number; M, male; F, female; SD, standard deviation; TB, tuberculosis; PTB, pulmonary tuberculosis; EPTB, extrapulmonary tuberculosis.

TABLE 2 | Comparison of allelic and genotypic frequencies of CCR5 gene between TB patients and controls.

Comparison		Control (n = 306) n (Freq.)	TB (n = 450) n (Freq.)	*P*	OR (95%CI)
rs2227010					
Allelic	**A**	501 (0.819)	734(0.816)		Ref.
	G	111 (0.181)	166(0.184)	0.879	1.021(0.783–1.332)
Genotypic	**A/A**	207 (0.676)	302(0.671)	0.988	Ref.
	G/A	87 (0.284)	130(0.289)		1.024(0.741–1.416)
	G/G	12 (0.039)	18(0.040)		1.028(0.485–2.180)
Dominant	**A/A**	207 (0.676)	302(0.671)		Ref.
	G/G-G/A	99 (0.324)	148 (0.329)	0.877	1.025(0.752–1.397)
Recessive	**A/A-G/A**	294 (0.961)	432 (0.960)		Ref.
	G/G	12 (0.039)	18(0.040)	0.957	1.021(0.484–2.151)
rs2734648					
Allelic	**T**	328 (0.536)	410(0.456)		Ref.
	G	284 (0.464)	490(0.544)	**0.002**	1.380(1.123–1.696)
Genotypic	**T/T**	83 (0.271)	118(0.262)	**1.07E-05**	Ref.
	G/T	162 (0.529)	174(0.387)		0.755(0.531–1.075)
	G/G	61 (0.199)	158(0.351)		1.822(1.212–2.739)
Dominant	**T/T**	83 (0.271)	118(0.262)		Ref.
	G/G-G/T	223 (0.729)	332 (0.738)	0.783	1.048(0.754–1.454)
Recessive	**G/T-T/T**	245 (0.801)	292 (0.649)		Ref.
	G/G	61 (0.199)	158(0.351)	**6.32E-06**	2.173(1.546–3.056)
rs1799987					
Allelic	**G**	365 (0.596)	516 (0.573)		Ref.
	A	247 (0.404)	384 (0.427)	0.372	1.100 (0.893–1.355)
Genotypic	**G/G**	110 (0.359)	174 (0.387)	**0.008**	Ref.
	G/A	145 (0.474)	168 (0.373)		0.732 (0.529–1.015)
	A/A	51 (0.167)	108 (0.240)		1.339 (0.889–2.017)
Dominant	**G/G**	110 (0.359)	174 (0.387)		Ref.
	A/A-A/G	196 (0.641)	276 (0.613)	0.449	0.890 (0.659–1.203)
Recessive	**G/G-A/G**	255 (0.833)	342 (0.760)		Ref.
	A/A	51 (0.167)	108(0.240)	0.015	1.579 (1.090–2.287)
rs1799988					
Allelic	**T**	358 (0.585)	532 (0.591)		Ref.
	C	254 (0.415)	368 (0.409)	0.8117	0.975 (0.791–1.201)
Genotypic	**T/T**	107 (0.350)	157 (0.349)	0.8806	Ref.
	C/T	144 (0.471)	218 (0.484)		1.032 (0.747–1.426)

(Continued)

TABLE 2 | Continued

Comparison		Control (n = 306) n (Freq.)	TB (n = 450) n (Freq.)	*P*	OR (95%CI)
	C/C	55 (0.180)	75 (0.167)		0.929 (0.607–1.423)
Dominant	T/T	107 (0.350)	157 (0.349)		Ref.
	C/C-C/T	199 (0.650)	293 (0.651)	0.982	1.003 (0.740–1.361)
Recessive	T/T-C/T	251 (0.820)	375 (0.833)		Ref.
	C/C	55 (0.180)	75 (0.167)	0.6401	0.913 (0.622–1.339)
rs1800023					
Allelic	G	336 (0.549)	482 (0.536)		Ref.
	A	276 (0.451)	418 (0.464)	0.6061	1.056 (0.859–1.297)
Genotypic	G/G	88 (0.288)	119 (0.264)	0.7798	Ref.
	A/G	160 (0.523)	244 (0.542)		1.128 (0.803–1.585)
	A/A	58 (0.190)	87 (0.193)		1.109 (0.720–1.708)
Dominant	G/G	88 (0.288)	119 (0.264)		Ref.
	A/A-A/G	218 (0.712)	331 (0.736)	0.4838	1.123 (0.812–1.553)
Recessive	A/G-G/G	248 (0.810)	363 (0.807)		Ref.
	A/A	58 (0.190)	87 (0.193)	0.8966	1.025 (0.708–1.483)
rs1800024					
Allelic	C	462 (0.755)	687 (0.763)		Ref.
	T	150 (0.245)	213 (0.237)	0.7064	0.955 (0.751–1.214)
Genotypic	C/C	170 (0.556)	268 (0.596)	0.1254	Ref.
	T/C	122 (0.399)	151 (0.336)		1.789 (0.911–3.513)
	T/T	14 (0.046)	31 (0.069)		1.405 (0.726–2.717)
Dominant	C/C	170 (0.556)	268 (0.596)		Ref.
	T/T-T/C	136 (0.444)	182 (0.404)	0.2742	0.849 (0.633–1.139)
Recessive	T/C-C/C	292 (0.954)	419 (0.931)		Ref.
	T/T	14 (0.046)	31 (0.069)	0.1869	1.543 (0.807–2.952)

Co, control; TB, tuberculosis; OR, odds ratio; CI, confidence interval.
The P-value, OR, and 95% CIs of pair-wise comparisons between TB and control groups were calculated based on the logistic regression model adjusted for age and gender. Bonferroni correction was applied, and the P-value was adjusted to 0.008 (0.05/6). And the P-value lower than 0.008 were marked in bold.

This study had powers over 80% to detect ORs of 1.021 for rs2227010, 0.725 for rs2734648, and 0.975 for rs1799988, and had power of 53.8% to detect with an OR of 1.1 for rs1799987, 60.6% to detect with an OR of 1.056 for rs1800023, and 72.6% to detect with a OR of 0.955 for rs1800024, respectively, in 450 TB patients compared with 306 controls.

Stratification Analysis of the Association Between TB and *CCR5* Promoter Polymorphisms

We performed stratification analysis to investigate the association of TB susceptibility with *CCR5* promoter SNPs. We stratified the TB patients into PTB and EPTB patients and compared the distribution of allelic and genotypic frequencies of the six SNPs among the stratification groups and the control group. The associations between SNPs and PTB or EPTB groups were adjusted for age and gender using multivariate logistic regression models. **Table 3** shows comparative results of rs2734648 and rs1799987. The results showed that the frequency of rs2734648-G was significantly higher in PTB patients as compared to controls ($P = 0.0013$, OR = 1.488, 95% CI: 1.192–1.858). Carriers of rs2734648-GG showed a notable increase in susceptibility to PTB in the recessive inheritance model ($P < 0.0001$, OR = 2.382, 95% CI: 1.663–3.413). Carriers of rs1799987-AA also showed a significant association with PTB in the recessive inheritance model ($P = 0.0078$, OR = 1.687, 95% CI: 1.141–2.495). However, significant associations of these two SNPs with EPTB in the recessive inheritance model were not detected (**Table 3**). For other SNPs, no significant differences were found between the PTB and control groups. It should be noted that the results from PTB (**Table 3**) simply reinforce the TB associations observed from **Table 2**, which is not surprising, since PTB represents 72.2% of the TB sample. Finally, no significant difference was found between the EPTB and control groups, and between the EPTB and PTB groups (**Supplementary Table 1**).

Additionally, we stratified the TB patients into IT and RT subgroups according to disease stage at the time of treatment, and analyzed allelic and genotypic distributions of the six SNPs. Associations between SNPs and disease recurrence were adjusted for age and gender using multivariate logistic regression models. We found rs2734648-G and rs2734648-GG to be significantly associated with TB recurrence (**Table 4**). After comparison between IT and control, RT and control, and RT and IT groups, we found that rs2734648-GG was significantly associated with TB recurrence in a dominant inheritance model ($P = 0.0032$, OR = 1.936, 95% CI: 1.221–3.068), while rs1799987 showed no significant association with disease recurrence (**Table 4** and **Supplementary Table 2**).

CCR5 Promoter SNP Combination Analysis and Association With TB

LD among eight SNPs (rs2227010, rs2856758, rs2734648, rs1799987, rs1799988, rs41469351, rs1800023, rs1800024) in the *CCR5* promoter was estimated, where the LD coefficient D (*D'*) was calculated. The *D'* value of these eight SNPs was >0.8,

TABLE 3 | Stratification analysis on the association between CCR5 promoter SNPs and clinical TB phenotypes.

Comparison		Control (n = 306)	PTB (n = 325)	EPTB (n = 125)	PTB vs Co.		EPTB vs Co.		EPTB vs PTB	
		n (Freq.)	n (Freq.)	n (Freq.)	*P*	OR (95%CI)	*P*	OR (95%CI)	*P*	OR (95%CI)
rs2734648										
Allelic	**T**	328(0.536)	284(0.437)	126(0.504)		Ref.		Ref.		Ref.
	G	284(0.464)	366(0.563)	124(0.496)	**1.3E-03**	1.488(1.192–1.858)	0.394	1.137(0.847–1.526)	0.700	0.764(0.570–1.023)
Genotypic	**T/T**	83(0.271)	80(0.246)	38 (0.304)	**5.20E-06**	Ref.	0.076	Ref.	0.256	Ref.
	G/T	162(0.530)	124(0.382)	50 (0.400)		0.794(0.540–1.168)		0.674(0.410–1.109)		0.849(0.511–1.409)
	G/G	61(0.199)	121(0.372)	37 (0.296)		2.058(1.332–3.179)		1.325(0.756–2.321)		0.644(0.378–1.098)
Dominant	**T/T**	83(0.271)	80(0.246)	38 (0.304)		Ref.		Ref.		Ref.
	G/G-G/T	223(0.729)	245(0.754)	87 (0.696)	0.5	1.140(0.798–1.628)	0.730	0.852(0.540–1.346)	0.211	0.748(0.473–1.181)
Recessive	**G/T-T/T**	245(0.801)	204(0.628)	88 (0.704)		Ref.		Ref.		Ref.
	G/G	61(0.199)	121(0.372)	37 (0.296)	**1.64E-06**	2.382(1.663–3.413)	0.049	1.689(1.050–2.717)	0.129	0.709(0.454–1.106)
rs1799987										
Allelic	**G**	365(0.596)	371(0.571)	145(0.580)		Ref.		Ref.		Ref.
	A	247(0.404)	279(0.429)	105(0.420)	0.519	1.111(0.888–1.390)	0.657	1.070(0.794–1.442)	0.802	0.963(0.717–1.294)
Genotypic	**G/G**	110(0.359)	128(0.394)	46 (0.368)	**0.0028**	Ref.	0.740	Ref.	0.353	Ref.
	G/A	145(0.474)	115(0.354)	53 (0.424)		0.682(0.479–0.970)		0.874(0.548–1.393)		1.282(0.803–2.049)
	A/A	51(0.167)	82(0.252)	26 (0.208)		1.382(0.897–2.130)		1.219(0.680–2.187)		0.882(0.506–1.537)
Dominant	**G/G**	110(0.359)	128(0.394)	46 (0.368)		Ref.		Ref.		Ref.
	A/A-A/G	196(0.641)	197(0.606)	79 (0.632)	0.373	0.864(0.626–1.193)	0.990	0.964(0.626–1.485)	0.614	1.116(0.729–1.709)
Recessive	**G/G-A/G**	255(0.833)	243(0.748)	99 (0.792)		Ref.		Ref.		Ref.
	A/A	51(0.167)	82(0.252)	26 (0.208)	**0.0078**	1.687(1.141–2.495)	0.470	1.313(0.776–2.223)	0.324	0.778(0.472–1.282)

Co, control; PTB, pulmonary tuberculosis; EPTB, extra pulmonary tuberculosis; OR, odds ratio; CI, confidence interval.
The P-value, OR, and 95% CIs of pair-wise comparisons between PTB and controls, and EPTB and controls, were calculated based on the logistic regression model adjusted for age and gender. Bonferroni correction was applied, and the P-value was adjusted to 0.008 (0.05/6). And the P-value lower than 0.008 were marked in bold.

indicating that these *CCR5* promoter SNPs were in LD (**Supplementary Figure 1**). Next, we constructed haplotypes of the eight SNPs (rs2227010-rs2856758-rs2734648-rs1799987-rs1799988-rs41469351-rs1800023-rs1800024) and compared haplotypes with frequencies over 0.01 between case and control groups, as listed in **Table 5**. The results revealed that haplotype H1 (A-A-T-G-T-C-G-C) was the most prevalent, both in control (50.3%) as well as TB patient groups (41.1%), and showed a significant resistance to TB disease (P = 1.17E-04, OR = 0.660, 95% CI: 0.535–0.816), with notable resistance to PTB (P = 1.05E-05, OR = 0.599, 95% CI: 0.477–0.753). In contrast, haplotype H5 (A-A-G-G-T-C-G-C) presented an extremely increased risk of susceptibility to TB by over 20-fold (P = 7.84E-10, OR = 21.877, 95% CI: 5.378–88.996), as well as a notably increased risk of susceptibility to PTB and EPTB (P = 6.33E-11, OR = 24.887, 95% CI: 6.081–101.841 and P = 8.35E-06, OR = 14.038, 95% CI: 3.088–63.804, respectively); whereas haplotype H7 (A-A-G-A-T-C-G-C) increased the risk of susceptibility to TB and PTB by 10-fold (P = 0.004, OR = 10.715, 95% CI: 1.421–80.796, and P = 0.002, OR = 12.196, 95% CI: 1.595–93.269, respectively). Additionally, both haplotypes H10 (A-A-T-A-T-C-G-C) and H11 (G-A-G-G-C-C-A-C) appeared only in the case group, mainly in the PTB cohort, and frequency differences between PTB and control groups were remarkable after Bonferroni correction (P = 7.63E-05 and P = 0.003, respectively). However, there was no difference between PTB and EPTB groups (**Supplementary Table 3**).

DISCUSSION

TB is a serious infectious disease caused by *M. tuberculosis*; however, only 5–10% of infected individuals actually develop the active form of disease with clinical symptoms, prompting researchers to identify the factors influencing susceptibility to TB. Understanding host immune responses to *M. tuberculosis* infection is critical in identifying the reasons behind varying outcomes after *M. tuberculosis* exposure (latent or active TB disease), and for the development of effective TB vaccines and immune therapeutics. There is substantial evidence to suggest that the onset of TB is influenced by host genetic factors (2, 9, 15, 24). CCR5 has been reported to play important roles in immune responses against *M. tuberculosis* infection by regulating and activating the recruitment of macrophages, and by further activation of T-cells. In the present study, we investigated

TABLE 4 | Association between CCR5 gene variants and TB recurrence.

Comparison		Co (n = 306)	IT (n = 279)	RT (n = 171)	*P*	IT vs Co	*P*	RT vs Co	*P*	IT vs RT
		n (freq.)	n (freq.)	n (freq.)		OR (95% CI)		OR (95% CI)		OR (95% CI)
rs2734648										
Allelic	T	328(0.536)	269(0.482)	141(0.412)		Ref.		Ref.		Ref.
	G	284(0.464)	289(0.518)	201(0.588)	0.0725	1.241(0.986–1.561)	**1.7E-04**	1.646(1.260–2.151)	0.0471	1.327(1.011–1.741)
Genotypic	T/T	83(0.271)	86(0.308)	32(0.187)	**1.0E-05**	Ref.	**2.0E-04**	Ref.	0.01	Ref.
	G/T	162(0.529)	97(0.348)	77(0.450)		0.578(0.390–0.856)		1.233(0.755–2.012)		2.133(1.289–3.532)
	G/G	61(0.199)	96(0.344)	62(0.363)		1.519(0.978–2.359)		2.636(1.537–4.522)		1.736(1.036–2.909)
Dominant	T/T	83(0.271)	86(0.308)	32(0.187)		Ref.		Ref.		Ref.
	G/G-G/T	223 (0.729)	193 (0.692)	139 (0.813)	0.35	0.835(0.584–1.195)	0.034	1.617(1.021–2.560)	**0.0032**	1.936(1.221–3.068)
Recessive	T/T-G/T	245 (0.801)	183 (0.656)	109(0.637)		Ref.		Ref.		Ref.
	G/G	61(0.199)	96(0.344)	62(0.363)	**1.00E-04**	2.107(1.450–3.062)	**1.00E-04**	2.285(1.502–3.475)	0.58	1.084(0.728–1.614)
rs1799987										
Allelic	G	365(0.596)	322(0.577)	194(0.567)		Ref.		Ref.		Ref.
	A	247(0.404)	236(0.423)	148(0.433)	0.555	1.803(0.858–1.367)	0.3848	1.127(0.862–1.474)	0.6775	1.041(0.793–1.366)
Genotypic	G/G	110(0.359)	115(0.412)	59(0.345)	**9.0E-04**	Ref.	0.51	Ref.	0.045	Ref.
	A/G	145(0.474)	92(0.330)	76(0.444)		0.607(0.419–0.878)		0.977(0.642–1.488)		1.610(1.040–2.492)
	A/A	51(0.167)	72(0.258)	36(0.211)		1.350(0.866–2.105)		1.316(0.774–1.577)		0.975(0.586–1.621)
Dominant	G/G	110(0.359)	115(0.412)	59(0.345)		Ref.		Ref.		Ref.
	A/A-A/G	196 (0.641)	164 (0.588)	112 (0.655)	0.19	0.800(0.573–1.117)	0.73	1.065(0.720–1.577)	0.11	1.331(0.897–1.976)
Recessive	A/G-G/G	255 (0.833)	207 (0.742)	135 (0.789)		Ref.		Ref.		Ref.
	A/A	51(0.167)	72(0.258)	36(0.211)	**7.9E-03**	1.739(1.162–2.602)	0.24	1.333(0.829–2.144)	0.3	0.767(0.486–1.208)

Co, control; IT, initial treatment; RT, retreatment; OR, odds ratio; CI, confidence interval.
The P-value, OR, and 95% CIs of pair-wise comparisons between IT and control, RT and control, and RT and IT groups were calculated on the basis of the logistic regression model adjusted for age and gender. Bonferroni correction was applied, and the P-value was adjusted to 0.008 (0.05/6). And the P-value lower than 0.008 were marked in bold.

associations between *CCR5* promoter polymorphisms and TB and discovered that *CCR5* promoter polymorphisms were significantly associated with PTB and TB progression in the Chinese Han population for the first time.

In this study, we found that the allelic frequency of rs2734648-G was significantly higher in the TB patient group, especially in the PTB group, as compared to the control group, and also that rs2734648-GG carriers had a 2.382-fold increased

TABLE 5 | *CCR5* promoter haplotype frequencies in case and control groups.

Haplotype[a,d]	Haplotype similarity[b]	Co (2n = 612)	TB patients (2n = 900)			PTB (2n = 650)			EPTB patients (2n = 250)		
		N (freq.)	N (freq.)	P[c]	OR (95%CI)	N (freq.)	P[c]	OR (95%CI)	N (freq.)	P[c]	OR (95%CI)
H1: AATGTCGC	HHC	307.60 (0.503)	370.30 (0.411)	**1.17E-04**	0.660 (0.535–0.816)	250.99 (0.386)	**1.05E-05**	0.599 (0.477–0.753)	121.5 (0.486)	0.6652	0.947(0.706–1.271)
H2: AAGACCAT	HHF*1	126.14 (0.206)	179.78 (0.200)	0.644	0.941 (0.728–1.217)	128.64 (0.198)	0.649	0.938 (0.711–1.237)	47.6 (0.190)	0.5996	0.917(0.633–1.328)
H3: GAGACCAC	HHE	97.75 (0.160)	143.12 (0.159)	0.863	0.975 (0.736–1.293)	95.95 (0.148)	0.499	0.899 (0.661–1.223)	45.9 (0.184)	0.3999	1.183(0.804–1.740)
H4: AAGGTCAC	HHA	29.97 (0.049)	46.68 (0.052)	0.857	1.044 (0.652–1.673)	38.87 (0.060)	0.421	1.223 (0.749–1.997)	9.8 (0.039)	0.5409	0.728(0.340–1.555)
H5: AAGGTCGC	unknown	2.03 (0.003)	61.78 (0.069)	**7.84E-10**	21.877 (5.378–88.996)	49.95 (0.077)	**6.33E-11**	24.887 (6.081–101.841)	11.2 (0.045)	**8.35E-06**	14.038(3.088–63.804)
H6: AAGGCCAT	unknown	1.95 (0.003)	14.47 (0.016)	0.019	5.030 (1.124–22.509)	13.46 (0.021)	0.005	6.551 (1.453–29.528)	1(0.004)	0.8396	1.225(0.111–13.570)
H7: AAGATCGC	unknown	1.00 (0.002)	15.81 (0.018)	**4.10E-03**	10.715 (1.421–80.796)	12.88 (0.020)	**0.002**	12.196 (1.595–93.269)	3(0.012)	0.0423	7.421(0.768–71.690)
H8: AAGACCGT	unknown	7.04 (0.012)	4.36 (0.005)	0.134	0.411 (0.124–1.365)	3.30 (0.005)	0.200	0.435 (0.117–1.614)	1.6 (0.006)	0.4821	0.697(0.144–3.379)
H9: AATGCCGC	unknown	7.07 (0.012)	1.01 (0.001)	0.006	0.094 (0.012–0.762)	1.01 (0.002)	0.025	0.131 (0.016–1.063)	0(0.000)	0.46	0.302(0.038–2.426)
H10: AATATCGC	unknown	0.00 (0.000)	20.04 (0.022)	**2.43E-04**	14.612(1.960–108.915)	17.24 (0.027)	**7.63E-05**	17.459(2.324–131.181)	3(0.012)	0.027	9.746(1.095–86.770)
H11: GAGGCCAC	unknown	0.00 (0.000)	10.48 (0.012)	0.034	7.576(0.976–58.835)	10.51 (0.016)	**0.003**	11.530(1.495–88.938)	0(0.000)	–	–

[a]Haplotypes were constructed with rs2227010-rs2856758-rs2734648-rs1799987-rs1799988-rs41469351-rs1800023-rs1800024.
[b]HHA, HHB, HHC, and HHF were previously reported (25–27).
[c]Bonferroni correction was applied, and the P-value was adjusted to 0.004 (0.05/11). And the P-value lower than 0.004 were marked in bold.
[d]Haplotypes with frequencies over 0.01 were compared and listed in this table.

risk of susceptibility to PTB in a recessive inheritance model. Additionally, rs2734648 was found to be significantly associated with TB recurrence. It has been reported that *CCR5* variants may alter the response of CCR5-chemokines, including altered ligand-binding properties (28), and *CCR5* promoter polymorphisms could differentially affect *CCR5* gene transcription. We constructed a predictive model involving potential binding sites of transcription factors in the *CCR5* promoter and discovered that SNPs in the *CCR5* promoter might differentially influence transcription factor binding, based on the nucleotide substitution(s) involved (20). Mummidi et al. demonstrated that G to T substitution in rs2734648 (-2554G>T) is associated with differences in binding avidity of the NF-κB family of transcription factors (the binding avidity of rs2734648-G is greater than that of rs2734648-T), which might affect the transcriptional activity of *CCR5*. rs2856758-G can bind to novel nuclear factor 1 (NF1), which can repress transcription of certain genes (29), whereas rs2856758-A cannot bind to NF1 (26). For another SNP in the *CCR5* promoter, rs1799987-AA, we found an increasing risk of susceptibility to PTB in a recessive inheritance model. McDremott et al. reported that rs1799987 (-2459A>G) influences the expression of *CCR5*, and rs1799987-G has 45% lower promoter activity than rs1799987-A *in vitro* (30). The latter authors also observed that rs1799987-A/rs1799988-C in combination stimulates *CCR5* promoter activity by 45% more than other rs1799987/rs1799988 allelic combinations (30). Li et al. showed that rs1799988 C to T substitution results in reduced expression of *CCR5*, which consequently correlated with slower AIDS progression. Furthermore, rs1799988-CC carriers display increased CCR5 expression on the surface of peripheral blood mononuclear cells (PBMCs), CD4+ cells, and CD4+ monocytes, as compared to two other *CCR5*-rs1799988 genotypes (31). Therefore, we deduced that SNPs in the *CCR5* promoter could influence *CCR5* gene and cell surface CCR5 protein expression by altering the binding of transcription factors, thereby affecting the function of CCR5. Hence, rs2734648-GG and rs1799987-AA were significantly associated with PTB and TB progression by possibly increased expression of CCR5.

We also analyzed the effects of combinations of the 8 *CCR5* promoter SNPs (rs2227010, rs2856758, rs2734648, rs1799987, rs1799988, rs41469351, rs1800023, rs1800024) on TB susceptibility and found that haplotype H1 (A-A-T-G-T-C-G-C)—constructed using the major alleles of the eight SNPs—was significantly associated with resistance to PTB; and haplotype H5 (A-A-G-G-T-C-G-C) increased the susceptibility to PTB by over 20-times. *CCR2-CCR5* haplogroups constructed using CCR2 (V>64I), rs2856758(-2733A>G), rs2734648(-2554G>T), rs1799987(-2459G>A), rs1799988(-2135T>C), rs41469351 (-2132C>T), rs1800023(-2086A>G), rs1800024(-1835C>T), and rs333(CCR5Δ32) have been characterized and described in earlier studies, and the haplogroups are termed HHA, HHB, HHC, HHD, HHE, HHF*1, HHF*2, HHG*1, and HHG*2, respectively (25, 26). CCR2-CCR5 haplogroups are correlated with differences in *CCR5* expression and transcriptional activity. HHA is associated with lower *CCR5* expression, whereas HHF and HHG are associated with higher *CCR5* expression (32). Similarly, K562 cells, HHA and HHC exhibit lower transcriptional activity, whereas in Jurkat T-cells, HHB, and HHD show higher transcriptional activity than HHA (33, 34). In 2011, Mamtani et al. found that the *CCR5* promoter haplogroup HHD was associated with susceptibility to TB, by increasing *CCR5* expression in either activated PBMCs, or surface expression on activated ($HLA\text{-}DR^+$) $CD4^+$ T cells (34). In our study, we constructed haplotypes with eight SNPs in the *CCR5* promoter, and only rs2227010 was not included in the defined CCR2-CCR5 haplogroups. Our results showed that H1 was similar to HHC (which exhibited lower transcriptional activity and lower *CCR5* expression), H2 was similar to HHF*1 (related to higher *CCR5* expression), H3 was similar to HHE, and H4 was similar to HHA. Therefore, the noticeable protection against PTB by the H1 haplotype in this study was likely due to the lower transcriptional activity of H1 (similar to HHC, which was associated with lower CCR5 expression). However, haplotype H5 was different from haplotype H1 at only one locus: rs2734648, which was T in haplotype H1 and G in H5. Note that H5 is a novel haplotype not previously detected in any other population. Based on the significant susceptibility of rs2734648-G to TB, and the extraordinarily high frequency of rs2734648-G in the Han population, rs2734648-G as well as haplotype H5 could provide crucial insights into immune responses to TB in the Chinese Han population. In this study, we also found one haplotype rs2856758A-rs2734648T-rs1799987G-rs1799988T-rs41469531C-rs1800023A-rs1800024C was most similar as HHD. However, the haplotype frequencies were very low (0.5 and 0.5% in control and TB group respectively, and data not showed) and with no difference between TB and control group. In addition, haplotype H1, which presented only two differences loci when compared with HHD (rs41469351-C and rs1800023-G in H1, whereas rs41469351-T and rs1800023-A in HHD), showed significant frequency difference between TB and control groups (P = 2.25E-04, OR = 0.674, 95% CI: 0.547–0.832). But haplotype HHD and H1 showed entirely opposite effects on the susceptibility to TB. The reason of this discrepancy could be the different frequency of rs41469351 and rs1800023. According to the 1000 Genomes database the rs41469351-T is only detected in African and American population with the frequencies of 26 and 2%, respectively, and were monomorphic (rs41469351-CC) in Chinese Han and European people (http://asia.ensembl.org/Homo_sapiens/Variation/Population?db=core;r=3:46370271-46371271;v=rs41469351;vdb=variation;vf=5860779). And for rs1800023, the A-allele frequencies in Chinese Han people is 43%, however, there are 91% in African, 63% in European (http://asia.ensembl.org/Homo_sapiens/Variation/Population?db=core;r=3:46370317-46371317;v=rs1800023;vdb=variation;vf=816197). So rs41469351 and rs1800023 maybe important loci which might affect the susceptibility of TB. Haplotypes H7, H10, and H11, which were unlike any reported haplogroups, also showed significantly higher frequencies in the TB group, as well as the PTB cohort. Hence, the combined functions of *CCR5* promoter SNPs might play important roles in *CCR5*-mediated immune responses to TB.

Associations of SNPs with diseases have always been inconsistent among different populations. Previous studies indicate that *CCR5* allelic frequencies are remarkably different among different populations (16, 35), which might influence the results of correlative studies. Among most populations in the world (including Africans, Americans, Europeans, Japanese, and South Asians), rs2734648-G is the major allele; however, in Chinese Han populations, rs2734648-T is the predominant allele (Han Chinese in Beijing, and Southern Han Chinese from the 1000 Genomes database, and Chinese Han in Yunnan in this study), indicating that the frequency differences in rs2734648 could account for the specific association with TB in Han Chinese people. However, the function of rs2734648 substitution is still unclear; therefore, functional studies regarding the role of rs2734648 in *M. tuberculosis* infection and TB progression need to be conducted in the future.

Hence, more studies involving more individuals from different populations are needed. Additionally, as discussed above, SNP combinations also play an important role in susceptibility to TB and in its progression. Hence, further studies regarding haplotype structure, especially in terms of combinations of rs2734648 with other SNPs in the *CCR5* promoter, are required.

CONCLUSIONS

SNP rs2734638-G of the *CCR5* promoter, as well as haplotype H5, consistent with rs2734648-G, are significantly associated with susceptibility to PTB and with TB recurrence by affecting the transcriptional activity and expression of *CCR5*.

ETHICS STATEMENT

The studies involving human participants were reviewed and approved by the institutional review board of the Third Hospital of Kunming (approval number is 2018030720). The patients/participants provided their written informed consent to participate in this study.

AUTHOR CONTRIBUTIONS

SL and LS conceived and designed the research. SL and NL mainly performed experiments and data analysis. HW and SZ did the clinical diagnosis. HW and XZ prepared samples for experiments and performed part of the experiments. SL wrote the manuscript. YY, SZ, and LS wrote parts of the manuscript and reviewed the manuscript. All authors contributed to the article and approved the submitted version.

ACKNOWLEDGMENTS

We thank all participants for their cooperation.

REFERENCES

1. Cliff JM, Kaufmann SHE, Mcshane H, Van Helden P, O'garra A. The human immune response to tuberculosis and its treatment: a view from the blood. *Immunol Rev* (2015) 264:88–102. doi: 10.1111/imr.12269
2. Abel L, El-Baghdadi J, Bousfiha AA, Casanova J-L, Schurr E. Human genetics of tuberculosis: a long and winding road. *Philos Trans R Soc Lond B Biol Sci* (2014) 369:20130428–20130428. doi: 10.1098/rstb.2013.0428
3. Pai M, Behr MA, Dowdy D, Dheda K, Divangahi M, Boehme CC, et al. Tuberculosis. *Nat Rev Dis Primers* (2016) 2:16076. doi: 10.1038/nrdp.2016.76
4. Dallmann-Sauer M, Correa-Macedo W, Schurr E. Human genetics of mycobacterial disease. *Mamm Genome Off J Int Mamm Genome Soc* (2018) 29:523–38. doi: 10.1007/s00335-018-9765-4
5. Lyadova IV, Tsiganov EN, Kapina MA, Shepelkova GS, Sosunov VV, Radaeva TV, et al. In mice, tuberculosis progression is associated with intensive inflammatory response and the accumulation of Gr-1 cells in the lungs. *PloS One* (2010) 5:e10469. doi: 10.1371/journal.pone.0010469
6. Aravindan PP. Host genetics and tuberculosis: Theory of genetic polymorphism and tuberculosis. *Lung India* (2019) 36:244–52. doi: 10.1016/j.ejcdt.2013.12.002
7. Azad AK, Sadee W, Schlesinger LS. Innate immune gene polymorphisms in tuberculosis. *Infect Immunity* (2012) 80:3343–59. doi: 10.1128/IAI.00443-12
8. Blanpain C, Migeotte I, Lee B, Vakili J, Doranz BJ, Govaerts C, et al. CCR5 Binds Multiple CC-chemokines: MCP-3 Acts as a Natural Antagonist. *Blood* (1999) 94:1899–905. doi: 10.1182/blood.V94.6.1899
9. Camargo JF, Quinones MP, Mummidi S, Srinivas S, Gaitan AA, Begum K, et al. CCR5 expression levels influence NFAT translocation, IL-2 production, and subsequent signaling events during T lymphocyte activation. *J Immunol (Baltimore Md 1950)* (2009) 182:171–82. doi: 10.4049/jimmunol.182.1.171
10. Pokkali S, Das SD. Augmented chemokine levels and chemokine receptor expression on immune cells during pulmonary tuberculosis. *Hum Immunol* (2009) 70:110–5. doi: 10.1016/j.humimm.2008.11.003
11. Qiu L, Huang D, Chen CY, Wang R, Shen L, Shen Y, et al. Severe tuberculosis induces unbalanced up-regulation of gene networks and overexpression of IL-22, MIP-1alpha, CCL27, IP-10, CCR4, CCR5, CXCR3, PD1, PDL2, IL-3, IFN-beta, TIM1, and TLR2 but low antigen-specific cellular responses. *J Infect Dis* (2008) 198:1514–9. doi: 10.1086/592448
12. Juffermans NP, Paxton WA, Dekkers PE, Verbon A, De Jonge E, Speelman P, et al. Up-regulation of HIV coreceptors CXCR4 and CCR5 on CD4(+) T cells during human endotoxemia and after stimulation with (myco)bacterial antigens: the role of cytokines. *Blood* (2000) 96:2649–54. doi: 10.1182/blood.V96.8.2649
13. Galkina E, Thatte J, Dabak V, Williams MB, Ley K, Braciale TJ. Preferential migration of effector CD8+ T cells into the interstitium of the normal lung. *J Clin Invest* (2005) 115:3473–83. doi: 10.1172/jci24482
14. Kohlmeier JE, Reiley WW, Perona-Wright G, Freeman ML, Yager EJ, Connor LM, et al. Inflammatory chemokine receptors regulate CD8+ T cell contraction and memory generation following infection. *J Exp Med* (2011) 208:1621–34. doi: 10.1084/jem.20102110
15. Kauffman KD, Sallin MA, Sakai S, Kamenyeva O, Kabat J, Weiner D, et al. Defective positioning in granulomas but not lung-homing limits CD4 T-cell interactions with Mycobacterium tuberculosis-infected macrophages in rhesus macaques. *Mucosal Immunol* (2018) 11:462–73. doi: 10.1038/mi.2017.60
16. Carpenter D, Taype C, Goulding J, Levin M, Eley B, Anderson S. M.-A. Shaw, and J.a.L. Armour. CCL3L1 copy number, CCR5genotype and susceptibility to tuberculosis. *BMC Med Genet* (2014) 15:5. doi: 10.1186/1471-2350-15-5
17. World Health Organization. Global tuberculosis report 2019. Geneva: World Health Organization (2019). Available at: https://apps.who.int/iris/handle/10665/329368.
18. National Health and Family Planning Commission of the People's Republic of China. Diagnosis for pulmonary tuberculosis(WS 288-2017). *Chin J Infect Control* (2018) 17:642–52. doi: 10.19871/j.cnki.xfcrbzz.2018.01.017
19. National Health and Family Planning Commission of the People's Republic of China. Classification of tuberculosis (WS 196-2017). *Chin J Infect Control* (2018) 17:367–8. doi: 10.19871/j.cnki.xfcrbzz.2018.03.018
20. Liu S, Chen J, Yan Z, Dai S, Li C, Yao Y, et al. Polymorphisms in the CCR5 promoter associated with cervical intraepithelial neoplasia in a Chinese Han population. *BMC Cancer* (2019) 19:525–5. doi: 10.1186/s12885-019-5738-6

21. Purcell S, Neale B, Todd-Brown K, Thomas L, Ferreira MA, Bender D, et al. PLINK: a tool set for whole-genome association and population-based linkage analyses. *Am J Hum Genet* (2007) 81:559–75. doi: 10.1086/519795
22. Barrett JC, Fry B, Maller J, Daly MJ. Haploview: analysis and visualization of LD and haplotype maps. *Bioinformatics* (2005) 21:263–5. doi: 10.1093/bioinformatics/bth457
23. Dupont W, Plummer WD Jr. Power and sample size calculations. A review and computer program. *Control Clin Trials* (1990) 11(2):116–28. doi: 10.1016/0197-2456(90)90005-m
24. Kalsdorf B, Skolimowska KH, Scriba TJ, Dawson R, Dheda K, Wood K, et al. Relationship between chemokine receptor expression, chemokine levels and HIV-1 replication in the lungs of persons exposed to Mycobacterium tuberculosis. *Eur J Immunol* (2013) 43:540–9. doi: 10.1002/eji.201242804
25. Martin MP, Dean M, Smith MW, Winkler C, Gerrard B, Michael NL, et al. Genetic acceleration of AIDS progression by a promoter variant of CCR5. *Sci (N Y NY)* (1998) 282:1907–11. doi: 10.1126/science.282.5395.1907
26. Mummidi S, Bamshad M, Ahuja SS, Gonzalez E, Feuillet PM, Begum K, et al. Evolution of human and non-human primate CC chemokine receptor 5 gene and mRNA. Potential roles for haplotype and mRNA diversity, differential haplotype-specific transcriptional activity, and altered transcription factor binding to polymorphic nucleotides in the pathogenesis of HIV-1 and simian immunodeficiency virus. *J Biol Chem* (2000) 275:18946–61. doi: 10.1074/jbc.M000169200
27. Picton AC, Paximadis M, Tiemessen CT. Genetic variation within the gene encoding the HIV-1 CCR5 coreceptor in two South African populations. *Infect Genet Evol J Mol Epidemiol Evolutionary Genet Infect Dis* (2010) 10:487–94. doi: 10.1016/j.meegid.2010.02.012
28. Blanpain C, Lee B, Tackoen M, Puffer B, Boom A, Libert F, et al. Multiple nonfunctional alleles of CCR5 are frequent in various human populations. *Blood* (2000) 96:1638 45. doi: 10.1182/blood.V96.5.1638
29. Rafty LA, Santiago FS, Khachigian LM. NF1/X represses PDGF A-chain transcription by interacting with Sp1 and antagonizing Sp1 occupancy of the promoter. *EMBO J* (2002) 21:334–43. doi: 10.1093/emboj/21.3.334
30. Mcdermott DH, Zimmerman PA, Guignard F, Kleeberger CA, Leitman SF, Murphy PM. CCR5 promoter polymorphism and HIV-1 disease progression. *Lancet* (1998) 352:866–70. doi: 10.1016/S0140-6736(98)04158-0
31. Li C, Lu SC, Hsieh PS, Huang YH, Huang HI, Ying TH, et al. Distribution of human chemokine (C-X3-C) receptor 1 (CX3CR1) gene polymorphisms and haplotypes of the CC chemokine receptor 5 (CCR5) promoter in Chinese people, and the effects of CCR5 haplotypes on CCR5 expression. *Int J Immunogenet* (2005) 32:99–106. doi: 10.1111/j.1744-313X.2005.00498.x
32. Gornalusse GG, Mummidi S, Gaitan AA, Jimenez F, Ramsuran V, Picton A, et al. Epigenetic mechanisms, T-cell activation, and CCR5 genetics interact to regulate T-cell expression of CCR5, the major HIV-1 coreceptor. *Proc Natl Acad Sci U S A* (2015) 112:E4762–71. doi: 10.1073/pnas.1423228112
33. Mummidi S, Ahuja SS, Mcdaniel BL, Ahuja SK. The human CC chemokine receptor 5 (CCR5) gene. Multiple transcripts with 5'-end heterogeneity, dual promoter usage, and evidence for polymorphisms within the regulatory regions and noncoding exons. *J Biol Chem* (1997) 272:30662–71. doi: 10.1074/jbc.272.49.30662
34. Mamtani M, Mummidi S, Ramsuran V, Pham M-H, Maldonado R, Begum K, et al. Influence of Variations in CCL3L1 and CCR5 on Tuberculosis in a Northwestern Colombian Population. *J Infect Dis* (2011) 203:1590–4. doi: 10.1093/infdis/jir145
35. Ometto L, Bertorelle R, Mainardi M, Zanchetta M, Tognazzo S, Rampon O, et al. Polymorphisms in the CCR5 promoter region influence disease progression in perinatally human immunodeficiency virus type 1-infected children. *J Infect Dis* (2001) 183:814–8. doi: 10.1086/318828

Permissions

All chapters in this book were first published by Frontiers; hereby published with permission under the Creative Commons Attribution License or equivalent. Every chapter published in this book has been scrutinized by our experts. Their significance has been extensively debated. The topics covered herein carry significant findings which will fuel the growth of the discipline. They may even be implemented as practical applications or may be referred to as a beginning point for another development.

The contributors of this book come from diverse backgrounds, making this book a truly international effort. This book will bring forth new frontiers with its revolutionizing research information and detailed analysis of the nascent developments around the world.

We would like to thank all the contributing authors for lending their expertise to make the book truly unique. They have played a crucial role in the development of this book. Without their invaluable contributions this book wouldn't have been possible. They have made vital efforts to compile up to date information on the varied aspects of this subject to make this book a valuable addition to the collection of many professionals and students.

This book was conceptualized with the vision of imparting up-to-date information and advanced data in this field. To ensure the same, a matchless editorial board was set up. Every individual on the board went through rigorous rounds of assessment to prove their worth. After which they invested a large part of their time researching and compiling the most relevant data for our readers.

The editorial board has been involved in producing this book since its inception. They have spent rigorous hours researching and exploring the diverse topics which have resulted in the successful publishing of this book. They have passed on their knowledge of decades through this book. To expedite this challenging task, the publisher supported the team at every step. A small team of assistant editors was also appointed to further simplify the editing procedure and attain best results for the readers.

Apart from the editorial board, the designing team has also invested a significant amount of their time in understanding the subject and creating the most relevant covers. They scrutinized every image to scout for the most suitable representation of the subject and create an appropriate cover for the book.

The publishing team has been an ardent support to the editorial, designing and production team. Their endless efforts to recruit the best for this project, has resulted in the accomplishment of this book. They are a veteran in the field of academics and their pool of knowledge is as vast as their experience in printing. Their expertise and guidance has proved useful at every step. Their uncompromising quality standards have made this book an exceptional effort. Their encouragement from time to time has been an inspiration for everyone.

The publisher and the editorial board hope that this book will prove to be a valuable piece of knowledge for researchers, students, practitioners and scholars across the globe.

List of Contributors

Lien Van Hoecke and Bert Schepens
VIB-UGent Center for Medical Biotechnology, VIB, Ghent, Belgium
Department of Biomedical Molecular Biology, Ghent University, Ghent, Belgium

Wim Nerinckx
VIB-UGent Center for Medical Biotechnology, VIB, Ghent, Belgium
Department of Biochemistry and Microbiology, Ghent University, Ghent, Belgium

Dorien De Vlieger, Marlies Ballegeer, Sarah Creytens and Xavier Saelens
VIB-UGent Center for Medical Biotechnology, VIB, Ghent, Belgium
Department of Biomedical Molecular Biology, Ghent University, Ghent, Belgium
Department of Biochemistry and Microbiology, Ghent University, Ghent, Belgium

Katja Hoffmann and Hartmut Hengel
Institute of Virology, Medical Center, Faculty of Medicine, University of Freiburg, Freiburg, Germany

Inge Van Molle and Han Remaut
Structural Biology Brussels, Vrije Universiteit Brussel, Brussels, Belgium
VIB-VUB Center for Structural Biology, Brussels, Belgium

Estelle M. Mewamba and Gustave Simo
Molecular Parasitology and Entomology Unit, Faculty of Science, University of Dschang, Dschang, Cameroon

Oscar A. Nyangiri and Enock Matovu
College of Veterinary Medicine Animal Resources and Biosecurity, Makerere University, Kampala, Uganda

Harry A. Noyes
Centre for Genomic Research, School of Biological Sciences, University of Liverpool, Liverpool, United Kingdom

Moses Egesa
Medical Research Council/Uganda Virus Research Institute and London School of Hygiene & Tropical Medicine Uganda Research Unit, Entebbe, Uganda
London School of Hygiene and Tropical Medicine, London, United Kingdom

Meng Qin, Lan Wang, YooJin Lee, Yiming Xie, Jing Wen and Irvin S. Y. Chen
Department of Microbiology, Immunology and Molecular Genetics, David Geffen School of Medicine at University of California, Los Angeles, Los Angeles, CA, United States
UCLA AIDS Institute, Los Angeles, CA, United States

Di Wu, Duo Xu and Yunfeng Lu
Department of Chemical and Biomolecular Engineering, School of Engineering, UCLA, Los Angeles, CA, United States

Christopher K. Williams and Harry V. Vinters
Departments of Pathology & Laboratory Medicine (Neuropathology) and Neurology, David Geffen School of Medicine at UCLA, Los Angeles, CA, United States

Emiko Kranz and Masakazu Kamata
UCLA AIDS Institute, Los Angeles, CA, United States
Division of Hematology-Oncology, David Geffen School of Medicine at UCLA, Los Angeles, CA, United States

Qi Guo
UCLA AIDS Institute, Los Angeles, CA, United States
School of Nursing, UCLA, Los Angeles, CA, United States

Jiaoqiong Guan and Zhanlong He
Institute of Medical Biology, Peking Union Medical College, Chinese Academy of Medical Sciences, Kunming, China

Yun Luo, Guibo Sun and Xiaobo Sun
Institute of Medicinal Plant Development, Peking Union Medical College, Chinese Academy of Medical Sciences, Beijing, China

Dhêmerson Souza De Lima, Vinícius N. C. Leal, Edione C. Reis, Jaíne L. S. Soares and Fernanda P. Fernandes
Laboratório de Imunogenética, Departamento de Imunologia, Instituto de Ciências Biomédicas, Universidade de São Paulo, São Paulo, Brazil

Caio C. B. Bomfim, Eduardo P. Amaral and Maria R. D'Imperio Lima
Laboratório de Imunologia das Doenças Infecciosas, Departamento de Imunologia, Instituto de Ciências Biomédicas, Universidade de São Paulo, São Paulo, Brazil

Flavio V. Loures
Instituto de Ciência e Tecnologia, Universidade Federal de São Paulo, São José dos Campos, Brazil

Mauricio M. Ogusku
Laboratório de Micobacteriologia, Instituto Nacional de Pesquisas da Amazônia, Manaus, Brazil

Alessandra Pontillo
Departament of Immunology, Instituto de Ciências Biomédicas (ICB), University of São Paulo, São Paulo, Brazil
Laboratório de Imunogenética, Departamento de Imunologia, Instituto de Ciências Biomédicas, Universidade de São Paulo, São Paulo, Brazil

Anna Rosa Garbuglia, Daniele Lapa, Catia Sias and Maria Rosaria Capobianchi
Laboratory of Virology, "Lazzaro Spallanzani" National Institute for Infectious Diseases, IRCCS, Rome, Italy

Paola Del Porto
Department of Biology and Biotechnology "C. Darwin," Sapienza University, Rome, Italy

Abdou Khadre Dit Jadir Fall, Celia Dechavanne, Audrey Sabbagh, Jacqueline Milet, André Garcia, David Courtin and Florence Migot-Nabias
Université de Paris, Institut de Recherche pour le Développement (IRD), UMR 261 MERIT, Paris, France

Evelyne Guitard and Jean-Michel Dugoujon
CNRS UMR 5288 Laboratoire d'Anthropologie Moléculaire et d'Imagerie de Synthèse (AMIS), Université Paul Sabatier Toulouse III, Toulouse, France

Ana Carolina Campi-Azevedo, Laise Rodrigues Reis, Vanessa Peruhype-Magalhães, Jordana Grazziela Coelho-dos-Reis, Lis Ribeiro Antonelli, Cristina Toscano Fonseca, Christiane Costa-Pereira, Ismael Artur da Costa-Rocha, Juliana Vaz de Melo Mambrini, Iramaya Rodrigues Caldas, Andréa Teixeira-Carvalho and Olindo Assis Martins-Filho
Instituto René Rachou, Fundação Oswaldo Cruz - FIOCRUZ-Minas, Belo Horizonte, Brazil

Elaine Maria Souza-Fagundes
Departamento de Fisiologia e Biofísica, Universidade Federal de Minas Gerais, Belo Horizonte, Brazil

Jandira Aparecida Campos Lemos
Secretaria Municipal de Saúde de Belo Horizonte, Belo Horizonte, Brazil

José Geraldo Leite Ribeiro
Secretaria do Estado de Saúde de Minas Gerais, Belo Horizonte, Brazil

Luiz Antônio Bastos Camacho
Escola Nacional de Saúde Pública - FIOCRUZ, Rio de Janeiro, Brazil

Maria de Lourdes de Sousa Maia, Tatiana Guimarães de Noronha, Sheila Maria Barbosa de Lima, Marisol Simões, Marcos da Silva Freire, Reinaldo de Menezes Martins and Akira Homma
Instituto de Tecnologia em Imunobiológicos Bio-Manguinhos - FIOCRUZ, Rio de Janeiro, Brazil

Pedro Luiz Tauil
Faculdade de Medicina, Universidade de Brasília, Brasilia, Brazil

Pedro Fernando Costa Vasconcelos
Instituto Evandro Chagas, Ananindeua, Brazil

Alessandro Pecego Martins Romano
Departamento de Imunização e Doenças Transmissíveis (DEIDT) - Secretaria de Vigilância em Saúde, Ministério da Saúde, Brasilia, Brazil

Carla Magda Domingues
Programa Nacional de Imunizações - Secretaria de Vigilância em Saúde, Ministério da Saúde, Brasilia, Brazil

Mariana Brasil de Andrade Figueira, Antonio Luiz Boechat and Aya Sadahiro
Laboratório de Imunologia Molecular, Departamento de Parasitologia, Universidade Federal do Amazonas (UFAM), Manaus, Brazil
Programa de Pós-Graduação em Imunologia Básica e Aplicada, Universidade Federal do Amazonas, Manaus, Brazil

Milton Gomes do Nascimento Filho, Thaís Rodrigues de Albuquerque Ribeiro, Luana Sousa Felix and Ariane Senna Fonseca Gonçalves
Laboratório de Imunologia Molecular, Departamento de Parasitologia, Universidade Federal do Amazonas (UFAM), Manaus, Brazil

Irineide Assumpção Antunes and Joycenéa da Silva Matsuda
Policlínica Cardoso Fontes - Secretaria de Estado da Saúde do Amazonas-SUSAM, Manaus, Brazil

Rajendranath Ramasawmy
Programa de Pós-Graduação em Imunologia Básica e Aplicada, Universidade Federal do Amazonas, Manaus, Brazil
Instituto de Pesquisa Clínica Carlos Borborema, Fundação de Medicina Tropical Dr. Heitor Vieira Dourado, Manaus, Brazil
Faculdade de Medicina Nilton Lins, Universidade Nilton Lins, Manaus, Brazil

Mauricio Morishi Ogusku
Laboratório de Micobacteriologia, Instituto Nacional de Pesquisas da Amazônia (INPA), Manaus, Brazil

Allyson Guimarães da Costa
Programa de Pós-Graduação em Imunologia Básica e Aplicada, Universidade Federal do Amazonas, Manaus, Brazil
Diretoria de Ensino e Pesquisa, Fundação Hospitalar de Hematologia e Hemoterapia do Amazonas (HEMOAM), Manaus, Brazil

Akiko Takaya
Laboratory of Microbiology and Molecular Genetics, Graduate School of Pharmaceutical Sciences, Chiba University, Chiba, Japan

Tomoko Yamamoto
Department of Infectious Diseases, Medical Mycology Research Center, Chiba University, Chiba, Japan

Koji Tokoyoda
Deutsches Rheuma-Forschungszentrum Berlin (DRFZ), A Leibniz Institute, Berlin, Germany

Paula Keiko Sato, Felipe Delatorre Busser and Constancia Lima Diogo
Laboratory of Medical Investigation in Immunology (LIM48), Faculdade de Medicina, Hospital das Clínicas, University of São Paulo, São Paulo, Brazil
Institute of Tropical Medicine, Faculdade de Medicina, University of São Paulo, São Paulo, Brazil

Flávia Mendes da Cunha Carvalho and Alexandra Gomes dos Santos
Laboratory of Medical Investigation in Immunology (LIM48), Faculdade de Medicina, Hospital das Clínicas, University of São Paulo, São Paulo, Brazil
Department of Infectious and Parasitic Diseases, Faculdade de Medicina, University of São Paulo, São Paulo, Brazil

Maria Aparecida Shikanai-Yasuda
Laboratory of Medical Investigation in Immunology (LIM48), Faculdade de Medicina, Hospital das Clínicas, University of São Paulo, São Paulo, Brazil
Institute of Tropical Medicine, Faculdade de Medicina, University of São Paulo, São Paulo, Brazil
Department of Infectious and Parasitic Diseases, Faculdade de Medicina, University of São Paulo, SãoPaulo, Brazil

Adriana Satie Gonçalves Kono
Infectious Diseases Division, Hospital das Clínicas, University of São Paulo, São Paulo, Brazil

Maria Luiza Moretti
Faculdade de Ciências Médicas, Hospital das Clínicas, State University of Campinas, Campinas, Brazil

Olinda do Carmo Luiz
Department of Preventive Medicine, Faculdade de Medicina, University of São Paulo, São Paulo, Brazil

Lulu Zhang, Xubiao Wei, Rijun Zhang, Dayong Si, Zhongxuan Li, Junhao Cheng and Mengsi Du
Laboratory of Feed Biotechnology, State Key Laboratory of Animal Nutrition, College of Animal Science and Technology, China Agricultural University, Beijing, China

Jim N. Petitte
Prestage Department of Poultry Science, North Carolina State University, Raleigh, NC, United States

Alexandra Gomes dos Santos, Jamille Oliveira and Claudia Silva Oliveira
Department of Infectious and Parasitic Diseases, Faculdade de Medicina, University of São Paulo, São Paulo, Brazil

Elieser Hitoshi Watanabe and Luiz Fernando Onuchic
Department of Medicine, Divisions of Molecular Medicine and Nephrology, Faculdade de Medicina, University of São Paulo, São Paulo, Brazil

Daiane Tomomi Ferreira, Érika Shimoda Nakanishi and Paula Keiko Sato
Laboratory of Immunology (LIM 48), Hospital das Cl´ınicas, Faculdade de Medicina, University of São Paulo, São Paulo, Brazil

Vera Lucia Teixeira de Freitas
Department of Infectious and Parasitic Diseases, Faculdade de Medicina, University of São Paulo, São Paulo, Brazil
Laboratory of Immunology (LIM 48), Hospital das Clínicas, Faculdade de Medicina, University of São Paulo, São Paulo, Brazil

Edimar Bocchi and Fatima Cruz
Heart Institute, Hospital das Cl´ınicas, Faculdade de Medicina, University of São Paulo, São Paulo, Brazil

Cristina Terra Gallafrio Novaes and Noemia Barbosa Carvalho
Division of Infectious Diseases, Hospital das Clinicas, Faculdade de Medicina, University of São Paulo, São Paulo, Brazil

Edite Hatsumi Yamashiro-Kanashiro
Laboratory of Immunology (LIM 48), Hospital das Cl´ınicas, Faculdade de Medicina, University of São Paulo, São Paulo, Brazil
Instituto de Medicina Tropical, University of São Paulo, São Paulo, Brazil

Monica C. Gestal, Hannah M. Johnson and Eric T. Harvill
Department of Infectious Diseases, College of Veterinary Sciences, University of Georgia, Athens, GA, United States

Barbara Maria Ianni, Paula Buck and Alexandre Costa Pereira
Heart Institute (InCor), University of São Paulo School of Medicine (FMUSP), São Paulo, Brazil

Sandrine Cabantous
Aix-Marseille Université, INSERM, GIMP UMR_S906, Marseille, France

Edecio Cunha-Neto
Heart Institute (InCor), University of São Paulo School of Medicine (FMUSP), São Paulo, Brazil
Institute for Investigation in Immunology (iii), INCT, São Paulo, Brazil
Division of Clinical Immunology and Allergy, University of São Paulo School of Medicine, São Paulo, Brazil

Jorge Kalil
Heart Institute (InCor), University of São Paulo School of Medicine (FMUSP), São Paulo, Brazil
Institute for Investigation in Immunology (iii), INCT, São Paulo, Brazil
Bioengineering Program, Instituto Tecnológico, Universidade Brasil, São Paulo, Brazil

Amanda Farage Frade-Barros
Heart Institute (InCor), University of São Paulo School of Medicine (FMUSP), São Paulo, Brazil
Institute for Investigation in Immunology (iii), INCT, São Paulo, Brazil
Aix-Marseille Université, INSERM, GIMP UMR_S906, Marseille, France
Division of Clinical Immunology and Allergy, University of São Paulo School of Medicine, São Paulo, Brazil
Bioengineering Program, Instituto Tecnológico, Universidade Brasil, São Paulo, Brazil

Cristina Wide Pissetti and Virmondes Rodrigues
Laboratory of Immunology, Universidade Federal Do Triângulo Mineiro (UFTM), Uberaba, Brazil

Bruno Saba, Hui Tzu Lin-Wang, Marcelo Sampaio and Abílio Fragata
Laboratório de Investigação Molecular em Cardiologia, Instituto de Cardiologia Dante Pazzanese (IDPC), São Paulo, Brazil

José Antonio Marin-Neto, André Schmidt, Fabrício Dias and Eduardo Donadi
School of Medicine of Ribeirão Preto (FMRP), University of São Paulo, Ribeirão Preto, Brazil

Mario Hiroyuki Hirata
Department of Clinical and Toxicological Analyses, Faculty of Pharmaceutical Sciences, University of São Paulo (USP), São Paulo, Brazil

Christophe Chevillard
Aix Marseille Université, INSERM, TAGC Theories and Approaches of Genomic Complexity, UMR_1090, Marseille, France

Mohammad Tarique, Chaman Saini and Alpana Sharma
Department of Biochemistry, All India Institute of Medical Sciences (AIIMS), New Delhi, India

Huma Naz
Centre for Interdisciplinary Research in Basic Sciences, Jamia Millia Islamia, New Delhi, India

Mohd Suhail
King Fahd Medical Research Center, King Abdulaziz University, Jeddah, Saudi Arabia
Department of Medical Laboratory Technology, Faculty of Applied Medical Sciences, King Abdulaziz University, Jeddah, Saudi Arabia

Hari Shankar
Parasite-Host Biology Group, ICMR - National Institute of Malaria Research, New Delhi, India

Neena Khanna
Department of Dermatovenerology, All India Institute of Medical Sciences (AIIMS), New Delhi, India

Nimitha R. Mathew and Davide Angeletti
Department of Microbiology and Immunology, Institute of Biomedicine, University of Gothenburg, Gothenburg, Sweden

Anna Stachyra, Anna Zawistowska-Deniziak, Katarzyna Basałaj, Sylwia Grzelak and Justyna Bień-Kalinowska
Witold Stefanski Institute of Parasitology, Polish Academy of Sciences, Warsaw, Poland

Michał Gondek
Department of Food Hygiene of Animal Origin, Faculty of Veterinary Medicine, University of Life Sciences in Lublin, Lublin, Poland

Shuyuan Liu, Nannan Liu, Xinwen Zhang and Li Shi
Institute of Medical Biology, Chinese Academy of Medical Sciences & Peking Union Medical College, Kunming, China

Hui Wang and Shuqiong Zhang
The Third People's Hospital of Kunming, Kunming, China

Yufeng Yao
Institute of Medical Biology, Chinese Academy of Medical Sciences & Peking Union Medical College, Kunming, China
Yunnan Key Laboratory of Vaccine Research and Development on Severe Infectious Diseases, Kunming, China

Index

www.ingramcontent.com/pod-product-compliance
Lightning Source LLC
LaVergne TN
LVHW082149200926
848484LV00008B/2130